# HEALTH SECURITY ACT

103D CONGRESS
1ST SESSION **H. R. /S.** _____

IN THE HOUSE OF REPRESENTATIVES /

IN THE SENATE OF THE UNITED STATES

Mr. _____ introduced the following bill; which was [read twice and] referred to the Committee on _____

# A BILL

To ensure individual and family security through health care coverage for all Americans in a manner that contains the rate of growth in health care costs and promotes responsible health insurance practices, to promote choice in health care, and to ensure and protect the health care of all Americans.

1   *Be it enacted by the Senate and House of Representa-*
2   *tives of the United States of America in Congress assembled,*

# SECTION 1. SHORT TITLE; TABLE OF TITLES AND SUBTITLES.

(a) SHORT TITLE.—This Act may be cited as the "Health Security Act".

(b) TABLE OF TITLES AND SUBTITLES IN ACT.—The following are the titles and subtitles contained in this Act:

### TITLE I—HEALTH CARE SECURITY

Subtitle A—Universal Coverage and Individual Responsibility
Subtitle B—Benefits
Subtitle C—State Responsibilities
Subtitle D—Health Alliances
Subtitle E—Health Plans
Subtitle F—Federal Responsibilities
Subtitle G—Employer Responsiblities
[Subtitle H—Reserved]
[Subtitle I—Reserved]
Subtitle J—General Definitions; Miscellaneous Provisions

### TITLE II—NEW BENEFITS

Subtitle A—Medicare Outpatient Prescription Drug Benefit
Subtitle B—Long-Term Care

### TITLE III—PUBLIC HEALTH INITIATIVES

Subtitle A—Workforce Priorities Under Federal Payments
Subtitle B—Academic Health Centers
Subtitle C—Health Research Initiatives
Subtitle D—Core Functions of Public Health Programs; National Initiatives Regarding Preventive Health
Subtitle E—Health Services for Medically Underserved Populations
Subtitle F—Mental Health; Substance Abuse
Subtitle G—Comprehensive School Health Education; School-Related Health Services
Subtitle H—Public Health Service Initiatives Fund
Subtitle I—Coordination With COBRA Continuation Coverage

### TITLE IV—MEDICARE AND MEDICAID

Subtitle A—Medicare and the Alliance System
Subtitle B—Savings in Medicare Program
Subtitle C—Medicaid
Subtitle D—Increase in SSI Personal Needs Allowance

### TITLE V—QUALITY AND CONSUMER PROTECTION

Subtitle A—Quality Management and Improvement
Subtitle B—Information Systems, Privacy, and Administrative Simplification
Subtitle C—Remedies and Enforcement

(A) health insurance and high quality health care should be secure, uninterrupted, and affordable for all individuals in the United States;

(B) comprehensive health care benefits that meet the full range of health needs, including primary, preventive, and specialized care, should be available to all individuals in the United States;

(C) the current high quality of health care in the United States should be maintained;

(D) individuals in the United States should be afforded a meaningful opportunity to choose among a range of health plans, health care providers, and treatments;

(E) regulatory and administrative burdens should be reduced;

(F) the rapidly escalating costs of health care should be contained without sacrificing high quality or impeding technological improvements;

(G) competition in the health care industry should ensure that health plans and health care providers are efficient and charge reasonable prices;

(H) a partnership between the Federal Government and each State should allow the State and its local communities to design an effective, high-quality system of care that serves the residents of the State;

(I) all individuals should have a responsibility to pay their fair share of the costs of health care coverage;

(J) a health care system should build on the strength of the employment-based coverage arrangements that now exist in the United States;

(K) the penalties for fraud and abuse should be swift and severe; and

(L) an individual's medical information should remain confidential and should be protected from unauthorized disclosure and use.

**SEC. 3. PURPOSES.**

The purposes of this Act are as follows:

(1) To guarantee comprehensive and secure health care coverage.

(2) To simplify the health care system for consumers and health care professionals.

(3) To control the cost of health care for employers, employees, and others who pay for health care coverage.

(4) To promote individual choice among health plans and health care providers.

(5) To ensure high quality health care.

(6) To encourage all individuals to take responsibility for their health care coverage.

# TITLE I—HEALTH CARE SECURITY

TABLE OF CONTENTS OF TITLE

## Subtitle A—Universal Coverage and Individual Responsibility

### PART 1—UNIVERSAL COVERAGE

Sec. 1001. Entitlement to health benefits.
Sec. 1002. Individual responsibilities.
Sec. 1003. Protection of consumer choice.
Sec. 1004. Applicable health plan providing coverage.
Sec. 1005. Treatment of other nonimmigrants.
Sec. 1006. Effective date of entitlement.

### PART 2—TREATMENT OF FAMILIES AND SPECIAL RULES

Sec. 1011. General rule of enrollment of family in same health plan.
Sec. 1012. Treatment of certain families.
Sec. 1013. Multiple employment situations.
Sec. 1014. Treatment of residents of States with Statewide single-payer systems.

## Subtitle B—Benefits

### PART 1—COMPREHENSIVE BENEFIT PACKAGE

Sec. 1101. Provision of comprehensive benefits by plans.

### PART 2—DESCRIPTION OF ITEMS AND SERVICES COVERED

Sec. 1111. Hospital services.
Sec. 1112. Services of health professionals.
Sec. 1113. Emergency and ambulatory medical and surgical services.
Sec. 1114. Clinical preventive services.
Sec. 1115. Mental health and substance abuse services.
Sec. 1116. Family planning services and services for pregnant women.
Sec. 1117. Hospice care.
Sec. 1118. Home health care.
Sec. 1119. Extended care services.
Sec. 1120. Ambulance services.
Sec. 1121. Outpatient laboratory, radiology, and diagnostic services.
Sec. 1122. Outpatient prescription drugs and biologicals.
Sec. 1123. Outpatient rehabilitation services.
Sec. 1124. Durable medical equipment and prosthetic and orthotic devices.
Sec. 1125. Vision care.
Sec. 1126. Dental care.
Sec. 1127. Health education classes.
Sec. 1128. Investigational treatments.

### PART 3—COST SHARING

Sec. 1131. Cost sharing.

**Health Security Act**  *Title I*

Sec. 1132. Lower cost sharing.
Sec. 1133. Higher cost sharing.
Sec. 1134. Combination cost sharing.
Sec. 1135. Table of copayments and coinsurance.
Sec. 1136. Indexing dollar amounts relating to cost sharing.

PART 4—EXCLUSIONS

Sec. 1141. Exclusions.

PART 5—ROLE OF THE NATIONAL HEALTH BOARD

Sec. 1151. Definition of benefits.
Sec. 1152. Acceleration of expanded benefits.
Sec. 1153. Authority with respect to clinical preventive services.
Sec. 1154. Establishment of standards regarding medical necessity.

PART 6—ADDITIONAL PROVISIONS RELATING TO HEALTH CARE PROVIDERS

Sec. 1161. Override of restrictive State practice laws.
Sec. 1162. Provision of items or services contrary to religious belief or moral conviction.

## Subtitle C—State Responsibilities

Sec. 1200. Participating State.

PART 1—GENERAL STATE RESPONSIBILITIES

Sec. 1201. General State responsibilities.
Sec. 1202. State responsibilities with respect to alliances.
Sec. 1203. State responsibilities relating to health plans.
Sec. 1204. Financial solvency; fiscal oversight; guaranty fund.
Sec. 1205. Restrictions on funding of additional benefits.

PART 2—REQUIREMENTS FOR STATE SINGLE-PAYER SYSTEMS

Sec. 1221. Single-payer system described.
Sec. 1222. General requirements for single-payer systems.
Sec. 1223. Special rules for States operating Statewide single-payer system.
Sec. 1224. Special rules for alliance-specific single-payer systems.

## Subtitle D—Health Alliances

Sec. 1300. Health alliance defined.

PART 1—ESTABLISHMENT OF REGIONAL AND CORPORATE ALLIANCES

SUBPART A—REGIONAL ALLIANCES

Sec. 1301. Regional alliance defined.
Sec. 1302. Board of directors.
Sec. 1303. Provider advisory boards for regional alliances.

SUBPART B—CORPORATE ALLIANCES

Sec. 1311. Corporate alliance defined; individuals eligible for coverage through corporate alliances; additional definitions.
Sec. 1312. Timing of elections.
Sec. 1313. Termination of alliance election.

## Part 2—General Responsibilities and Authorities of Regional Alliances

Sec. 1321. Contracts with health plans.
Sec. 1322. Offering choice of health plans for enrollment; establishment of fee-for-service schedule.
Sec. 1323. Enrollment rules and procedures.
Sec. 1324. Issuance of health security cards.
Sec. 1325. Consumer information and marketing.
Sec. 1326. Ombudsman.
Sec. 1327. Data collection; quality.
Sec. 1328. Additional duties.
Sec. 1329. Additional authorities for regional alliances to address needs in areas with inadequate health services; prohibition of insurance role.
Sec. 1330. Prohibition against self-dealing and conflicts of interest.

## Part 3—Authorities and Responsibilities Relating to Financing and Income Determinations

### Subpart A—Collection of Funds

Sec. 1341. Information and negotiation and acceptance of bids.
Sec. 1342. Amount of premiums charged.
Sec. 1343. Determination of family obligation for family share and alliance credit amount.
Sec. 1344. Notice of family payments due.
Sec. 1345. Collection of premium payments.
Sec. 1346. Coordination among regional alliances.

### Subpart B—Payments

Sec. 1351. Payment to regional alliance health plans.
Sec. 1352. Alliance administrative allowance percentage.
Sec. 1353. Payments for graduate medical education and academic health centers.

### Subpart C—Financial Management

Sec. 1361. Management of finances and records.

### Subpart D—Reductions in Cost Sharing; Income Determinations

Sec. 1371. Reduction in cost sharing for low-income families.
Sec. 1372. Application process for cost sharing reductions.
Sec. 1373. Application for premium reductions and reduction in liability to alliance.
Sec. 1374. General provisions relating to application process.
Sec. 1375. End-of-year reconciliation for premium discount and repayment reduction with actual income.

## Part 4—Responsibilities and Authorities of Corporate Alliances

Sec. 1381. Contracts with health plans.
Sec. 1382. Offering choice of health plans for enrollment.
Sec. 1383. Enrollment; issuance of health security card.
Sec. 1384. Community-rated premiums within premium areas.
Sec. 1385. Assistance for low-wage families.

Sec. 1386. Consumer information and marketing; consumer assistance; data collection and quality; additional duties.
Sec. 1387. Plan and information requirements.
Sec. 1388. Management of funds; relations with employees.
Sec. 1389. Cost control.
Sec. 1390. Payments by corporate alliance employers to corporate alliances.
Sec. 1391. Coordination of payments.
Sec. 1392. Applicability of ERISA enforcement mechanisms for enforcement of certain requirements.
Sec. 1393. Applicability of certain ERISA protections to covered individuals.
Sec. 1394. Disclosure and reserve requirements.
Sec. 1395. Trusteeship by the Secretary of insolvent corporate alliance health plans.
Sec. 1396. Guaranteed benefits under trusteeship of the secretary.
Sec. 1397. Imposition and collection of periodic assessments on self-insured corporate alliance plans.

## Subtitle E—Health Plans

Sec. 1400. Health plan defined.

### Part 1—Requirements Relating to Comprehensive Benefit Package

Sec. 1401. Application of requirements.
Sec. 1402. Requirements relating to enrollment and coverage.
Sec. 1403. Community rating.
Sec. 1404. Marketing of health plans; information.
Sec. 1405. Grievance procedure.
Sec. 1406. Health plan arrangements with providers.
Sec. 1407. Preemption of certain State laws relating to health plans.
Sec. 1408. Financial solvency.
Sec. 1409. Requirement for offering cost sharing policy.
Sec. 1410. Quality assurance.
Sec. 1411. Provider verification.
Sec. 1412. Consumer disclosures of utilization management protocols.
Sec. 1413. Confidentiality, data management, and reporting.
Sec. 1414. Participation in reinsurance system.

### Part 2—Requirements Relating to Supplemental Insurance

Sec. 1421. Imposition of requirements on supplemental insurance.
Sec. 1422. Standards for supplemental health benefit policies.
Sec. 1423. Standards for cost sharing policies.

### Part 3—Requirements Relating to Essential Community Providers

Sec. 1431. Health plan requirement.
Sec. 1432. Sunset of requirement.

### Part 4—Requirements Relating to Workers' Compensation and Automobile Medical Liability Coverage

Sec. 1441. Reference to requirements relating to workers compensation services.
Sec. 1442. Reference to requirements relating to automobile medical liability services.

## Subtitle F—Federal Responsibilities

## PART 1—NATIONAL HEALTH BOARD

### SUBPART A—ESTABLISHMENT OF NATIONAL HEALTH BOARD

Sec. 1501. Creation of National Health Board; membership.
Sec. 1502. Qualifications of board members.
Sec. 1503. General duties and responsibilities.
Sec. 1504. Annual report.
Sec. 1505. Powers.
Sec. 1506. Funding.

### SUBPART B—RESPONSIBILITIES RELATING TO REVIEW AND APPROVAL OF STATE SYSTEMS

Sec. 1511. Federal review and action on State systems.
Sec. 1512. Failure of participating States to meet conditions for compliance.
Sec. 1513. Reduction in payments for health programs by secretary of health and human services.
Sec. 1514. Review of Federal determinations.
Sec. 1515. Federal support for State implementation.

### SUBPART C—RESPONSIBILITIES IN ABSENCE OF STATE SYSTEMS

Sec. 1521. Application of subpart.
Sec. 1522. Federal assumption of responsibilities in non-participating States.
Sec. 1523. Imposition of surcharge on premiums under federally-operated system.
Sec. 1524. Return to State operation.

### SUBPART D—ESTABLISHMENT OF CLASS FACTORS FOR CHARGING PREMIUMS

Sec. 1531. Premium class factors.

### SUBPART E—RISK ADJUSTMENT AND REINSURANCE METHODOLOGY FOR PAYMENT OF PLANS

Sec. 1541. Development of a risk adjustment and reinsurance methodology.
Sec. 1542. Incentives to enroll disadvantaged groups.
Sec. 1543. Advisory committee.
Sec. 1544. Research and demonstrations.
Sec. 1545. Technical assistance to States and alliances.

### SUBPART F—RESPONSIBILITIES FOR FINANCIAL REQUIREMENTS

Sec. 1551. Capital standards for regional alliance health plan.
Sec. 1552. Standard for guaranty funds.

## PART 2—RESPONSIBILITIES OF DEPARTMENT OF HEALTH AND HUMAN SERVICES

### SUBPART A—GENERAL RESPONSIBILITIES

Sec. 1571. General responsibilities of Secretary of Health and Human Services.
Sec. 1572. Establishment of breakthrough drug committee.

### SUBPART B—CERTIFICATION OF ESSENTIAL COMMUNITY PROVIDERS

Sec. 1581. Certification.
Sec. 1582. Categories of providers automatically certified.
Sec. 1583. Standards for additional providers.

Sec. 1584. Certification process; review; termination of certifications.
Sec. 1585. Notification of health alliances and participating States.

PART 3—SPECIFIC RESPONSIBILITIES OF SECRETARY OF LABOR.

Sec. 1591. Responsibilities of Secretary of Labor.

### Subtitle G—Employer Responsiblities

Sec. 1601. Payment requirement.
Sec. 1602. Requirement for information reporting.
Sec. 1603. Requirements relating to new employees.
Sec. 1604. Auditing of records.
Sec. 1605. Prohibition of certain employer discrimination.
Sec. 1606. Obligation relating to retiree health benefits.
Sec. 1607. Prohibition on self-funding of cost sharing benefits by regional alliance employers.

[Subtitle H—Reserved]

[Subtitle I—Reserved]

### Subtitle J—General Definitions; Miscellaneous Provisions

PART 1—GENERAL DEFINITIONS

Sec. 1901. Definitions relating to employment and income.
Sec. 1902. Other general definitions.

PART 2—MISCELLANEOUS PROVISIONS

Sec. 1911. Use of interim, final regulations.

# TITLE I—HEALTH CARE SECURITY

## Subtitle A—Universal Coverage and Individual Responsibility

### PART 1—UNIVERSAL COVERAGE

**SEC. 1001. ENTITLEMENT TO HEALTH BENEFITS.**

(a) IN GENERAL.—In accordance with this part, each eligible individual is entitled to the comprehensive benefit package under subtitle B through the applicable health plan in which the individual is enrolled consistent with this title.

(b) HEALTH SECURITY CARD.—Each eligible individual is entitled to a health security card to be issued by the alliance or other entity that offers the applicable health plan in which the individual is enrolled.

(c) ELIGIBLE INDIVIDUAL DEFINED.—In this Act, the term "eligible individual" means an individual who is residing in the United States and who is—

    (1) a citizen or national of the United States;

    (2) an alien permanently residing in the United States under color of law (as defined in section 1902(1)); or

    (3) a long-term nonimmigrant (as defined in section 1902(19)).

(d) TREATMENT OF MEDICARE-ELIGIBLE INDIVIDUALS.—Subject to section 1012(a), a medicare-eligible individual is entitled to health benefits under the medicare program instead of the entitlement under subsection (a).

(e) TREATMENT OF PRISONERS.—A prisoner (as defined in section 1902(26)) is entitled to health care services provided by the authority responsible for the prisoner instead of the entitlement under subsection (a).

**SEC. 1002. INDIVIDUAL RESPONSIBILITIES.**

(a) IN GENERAL.—In accordance with this Act, each eligible individual (other than a medicare-eligible individual)—

(1) must enroll in an applicable health plan for the individual, and

(2) must pay any premium required, consistent with this Act, with respect to such enrollment.

(b) LIMITATION ON DISENROLLMENT.—No eligible individual shall be disenrolled from an applicable health plan until the individual—

(1) is enrolled under another applicable health plan, or

(2) becomes a medicare-eligible individual.

**SEC. 1003. PROTECTION OF CONSUMER CHOICE.**

Nothing in this Act shall be construed as prohibiting the following:

(1) An individual from purchasing any health care services.

(2) An individual from purchasing supplemental insurance (offered consistent with this Act) to cover health care services not included within the comprehensive benefit package.

(3) An individual who is not an eligible individual from purchasing health insurance (other than through a regional alliance).

(4) Employers from providing coverage for benefits in addition to the comprehensive benefit package (subject to part 2 of subtitle E).

## SEC. 1004. APPLICABLE HEALTH PLAN PROVIDING COVERAGE.

(a) SPECIFICATION OF APPLICABLE HEALTH PLAN.—Except as otherwise provided:

(1) GENERAL RULE: REGIONAL ALLIANCE HEALTH PLANS.—The applicable health plan for a family is a regional alliance health plan for the alliance area in which the family resides.

(2) CORPORATE ALLIANCE HEALTH PLANS.—In the case of a family member that is eligible to enroll in a corporate alliance health plan under section 1311(c), the applicable health plan for the family is such a corporate alliance health plan.

(b) CHOICE OF PLANS FOR CERTAIN GROUPS.—

(1) MILITARY PERSONNEL AND FAMILIES.—For military personnel and families who elect a Uniformed Services Health Plan of the Department of Defense under section 1073a(d) of title 10, United States Code, as inserted by section 8001(a) of this Act, that plan shall be the applicable health plan.

(2) VETERANS.—For veterans and families who elect to enroll in a veterans health plan under section 1801 of title 38, United States Code, as inserted by section 8101(a) of this Act, that plan shall be the applicable health plan.

(3) INDIANS.—For those individuals who are eligible to enroll, and who elect to enroll, in a health program of the Indian Health Service under section 8302(b), that program shall be the applicable health plan.

SEC. 1005. TREATMENT OF OTHER NONIMMIGRANTS.

(a) UNDOCUMENTED ALIENS INELIGIBLE FOR BENEFITS.—An undocumented alien is not eligible to obtain the comprehensive benefit package through enrollment in a health plan pursuant to this Act.

(b) DIPLOMATS AND OTHER FOREIGN GOVERNMENT OFFICIALS.—Subject to conditions established by the National Health Board in consultation with the Secretary of State, a nonimmigrant under subparagraph (A) or (G) of section 101(a)(15) of the Immigration and Nationality Act may obtain the comprehensive benefit package through enrollment in the regional alliance health plan for the alliance area in which the nonimmigrant resides.

(c) RECIPROCAL TREATMENT OF OTHER NONIMMIGRANTS.—With respect to those classes of individuals who are lawful nonimmigrants but who are not long-term nonimmigrants (as defined in section 1902(19)) or described in subsection (b), such individuals may obtain such benefits through enrollment with regional alliance health plans only in accordance with such reciprocal agreements between the United States and foreign states as may be entered into.

**SEC. 1006. EFFECTIVE DATE OF ENTITLEMENT.**

(a) REGIONAL ALLIANCE ELIGIBLE INDIVIDUALS.—

(1) IN GENERAL.—In the case of regional alliance eligible individuals residing in a State, the entitlement under this part (and requirements under section 1002) shall not take effect until the State becomes a participating State (as defined in section 1200).

(2) TRANSITIONAL RULE FOR CORPORATE ALLIANCES.—

(A) IN GENERAL.—In the case of a State that becomes a participating State before the general effective date (as defined in subsection (c)) and for periods before such date, under rules established by the Board, an individual who is covered under an employee benefit plan (described in subparagraph (C)) based on the individual (or the individual's spouse) being a qualifying employee of a qualifying employer, the individual shall not be treated under this Act as a regional alliance eligible individual.

(B) QUALIFYING EMPLOYER DEFINED.—In subparagraph (A), the term "qualifying employer" means an employer that—

 (i) is described in section 1311(b)(1)(A), or is participating in a multiemployer plan described in section 1311(b)(1)(B) or arrangement described in section 1311(b)(1)(C), and

 (ii) provides such notice to the regional alliance involved as the Board specifies.

(C) BENEFITS PLAN DESCRIBED.—A plan described in this subparagraph is an employee benefit plan that—

 (i) provides (through insurance or otherwise) the comprehensive benefit package, and

 (ii) provides an employer contribution of at least 80 percent of the premium (or premium equivalent) for coverage

(b) CORPORATE ALLIANCE ELIGIBLE INDIVIDUALS.—

(1) IN GENERAL.—In the case of corporate alliance eligible individuals, the entitlement under this

part shall not take effect until the general effective date.

(2) TRANSITION.—For purposes of this Act and before the general effective date, in the case of an eligible individual who resides in a participating State, the individual is deemed a regional alliance eligible individual until the individual becomes a corporate alliance eligible individual, unless paragraph (2)(A) applies to the individual.

(c) GENERAL EFFECTIVE DATE DEFINED.—In this Act, the term "general effective date" means January 1, 1998.

## PART 2—TREATMENT OF FAMILIES AND SPECIAL RULES

### SEC. 1011. GENERAL RULE OF ENROLLMENT OF FAMILY IN SAME HEALTH PLAN.

(a) IN GENERAL.—Except as provided in this part or otherwise, all members of the same family (as defined in subsection (b)) shall be enrolled in the same applicable health plan.

(b) FAMILY DEFINED.—In this Act, unless otherwise provided, the term "family"—

(1) means, with respect to an eligible individual who is not a child (as defined in subsection (c)), the individual; and

(2) includes the following persons (if any):

(A) The individual's spouse if the spouse is an eligible individual.

(B) The individual's children (and, if applicable, the children of the individual's spouse) if they are eligible individuals.

(c) CLASSES OF FAMILY ENROLLMENT; TERMINOLOGY.—

(1) IN GENERAL.—In this Act, each of the following is a separate class of family enrollment under this Act:

(A) Coverage only of an individual (referred to in this Act as the "individual" class of enrollment).

(B) Coverage of a married couple without children (referred to in this Act as the "couple-only" class of enrollment).

(C) Coverage of an unmarried individual and one or more children (referred to in this Act as the "single parent" class of enrollment).

(D) Coverage of a married couple and one or more children (referred to in this Act as the "dual parent" class of enrollment).

(2) REFERENCES TO FAMILY AND COUPLE CLASSES OF ENROLLMENT.—In this Act:

(A) FAMILY.—The term "family", with respect to a class of enrollment, refers to enrollment in a class of enrollment described in subparagraph (B), (C), or (D) of paragraph (1).

(B) COUPLE.—The term "couple", with respect to a class of enrollment, refers to enrollment in a class of enrollment described in subparagraph (B) or (D) of paragraph (1).

(d) SPOUSE; MARRIED; COUPLE.—

(1) IN GENERAL.—In this Act, the terms "spouse" and "married" mean, with respect to a person, another individual who is the spouse of the person or married to the person, as determined under applicable State law.

(2) COUPLE.—The term "couple" means an individual and the individual's spouse.

(e) CHILD DEFINED.—

(1) IN GENERAL.—In this Act, except as otherwise provided, the term "child" means an eligible individual who (consistent with paragraph (3))—

(A) is under 18 years of age (or under 24 years of age in the case of a full-time student), and

(B) is a dependent of an eligible individual.

(2) APPLICATION OF STATE LAW.—Subject to paragraph (3), determinations of whether a person is the child of another person shall be made in accordance with applicable State law.

(3) NATIONAL RULES.—The National Health Board may establish such national rules respecting individuals who will be treated as children as the Board determines to be necessary. Such rules shall be consistent with the following principles:

    (A) STEP AND FOSTER CHILD.—A child includes a step child or foster child who is an eligible individual living with an adult in a regular parent-child relationship.

    (B) DISABLED CHILD.—A child includes an unmarried dependent eligible individual regardless of age who is incapable of self-support because of mental or physical disability which existed before age 21.

    (C) CERTAIN 3-GENERATION FAMILIES.—A child includes the grandchild of an individual, if the parent of the grandchild is a child and the parent and grandchild are living with the grandparent.

    (D) TREATMENT OF EMANCIPATED MINORS AND MARRIED INDIVIDUALS.—An emancipated minor or married individual shall not be treated as a child.

(f) ADDITIONAL RULES.—The Board shall provide for such additional exceptions and special rules, including rules relating to—

(1) families in which members are not residing in the same area,

(2) the treatment of individuals who are under 19 years of age and who are not a dependent of an eligible individual, and

(3) changes in family composition occurring during a year,

as the Board finds appropriate.

SEC. 1012. TREATMENT OF CERTAIN FAMILIES.

(a) TREATMENT OF MEDICARE-ELIGIBLE INDIVIDUALS WHO ARE QUALIFIED EMPLOYEES OR SPOUSES OF QUALIFIED EMPLOYEES.—

(1) IN GENERAL.—Except as specifically provided, in the case of an individual who is an individual described in paragraph (2) with respect to 2 consecutive months in a year (and it is anticipated would be in the following month), the individual shall not be treated as a medicare-eligible individual under this Act during the following month and the remainder of the year.

(2) INDIVIDUAL DESCRIBED.—An individual described in this paragraph with respect to a month is a medicare-eligible individual (determined without regard to paragraph (1)) who is a qualifying employee or the spouse or family member of a qualifying employee in the month.

(3) EXCEPTION.—Paragraph (1) shall not apply, in the case of an individual, if the individual described in paragraph (2) terminates qualifying employment in the month preceding the first month in which paragraph (1) applies. The previous sentence shall apply until with respect to qualifying employment occurring before such first month.

(b) SEPARATE TREATMENT FOR CERTAIN GROUPS OF INDIVIDUALS.—In the case of a family that includes one or more individuals in a group described in subsection (c)—

(1) all the individuals in each such group within the family shall be treated as a separate family, and

(2) all the individuals not described in any such group shall be treated collectively as a separate family.

(c) GROUPS OF INDIVIDUALS DESCRIBED.—Each of the following is a group of individuals described in this subsection:

(1) AFDC recipients (as defined in section 1902(3)).

(2) Disabled SSI recipients (as defined in section 1902(13)).

(3) SSI recipients who are not disabled SSI recipients.

(4) Electing veterans (as defined in subsection (d)(1)).

(5) Active duty military personnel (as defined in subsection (d)(2)).

(6) Electing Indians (as defined in subsection (d)(3)).

(7) Prisoners (as defined in section 1902(26)).

(d) SPECIAL RULES.—In this Act:

(1) ELECTING VETERANS.—

(A) DEFINED.—Subject to subparagraph (B), the term "electing veteran" means a veteran who makes an election to enroll with a health plan of the Department of Veterans Affairs under chapter 18 of title 38, United States Code.

(B) FAMILY EXCEPTION.—Subparagraph (A) shall not apply with respect to coverage under a health plan referred to in such subparagraph if, for the area in which the electing veteran resides, such health plan offers coverage to family members of an electing veteran and the veteran elects family enrollment under such plan (instead of individual enrollment).

(2) ACTIVE DUTY MILITARY PERSONNEL.—

(A) IN GENERAL.—Subject to subparagraph (B), the term "active duty military personnel" means an individual on active duty in the Uniformed Services of the United States.

(B) EXCEPTION.—If an individual described in subparagraph (A) elects family coverage under section 1073a(d)(1) of title 10, United States Code, then paragraph (5) of subsection (c) shall not apply with respect to such coverage.

(3) ELECTING INDIANS.—

(A) IN GENERAL.—Subject to subparagraph (B), the term "electing Indian" means an eligible individual who makes an election under section 8302(b) of this Act.

(B) FAMILY ELECTION FOR ALL INDIVIDUALS ELIGIBLE TO ELECT.—No such election shall be made with respect to an individual in a family (as defined without regard to this section) unless such election is made for all eligible individuals (described in section 8302(a)) who are family members of the family.

(4) MULTIPLE CHOICE.—Eligible individuals who are permitted to elect coverage under more than one health plan or program referred to in this subsection may elect which of such plans or programs will be the applicable health plan under this Act.

(e) QUALIFYING STUDENTS.—

(1) IN GENERAL.—In the case of a qualifying student (described in paragraph (2)), the individual may elect to enroll in a regional alliance health plan offered by the regional alliance for the area in which the school is located.

(2) QUALIFYING STUDENT.—In paragraph (1), the term "qualifying student" means an individual who—

(A) but for this subsection would receive coverage under a health plan as a child of another person, and

(B) is a full-time student at a school in an alliance area that is different from the alliance area (or, in the case of a corporate alliance, such coverage area as the Board may specify) providing the coverage described in subparagraph (A).

(3) PAYMENT RULES.—

(A) CONTINUED TREATMENT AS FAMILY.—Except as provided in subparagraph (B), nothing in this subsection shall be construed as affecting the payment liabilities between families and health alliances or between health alliances and health plans.

(B) TRANSFER PAYMENT.—In the case of an election under paragraph (1), the health plan described in paragraph (2)(A) shall make payment to the health plan referred to in paragraph (1) in accordance with rules specified by the Board.

(f) SPOUSES LIVING IN DIFFERENT ALLIANCE AREAS.—The Board shall provide for such special rules in applying this Act in the case of a couple in which the spouses reside in different alliance areas as the Board finds appropriate.

SEC. 1013. MULTIPLE EMPLOYMENT SITUATIONS.

(a) MULTIPLE EMPLOYMENT OF AN INDIVIDUAL.—In the case of an individual who—

(1)(A) is not married or (B) is married and whose spouse is not a qualifying employee (as defined in section 6121(c)(1)),

(2) is not a child, and

(3) who is a qualifying employee both of a regional alliance employer and of a corporate alliance employer (or of 2 corporate alliance employers),

the individual may elect the applicable health plan to be either a regional alliance health plan (for the alliance area in which the individual resides) or a corporate alliance health plan (for an employer employing the individual).

(b) MULTIPLE EMPLOYMENT WITHIN A FAMILY.—

(1) MARRIED COUPLE WITH EMPLOYMENT WITH A REGIONAL ALLIANCE EMPLOYER AND WITH A CORPORATE ALLIANCE EMPLOYER.—In the case of a married individual—

(A) who is a qualifying employee of a regional alliance employer and whose spouse is an qualifying employee of a corporate alliance employer, or

(B) who is a qualifying employee of a corporate alliance employer and whose spouse is an qualifying employee of a regional alliance employer,

the individual and the individual's spouse may elect the applicable health plan to be either a regional alliance health plan (for the alliance area in which the couple resides) or a corporate alliance health plan (for an employer employing the individual or the spouse).

(2) MARRIED COUPLE WITH DIFFERENT CORPORATE ALLIANCE EMPLOYERS.—In the case of a married individual—

 (A) who is a qualifying employee of a corporate alliance employer, and

 (B) whose spouse is a qualifying employee of a different corporate alliance employer,

the individual and the individual's spouse may elect the applicable health plan to be a corporate alliance health plan for an employer employing either the individual or the spouse.

## SEC. 1014. TREATMENT OF RESIDENTS OF STATES WITH STATEWIDE SINGLE-PAYER SYSTEMS.

(a) UNIVERSAL COVERAGE.—Notwithstanding the previous provisions of this title, except as provided in part 2 of subtitle C, in the case of an individual who resides in a State that has a Statewide single-payer system under section 1223, universal coverage shall be provided consistent with section 1222(3).

(b) INDIVIDUAL RESPONSIBILITIES.—In the case of an individual who resides in a single-payer State, the responsibilities of such individual under such system shall supersede the obligations of the individual under section 1002.

## Subtitle B—Benefits

### PART 1—COMPREHENSIVE BENEFIT PACKAGE

### SEC. 1101. PROVISION OF COMPREHENSIVE BENEFITS BY PLANS.

(a) IN GENERAL.—The comprehensive benefit package shall consist of the following items and services (as described in part 2), subject to the cost sharing requirements described in part 3, the exclusions described in part 4, and the duties and authority of the National Health Board described in part 5:

   (1) Hospital services (described in section 1111).

   (2) Services of health professionals (described in section 1112).

   (3) Emergency and ambulatory medical and surgical services (described in section 1113).

   (4) Clinical preventive services (described in section 1114).

   (5) Mental health and substance abuse services (described in section 1115).

   (6) Family planning services and services for pregnant women (described in section 1116).

   (7) Hospice care (described in section 1117).

(8) Home health care (described in section 1118).

(9) Extended care services (described in section 1119).

(10) Ambulance services (described in section 1120).

(11) Outpatient laboratory, radiology, and diagnostic services (described in section 1121).

(12) Outpatient prescription drugs and biologicals (described in section 1122).

(13) Outpatient rehabilitation services (described in section 1123).

(14) Durable medical equipment and prosthetic and orthotic devices (described in section 1124).

(15) Vision care (described in section 1125).

(16) Dental care (described in section 1126).

(17) Health education classes (described in section 1127).

(18) Investigational treatments (described in section 1128).

(b) NO OTHER LIMITATIONS OR COST SHARING.—The items and services in the comprehensive benefit package shall not be subject to any duration or scope limitation or any deductible, copayment, or coinsurance amount that is not required or authorized under this Act.

(c) HEALTH PLAN.—Unless otherwise provided in this subtitle, for purposes of this subtitle, the term "health plan" has the meaning given such term in section 1400.

## PART 2—DESCRIPTION OF ITEMS AND SERVICES COVERED

### SEC. 1111. HOSPITAL SERVICES.

(a) COVERAGE.—The hospital services described in this section are the following items and services:

    (1) Inpatient hospital services.

    (2) Outpatient hospital services.

    (3) 24-hour a day hospital emergency services.

(b) LIMITATION.—The hospital services described in this section do not include hospital services provided for the treatment of a mental or substance abuse disorder (which are subject to section 1115), except for medical detoxification as required for the management of medical conditions associated with withdrawal from alcohol or drugs (which is not covered under such section).

(c) DEFINITIONS.—For purposes of this subtitle:

    (1) HOSPITAL.—The term "hospital" has the meaning given such term in section 1861(e) of the Social Security Act, except that such term shall include—

        (A) in the case of an item or service provided to an individual whose applicable health plan is specified pursuant to section 1004(b)(1), a facility of the uniformed services under title 10, United States Code, that is primarily engaged in providing services to inpatients that are equivalent to the services provided by a hospital defined in section 1861(e);

(B) in the case of an item or service provided to an individual whose applicable health plan is specified pursuant to section 1004(b)(2), a facility operated by the Department of Veterans Affairs that is primarily engaged in providing services to inpatients that are equivalent to the services provided by a hospital defined in section 1861(e); and

(C) in the case of an item or service provided to an individual whose applicable health plan is specified pursuant to section 1004(b)(3), a facility operated by the Indian Health Service that is primarily engaged in providing services to inpatients that are equivalent to the services provided by a hospital defined in section 1861(e).

(2) INPATIENT HOSPITAL SERVICES.—The term "inpatient hospital services" means items and services described in paragraphs (1) through (3) of sec-

tion 1861(b) of the Social Security Act when provided to an inpatient of a hospital. The National Health Board shall specify those health professional services described in section 1112 that shall be treated as inpatient hospital services when provided to an inpatient of a hospital.

**SEC. 1112. SERVICES OF HEALTH PROFESSIONALS.**

(a) COVERAGE.—The items and services described in this section are—

　(1) inpatient and outpatient health professional services, including consultations, that are provided in—

　　(A) a home, office, or other ambulatory care setting; or

　　(B) an institutional setting; and

　(2) services and supplies (including drugs and biologicals which cannot be self-administered) furnished as an incident to such health professional services, of kinds which are commonly furnished in the office of a health professional and are commonly either rendered without charge or included in the bill of such professional.

(b) LIMITATION.—The items and services described in this section do not include items or services that are described in any other section of this part. An item or service that is described in section 1114 but is not provided consistent with a periodicity schedule for such item or service specified in such section or under section 1153 may be covered under this section if the item or service otherwise meets the requirements of this section.

(c) DEFINITIONS.—Unless otherwise provided in this Act, for purposes of this Act:

(1) HEALTH PROFESSIONAL.—The term "health professional" means an individual who provides health professional services.

(2) HEALTH PROFESSIONAL SERVICES.—The term "health professional services" means professional services that—

(A) are lawfully provided by a physician; or

(B) would be described in subparagraph (A) if provided by a physician, but are provided by another person who is legally authorized to provide such services in the State in which the services are provided.

## SEC. 1113. EMERGENCY AND AMBULATORY MEDICAL AND SURGICAL SERVICES.

The emergency and ambulatory medical and surgical services described in this section are the following items and services provided by a health facility that is not a hospital and that is legally authorized to provide the services in the State in which they are provided:

(1) 24-hour a day emergency services.

(2) Ambulatory medical and surgical services.

SEC. 1114. CLINICAL PREVENTIVE SERVICES.

(a) COVERAGE.—The clinical preventive services described in this section are—

(1) an item or service for high risk populations (as defined by the National Health Board) that is specified and defined by the Board under section 1153, but only when the item or service is provided consistent with any periodicity schedule for the item or service promulgated by the Board;

(2) except as modified by the National Health Board under section 1153, an age-appropriate immunization, test, or clinician visit specified in one of subsections (b) through (h) that is provided consistent with any periodicity schedule for the item or service specified in the applicable subsection or by the National Health Board under section 1153; and

(3) an immunization, test, or clinician visit that is provided to an individual during an age range other than the age range for such immunization, test, or clinician visit that is specified in one of subsections (b) through (h), but only when provided

consistent with any requirements for such immunizations, tests, and clinician visits established by the National Health Board under section 1153.

(b) INDIVIDUALS UNDER 3.—For an individual under 3 years of age:

(1) IMMUNIZATIONS.—The immunizations specified in this subsection are age-appropriate immunizations for the following illnesses:

(A) Diphtheria.
(B) Tetanus.
(C) Pertussis.
(D) Polio.
(E) Haemophilus influenzae type B.
(F) Measles.
(G) Mumps.
(H) Rubella.
(I) Hepatitis B.

(2) TESTS.—The tests specified in this subsection are as follows:

(A) 1 hematocrit.
(B) 2 blood tests to screen for blood lead levels for individuals who are at risk for lead exposure.

(3) CLINICIAN VISITS.—The clinician visits specified in this subsection are 1 clinician visit for

an individual who is newborn and 7 other clinician visits.

(c) INDIVIDUALS AGE 3 TO 5.—For an individual at least 3 years of age, but less than 6 years of age:

    (1) IMMUNIZATIONS.—The immunizations specified in this subsection are age-appropriate immunizations for the following illnesses:

        (A) Diphtheria.

        (B) Tetanus.

        (C) Pertussis.

        (D) Polio.

        (E) Measles.

        (F) Mumps.

        (G) Rubella.

    (2) TESTS.—The tests specified in this subsection are 1 urinalysis.

    (3) CLINICIAN VISITS.—The clinician visits specified in this subsection are 3 clinician visits.

(d) INDIVIDUALS AGE 6 TO 19.—For an individual at least 6 years of age, but less than 20 years of age:

    (1) IMMUNIZATIONS.—The immunizations specified in this subsection are age-appropriate immunizations for the following illnesses:

        (A) Tetanus.

        (B) Diphtheria.

(2) TESTS.—The tests specified in this subsection are as follows:

(A) Papanicolaou smears and pelvic exams for females who have reached childbearing age and are at risk for cervical cancer every 3 years, but—

(i) annually until 3 consecutive negative smears have been obtained; and

(ii) annually for females who are at risk for fertility related infectious illnesses.

(B) Annual screening for chlamydia and gonorrhea for females who have reached childbearing age and are at risk for fertility related infectious illnesses.

(3) CLINICIAN VISITS.—The clinician visits specified in this subsection are 5 clinician visits.

(e) INDIVIDUALS AGE 20 TO 39.—For an individual at least 20 years of age, but less than 40 years of age:

(1) IMMUNIZATIONS.—The immunizations specified in this subsection are booster immunizations against tetanus and diphtheria every 10 years.

(2) TESTS.—The tests specified in this subsection are as follows:

(A) Papanicolaou smears and pelvic exams for females every 3 years, but—

(i) annually if an abnormal smear has been obtained, until 3 consecutive negative smears have been obtained; and

(ii) annually for females who are at risk for fertility related infectious illnesses.

(B) Annual screening for chlamydia and gonorrhea for females who are at risk for fertility related infectious illnesses.

(C) Cholesterol every 5 years.

(3) CLINICIAN VISITS.—The clinician visits specified in this subsection are 1 clinician visit every 3 years.

(f) INDIVIDUALS AGE 40 TO 49.—For an individual at least 40 years of age, but less than 50 years of age:

(1) IMMUNIZATIONS.—The immunizations specified in this subsection are booster immunizations against tetanus and diphtheria every 10 years.

(2) TESTS.—The tests specified in this subsection are as follows:

(A) Papanicolaou smears and pelvic exams for females every 2 years, but—

(i) annually if an abnormal smear has been obtained, until 3 consecutive negative smears have been obtained; and

(ii) annually for females who are at risk for fertility related infectious illnesses.

(B) Annual screening for chlamydia and gonorrhea for females who are at risk for fertility related infectious illnesses.

(C) Cholesterol every 5 years.

(3) CLINICIAN VISITS.—The clinician visits specified in this subsection are 1 clinician visit every 2 years.

(g) INDIVIDUALS AGE 50 TO 65.—For an individual at least 50 years of age, but less than 65 years of age:

(1) IMMUNIZATIONS.—The immunizations specified in this subsection are booster immunizations against tetanus and diphtheria every 10 years.

(2) TESTS.—The tests specified in this subsection are as follows:

(A) Papanicolaou smears and pelvic exams for females every 2 years.

(B) Mammograms for females every 2 years.

(C) Cholesterol every 5 years.

(3) CLINICIAN VISITS.—The clinician visits specified in this subsection are 1 clinician visit every 2 years.

(h) INDIVIDUALS AGE 65 OR OLDER.—For an individual at least 65 years of age who is enrolled under a health plan:

>(1) IMMUNIZATIONS.—The immunizations specified in this subsection are as follows:
>>(A) Booster immunizations against tetanus and diphtheria every 10 years.
>>(B) Age-appropriate immunizations for the following illnesses:
>>>(i) Influenza.
>>>(ii) Pneumococcal invasive disease.
>
>(2) TESTS.—The tests specified in this subsection are as follows:
>>(A) Papanicolaou smears and pelvic exams for females who are at risk for cervical cancer every 2 years.
>>(B) Mammograms for females every 2 years.
>>(C) Cholesterol every 5 years.
>
>(3) CLINICIAN VISITS.—The clinician visits specified in this subsection are 1 clinician visit every year.

(i) CLINICIAN VISIT.—For purposes of this section, the term "clinician visit" includes the following health professional services (as defined in section 1112(c)):

(1) A complete medical history.

(2) An appropriate physical examination.

(3) Risk assessment.

(4) Targeted health advice and counseling, including nutrition counseling.

(5) The administration of age-appropriate immunizations and tests specified in subsections (b) through (h).

(j) IMMUNIZATIONS AND TESTS NOT ADMINISTERED DURING CLINICIAN VISIT.—Notwithstanding subsection (i)(5), the clinical preventive services described in this section include an immunization or test described in this section that is administered to an individual consistent with any periodicity schedule for the immunization or test during the age range specified for the immunization or test, and any administration fee for such immunization or test, even if the immunization or test is not administered during a clinician visit.

### SEC. 1115. MENTAL HEALTH AND SUBSTANCE ABUSE SERVICES.

(a) COVERAGE.—The mental health and substance abuse services that are described in this section are the following items and services for eligible individuals, as defined in section 1001(c), who satisfy the eligibility requirements in subsection (b):

(1) Inpatient and residential mental health and substance abuse treatment.

(2) Intensive nonresidential mental health and substance abuse treatment.

(3) Outpatient mental health and substance abuse treatment, including case management, screening and assessment, crisis services, and collateral services.

(b) ELIGIBILITY.—The eligibility requirements referred to in subsection (a) are as follows:

(1) INPATIENT, RESIDENTIAL, NONRESIDENTIAL, AND OUTPATIENT TREATMENT.—An eligible individual is eligible to receive coverage for inpatient and residential mental health and substance abuse treatment, intensive nonresidential mental health and substance abuse treatment, or outpatient mental health and substance abuse treatment (except case management and collateral services) if the individual—

(A) has, or has had during the 1-year period preceding the date of such treatment, a diagnosable mental or substance abuse disorder; and

(B) is experiencing, or is at significant risk of experiencing, functional impairment in family, work, school, or community activities.

For purposes of this paragraph, an individual who has a diagnosable mental or substance abuse disorder, is receiving treatment for such disorder, but does not satisfy the functional impairment criterion in subparagraph (B) shall be treated as satisfying such criterion if the individual would satisfy such criterion without such treatment.

(2) CASE MANAGEMENT.—An eligible individual is eligible to receive coverage for case management if—

    (A) the health plan in which the individual is enrolled has elected to offer case management and determines that the individual should receive such services; and

    (B) the individual is eligible to receive coverage for, and is receiving, outpatient mental health and substance abuse treatment.

(3) SCREENING AND ASSESSMENT AND CRISIS SERVICES.—All eligible individuals enrolled under a health plan are eligible to receive coverage for outpatient mental health and substance abuse treat-

ment consisting of screening and assessment and crisis services.

(4) COLLATERAL SERVICES.—An eligible individual is eligible to receive coverage for outpatient mental health and substance abuse treatment consisting of collateral services if the individual is a family member (as defined in section 1011(b)) of an individual who is receiving inpatient and residential mental health and substance abuse treatment, intensive nonresidential mental health and substance abuse treatment, or outpatient mental health and substance abuse treatment.

(c) INPATIENT AND RESIDENTIAL TREATMENT.—

(1) DEFINITION.—For purposes of this subtitle, the term "inpatient and residential mental health and substance abuse treatment" means the items and services described in paragraphs (1) through (3) of section 1861(b) of the Social Security Act when provided with respect to a diagnosable mental or substance abuse disorder to—

> (A) an inpatient of a hospital, psychiatric hospital, residential treatment center, residential detoxification center, crisis residential program, or mental health residential treatment program; or

(B) a resident of a therapeutic family or group treatment home or community residential treatment and recovery center for substance abuse.

The National Health Board shall specify those health professional services described in section 1112 that shall be treated as inpatient and residential mental health and substance abuse treatment when provided to such an inpatient or resident.

(2) LIMITATIONS.—Coverage for inpatient and residential mental health and substance abuse treatment is subject to the following limitations:

(A) LEAST RESTRICTIVE SETTING.—Such treatment is covered only when—

(i) provided to an individual in the least restrictive inpatient or residential setting that is effective and appropriate for the individual; and

(ii) less restrictive intensive nonresidential or outpatient treatment would be ineffective or inappropriate.

(B) LICENSED FACILITY.—Such treatment is only covered when provided by a facility described in paragraph (1) that is legally authorized to provide the treatment in the State in which the facility is located.

(C) DAY LIMITS.—Subject to subparagraph (D), such treatment is covered for each period beginning on the date an episode of inpatient or residential treatment begins and ending on the date the episode ends, except that, prior to January 1, 2001, such treatment is not covered after such an episode exceeds 30 days unless the individual receiving treatment poses a threat to their own life or the life of another individual. Whether such a threat exists shall be determined by a health professional designated by the health plan in which the individual receiving treatment is enrolled. For purposes of this subtitle, an episode of inpatient and residential mental health and substance abuse treatment shall be considered to begin on the date an individual is admitted to a facility for such treatment and to end on the date the individual is discharged from the facility.

(D) ANNUAL LIMIT.—Prior to January 1, 2001, such treatment in all settings is subject to an aggregate annual limit of 60 days.

(E) INPATIENT HOSPITAL TREATMENT FOR SUBSTANCE ABUSE.—Substance abuse treatment, when provided to an inpatient of a hospital or psychiatric hospital, is covered under this section only for medical detoxification associated with withdrawal from alcohol or drugs.

(d) INTENSIVE NONRESIDENTIAL TREATMENT.—

(1) DEFINITION.—For purposes of this subtitle, the term "intensive nonresidential mental health and substance abuse treatment" means diagnostic or therapeutic items or services provided with respect to a diagnosable mental or substance abuse disorder to an individual—

(A) participating in a partial hospitalization program, a day treatment program, a psychiatric rehabilitation program, or an ambulatory detoxification program; or

(B) receiving home-based mental health services or behavioral aide mental health services.

The National Health Board shall specify those health professional services described in section 1112 that shall be treated as intensive nonresidential mental health and substance abuse treatment when provided to such an individual.

(2) LIMITATIONS.—Coverage for intensive nonresidential mental health and substance abuse treatment is subject to the following limitations:

(A) DISCRETION OF PLAN.—A health plan may cover intensive nonresidential mental health and substance abuse treatment at its discretion.

(B) TREATMENT PURPOSES.—Such treatment is covered only when provided—

(i) to avert the need for, or as an alternative to, treatment in residential or inpatient settings;

(ii) to facilitate the earlier discharge of an individual receiving inpatient or residential care;

(iii) to restore the functioning of an individual with a diagnosable mental health or substance abuse disorder; or

(iv) to assist the individual to develop the skills and gain access to the support services the individual needs to achieve the maximum level of functioning of the individual within the community.

(C) ANNUAL LIMIT.—

(i) IN GENERAL.—Prior to January 1, 2001, such treatment in all settings is subject to an aggregate annual limit of 120 days.

(ii) RELATIONSHIP TO OTHER ANNUAL LIMITS.—For each 2 days of intensive nonresidential mental health and substance abuse treatment provided to an individual, the number of treatment days available to the individual before the annual aggregate limit on inpatient and residential mental health and substance abuse treatment described in subsection (c)(2)(D) is exceeded shall be reduced by 1 day. The preceding sentence shall not apply after an individual has received 60 days of intensive nonresidential mental health and substance abuse treatment in a year.

(iii) ADDITIONAL DAYS.—A maximum of 60 additional days of intensive nonresidential mental health and substance abuse treatment may be provided to an individual if a health professional designated by the health plan in which the individual receiving treatment is enrolled determines that such additional treatment is medically necessary or appropriate.

(D) OUT-OF-POCKET MAXIMUM.—Prior to January 1, 2001, expenses for intensive nonresidential mental health and substance abuse treatment that an individual incurs prior to satisfying a deductible applicable to such treatment, and copayments and coinsurance paid by or on behalf of the individual for such treatment, that substitute for inpatient and residential mental health and substance abuse treatment (up to 60 days) may be applied toward the annual out-of-pocket limit on cost sharing under any cost sharing schedule described in part 3 of this subtitle.

(e) OUTPATIENT TREATMENT.—

(1) DEFINITION.—For purposes of this subtitle, the term "outpatient mental health and substance abuse treatment" means the following services provided with respect to a diagnosable mental or substance abuse disorder in an outpatient setting:

(A) Screening and assessment.

(B) Diagnosis.

(C) Medical management.

(D) Substance abuse counseling and relapse prevention.

(E) Crisis services.

(F) Somatic treatment services.

(G) Psychotherapy.

(H) Case management.

(I) Collateral services.

(2) LIMITATIONS.—Coverage for outpatient mental health and substance abuse treatment is subject to the following limitations:

(A) HEALTH PROFESSIONAL SERVICES.—Such treatment is covered only when it constitutes health professional services (as defined in section 1112(c)(2)).

(B) SUBSTANCE ABUSE COUNSELING.—Substance abuse counseling and relapse prevention is covered only when provided by a substance abuse treatment provider who—

(i) is legally authorized to provide such services in the State in which the services are provided; and

(ii) provides no items or services other than substance abuse counseling and relapse prevention, medical management, or laboratory and diagnostic tests for individuals with substance abuse disorders.

(C) ANNUAL LIMITS.—

(i) PYCHOTHERAPY AND COLLATERAL SERVICES.—Prior to January 1, 2001, psychotherapy and collateral services are subject to annual limits of 30 visits for each type of service. Additional visits may be covered, at the discretion of the health plan in which the individual receiving treatment is enrolled, to prevent hospitalization or to facilitate earlier hospital release, for which the annual aggregate limit on inpatient and residential mental health and substance abuse treatment described in subsection (c)(2)(D) shall be reduced by 1 day for each 4 visits.

(ii) SUBSTANCE ABUSE.—At the discretion of the health plan in which an individual receiving outpatient substance abuse treatment is enrolled, the annual aggregate limit on inpatient and residential mental health and substance abuse treatment described in subsection (c)(2)(D) may be reduced by 1 day for each 4 outpatient visits.

Within 12 months after inpatient and residential treatment or intensive nonresidential treatment, 30 visits in group therapy shall be covered for substance abuse counseling and relapse prevention. For individuals who were not initially treated in an inpatient, residential, or intensive nonresidential setting, additional visits shall be covered for which the annual aggregate limit on inpatient and residential mental health and substance abuse treatment described in subsection (c)(2)(D) shall be reduced by 1 day for each 4 visits.

(D) OUT-OF-POCKET MAXIMUM.—Prior to January 1, 2001, expenses for outpatient mental health and substance abuse treatment that an individual incurs prior to satisfying a deductible applicable to such treatment, and copayments and coinsurance paid by or on behalf of the individual for such treatment, may not be applied toward any annual out-of-pocket limit on cost sharing under any cost sharing schedule described in part 3 of this subtitle.

(E) DETOXIFICATION.—Outpatient detoxification shall be provided only in the context of a treatment program. If the first detoxification treatment is unsuccessful, subsequent treatments are covered if a health professional designated by the health plan in which the individual receiving treatment is enrolled determines that there is a substantial chance of success.

(f) OTHER DEFINITIONS.—For purposes of this subtitle:

(1) CASE MANAGEMENT.—The term "case management" means services that assist individuals in gaining access to needed medical, social, educational, and other services.

(2) DIAGNOSABLE MENTAL OR SUBSTANCE ABUSE DISORDER.—The term "diagnosable mental or substance abuse disorder" means a disorder that is listed in any authoritative text specifying diagnostic criteria for mental or substance abuse disorders that is identified by the National Health Board.

(3) PSYCHIATRIC HOSPITAL.—The term "psychiatric hospital" has the meaning given such term in section 1861(f) of the Social Security Act, except that such term shall include—

(A) in the case of an item or service provided to an individual whose applicable health plan is specified pursuant to section 1004(b)(1), a facility of the uniformed services under title 10, United States Code, that is engaged in providing services to inpatients that are equivalent to the services provided by a psychiatric hospital;

(B) in the case of an item or service provided to an individual whose applicable health plan is specified pursuant to section 1004(b)(2), a facility operated by the Department of Veterans Affairs that is engaged in providing services to inpatients that are equivalent to the services provided by a psychiatric hospital; and

(C) in the case of an item or service provided to an individual whose applicable health plan is specified pursuant to section 1004(b)(3), a facility operated by the Indian Health Service that is engaged in providing services to inpatients that are equivalent to the services provided by a psychiatric hospital.

## SEC. 1116. FAMILY PLANNING SERVICES AND SERVICES FOR PREGNANT WOMEN.

The services described in this section are the following items and services:

(1) Voluntary family planning services.

(2) Contraceptive devices that—

(A) may only be dispensed upon prescription; and

(B) are subject to approval by the Secretary of Health and Human Services under the Federal Food, Drug, and Cosmetic Act.

(3) Services for pregnant women.

## SEC. 1117. HOSPICE CARE.

The hospice care described in this section is the items and services described in paragraph (1) of section 1861(dd) of the Social Security Act, as defined in paragraphs (2), (3), and (4)(A) of such section (with the exception of paragraph (2)(A)(iii)), except that all references to the Secretary of Health and Human Services in such paragraphs shall be treated as references to the National Health Board.

## SEC. 1118. HOME HEALTH CARE.

(a) COVERAGE.—The home health care described in this section is—

(1) the items and services described in section 1861(m) of the Social Security Act; and

(2) home infusion drug therapy services described in section 1861(ll) of the Social Security Act (as added by section 2006).

(b) LIMITATIONS.—Coverage for home health care is subject to the following limitations:

(1) INPATIENT TREATMENT ALTERNATIVE.—Such care is covered only as an alternative to inpatient treatment in a hospital, skilled nursing facility, or rehabilitation facility after an illness or injury.

(2) REEVALUATION.—At the end of each 60-day period of home health care, the need for continued care shall be reevaluated by the person who is primarily responsible for providing the home health care. Additional periods of care are covered only if such person determines that the requirement in paragraph (1) is satisfied.

## SEC. 1119. EXTENDED CARE SERVICES.

(a) COVERAGE.—The extended care services described in this section are the items and services described in section 1861(h) of the Social Security Act when provided to an inpatient of a skilled nursing facility or a rehabilitation facility.

(b) LIMITATIONS.—Coverage for extended care services is subject to the following limitations:

(1) HOSPITAL ALTERNATIVE.—Such services are covered only as an alternative to inpatient treatment in a hospital after an illness or injury.

(2) ANNUAL LIMIT.—Such services are subject to an aggregate annual limit of 100 days.

(c) DEFINITIONS.—For purposes of this subtitle:

(1) REHABILITATION FACILITY.—The term "rehabilitation facility" means an institution (or a distinct part of an institution) which is established and operated for the purpose of providing diagnostic, therapeutic, and rehabilitation services to individuals for rehabilitation from illness or injury.

(2) SKILLED NURSING FACILITY.—The term "skilled nursing facility" means an institution (or a distinct part of an institution) which is primarily engaged in providing to residents—

(A) skilled nursing care and related services for residents who require medical or nursing care; or

(B) rehabilitation services to residents for rehabilitation from illness or injury.

**SEC. 1120. AMBULANCE SERVICES.**

(a) COVERAGE.—The ambulance services described in this section are the following items and services:

(1) Ground transportation by ambulance.

(2) Air transportation by an aircraft equipped for transporting an injured or sick individual.

(3) Water transportation by a vessel equipped for transporting an injured or sick individual.

(b) LIMITATIONS.—Coverage for ambulance services is subject to the following limitations:

(1) MEDICAL INDICATION.—Ambulance services are covered only in cases in which the use of an ambulance is indicated by the medical condition of the individual concerned.

(2) AIR TRANSPORT.—Air transportation is covered only in cases in which there is no other method of transportation or where the use of another method of transportation is contra-indicated by the medical condition of the individual concerned.

(3) WATER TRANSPORT.—Water transportation is covered only in cases in which there is no other method of transportation or where the use of another method of transportation is contra-indicated by the medical condition of the individual concerned.

SEC. 1121. OUTPATIENT LABORATORY, RADIOLOGY, AND DIAGNOSTIC SERVICES.

The items and services described in this section are laboratory, radiology, and diagnostic services provided upon prescription to individuals who are not inpatients of a hospital, hospice, skilled nursing facility, or rehabilitation facility.

SEC. 1122. OUTPATIENT PRESCRIPTION DRUGS AND BIOLOGICALS.

(a) COVERAGE.—The items described in this section are the following:

(1) Covered outpatient drugs described in section 1861(t) of the Social Security Act (as amended by section 2001(b))—

(A) except that, for purposes of this section, a medically accepted indication with respect to the use of a covered outpatient drug includes any use which has been approved by the Food and Drug Administration for the drug, and includes another use of the drug if—

(i) the drug has been approved by the Food and Drug Administration; and

(ii) such use is supported by one or more citations which are included (or approved for inclusion) in one or more of the following compendia: the American Hospital Formulary Service-Drug Information, the American Medical Association Drug Evaluations, the United States Pharmacopoeia-Drug Information, and other authoritative compendia as identified by the National Health Board, unless the Board has determined that the use is not medically appropriate or the use is identified as not indicated in one or more such compendia; or

(iii) such use is medically accepted based on supportive clinical evidence in peer reviewed medical literature appearing in publications which have been identified for purposes of this clause by the Board; and

(B) notwithstanding any exclusion from coverage that may be made with respect to such a drug under title XVIII of such Act pursuant to section 1862(a)(18) of such Act.

(2) Blood clotting factors when provided on an outpatient basis.

(b) REVISION OF COMPENDIA LIST.—The National Health Board may revise the list of compendia in subsection (a)(1)(A)(ii) designated as appropriate for identifying medically accepted indications for drugs.

(c) BLOOD CLOTTING FACTORS.—For purposes of this subtitle, the term "blood clotting factors" has the meaning given such term in section 1861(s)(2)(I) of the Social Security Act.

### SEC. 1123. OUTPATIENT REHABILITATION SERVICES.

(a) COVERAGE.—The outpatient rehabilitation services described in this section are—

(1) outpatient occupational therapy;

(2) outpatient physical therapy; and

(3) outpatient speech pathology services for the purpose of attaining or restoring speech.

(b) LIMITATIONS.—Coverage for outpatient rehabilitation services is subject to the following limitations:

(1) RESTORATION OF CAPACITY OR MINIMIZATION OF LIMITATIONS.—Such services include only items or services used to restore functional capacity or minimize limitations on physical and cognitive functions as a result of an illness or injury.

(2) REEVALUATION.—At the end of each 60-day period of outpatient rehabilitation services, the need for continued services shall be reevaluated by the person who is primarily responsible for providing the services. Additional periods of services are covered only if such person determines that functioning is improving.

### SEC. 1124. DURABLE MEDICAL EQUIPMENT AND PROSTHETIC AND ORTHOTIC DEVICES.

(a) COVERAGE.—The items and services described in this section are—

(1) durable medical equipment, including accessories and supplies necessary for repair and maintenance of such equipment;

(2) prosthetic devices (other than dental) which replace all or part of the function of an internal body organ (including colostomy bags and supplies directly related to colostomy care), including replacement of such devices;

(3) accessories and supplies which are used directly with a prosthetic device to achieve the therapeutic benefits of the prosthesis or to assure the proper functioning of the device;

(4) leg, arm, back, and neck braces;

(5) artificial legs, arms, and eyes, including replacements if required because of a change in the patient's physical condition; and

(6) fitting and training for use of the items described in paragraphs (1) through (5).

(b) LIMITATION.—An item or service described in this section is covered only if it improves functional ability or prevents further deterioration in function.

(c) DURABLE MEDICAL EQUIPMENT.—For purposes of this subtitle, the term "durable medical equipment" has the meaning given such term in section 1861(n) of the Social Security Act.

### SEC. 1125. VISION CARE.

(a) COVERAGE.—The vision care described in this section is diagnosis and treatment for defects in vision.

(b) LIMITATION.—Eyeglasses and contact lenses are covered only for individuals less than 18 years of age.

### SEC. 1126. DENTAL CARE.

(a) COVERAGE.—The dental care described in this section is the following:

(1) Emergency dental treatment, including simple extractions, for acute infections, bleeding, and injuries to natural teeth and oral structures for conditions requiring immediate attention to prevent risks to life or significant medical complications, as specified by the National Health Board.

(2) Prevention and diagnosis of dental disease, including oral dental examinations, radiographs, dental sealants, fluoride application, and dental prophylaxis.

(3) Treatment of dental disease, including routine fillings, prosthetics for genetic defects, periodontal maintenance, and endodontic services.

(4) Space maintenance procedures to prevent orthodontic complications.

(5) Interceptive orthodontic treatment to prevent severe malocclusion.

(b) LIMITATIONS.—Coverage for dental care is subject to the following limitations:

(1) PREVENTION AND DIAGNOSIS.—Prior to January 1, 2001, the items and services described in subsection (a)(2) are covered only for individuals less than 18 years of age. On or after such date, such items and services are covered for all eligible individuals enrolled under a health plan, except that dental sealants are not covered for individuals 18 years of age or older.

(2) TREATMENT OF DENTAL DISEASE.—Prior to January 1, 2001, the items and services described in subsection (a)(3) are covered only for individuals less than 18 years of age. On or after such date, such items and services are covered for all eligible individuals enrolled under a health plan, except that endodontic services are not covered for individuals 18 years of age or older.

(3) SPACE MAINTENANCE.—The items and services described in subsection (a)(4) are covered

only for individuals at least 3 years of age, but less than 13 years of age and—

 (A) are limited to posterior teeth;

 (B) involve maintenance of a space or spaces for permanent posterior teeth that would otherwise be prevented from normal eruption if the space were not maintained; and

 (C) do not include a space maintainer that is placed within 6 months of the expected eruption of the permanent posterior tooth concerned.

 (4) INTERCEPTIVE ORTHODONTIC TREATMENT.—Prior to January 1, 2001, the items and services described in subsection (a)(5) are not covered. On or after such date, such items and services are covered only for individuals at least 6 years of age, but less than 12 years of age.

SEC. 1127. HEALTH EDUCATION CLASSES.

(a) COVERAGE.—Subject to subsection (b), the items and services described in this section are health education and training classes to encourage the reduction of behavioral risk factors and to promote healthy activities. Such education and training classes may include smoking cessation, nutrition counseling, stress management, support groups, and physical training classes.

(b) DISCRETION OF PLAN.—A health plan may offer education and training classes at its discretion.

(c) CONSTRUCTION.—This section shall not be construed to include or limit education or training that is provided in the course of the delivery of health professional services (as defined in section 1112(c)).

SEC. 1128. INVESTIGATIONAL TREATMENTS.

(a) COVERAGE.—Subject to subsection (b), the items and services described in this subsection are qualifying investigational treatments that are administered for a life-threatening disease, disorder, or other health condition (as defined by the National Health Board).

(b) DISCRETION OF PLAN.—A health plan may cover an investigational treatment described in subsection (a) at its discretion.

(c) ROUTINE CARE DURING INVESTIGATIONAL TREATMENTS.—The comprehensive benefit package includes an item or service described in any other section of this part, subject to the limitations and cost sharing requirements applicable to the item or service, when the item or service is provided to an individual in the course of an investigational treatment, if—

(1) the treatment is a qualifying investigational treatment; and

(2) the item or service would have been provided to the individual even if the individual were not receiving the investigational treatment.

(d) DEFINITIONS.—For purposes of this subtitle:

(1) QUALIFYING INVESTIGATIONAL TREATMENT.—The term "qualifying investigational treatment" means a treatment—

(A) the effectiveness of which has not been determined; and

(B) that is under clinical investigation as part of an approved research trial.

(2) APPROVED RESEARCH TRIAL.—The term "approved research trial" means—

(A) a research trial approved by the Secretary of Health and Human Services, the Director of the National Institutes of Health, the Commissioner of the Food and Drug Administration, the Secretary of Veterans Affairs, the Secretary of Defense, or a qualified nongovernmental research entity as defined in guidelines of the National Institutes of Health; or

(B) a peer-reviewed and approved research program, as defined by the Secretary of Health and Human Services, conducted for the primary purpose of determining whether or not a treatment is safe, efficacious, or having any other characteristic of a treatment which must be demonstrated in order for the treatment to be medically necessary or appropriate.

## PART 3—COST SHARING

### SEC. 1131. COST SHARING.

(a) IN GENERAL.—Each health plan shall offer to individuals enrolled under the plan one of the following cost sharing schedules, which schedule shall be offered to all such enrollees:

　　(1) lower cost sharing (described in section 1132);

　　(2) higher cost sharing (described in section 1133); or

　　(3) combination cost sharing (described in section 1134).

(b) COST SHARING FOR LOW-INCOME FAMILIES.—For provisions relating to reducing cost sharing for certain low-income families, see section 1371.

(c) DEDUCTIBLES, COST SHARING, AND OUT-OF-POCKET LIMITS ON COST SHARING.—

　　(1) APPLICATION ON AN ANNUAL BASIS.—The deductibles and out-of-pocket limits on cost sharing for a year under the schedules referred to in sub-

section (a) shall be applied based upon expenses incurred for items and services furnished in the year.

(2) INDIVIDUAL AND FAMILY GENERAL DEDUCTIBLES.—

(A) INDIVIDUAL.—Subject to subparagraph (B), with respect to an individual enrolled under a health plan (regardless of the class of enrollment), any individual general deductible in the cost sharing schedule offered by the plan represents the amount of countable expenses (as defined in subparagraph (C)) that the individual may be required to incur in a year before the plan incurs liability for expenses for such items and services furnished to the individual.

(B) FAMILY.—In the case of an individual enrolled under a health plan under a family class of enrollment (as defined in section 1011(c)(2)(A)), the individual general deductible under subparagraph (A) shall not apply to countable expenses incurred by any member of the individual's family in a year at such time as the family has incurred, in the aggregate, countable expenses in the amount of the family general deductible for the year.

(C) COUNTABLE EXPENSE.—In this paragraph, the term "countable expense" means, with respect to an individual for a year, an expense for an item or service covered by the comprehensive benefit package that is subject to the general deductible and for which, but for such deductible and other cost sharing under this subtitle, a health plan is liable for payment. The amount of countable expenses for an individual for a year under this paragraph shall not exceed the individual general deductible for the year.

(3) COINSURANCE AND COPAYMENTS.—After a general or separate deductible that applies to an item or service covered by the comprehensive benefit package has been satisfied for a year, subject to paragraph (4), coinsurance and copayments are amounts that an individual may be required to pay with respect to the item or service.

(4) INDIVIDUAL AND FAMILY LIMITS ON COST SHARING.—

(A) INDIVIDUAL.—Subject to subparagraph (B), with respect to an individual enrolled under a health plan (regardless of the class of enrollment), the individual out-of-pocket limit on cost sharing in the cost sharing schedule offered by the plan represents the amount of expenses that the individual may be required to incur under the plan in a year because of a general deductible, separate deductibles, copayments, and coinsurance before the plan may no longer impose any cost sharing with respect to items or services covered by the comprehensive benefit package that are provided to the individual, except as provided in subsections (d)(2)(D) and (e)(2)(D) of section 1115.

(B) FAMILY.—In the case of an individual enrolled under a health plan under a family class of enrollment (as defined in section 1011(c)(2)(A)), the family out-of-pocket limit on cost sharing in the cost sharing schedule offered by the plan represents the amount of expenses that members of the individual's family, in the aggregate, may be required to incur under the plan in a year because of a general deductible, separate deductibles, copayments, and coinsurance before the plan may no longer impose any cost sharing with respect to items or services covered by the comprehensive benefit package that are provided to any member of the individual's family, except as provided in subsections (d)(2)(D) and (e)(2)(D) of section 1115.

### SEC. 1132. LOWER COST SHARING.

(a) IN GENERAL.—The lower cost sharing schedule referred to in section 1131 that is offered by a health plan—

    (1) may not include a deductible;

    (2) shall have—

        (A) an annual individual out-of-pocket limit on cost sharing of $1500; and

        (B) an annual family out-of-pocket limit on cost sharing of $3000;

    (3) except as provided in paragraph (4)—

        (A) shall prohibit payment of any coinsurance; and

        (B) subject to section 1152, shall require payment of the copayment for an item or service (if any) that is specified for the item or service in the table under section 1135; and

    (4) shall require payment of coinsurance for an out-of-network item or service (as defined in section 1402(f)) in an amount that is a percentage (determined under subsection (b)) of the applicable pay-

ment rate for the item or service established under section 1322(c), but only if the item or service is subject to coinsurance under the higher cost sharing schedule described in section 1133.

(b) OUT-OF-NETWORK COINSURANCE PERCENTAGE.—

(1) IN GENERAL.—The National Health Board shall determine a percentage referred to in subsection (a)(4). The percentage—

(A) may not be less than 20 percent; and

(B) shall be the same with respect to all out-of-network items and services that are subject to coinsurance, except as provided in paragraph (2).

(2) EXCEPTION.—The National Health Board may provide for a percentage that is greater than a percentage determined under paragraph (1) in the case of an out-of-network item or service for which the coinsurance is greater than 20 percent of the applicable payment rate under the higher cost sharing schedule described in section 1133.

**SEC. 1133. HIGHER COST SHARING.**

The higher cost sharing schedule referred to in section 1131 that is offered by a health plan—

(1) shall have an annual individual general deductible of $200 and an annual family general deductible of $400 that apply with respect to expenses incurred for all items and services in the comprehensive benefit package except—

　(A) an item or service with respect to which a separate individual deductible applies under paragraph (2), (3), or (4); or

　(B) an item or service described in paragraph (5), (6), or (7) with respect to which a deductible does not apply;

(2) shall require an individual to incur expenses during each episode of inpatient and residential mental health and substance abuse treatment (described in section 1115) equal to the cost of one day of such treatment before the plan provides benefits for such treatment to the individual;

(3) shall require an individual to incur expenses in a year for outpatient prescription drugs and biologicals (described in section 1122) equal to $250 before the plan provides benefits for such items to the individual;

(4) shall require an individual to incur expenses in a year for dental care described in section 1126, except the items and services for prevention and di-

agnosis of dental disease described in section 1126(a)(2), equal to $50 before the plan provides benefits for such care to the individual;

(5) may not require any deductible for clinical preventive services (described in section 1114);

(6) may not require any deductible for clinician visits and associated services related to prenatal care or 1 post-partum visit under section 1116;

(7) may not require any deductible for the items and services for prevention and diagnosis of dental disease described in section 1126(a)(2);

(8) shall have—

    (A) an annual individual out-of-pocket limit on cost sharing of $1500; and

    (B) an annual family out-of-pocket limit on cost sharing of $3000;

(9) shall prohibit payment of any copayment; and

(10) subject to section 1152, shall require payment of the coinsurance for an item or service (if any) that is specified for the item or service in the table under section 1135.

# SEC. 1134. COMBINATION COST SHARING.

(a) IN GENERAL.—The combination cost sharing schedule referred to in section 1131 that is offered by a health plan—

    (1) shall have—

        (A) an annual individual out-of-pocket limit on cost sharing of $1500; and

        (B) an annual family out-of-pocket limit on cost sharing of $3000; and

    (2) otherwise shall require different cost sharing for in-network items and services than for out-of-network items and services.

(b) IN-NETWORK ITEMS AND SERVICES.—With respect to an in-network item or service (as defined in section 1402(f)(1)), the combination cost sharing schedule that is offered by a health plan—

    (1) may not apply a deductible;

    (2) shall prohibit payment of any coinsurance; and

    (3) shall require payment of a copayment in accordance with the lower cost sharing schedule described in section 1132.

(c) OUT-OF-NETWORK ITEMS AND SERVICES.—With respect to an out-of-network item or service (as defined in section 1402(f)(2)), the combination cost sharing schedule that is offered by a health plan—

(1) shall require an individual and a family to incur expenses before the plan provides benefits for the item or service in accordance with the deductibles under the higher cost sharing schedule described in section 1133;

(2) shall prohibit payment of any copayment; and

(3) shall require payment of coinsurance in accordance with such schedule.

## SEC. 1135. TABLE OF COPAYMENTS AND COINSURANCE.

(a) IN GENERAL.—The following table specifies, for different items and services, the copayments and coinsurance referred to in sections 1132 and 1133:

Copayments and Coinsurance for Items and Services

| Benefit | Section | Lower Cost Sharing Schedule | Higher Cost Sharing Schedule |
|---|---|---|---|
| Inpatient hospital services | 1111 | No copayment | 20 percent of applicable payment rate |
| Outpatient hospital services | 1111 | $10 per visit | 20 percent of applicable payment rate |
| Hospital emergency room services | 1111 | $25 per visit (unless patient has an emergency medical condition as defined in section 1867(e)(1) of the Social Security Act) | 20 percent of applicable payment rate |
| Services of health professionals | 1112 | $10 per visit | 20 percent of applicable payment rate |

# Health Security Act

*Title I, Subtitle B*

## Copayments and Coinsurance for Items and Services—Continued

| Benefit | Section | Lower Cost Sharing Schedule | Higher Cost Sharing Schedule |
|---|---|---|---|
| Emergency services other than hospital emergency room services | 1113 | $25 per visit (unless patient has an emergency medical condition as defined in section 1867(e)(1) of the Social Security Act) | 20 percent of applicable payment rate |
| Ambulatory medical and surgical services | 1113 | $10 per visit | 20 percent of applicable payment rate |
| Clinical preventive services | 1114 | No copayment | No coinsurance |
| Inpatient and residential mental health and substance abuse treatment | 1115 | No copayment | 20 percent of applicable payment rate |
| Intensive nonresidential mental health and substance abuse treatment | 1115 | No copayment | 20 percent of applicable payment rate |
| Outpatient mental health and substance abuse treatment (except psychotherapy, collateral services, and case management) | 1115 | $10 per visit | 20 percent of applicable payment rate |
| Outpatient psychotherapy and collateral services | 1115 | $25 per visit until January 1, 2001, and $10 per visit thereafter | 50 percent of applicable payment rate until January 1, 2001, and 20 percent thereafter |
| Case management | 1115 | No copayment | No coinsurance |
| Family planning and services for pregnant women (except clinician visits and associated services related to prenatal care and 1 post-partum visit) | 1116 | $10 per visit | 20 percent of applicable payment rate |
| Clinician visits and associated services related to prenatal care and 1 post-partum visit | 1116 | No copayment | No coinsurance |
| Hospice care | 1117 | No copayment | 20 percent of applicable payment rate |
| Home health care | 1118 | No copayment | 20 percent of applicable payment rate |
| Extended care services | 1119 | No copayment | 20 percent of applicable payment rate |

**Copayments and Coinsurance for Items and Services—Continued**

| Benefit | Section | Lower Cost Sharing Schedule | Higher Cost Sharing Schedule |
|---|---|---|---|
| Ambulance services | 1120 | No copayment | 20 percent of applicable payment rate |
| Outpatient laboratory, radiology, and diagnostic services | 1121 | No copayment | 20 percent of applicable payment rate |
| Outpatient prescription drugs and biologicals | 1122 | $5 per prescription | 20 percent of applicable payment rate |
| Outpatient rehabilitation services | 1123 | $10 per visit | 20 percent of applicable payment rate |
| Durable medical equipment and prosthetic and orthotic devices | 1124 | No copayment | 20 percent of applicable payment rate |
| Vision care | 1125 | $10 per visit (No additional charge for 1 set of necessary eyeglasses for an individual less than 18 years of age) | 20 percent of applicable payment rate |
| Dental care (except space maintenance procedures and interceptive orthodontic treatment) | 1126 | $10 per visit | 20 percent of applicable payment rate |
| Space maintenance procedures and interceptive orthodontic treatment | 1126 | $20 per visit | 40 percent of applicable payment rate |
| Health education classes | 1127 | All cost sharing rules determined by plans | All cost sharing rules determined by plans |
| Investigational treatment for life-threatening condition | 1128 | All cost sharing rules determined by plans | All cost sharing rules determined by plans |

(b) APPLICABLE PAYMENT RATE.—For purposes of this section, the term "applicable payment rate", when used with respect to an item or service, means the applicable payment rate for the item or service established under section 1322(c).

## SEC. 1136. INDEXING DOLLAR AMOUNTS RELATING TO COST SHARING.

(a) IN GENERAL.—Any deductible, copayment, out-of-pocket limit on cost sharing, or other amount expressed in dollars in this subtitle for items or services provided in a year after 1994 shall be such amount increased by the percentage specified in subsection (b) for the year.

(b) PERCENTAGE.—The percentage specified in this subsection for a year is equal to the product of the factors described in subsection (d) for the year and for each previous year after 1994.

(c) ROUNDING.—Any increase (or decrease) under subsection (a) shall be rounded, in the case of an amount specified in this subtitle of—

  (1) $200 or less, to the nearest multiple of $1,

  (2) more than $200, but less $500, to the nearest multiple of $5, or

  (3) $500 or more, to the nearest multiple of $10.

(d) FACTOR.—

  (1) IN GENERAL.—The factor described in this subsection for a year is 1 plus the general health care inflation factor (as specified in section 6001(a)(3) and determined under paragraph (2)) for the year.

(2) DETERMINATION.—In computing such factor for a year, the percentage increase in the CPI for a year (referred to in section 6001(b)) shall be determined based upon the percentage increase in the average of the CPI for the 12-month period ending with August 31 of the previous year over such average for the preceding 12-month period.

## PART 4—EXCLUSIONS

**SEC. 1141. EXCLUSIONS.**

(a) MEDICAL NECESSITY.—The comprehensive benefit package does not include—

(1) an item or service (other than services referred to in paragraph (2)) that is not medically necessary or appropriate; or

(2) an item or service that the National Health Board may determine is not medically necessary or appropriate in a regulation promulgated under section 1154.

(b) ADDITIONAL EXCLUSIONS.—The comprehensive benefit package does not include the following items and services:

(1) Custodial care, except in the case of hospice care under section 1117.

(2) Surgery and other procedures performed solely for cosmetic purposes and hospital or other services incident thereto, unless—

    (A) required to correct a congenital anomaly; or

    (B) required to restore or correct a part of the body that has been altered as a result of—

        (i) accidental injury;

        (ii) disease; or

        (iii) surgery that is otherwise covered under this subtitle.

(3) Hearing aids.

(4) Eyeglasses and contact lenses for individuals at least 18 years of age.

(5) In vitro fertilization services.

(6) Sex change surgery and related services.

(7) Private duty nursing.

(8) Personal comfort items, except in the case of hospice care under section 1117.

(9) Any dental procedures involving orthodontic care, inlays, gold or platinum fillings, bridges, crowns, pin/post retention, dental implants, surgical periodontal procedures, or the preparation of the mouth for the fitting or continued use of dentures, except as specifically described in section 1126.

# PART 5—ROLE OF THE NATIONAL HEALTH BOARD

SEC. 1151. DEFINITION OF BENEFITS.

(a) IN GENERAL.—The National Health Board may promulgate such regulations or establish such guidelines as may be necessary to assure uniformity in the application of the comprehensive benefit package across all health plans.

(b) FLEXIBILITY IN DELIVERY.—The regulations or guidelines under subsection (a) shall permit a health plan to deliver covered items and services to individuals enrolled under the plan using the providers and methods that the plan determines to be appropriate.

SEC. 1152. ACCELERATION OF EXPANDED BENEFITS.

(a) IN GENERAL.—Subject to subsection (b), at any time prior to January 1, 2001, the National Health Board, in its discretion, may by regulation expand the comprehensive benefit package by—

(1) adding any item or service that is added to the package as of January 1, 2001; and

(2) requiring that a cost sharing schedule described in part 3 of this subtitle reflect (wholly or in part) any of the cost sharing requirements that apply to the schedule as of January 1, 2001.

No such expansion shall be effective except as of January 1 of a year.

(b) CONDITION.—The Board may not expand the benefit package under subsection (a) which is to become effective with respect to a year, by adding any item or service or altering any cost sharing schedule, unless the Board estimates that the additional increase in per capita health care expenditures resulting from the addition or alteration, for each regional alliance for the year, will not cause any regional alliance to exceed its per capita target (as determined under section 6003(a)).

## SEC. 1153. AUTHORITY WITH RESPECT TO CLINICAL PREVENTIVE SERVICES.

(a) IN GENERAL.—With respect to clinical preventive services described in section 1114, the National Health Board—

    (1) shall specify and define specific items and services as clinical preventive services for high risk populations and shall establish and update a periodicity schedule for such items and services;

    (2) shall update the periodicity schedules for the age-appropriate immunizations, tests, and clinician visits specified in subsections (b) through (h) of such section;

    (3) shall establish rules with respect to coverage for an immunization, test, or clinician visit that is not provided to an individual during the age range

for such immunization, test, or clinician visit that is specified in one of subsections (b) through (h) of such section; and

(4) may otherwise modify the items and services described in such section, taking into account age and other risk factors, but may not modify the cost sharing for any such item or service.

(b) CONSULTATION.—In performing the functions described in subsection (a), the National Health Board shall consult with experts in clinical preventive services.

## SEC. 1154. ESTABLISHMENT OF STANDARDS REGARDING MEDICAL NECESSITY.

The National Health Board may promulgate such regulations as may be necessary to carry out section 1141(a)(2) (relating to the exclusion of certain services that are not medically necessary or appropriate).

## PART 6—ADDITIONAL PROVISIONS RELATING TO HEALTH CARE PROVIDERS

## SEC. 1161. OVERRIDE OF RESTRICTIVE STATE PRACTICE LAWS.

No State may, through licensure or otherwise, restrict the practice of any class of health professionals beyond what is justified by the skills and training of such professionals.

### SEC. 1162. PROVISION OF ITEMS OR SERVICES CONTRARY TO RELIGIOUS BELIEF OR MORAL CONVICTION.

A health professional or a health facility may not be required to provide an item or service in the comprehensive benefit package if the professional or facility objects to doing so on the basis of a religious belief or moral conviction.

## Subtitle C—State Responsibilities

### SEC. 1200. PARTICIPATING STATE.

(a) IN GENERAL.—For purposes of the approval of a State health care system by the Board under section 1511, a State is a "participating State" if the State meets the applicable requirements of this subtitle.

(b) SUBMISSION OF SYSTEM DOCUMENT.—

(1) IN GENERAL.—In order to be approved as a participating State under section 1511, a State shall submit to the National Health Board a document (in a form and manner specified by the Board) that describes the State health care system that the State is establishing (or has established).

(2) DEADLINE.—If a State is not a participating State with a State health care system in operation by January 1, 1998, the provisions of subpart B of part 2 of subtitle F (relating to Federal operation of a State health care system) shall take effect.

(3) SUBMISSION OF INFORMATION SUBSEQUENT TO APPROVAL.—A State approved as a participating State under section 1511 shall submit to the Board an annual update to the State health care system not later than February 15 of each year following the first year for which the State is a participating State that contains—

    (A) such information as the Board may require to determine that the system shall meet the applicable requirements of subtitle C for the succeeding year; and

    (B) such information as the Board may require to determine that the State operated the system during the previous year in accordance with the Board's approval of the system for such previous year.

## PART 1—GENERAL STATE RESPONSIBILITIES

**SEC. 1201. GENERAL STATE RESPONSIBILITIES.**

The responsibilities for a participating State are as follows:

    (1) REGIONAL ALLIANCES.—Establishing one or more regional alliances (in accordance with section 1202).

    (2) HEALTH PLANS.—Certifying health plans (in accordance with section 1203).

(3) FINANCIAL SOLVENCY OF PLANS.—Assuring the financial solvency of health plans (in accordance with section 1204).

(4) ADMINISTRATION.—Designating an agency or official charged with coordinating the State responsibilities under Federal law.

(5) WORKERS COMPENSATION AND AUTOMOBILE INSURANCE.—Conforming State laws to meet the requirements of title X (relating to medical benefits under workers compensation and automobile insurance).

(6) OTHER RESPONSIBILITIES.—Carrying out other responsibilities of participating States specified under this Act.

## SEC. 1202. STATE RESPONSIBILITIES WITH RESPECT TO ALLIANCES.

(a) ESTABLISHMENT OF ALLIANCES.—

(1) IN GENERAL.—A participating State shall—

(A) establish and maintain one or more regional alliances in accordance with this section and subtitle D, and ensure that such alliances meet the requirements of this Act; and

(B) designate alliance areas in accordance with subsection (b).

(2) DEADLINE.—A State may not be a participating State for a year unless the State has established such alliances by March 1 of the previous year.

(b) ALLIANCE AREAS.—

(1) IN GENERAL.—In accordance with this subsection, each State shall designate a geographic area assigned to each regional alliance. Each such area is referred to in this Act as an "alliance area".

(2) POPULATION REQUIRED.—

(A) IN GENERAL.—Each alliance area shall encompass a population large enough to ensure that the alliance has adequate market share to negotiate effectively with health plans providing the comprehensive benefit package to eligible individuals who reside in the area.

(B) TREATMENT OF CONSOLIDATED METROPOLITAN STATISTICAL AREAS.—An alliance area that includes a Consolidated Metropolitan Statistical Area within a State is presumed to meet the requirements of subparagraph (A).

(3) SINGLE ALLIANCE IN EACH AREA.—No geographic area may be assigned to more than one regional alliance.

(4) BOUNDARIES.—In establishing boundaries for alliance areas, the State may not discriminate on the basis of or otherwise take into account race, ethnicity, language, religion, national origin, socio-economic status, disability, or perceived health status.

(5) TREATMENT OF METROPOLITAN AREAS.—The entire portion of a metropolitan statistical area located in a State shall be included in the same alliance area.

(6) NO PORTIONS OF STATE PERMITTED TO BE OUTSIDE ALLIANCE AREA.—Each portion of the State shall be assigned to a regional alliance under this subsection.

(c) STATE COORDINATION OF REGIONAL ALLIANCES.—One or more States may allow or require two or more regional alliances to coordinate their operations, whether such alliances are in the same or different States. Such coordination may include adoption of joint operating rules, contracting with health plans, enforcement activities, and establishment of fee schedules for health providers.

(d) ASSISTANCE IN COLLECTION OF AMOUNTS OWED TO ALLIANCES.—Each State shall assure that the amounts owed to regional alliances in the State are collected and paid to such alliances.

(e) ASSISTANCE IN ELIGIBILITY VERIFICATIONS.—

(1) IN GENERAL.—Each State shall assure that the determinations of eligibility for cost sharing assistance (and premium discounts and cost sharing reductions for families) are made by regional alliances in the State on the basis of the best information available to the alliances and the State.

(2) PROVISION OF INFORMATION.—Each State shall use the information available to the State under section 6103(l)(7)(D)(x) of the Internal Revenue Code of 1986 to assist regional alliances in verifying such eligibility status.

(f) SPECIAL REQUIREMENTS FOR ALLIANCES WITH SINGLE-PAYER SYSTEM.—If the State operates an alliance-specific single-payer system (as described in part 2), the State shall assure that the regional alliance in which the system is operated meets the requirements for such an alliance described in section 1224(b).

(g) PAYMENT OF SHORTFALLS FOR CERTAIN ADMINISTRATIVE ERRORS.—Each participating State is financially responsible, under section 9201(c)(2), for administrative errors described in section 9201(e)(2).

SEC. 1203. STATE RESPONSIBILITIES RELATING TO HEALTH PLANS.

(a) CRITERIA FOR CERTIFICATION.—

(1) IN GENERAL.—For purposes of this section, a participating State shall establish and publish the criteria that are used in the certification of health plans under this section.

(2) REQUIREMENTS.—Such criteria shall be established with respect to—

    (A) the quality of the plan,

    (B) the financial stability of the plan,

    (C) the plan's capacity to deliver the comprehensive benefit package in the designated service area,

    (D) other applicable requirements for health plans under parts 1, 3, and 4 of subtitle E, and

    (E) other requirements imposed by the State consistent with this part.

(b) CERTIFICATION OF HEALTH PLANS.—A participating State shall certify each plan as a regional alliance health plan that it determines meet the criteria for certification established and published under subsection (a).

(c) MONITORING.—A participating State shall monitor the performance of each State-certified regional alliance health plan to ensure that it continues to meet the criteria for certification.

(d) LIMITATIONS ON AUTHORITY.—A participating State may not—

    (1) discriminate against a plan based on the domicile of the entity offering of the plan; and

    (2) regulate premium rates charged by health plans, except as may be required under title VI (relating to the enforcement of cost containment rules for plans in the State) or as may be necessary to ensure that plans meet financial solvency requirements under section 1408.

(e) ASSURING ADEQUATE ACCESS TO A CHOICE OF HEALTH PLANS.—

    (1) GENERAL ACCESS.—

        (A) IN GENERAL.—Each participating State shall ensure that—

            (i) each regional alliance eligible family has adequate access to enroll in a choice of regional alliance health plans providing services in the area in which the individual resides, including (to the maximum extent practicable) adequate access to a plan whose premium is at or below the weighted average premium for plans in the regional alliance, and

(ii) each such family that is eligible for a premium discount under section 6104(b) is provided a discount in accordance with such section (including an increase in such discount described in section 6104(b)(2)).

(B) AUTHORITY.—In order to carry out its responsibility under subparagraph (A), a participating State may require, as a condition of entering into a contract with a regional alliance under section 1321, that one or more certified regional alliance health plans cover all (or selected portions) of the alliance area.

(2) ACCESS TO PLANS USING CENTERS OF EXCELLENCE.—Each participating State may require, as a condition of entering into a contract with a regional alliance under section 1321, that one or more certified health plans provide access (through reimbursement, contracts, or otherwise) of enrolled individuals to services of centers of excellence (as designated by the State in accordance with rules promulgated by the Secretary).

(3) USE OF INCENTIVES TO ENROLL AND SERVE DISADVANTAGED GROUPS.—A State may provide—

(A) for an adjustment to the risk-adjustment methodology under section 1542(c) and other financial incentives to regional alliance health plans to ensure that such plans enroll individuals who are members of disadvantaged groups, and

(B) for appropriate extra services, such as outreach to encourage enrollment and transportation and interpreting services to ensure access to care, for certain population groups that face barriers to access because of geographic location, income levels, or racial or cultural differences.

(f) COORDINATION OF WORKERS' COMPENSATION SERVICES AND AUTOMOBILE INSURANCE.—Each participating State shall comply with the responsibilities regarding workers' compensation and automobile insurance specified in title X.

(g) IMPLEMENTATION OF MANDATORY REINSURANCE SYSTEM.—If the risk adjustment and reinsurance methodology developed under section 1541 includes a mandatory reinsurance system, each participating State shall establish a reinsurance program consistent with such methodology and any additional standards established by the Board.

(h) REQUIREMENTS FOR PLANS OFFERING SUPPLEMENTAL INSURANCE.—Notwithstanding any other provision of this Act a State may not certify a regional alliance health plan under this section if—

    (1) the plan (or any entity with which the plan is affiliated under such rules as the Board may establish) offers a supplemental health benefit policy (as defined in section 1421(a)(1)) that fails to meet the applicable requirements for such a policy under part 2 of subtitle E (without regard to the State in which the policy is offered); or

    (2) the plan offers a cost sharing policy (as defined in section 1421(a)(2)) that fails to meet the applicable requirements for such a policy under part 2 of subtitle E.

### SEC. 1204. FINANCIAL SOLVENCY; FISCAL OVERSIGHT; GUARANTY FUND.

(a) CAPITAL STANDARDS.—A participating State shall establish capital standards for health plans that meet minimum Federal requirements established by the National Health Board under section 1505(i).

(b) REPORTING AND AUDITING REQUIREMENTS.—Each participating State shall define financial reporting and auditing requirements and requirements for fund reserves adequate to monitor the financial status of plans.

(c) GUARANTY FUND.—

(1) ESTABLISHMENT.—Each participating State shall ensure that there is a guaranty fund that meets the requirements established by the Board under section 1505(j)(2), in order to provide financial protection to health care providers and others in the case of a failure of a regional alliance health plan.

(2) ASSESSMENTS TO PROVIDE FUNDS.—In the case of a failure of one or more regional alliance health plans, the State may require each regional alliance health plan within the State to pay an assessment to the State in an amount not to exceed 2 percent of the premiums of such plans paid by or on behalf of regional alliance eligible individuals during a year for so long as necessary to generate sufficient revenue to cover any outstanding claims against the failed plan.

(d) PROCEDURES IN EVENT OF PLAN FAILURE.—

(1) IN GENERAL.—A participating State shall assure that, in the event of the failure of a regional alliance health plan in the State, eligible individuals enrolled in the plan will be assured continuity of coverage for the comprehensive benefit package.

(2) DESIGNATION OF STATE AGENCY.—A participating State shall designate an agency of State government that supervises or assumes control of the operation of a regional alliance health plan in the case of the failure of the plan.

(3) PROTECTIONS FOR HEALTH CARE PROVIDERS AND ENROLLEES.—Each participating State shall assure that in the case of a plan failure—

>(A) the guaranty fund shall pay health care providers for items and services covered under the comprehensive benefit package for enrollees of the plan for which the plan is otherwise obligated to make payment;

>(B) after making all payments required to be made to providers under subparagraph (A), the guaranty fund shall make payments for the operational, administrative, and other costs and debts of the plan (in accordance with requirements imposed by the State based on rules promulgated by the Board);

>(C) such health care providers have no legal right to seek payment from eligible individuals enrolled in the plan for any such covered items or services (other than the enrollees'

obligations under cost sharing arrangements); and

> (D) health care providers are required to continue caring for such eligible individuals until such individuals are enrolled in a new health plan.

(4) PLAN FAILURE.—For purposes of this section, the failure of a health plan means the current or imminent inability to pay claims.

## SEC. 1205. RESTRICTIONS ON FUNDING OF ADDITIONAL BENEFITS.

If a participating State provides benefits (either directly or through regional alliance health plans or otherwise) in addition to those covered under the comprehensive benefit package, the State may not provide for payment for such benefits through funds provided under this Act.

## PART 2—REQUIREMENTS FOR STATE SINGLE-PAYER SYSTEMS

### SEC. 1221. SINGLE-PAYER SYSTEM DESCRIBED.

The Board shall approve the application of a State to operate a single-payer system if the Board finds that the system—

(1) meets the requirements of section 1222;

(2) meets the requirements for a Statewide single-payer system under section 1223, in the case of a system offered throughout a State; and

(3) meets the requirements for an alliance-specific single-payer system under section 1224, in the case of a system offered in a single alliance of a State.

### SEC. 1222. GENERAL REQUIREMENTS FOR SINGLE-PAYER SYSTEMS.

Each single-payer system shall meet the following requirements:

(1) ESTABLISHMENT BY STATE.—The system is established under State law, and State law provides for mechanisms to enforce the requirements of the plan.

(2) OPERATION BY STATE.—The system is operated by the State or a designated agency of the State.

(3) ENROLLMENT OF ELIGIBLE INDIVIDUALS.—

(A) MANDATORY ENROLLMENT OF ALL REGIONAL ALLIANCE INDIVIDUALS.—The system provides for the enrollment of all eligible individuals residing in the State (or, in the case of an alliance-specific single-payer system, in the alliance area) for whom the applicable health plan would otherwise be a regional alliance health plan.

(B) OPTIONAL ENROLLMENT OF MEDICARE-ELIGIBLE INDIVIDUALS.—At the option of the State, the system may provide for the enrollment of medicare-individuals residing in the State (or, in the case of an alliance-specific single-payer system, in the alliance area) if the Secretary of Health and Human Services has approved an application submitted by the State under section 1893 of the Social Security Act (as added by section 4001(a)) for the integration of medicare beneficiaries into plans of the State. Nothing in this subparagraph shall be construed as requiring that a State have a single-payer system in order to provide for such integration.

(C) OPTIONAL ENROLLMENT OF CORPORATE ALLIANCE INDIVIDUALS IN STATEWIDE PLANS.—At the option of the State, a Statewide single-payer system may provide for the enrollment of individuals residing in the State who are otherwise eligible to enroll in a corporate alliance health plan under section 1311.

(D) OPTIONS INCLUDED IN STATE SYSTEM DOCUMENT.—A State may not exercise any of the options described in subparagraphs (A) or (B) for a year unless the State included a description of the option in the submission of its system document to the Board for the year under section 1200(b).

(E) EXCLUSION OF CERTAIN INDIVIDUALS.—A single-payer system may not require the enrollment of electing veterans, active duty military personnel, and electing Indians (as defined in 1012(d)).

(4) DIRECT PAYMENT TO PROVIDERS.—

(A) IN GENERAL.—With respect to providers who furnish items and services included in the comprehensive benefit package to individuals enrolled in the system, the State shall make payments directly to such providers and assume (subject to subparagraph (B)) all financial risk associated with making such payments.

(B) CAPITATED PAYMENTS PERMITTED.—Nothing in subparagraph (A) shall be construed to prohibit providers furnishing items and services under the system from receiving payments from the plan on a capitated, at-risk basis based on prospectively determined rates.

(5) PROVISION OF COMPREHENSIVE BENEFIT PACKAGE.—

(A) IN GENERAL.—The system shall provide for coverage of the comprehensive benefit package, including the cost sharing provided under the package (subject to subparagraph (B)), to all individuals enrolled in the system.

(B) IMPOSITION OF REDUCED COST SHARING.—The system may decrease the cost sharing otherwise provided in the comprehensive benefit package with respect to any class of individuals enrolled in the system or any class of services included in the package, so long as the system does not increase the cost sharing otherwise imposed with respect to any other class of individuals or services.

(6) COST CONTAINMENT.—The system shall provide for mechanisms to ensure, in a manner satisfactory to the Board, that—

(A) per capita expenditures for items and services in the comprehensive benefit package under the system for a year (beginning with the first year) do not exceed an amount equivalent to the regional alliance per capita premium target that is determined under section 6003 (based on the State being a single regional alliance) for the year;

  (B) the per capita expenditures described in subparagraph (A) are computed and effectively monitored; and

  (C) automatic, mandatory, nondiscretionary reductions in payments to health care providers will be imposed to the extent required to assure that such per capita expenditures do not exceed in the applicable target referred to in subparagraph (A).

 (7) REQUIREMENTS GENERALLY APPLICABLE TO HEALTH PLANS.—The system shall meet the requirements applicable to a health plan under section 1400(a), except that—

  (A) the system does not have the authority provided to health plans under section 1402(a)(2) (relating to permissible limitations on the enrollment of eligible individuals on the basis of limits on the plan's capacity);

  (B) the system is not required to meet the requirements of section 1404(a) (relating to restrictions on the marketing of plan materials); and

(C) the system is not required to meet the requirements of section 1408 (relating to plan solvency).

## SEC. 1223. SPECIAL RULES FOR STATES OPERATING STATEWIDE SINGLE-PAYER SYSTEM.

(a) IN GENERAL.—In the case of a State operating a Statewide single-payer system—

(1) the State shall operate the system throughout the State through a single alliance;

(2) except as provided in subsection (b), the State shall meet the requirements for participating States under part 1; and

(3) the State shall assume the functions described in subsection (c) that are otherwise required to be performed by regional alliances in participating States that do not operate a Statewide single-payer system.

(b) EXCEPTIONS TO CERTAIN REQUIREMENTS FOR PARTICIPATING STATES.—In the case of a State operating a Statewide single-payer system, the State is not required to meet the following requirements otherwise applicable to participating States under part 1:

(1) ESTABLISHMENT OF ALLIANCES.—The requirements of section 1202 (relating to the establishment of alliances).

(2) HEALTH PLANS.—The requirements of section 1203 (relating to health plans), other than the requirement of subsection (f) of such section (relating to coordination of workers' compensation services and automobile liability insurance).

(3) FINANCIAL SOLVENCY.—The requirements of section 1204 (relating to the financial solvency of health plans in the State).

(c) ASSUMPTION BY STATE OF CERTAIN REQUIREMENTS APPLICABLE TO REGIONAL ALLIANCES.—A State operating a Statewide single-payer system shall be subject to the following requirements otherwise applicable to regional alliances in other participating States:

(1) ENROLLMENT; ISSUANCE OF HEALTH SECURITY CARDS.—The requirements of subsections (a) and (c) of section 1323 and section 1324 shall apply to the State, eligible individuals residing in the State, and the single-payer system operated by the State in the same manner as such requirements apply to a regional alliance, alliance eligible individuals, and regional alliance plans.

(2) REDUCTIONS IN COST SHARING FOR LOW-INCOME INDIVIDUALS.—The requirement of section 1371 shall apply to the State in the same manner as such requirement applies to a regional alliance.

(3) DATA COLLECTION; QUALITY.—The requirements of section 1327(a) shall apply to the State and the single-payer system operated by the State in the same manner as such requirement applies to a regional alliance and health plans offered through a regional alliance.

(4) ANTI-DISCRIMINATION; COORDINATION.—The requirements of section 1328 shall apply to the State in the same manner as such requirements apply with respect to a regional alliance.

(d) FINANCING.—

(1) IN GENERAL.—A State operating a State-wide single-payer system shall provide for the financing of the system using, at least in part, a payroll-based financing system that requires employers to pay at least the amount that the employers would be required to pay if the employers were subject to the requirements of subtitle B of title VI.

(2) USE OF FINANCING METHODS.—Such a State may use, consistent with paragraph (1), any other method of financing.

(e) SINGLE-PAYER STATE DEFINED.—In this Act, the term "single-payer State" means a State with a State-wide single-payer system in effect that has been approved by the Board in accordance with this part.

## SEC. 1224. SPECIAL RULES FOR ALLIANCE-SPECIFIC SINGLE-PAYER SYSTEMS.

(a) IN GENERAL.—In the case of a State operating an alliance-specific single-payer system—

(1) the State shall meet the requirements for participating States under part 1, except that in establishing the regional alliance through which the system is offered, the requirement of section 1202(a)(1)(A) shall not apply to the extent necessary for the alliance to meet the requirements of section 1242; and

(2) the regional alliance in which the system is operated shall meet the requirements of subsection (b).

(b) REQUIREMENTS FOR ALLIANCE IN WHICH SYSTEM OPERATES.—A regional alliance in which an alliance-specific single payer system is operated shall meet the requirements applicable to regional alliances under subtitle D, except that the alliance is not required to meet the following requirements of such subtitle:

(1) CONTRACTS WITH HEALTH PLANS.—The requirements of section 1321 (relating to contracts with health plans).

(2) CHOICE OF HEALTH PLANS OFFERED.—The requirements of subsections (a) or (b) of section 1322 (relating to offering a choice of health plans to eligible enrollees).

(4) ESTABLISHMENT OF PROCESS FOR CONSUMER COMPLAINTS.—The requirements of section 1326(a) (relating to the establishment of a process for the hearing and resolution of consumer complaints against plans offered through the alliance).

(5) ADDRESSING NEEDS OF AREAS WITH INADEQUATE HEALTH SERVICES.—The regional alliance does not have any of the authorities described in subsections (a) and (b) of section 1329 (relating to adjusting payments to plans and encouraging the establishment of new plans).

## Subtitle D—Health Alliances

SEC. 1300. HEALTH ALLIANCE DEFINED.

In this Act, the term "health alliance" means a regional alliance (as defined in section 1301) and a corporate alliance (as defined in section 1311).

# PART 1—ESTABLISHMENT OF REGIONAL AND CORPORATE ALLIANCES

## Subpart A—Regional Alliances

SEC. 1301. REGIONAL ALLIANCE DEFINED.

In this Act, the term "regional alliance" means a non-profit organization, an independent state agency, or an agency of the State which—

    (1) meets the applicable organizational requirements of this subpart, and

    (2) is carrying out activities consistent with part 2.

SEC. 1302. BOARD OF DIRECTORS.

    (a) IN GENERAL.—A regional alliance must be governed by a Board of Directors appointed consistent with the provisions of this title. All powers vested in a regional alliance under this Act shall be vested in the Board of Directors.

    (b) MEMBERSHIP.—

        (1) IN GENERAL.—Such a Board of Directors shall consist of—

            (A) members who represent employers whose employees purchase health coverage through the alliance, including self-employed individuals who purchase such coverage; and

(B) members who represent individuals who purchase such coverage, including employees who purchase such coverage.

(2) EQUAL REPRESENTATION OF EMPLOYERS AND CONSUMERS.—The number of members of the Board described under subparagraph (A) of paragraph (1) shall be the same as the number of members described in subparagraph (B) of such paragraph.

(c) NO CONFLICT OF INTEREST PERMITTED.—An individual may not serve as a member of the Board of Directors if the individual is one of the following (or an immediate family member of one of the following):

(1) A health care provider.

(2) An individual who is an employee or member of the Board of Directors of, has a substantial ownership in, or derives substantial income from, a health care provider, health plan, pharmaceutical company, or a supplier of medical equipment, devices, or services.

(3) A person who derives substantial income from the provision of health care.

(4)(A) A member or employee of an association, law firm, or other institution or organization that represents the interests of one or more health care providers, health plans or others involved in the health care field, or (B) an individual who practices as a professional in an area involving health care.

## SEC. 1303. PROVIDER ADVISORY BOARDS FOR REGIONAL ALLIANCES.

Each regional alliance must establish a provider advisory board consisting of representatives of health care providers and professionals who provide covered services through health plans offered by the alliance.

### Subpart B—Corporate Alliances

## SEC. 1311. CORPORATE ALLIANCE DEFINED; INDIVIDUALS ELIGIBLE FOR COVERAGE THROUGH CORPORATE ALLIANCES; ADDITIONAL DEFINITIONS.

(a) CORPORATE ALLIANCE DEFINED.—In this Act, the term "corporate alliance" means an eligible sponsor (as defined in subsection (b)) if—

(1) the sponsor elects, in a form and manner specified by the Secretary of Labor consistent with this subpart, to be treated as a corporate alliance under this title and such election has not been terminated under section 1313; and

(2) the sponsor has filed with the Secretary of Labor a document describing how the sponsor shall

carry out activities as such an alliance consistent with part 3.

(b) ELIGIBLE SPONSORS.—

(1) IN GENERAL.—In this subpart, each of the following is an eligible sponsor of a corporate alliance:

　(A) LARGE EMPLOYER.—An employer that—

　　(i) is a large employer (as defined in subsection (e)(3)) as of the date of an election under subsection (a)(1), and

　　(ii) is not an excluded employer described in paragraph (2).

　(B) PLAN SPONSOR OF A MULTIEMPLOYER PLAN.—A plan sponsor described in section 3(16)(B)(iii) of Employee Retirement Income Security Act of 1974, but only with respect to a group health plan that is a multiemployer plan (as defined in subsection (e)(4)) maintained by the sponsor and only if—

　　(i) such plan offered health benefits as of September 1, 1993, and

　　(ii) as of both September 1, 1993, and January 1, 1996, such plan has more than 5,000 active participants in the United

States, or the plan is affiliated with a national labor agreement covering more than 5,000 employees.

(C) RURAL ELECTRIC COOPERATIVE AND RURAL TELEPHONE COOPERATIVE ASSOCIATION.—A rural electric cooperative or a rural telephone cooperative association, but only with respect to a group health plan that is maintained by such cooperative or association (or members of such cooperative or association) and only if such plan—

(i) offered health benefits as of September 1, 1993, and

(ii) as of both September 1, 1993, and January 1, 1996, has more than 5,000 full-time employees in the United States entitled to health benefits under the plan.

(2) EXCLUDED EMPLOYERS.—For purposes of paragraph (1)(A), any of the following are excluded employers described in this paragraph:

(A) An employer whose primary business is employee leasing.

(B) The Federal government (other than the United States Postal Service).

(C) A State government, a unit of local government, and an agency or instrumentality of government, including any special purpose unit of government.

(c) INDIVIDUALS ELIGIBLE TO ENROLL IN CORPORATE ALLIANCE HEALTH PLANS.—For purposes of part 1 of subtitle A, subject to subsection (d)—

    (1) LARGE EMPLOYER ALLIANCES.—

        (A) FULL-TIME EMPLOYEES.—Each eligible individual who is a full-time employee of a large employer that has an election in effect as a corporate alliance is eligible to enroll in a corporate alliance health plan offered by such corporate alliance.

        (B) ONE-TIME OPTION TO EXEMPT EMPLOYEES IN SMALL ESTABLISHMENTS.—At the time of making an election to become a corporate alliance under this subpart, a large employer may exercise an option to make ineligible for enrollment all full-time employees of the employer employed in any establishment of the employer which has (at the time of the election) fewer than 100 full-time employees. The option under this subparagraph may be exercised separately with respect to each establishment of the employer.

(2) MULTIEMPLOYER ALLIANCES.—

(A) PARTICIPANTS.—Each participant and beneficiary (as defined in subparagraph (B)) under a multiemployer plan, with respect to which an eligible sponsor of the plan described in subsection (b)(1)(B) has an election in effect as a corporate alliance, is eligible to enroll in a corporate alliance health plan offered by such corporate alliance.

(B) PARTICIPANT AND BENEFICIARY DEFINED.—In subparagraph (A), the terms "participant" and "beneficiary" have the meaning given such terms in section 3 of the Employee Retirement Income Security Act of 1974.

(3) FULL-TIME EMPLOYEES OF RURAL COOPERATIVE ALLIANCES.—Each full-time employee of a rural electric cooperative or rural telephone cooperative association (or of a member of such a cooperative or association) which has an election in effect as a corporate alliance is eligible to enroll in a corporate alliance health plan offered by such corporate alliance.

(4) INELIGIBLE TO ENROLL IN REGIONAL ALLIANCE HEALTH PLAN.—Except as provided in section 1013(b), a corporate alliance eligible individual is not eligible to enroll under a regional alliance health plan.

(d) EXCLUSION OF CERTAIN INDIVIDUALS.—In accordance with rules of the Board, the following individuals shall not be treated as corporate alliance eligible individuals:

(1) AFDC recipients.

(2) SSI recipients.

(3) Individuals who are described in section 1004(b) (relating to veterans, military personnel, and Indians) and who elect an applicable health plan described in such section.

(4) Employees who are seasonal or temporary workers (as defined by the Board), other than such workers who are treated as corporate alliance eligible individuals pursuant to a collective bargaining agreement (as defined by the Secretary of Labor).

(e) DEFINITIONS RELATING TO CORPORATE ALLIANCES.—In this subtitle, except as otherwise provided:

(1) ESTABLISHMENT.—The term "establishment" shall be defined by the Secretary of Labor.

(2) GROUP HEALTH PLAN.—The term "group health plan" means an employee welfare benefit plan (as defined in section 3(1) of the Employee Retirement Income Security Act of 1974) providing medical care (as defined in section 213(d) of the Internal Revenue Code of 1986) to participants or beneficiaries (as defined in section 3 of the Employee Retirement Income Security Act of 1974) directly or through insurance, reimbursement, or otherwise.

(3) LARGE EMPLOYER.—The term "large employer" means an employer that has more than 5,000 full-time employees in the United States, not including (subject to section 1312(a)(3)) any employee located at an establishment for which the option described in subsection (c)(1)(B) is in effect. Such term includes the United States Postal Service.

(4) MULTIEMPLOYER PLAN.—The term "multiemployer plan" has the meaning given such term in section 3(37) of the Employee Retirement Income Security Act of 1974, and includes any plan that is treated as such a plan under title I of such Act.

(5) RURAL ELECTRIC COOPERATIVE.—The term "rural electric cooperative" has the meaning given such term in section 3(40)(A)(iv) of the Employee Retirement Income Security Act of 1974.

(6) RURAL TELEPHONE COOPERATIVE ASSOCIATIONS.—The term "rural telephone cooperative association" has the meaning given such term in section 3(40)(A)(v) of the Employee Retirement Income Security Act of 1974.

SEC. 1312. TIMING OF ELECTIONS.

(a) FOR LARGE EMPLOYERS.—

(1) CURRENT LARGE EMPLOYERS.—

(A) IN GENERAL.—In the case of an employer that is an eligible sponsor described in section 1311(b)(1)(A) as of the most recent January 1 prior to the general effective date, the sponsor's election to be a corporate alliance under such section must be made and filed with the Secretary of Labor not later than the date specified in subparagraph (B).

(B) DEADLINE FOR NOTICE.—The date specified in this subparagraph is January 1 of the second year preceding the general effective date or, in the case of a State that elects to become a participating State before the general effective date, not later than one month later than the date specified for States to provide notice of their intent under section 1202(a)(2).

(2) NEW LARGE EMPLOYERS.—In the case of an employer that is not an eligible sponsor described in section 1311(b)(1)(A) as of the most recent January 1 prior to the general effective date, but first becomes such a sponsor as of a subsequent date, the election to be a corporate alliance under such section must be made and filed with the Secretary of Labor not later than March 1 of the year following the year in such report is submitted.

(3) APPLICATION OF OPTION.—The Secretary of Labor shall promulgate rules regarding how the option described in section 1311(c)(1)(B) will be applied to the determination of whether an employer is a large employer before an election is made under section 1311.

(b) FOR MULTIEMPLOYER PLANS AND RURAL COOPERATIVES.—In the case of an eligible sponsor described in section 1311(b)(1)(B) or (C), the sponsor's election to be a corporate alliance under such section must be made and filed with the Secretary of Labor not later than the second most recent March 1 prior to the general effective date.

(c) EFFECTIVE DATE OF ELECTION.—An election made under subsection (a) or (b) shall be effective for coverage provided under health plans on and after January

1 of the year following the year in which the election is made.

(d) ONE-TIME ELECTION.—If an eligible sponsor fails to make the election on a timely manner under subsection (a) or (b), the sponsor may not make such election at any other time.

SEC. 1313. TERMINATION OF ALLIANCE ELECTION.

(a) TERMINATION FOR INSUFFICIENT NUMBER OF FULL-TIME EMPLOYEES OR PARTICIPANTS.—If a corporate alliance reports under section 1387(c), that there were fewer than 4,800 full-time employees (or, active participants, in the case of one or more plans offered by a corporate alliance which is an eligible sponsor described in section 1311(b)(1)(B)) who are enrolled in a health plan through the alliance, the election under this part with respect to the alliance shall terminate.

(b) TERMINATION FOR FAILURE TO MEET REQUIREMENTS.—

(1) IN GENERAL.—If the Secretary of Labor finds that a corporate alliance has failed substantially to meet the applicable requirements of this subtitle, the Secretary shall terminate the election under this part with respect to the alliance

(2) EXCESS INCREASE IN PREMIUM EQUIVALENT.—If the Secretary of Labor finds that the alli-

ance is in violation of the requirements of section 6022 (relating to prohibition against excess increase in premium expenditures), the Secretary shall terminate the alliance in accordance with such section.

(c) ELECTIVE TERMINATION.—A corporate alliance may terminate an election under this part by filing with the National Health Board and the Secretary of Labor a notice of intent to terminate.

(d) EFFECTIVE DATE OF TERMINATION.—In the case of a termination of an election under this section, in accordance with rules established by the Secretary of Labor—

(1) the termination shall take effect as of the effective date of enrollments in regional alliance health plans made during the next open enrollment period (as provided in section 1323(d)), and

(2) the enrollment of eligible individuals in corporate alliance health plans of the corporate alliance shall be terminated as of such date and such individuals shall be enrolled in other applicable health plans effective on such date.

(e) NOTICE TO BOARD.—If an election with respect to a corporate alliance is terminated pursuant to subsection (a) or subsection (b), the Secretary of Labor shall notify the National Health Board of the termination of the election.

## PART 2—GENERAL RESPONSIBILITIES AND AUTHORITIES OF REGIONAL ALLIANCES

### SEC. 1321. CONTRACTS WITH HEALTH PLANS.

(a) CONTRACTS WITH PLANS.—

(1) IN GENERAL.—In order to assure the availability of the comprehensive benefit package to eligible individuals residing in the alliance area in a cost-effective manner, except as provided in this section, each regional alliance shall negotiate with any willing State-certified health plan to enter into a contract with the alliance for the enrollment under the plan of eligible individuals in the alliance area. Subject to paragraph (2), a regional alliance shall not enter into any such contract with a health plan that is not a State-certified health plan.

(2) TREATMENT OF CERTAIN PLANS.—Each regional alliance shall enter into a contract under this section with any veterans health plan of the Department of Veterans Affairs and with a Uniformed Services Health Plan of the Department of Defense, that offers the comprehensive benefit package to eligible individuals residing in the alliance area if the

appropriate official requests to enter into such a contract.

(b) GENERAL CONDITIONS FOR DENIAL OF CONTRACT BY A REGIONAL ALLIANCE.—A regional alliance is not required under this section to offer a contract with a health plan if—

> (1) the alliance finds that the proposed premium exceeds 120 percent of the weighted-average premium within the alliance; or
>
> (2) the plan has failed to comply with requirements under prior contracts with the alliance, including failing to offer coverage for all the services in the comprehensive benefit package in the entire service area of the plan.

## SEC. 1322. OFFERING CHOICE OF HEALTH PLANS FOR ENROLLMENT; ESTABLISHMENT OF FEE-FOR-SERVICE SCHEDULE.

(a) IN GENERAL.—Each health alliance must provide to each eligible enrollee with respect to the alliance a choice of health plans among the plans which have contracts in effect with the alliance under section 1321 (in the case of a regional alliance) or section 1341 (in the case of a corporate alliance).

(b) OFFERING OF PLANS BY ALLIANCES.—

(1) IN GENERAL.—Each regional alliance shall include among its health plan offerings at least one fee-for-service plan (as defined in paragraph (2)).

(2) FEE-FOR-SERVICE PLAN DEFINED.—

(A) IN GENERAL.—For purposes of this Act, the term "fee-for-service plan" means a health plan that—

(i) provides coverage for all items and services included in the comprehensive benefit package that are furnished by any lawful health care provider of the enrollee's choice, subject to reasonable restrictions (described in subparagraph (B)), and

(ii) makes payment to such a provider without regard to whether or not there is a contractual arrangement between the plan and the provider.

(B) REASONABLE RESTRICTIONS DESCRIBED.—The reasonable restrictions on coverage permitted under a fee-for-service plan (as specified by the National Health Board) are as follows:

(i) Utilization review.

(ii) Prior approval for specified services.

(iii) Exclusion of providers on the basis of poor quality of care, based on evidence obtainable by the plan.

Clause (ii) shall not be construed as permitting a plan to require prior approval for non-primary health care services through a gatekeeper or other process.

(c) ESTABLISHMENT OF FEE-FOR-SERVICE SCHEDULE.—

(1) IN GENERAL.—Except in the case of regional alliances of a State that has established a Statewide fee schedule under paragraph (3), each regional alliance shall establish a fee schedule setting forth the payment rates applicable to services furnished during a year to individuals enrolled in fee-for-service plans (or to services furnished under the fee-for-service component of any regional alliance health plan) for use by regional alliance health plans under section 1406(c) and corporate alliance health plans providing services subject to the schedule in the regional alliance area.

(2) NEGOTIATION WITH PROVIDERS.—The fee schedule under paragraph (1) shall be established after negotiations with providers, and (subject to

paragraphs (5) and (6)) providers may collectively negotiate the fee schedule with the regional alliance.

(3) USE OF STATEWIDE SCHEDULE.—At the option of a State, the State may establish its own statewide fee schedule which shall apply to all fee-for-service plans offered by regional alliances and corporate alliances in the State instead of alliance-specific schedules established under paragraph (1).

(4) ANNUAL REVISION.—A regional alliance or State (as the case may be) shall annually update the payment rates provided under the fee schedule established pursuant to paragraph (1) or paragraph (3).

(5) ACTIVITIES TREATED AS STATE ACTION OR EFFORTS INTENDED TO INFLUENCE GOVERNMENT ACTION.—The establishment of a fee schedule under this subsection by a regional alliance of a State shall be considered to be pursuant to a clearly articulated and affirmatively expressed State policy to displace competition and actively supervised by the State, and conduct by providers respecting the establishment of the fee schedule, including collective negotiations by providers with the regional alliance (or the State) pursuant to paragraph (2), shall be con-

sidered as efforts intended to influence governmental action.

(6) NO BOYCOTT PERMITTED.—Nothing in this subsection shall be construed to permit providers to threaten or engage in any boycott.

(7) NEGOTIATIONS DEFINED.—In this subsection, "negotiations" are the process by which providers collectively and jointly meet, confer, consult, discuss, share information, among and between themselves in order to agree on information to be provided, presentations to be made, and other such activities with respect to regional alliances (or States) relating to the establishment of the fee schedule (but not including any activity that constitutes engaging in or threatening to engage in a boycott), as well as any and all collective and joint meetings, discussions, presentations, conferences, and consultations between or among providers and any regional alliance (or State) for the purpose of establishing the fee schedule described in this subsection.

(d) PROSPECTIVE BUDGETING OF FEE-FOR-SERVICE.—

(1) IN GENERAL.—The fee schedule established by a regional alliance or a State under subsection (c)

may be based on prospective budgeting described in paragraph (2).

(2) PROSPECTIVE BUDGETING DESCRIBED.—Under prospective budgeting—

>(A) the regional alliance or State (as the case may be) shall negotiate with health providers annually to develop a budget for the designated fee-for-service plan;

>(B) the negotiated budget shall establish spending targets for each sector of health expenditures made by the plan; and

>(C) if the regional alliance or State (as the case may be) determines that the utilization of services under the plan is at a level that will result in expenditures under the plan exceeding the negotiated budget, the plan shall reduce the amount of payments otherwise made to providers (through a withhold or delay in payments or adjustments) in such a manner and by such amounts as necessary to assure that expenditures will not exceed the budget.

(3) USE OF PROSPECTIVE BUDGETING EXCLUSIVE.—If a regional alliance or State establishes the fee schedule for fee-for-service plans on the basis of prospective budgeting under this subsection, pay-

ment for all services provided by fee-for-service plans in the alliance or State shall be determined on such basis.

**SEC. 1323. ENROLLMENT RULES AND PROCEDURES.**

(a) IN GENERAL.—Each regional alliance shall assure that each regional alliance eligible individual who resides in the alliance area is enrolled in a regional alliance health plan and shall establish and maintain methods and procedures, consistent with this section, sufficient to assure such enrollment. Such methods and procedures shall assure the enrollment of alliance eligible individuals at the time they first become eligible enrollees in the alliance area, including individuals at the time of birth, at the time they move into the alliance area, and at the time of reaching the age of individual eligibility as an eligible enrollee (and not merely as a family member). Each regional alliance shall establish procedures, consistent with subtitle A, for the selection of a single health plan in which all members of a family are enrolled.

(b) POINT OF SERVICE ENROLLMENT MECHANISM.—

(1) IN GENERAL.—Each regional alliance shall establish a point-of-service enrollment mechanism (meeting the requirements of this subsection) for enrolling eligible individuals who are not enrolled in a

health plan of the alliance when the individual seeks health services.

(2) REQUIREMENTS OF MECHANISM.—Under such a mechanism, if an eligible individual seeks to receive services (included in the comprehensive benefit package) from a provider in an alliance area and does not present evidence of enrollment under any applicable health plan, or if the provider has no evidence of the individual's enrollment under any such plan, the following rules shall apply:

(A) NOTICE TO ALLIANCE.—The provider—

(i) shall provide the regional alliance with information relating to the identity of the eligible individual, and

(ii) may request payment from the regional alliance for the furnishing of such services.

(B) INITIAL DETERMINATION OF ELIGIBILITY AND ENROLLMENT STATUS.—The regional alliance shall determine—

(i) if the individual is an alliance eligible individual for the alliance, and

(ii) if the individual is enrolled under an applicable health plan (including a corporate alliance health plan).

(C) TREATMENT OF ALLIANCE ELIGIBLE INDIVIDUALS.—If the regional alliance determines that the individual is an alliance eligible individual with respect to the alliance and—

(i) is enrolled under a regional alliance health plan of the alliance, the alliance shall forward the claim to the health plan involved and shall notify the provider (and the individual) of the fact of such enrollment and the forwarding of such claim (and the plan shall make payment to the provider for the services furnished to the individual as described in paragraph (3)(C));

(ii) is not enrolled under a regional alliance health plan of the alliance but is required to be so enrolled in a specific health plan as a family member under section 1021, the alliance shall record the individual's enrollment under such specific plan, shall forward the claim to such plan, and shall notify the provider (and the individual) of the fact of such enrollment and the forwarding of such claim (and the plan shall make payment to the provider for the services furnished to the individual as described in paragraph (3)(C)); or

>(iii) is not enrolled under such a plan and is not described in clause (ii), the point-of-service enrollment procedures described in paragraph (3) shall apply.

(D) TREATMENT OF INDIVIDUALS ENROLLED UNDER HEALTH PLANS OF OTHER ALLIANCES.—If the regional alliance determines that the individual is not an alliance eligible individual with respect to the alliance but the individual is enrolled—

>(i) under a regional alliance health plan of another alliance, the alliance shall forward the claim to the other regional alliance and shall notify the provider (and the individual) of the fact of such enrollment and the forwarding of such claim (and the plan shall make payment to the provider for the services furnished to the individual as described in paragraph (3)(C)); or

(ii) under a corporate alliance health plan, the alliance shall forward the claim to the corporate alliance involved and shall notify the provider (and the individual) of the fact of such enrollment and the forwarding of such claim (and the plan shall make payment to the provider for the services furnished to the individual as described in section 1383(b)(2)(B)).

(E) TREATMENT OF OTHER ALLIANCE ELIGIBLE INDIVIDUALS NOT ENROLLED IN HEALTH PLAN.—If the regional alliance determines that the individual is not an alliance eligible individual with respect to the alliance and the individual is an alliance eligible individual with respect to another health alliance but is not enrolled in a health plan of such alliance, the regional alliance shall forward the claim to the other alliance involved and shall notify the provider (and the individual) of the forwarding of such claim and the requirement for prompt enrollment of the individual under an applicable health plan of such alliance pursuant to the procedures described in paragraph (3) (in the case of a regional alliance) or in section 1383(b) (in the case of a corporate alliance).

(F) TREATMENT OF ALL OTHER INDIVIDUALS.—The National Board shall promulgate rules regarding the responsibilities of regional alliances relating to individuals whose applicable health plan is not an alliance plan and other individuals the alliance is unable to identify as eligible individuals.

(3) POINT-OF-SERVICE ENROLLMENT PROCEDURES DESCRIBED.—The point-of-service enrollment procedures under this paragraph are as follows:

(A) Not later than 10 days after the date an alliance is notified of the receipt of services by an unenrolled individual, the alliance provides the individual with materials describing health plans offered through the alliance.

(B) The individual shall be provided a period of 30 days in which to enroll in a health plan of the individual's choice. If the individual fails to so enroll during such period, the alliance shall enroll the individual in a health plan of the alliance selected on a random basis.

(C) Using the fee-for-service schedule adopted by the alliance under section, the health plan in which the individual is enrolled under this subparagraph shall reimburse the provider who provided the services referred to in subparagraph (A) to the same extent as if the individual had been enrolled under the plan at the time of provision of the services.

(c) ENROLLMENT OF NEW RESIDENTS.—

(1) IN GENERAL.—Each regional alliance shall establish procedures for enrolling regional alliance eligible individuals who move into the alliance area.

(2) LONG-TERM RESIDENTS.—Such procedures shall assure that regional alliance eligible individuals who intend to reside in the alliance area for longer than 6 months shall register with the regional alliance for the area and shall enroll in a regional alliance health plan offered by the alliance.

(3) SHORT-TERM RESIDENTS.—Such procedures shall permit eligible individuals who intend to reside in the alliance area for more than 3 months but less than 6 months to choose among the following options:

(A) To continue coverage through the health plan in which such individual is previously enrolled, in which case coverage for care in the area of temporary residence may be limited to emergency services and urgent care.

        (B) To register with the regional alliance and enroll in a regional alliance health plan offered by the alliance.

        (C) To change enrollment in the previous alliance area to enrollment in a health plan of such alliance that provides for coverage on a fee-for-service basis of services provided outside the area of that alliance.

(d) CHANGES IN ENROLLMENT.—

    (1) ANNUAL OPEN ENROLLMENT PERIOD TO CHANGE PLAN ENROLLMENT.—Each regional alliance shall hold an annual open enrollment period during which each eligible enrollee in the alliance has the opportunity to choose among health plans offered through the alliance, according to rules to be promulgated by the National Health Board.

    (2) DISENROLLMENT FOR CAUSE.—In addition to the annual open enrollment period held under paragraph (1), each regional alliance shall establish procedures under which alliance eligible individuals enrolled in a plan may disenroll from the plan for good cause at any time during a year and enroll in another plan of the alliance. Such procedures shall

be implemented in a manner that ensures continuity of coverage for the comprehensive benefit package for such individuals during the year.

(e) ENROLLMENT OF FAMILY MEMBERS.—Each regional alliance shall provide for the enrollment of all family members in the same plan, consistent with part 2 of subtitle A.

(f) OVERSUBSCRIPTION OF PLANS.—

(1) IN GENERAL.—Each regional alliance shall establish a method for establishing enrollment priorities in the case of a health plan that does not have sufficient capacity to enroll all eligible individuals seeking enrollment.

(2) PREFERENCE FOR CURRENT MEMBERS.—Such method shall provide that in the case of such an oversubscribed plan—

(A) individuals already enrolled in the plan are given priority in continuing enrollment in the plan, and

(B) other individuals who seek enrollment during an applicable enrollment period are permitted to enroll in accordance with a random selection method, up to the enrollment capacity of the plan.

(g) TERMINATION OF ENROLLMENT.—

(1) IN GENERAL.—Each regional alliance shall establish special enrollment procedures to permit alliance eligible individuals to change the plan in which they are enrolled in the case of the termination of coverage under a plan, in a manner that ensures the individuals' continuation of coverage for the comprehensive benefit package.

(2) FAILURE OF A CORPORATE ALLIANCE.—Each regional alliance shall establish special enrollment procedures to permit individuals, who become alliance eligible individuals as a result of the failure of a corporate alliance, to enroll promptly in regional alliance health plans in a manner that ensures the individuals' continuation of coverage for the comprehensive benefit package.

(h) LIMITATION ON OFFERING OF COVERAGE TO INELIGIBLE INDIVIDUALS.—A regional alliance may not knowingly offer coverage under a regional alliance health plan or other health insurance or health benefits to an individual who is not an eligible individual. Nothing in this section shall be construed as affecting the ability of a regional alliance health plan or other health plan to offer coverage to such individuals without any financial payment by a regional alliance.

(i) ENFORCEMENT OF ENROLLMENT REQUIREMENT.—In the case of a regional alliance eligible individual who fails to enroll in an applicable health plan as required under section 1002(a)—

> (1) the applicable regional alliance shall enroll the individual in a regional alliance health plan (selected by the alliance consistent with this Act and with any rules established by the Board), and
>
> (2) such alliance shall require the payment of twice the amount of the family share of premiums that would have been payable under subtitle B of title VI if the individual had enrolled on a timely basis in the plan, unless the individual has established to the satisfaction of the alliance good cause for the failure to enroll on a timely basis.

### SEC. 1324. ISSUANCE OF HEALTH SECURITY CARDS.

A regional alliance is responsible for the issuance of health security cards to regional alliance eligible individuals under section 1001(b).

### SEC. 1325. CONSUMER INFORMATION AND MARKETING.

(a) CONSUMER INFORMATION.—

> (1) IN GENERAL.—Each regional alliance shall make available to eligible enrollees information, in an easily understood and useful form, that allows such enrollees (and other alliance eligible individ-

uals) to make valid comparisons among health plans offered by the alliance. Such information shall be made available in a brochure, published not less often than annually.

(2) INFORMATION TO BE INCLUDED.—Such information must include, in the same format for each plan, such information as the National Health Board shall require, including at least the following:

(A) The cost of the plan, including premiums and average out-of-pocket expenses.

(B) The characteristics and availability of health care professionals and institutions participating in the plan.

(C) Any restrictions on access to providers and services under the plan.

(D) A summary of the annual quality performance report, established pursuant to section 5005(d)(1), which contains measures of quality presented in a standard format.

(b) MARKETING.—Each regional alliance shall review and approve or disapprove the distribution of any materials used to market health plans offered through the alliance.

### SEC. 1326. OMBUDSMAN.

(a) ESTABLISHMENT.—Each regional alliance must establish and maintain an office of an ombudsman to assist consumers in dealing with problems that arise with health plans and the alliance.

(b) OPTIONAL FINANCING THROUGH VOLUNTARY CONTRIBUTION.—At the option of State in which a regional alliance is located, the alliance—

> (1) shall permit alliance eligible individuals to designate that one dollar of the premium paid for enrollment in the individual's regional alliance health plan for the operation of the office of the alliance's ombudsman; and
>
> (2) shall apply any such amounts towards the establishment and operation of such office.

### SEC. 1327. DATA COLLECTION; QUALITY.

Each regional alliance shall comply with requirements of subtitles A and B of title V (relating to quality, information systems, and privacy), and shall take appropriate steps to ensure that health plans offered through the alliance comply with such requirements.

### SEC. 1328. ADDITIONAL DUTIES.

(a) ANTI-DISCRIMINATION.—In carrying out its activities under this part, a health alliance may not discriminate against health plans on the basis of race, gender, ethnicity, religion, mix of health professionals, location of the plan's headquarters, or (except as specifically provided in this part) organizational arrangement.

(b) COORDINATION OF ENROLLMENT ACTIVITIES.—Each regional alliance shall coordinate, in a manner specified by the National Health Board, with other health alliances its activities, including enrollment and disenrollment activities, in a manner that ensures continuous, nonduplicative coverage of alliance eligible individuals in health plans and that minimizes administrative procedures and paperwork.

SEC. 1329. ADDITIONAL AUTHORITIES FOR REGIONAL ALLIANCES TO ADDRESS NEEDS IN AREAS WITH INADEQUATE HEALTH SERVICES; PROHIBITION OF INSURANCE ROLE.

(a) PAYMENT ADJUSTMENT.—In order to ensure that plans are available to all eligible individuals residing in all portions of the alliance area, a regional alliance may adjust payments to plans or use other financial incentives to encourage health plans to expand into areas that have inadequate health services.

(b) ENCOURAGING NEW PLANS.—Subject to subsection (c), in order to encourage the establishment of a new health plan in an area that has inadequate health services, an alliance may—

(1) organize health providers to create such a plan in such an area a new health plan targeted at such an area,

(2) provide assistance with setting up and administering such a plan, and

(3) arrange favorable financing for such a plan.

(c) PROHIBITION OF REGIONAL ALLIANCES BEARING RISK.—A regional alliance may not bear insurance risk.

**SEC. 1330. PROHIBITION AGAINST SELF-DEALING AND CONFLICTS OF INTEREST.**

(a) PROMULGATION OF STANDARDS.—The Board shall promulgate standards of conduct in accordance with subsection (b) for any administrator, officer, trustee, fiduciary, custodian, counsel, agent, or employee of any regional alliance.

(b) REQUIREMENTS FOR STANDARDS.—The standards of conduct shall referred to in subsection (a) shall set forth—

(1) the types of investment interests, ownership interests, affiliations or other employment that would be improper for an individual described in subsection (a) to hold during the time of the individual's service or employment with an alliance; and

(2) the circumstances that will constitute impermissible conflicts of interest or self-dealing by

such employees in performing their official duties and functions for any regional alliance.

(c) CIVIL MONETARY PENALTY.—Any individual who engages in an activity that the individual knows or has reason to know is in violation of the regulations and standards promulgated by the Board pursuant to paragraphs (a) and (b) shall be subject, in addition to any other penalties that may be prescribed by law, to a civil money penalty of not more than $10,000 for each such violation.

# PART 3—AUTHORITIES AND RESPONSIBILITIES RELATING TO FINANCING AND INCOME DETERMINATIONS

## Subpart A—Collection of Funds

### SEC. 1341. INFORMATION AND NEGOTIATION AND ACCEPTANCE OF BIDS.

(a) INFORMATION PROVIDED TO PLANS BEFORE SOLICITING BIDS.—

(1) IN GENERAL.—Each regional alliance shall make available, by April 1 of each year, to each plan that indicates an interest in submitting a premium bid under section 6004 in the year, information (including information described in paragraph (2)) that the Board specifies as being necessary to enable a plan to estimate, based upon an accepted bid, the amounts payable to such a plan under section 1351.

(2) INFORMATION TO BE INCLUDED.—Such information shall include the following:

(A) The demographic and other characteristics of regional alliance eligible individuals for the regional alliance.

(B) The uniform per capita conversion factor for the regional alliance (established under subsection (b)).

(C) The premium class factors (established by the Board under section 1531).

(D) The regional alliance inflation factor (determined under section 6001(a)).

(E) The risk-adjustment factors and reinsurance methodology and payment amounts (published under subsection (c)) to be used by the regional alliance in computing blended plan per capita rates (in accordance with section 6201).

(F) The plan bid proportion, the AFDC proportion, the SSI proportion, the AFDC per capita premium amount, and the SSI per capita premium amount, for the year, as computed under subtitle D of title VI.

(G) The alliance administrative allowance percentage, computed under section 1352(b).

(b) DETERMINATION OF UNIFORM PER CAPITA CONVERSION FACTOR.—Each regional alliance shall specify, not later than April 1 of each year (beginning with the year before the first year) a uniform per capita conversion factor to be used under section 6102(a)(2) in converting the accepted bid for each plan for the year into the premium for an individual enrollment for such plan for the year. SSI or AFDC recipients shall not be included for purposes of computing the conversion factor.

(c) DETERMINATION OF RISK-ADJUSTMENT FACTORS AND REINSURANCE PAYMENT AMOUNTS.—Each regional alliance shall compute and publish the risk-adjustment factors and reinsurance payment amounts to be used by the regional alliance in computing blended plan per capita rates under section 6201.

(d) SOLICITATION OF BIDS.—Each regional alliance shall solicit and negotiate, consistent with section 6004, with each regional alliance health plan a bid for the payment rate on a per capita basis for the comprehensive benefit package for all alliance eligible individuals in the alliance area.

# SEC. 1342. CALCULATION AND PUBLICATION OF GENERAL FAMILY SHARE AND GENERAL EMPLOYER PREMIUM AMOUNTS.

(a) CALCULATION OF COMPONENTS IN GENERAL FAMILY SHARE AND GENERAL EMPLOYER PREMIUMS.—

(1) FAMILY SHARE.—Each regional alliance shall compute the following components of the general family share of premiums:

(A) PLAN PREMIUMS.—For each plan offered, the premium for the plan for each class of family enrollment (including the amount of any family collection shortfall).

(B) ALLIANCE CREDIT.—The alliance credit amount for each class of family enrollment, under section 6103.

(C) EXCESS PREMIUM CREDIT.—The amount of any excess premium credit provided under section 6105 for each class of family enrollment.

(D) CORPORATE ALLIANCE OPT-IN CREDIT.—The amount of any corporate alliance opt-in credit provided under section 6106 for each class of family enrollment.

(2) EMPLOYER PREMIUMS.—Each regional alliance shall compute the following components of the general employer premium payment:

(A) BASE EMPLOYER MONTHLY PREMIUM PER WORKER.—The base employer monthly premium determined under section 6122 for each class of family enrollment.

(B) EMPLOYER COLLECTION SHORTFALL ADD-ON.—The employer collection shortfall add-on computed under section 6125(b).

(b) PUBLICATION.—

(1) FAMILY SHARE.—

(A) IN GENERAL.—Each regional alliance shall publish, before the open enrollment period in each year, the general family share of the premium (as defined in subparagraph (B)) for each class of family enrollment for each regional alliance health plan to be offered by the alliance in the following year.

(B) GENERAL FAMILY SHARE OF PREMIUM DEFINED.—In this subpart, the term "general family share of premium" means the family share of premium under section 6101 computed without regard to section 6104 and without regard to section 6101(b)(2)(C)(v).

(2) EMPLOYER PREMIUM.—

(A) IN GENERAL.—Each regional alliance shall publish, in December before each year (beginning with December before the first year) the general employer premium payment amount (as defined in subparagraph (B)) for each class of family enrollment for the following year.

(B) GENERAL EMPLOYER PREMIUM PAYMENT AMOUNT DEFINED.—In this subpart, the term "general employer premium payment amount" means the employer premium payment under section 6121 computed, as an amount per full-time equivalent worker, without regard to sections 6124, 6125, 6126.

## SEC. 1343. DETERMINATION OF FAMILY SHARE FOR FAMILIES.

(a) AMOUNT OF FAMILY SHARE.—The amount charged by a regional alliance to a family for a class of family enrollment (specified under section 1011(c)) under a regional alliance health plan is equal to the family share of premium established under section 6101(a) for the family. Based upon the information described in this section, each regional alliance shall determine the amount required to be paid under section 6101 and under section 6111 for each year for families enrolling in regional alliance health plans.

(b) FAMILY SHARE AMOUNT.—The amount required to be paid under section 6101, with respect to each family, takes into account—

    (1) the general family share of premium (as defined in section 1342(b)(1)(B)) for the class of enrollment involved;

    (2) any income-related discount provided under section 6104(a)(1) for the family; and

    (3) whether or not the family is an SSI or AFDC family.

(c) ALLIANCE CREDIT AMOUNT.—The amount of the alliance credit under section 6111, with respect to each family, takes into account the following:

    (1) The number of months of enrollment, and class of enrollment, in regional alliance health plans, used in determining the amount of the alliance credit under section 6103 for the family.

    (2) Reductions in liability under section 6111(b) based on employer premium payments based on net earnings from self-employment for the family.

    (3) Reductions in liability under section 6112 based on months of employment for the family.

(4) Limitations in liability under section 6113 on the basis of the adjusted family income for the family.

(5) The elimination of liability in the case of certain retirees and qualified spouses and children under section 6114.

(6) The elimination of liability in the case of certain working medicare beneficiaries under section 6115.

(d) ACCESS TO NECESSARY INFORMATION TO MAKE DETERMINATION.—Information required for an alliance to make the determination under subsection (a) shall be based on information obtained or maintained by the alliance in the conduct of its business, including the following:

(1) Information required for income-related determinations shall be obtained under subpart B.

(2) Information on SSI and AFDC recipients under subsection (e).

(3) Information submitted on a monthly and annual basis by employers under section 1602.

(4) Information submitted by self-employed individuals on net earnings from self-employment under section 1602(d).

(5) Applications for premium reductions under section 6114.

(6) Information concerning medicare-eligible individuals under subsection (f).

(7) Any income-related discount provided under section 6104(a)(1) for the family.

(8) Whether or not the family is an SSI or AFDC family.

(e) INFORMATION CONCERNING CASH ASSISTANCE STATUS.—Each participating State and the Secretary shall make available (in a time and manner specified by the Secretary) to each regional alliance such information as may be necessary to determine and verify whether an individual is an AFDC or SSI recipient for a month in a year.

(f) INFORMATION CONCERNING MEDICARE-ELIGIBLE INDIVIDUALS.—

(1) INFORMATION TO REGIONAL ALLIANCES.—The Secretary shall make available to regional alliances (through regional information centers or otherwise) information necessary to determine—

(A) whether an individual is a medicare-eligible individual,

(B) the eligibility of individuals for the special treatment under section 6115,

(C) if medicare-eligible individuals are described in section 1012(a), and

(D) the amounts of payments owed the alliance under section 1895 of the Social Security Act.

(2) INFORMATION TO SECRETARY.—Each regional alliance shall make available to the Secretary (through the national information system under section 5101 or otherwise) information relating to the enrollment of individuals who would be medicare-eligible individuals but for section 1012(a).

(g) ALLIANCE ACCOUNTING SYSTEM.—

(1) IN GENERAL.—Each regional alliance shall establish an accounting system that meets standards established by the Secretary.

(2) SPECIFICS.—Such system shall collect information, on a timely basis for each individual enrolled (and, to the extent required by the Secretary, identified and required to be enrolled) in a regional alliance health plan regarding—

(A) the applicable premium for such enrollment,

(B) family members covered under such enrollment,

(C) the premium payments made by (or on behalf of) the individual for such enrollment,

(D) employer premium payments made respecting the employment of the individual and other employer contributions made respecting such enrollment, and

(E) any government contributions made with respect to such enrollment (including contributions for electing veterans and active duty military personnel).

(3) END-OF-YEAR REPORTING.—Such system shall provide for a report, at the end of each year, regarding the total premiums imposed, and total amounts collected, for individuals enrolled under regional health alliance plans, in such manner as identifies net amounts that may be owed to the regional alliance.

**SEC. 1344. NOTICE OF FAMILY PAYMENTS DUE.**

(a) FAMILY STATEMENTS.—

(1) NOTICE OF NO AMOUNT OWED.—If the regional alliance determines under section 1343 that a family has paid any family share required under section 6101 and is not required to repay any amount under section 6111 for a year, the alliance shall mail notice of such determination to the family. Such notice shall include a prominent statement that the family is not required to make any additional pay-

ment and is not required to file any additional information with the regional alliance.

(2) NOTICE OF AMOUNT OWED.—

(A) IN GENERAL.—If the regional alliance determines that a family has not paid the entire family share required under section 6101 or is required to repay an amount under section 6111 for a year, the alliance shall mail to the family a notice of such determination.

(B) INFORMATION ON AMOUNT DUE.—Such notice shall include detailed information regarding the amount owed, the basis for the computation (including the amount of any reductions that have been made in the family's liability under subtitle B of title VI), and the date the amount is due and the manner in which such amount is payable.

(C) INFORMATION ON DISCOUNTS AND REDUCTIONS AVAILABLE.—Such notice shall include—

(i) information regarding the discounts and reductions available (under sections 6104, 6112, 6113, 6114, and 6115) to reduce or eliminate any liability, and

(ii) a worksheet which may be used to calculate reductions in liability based on income under sections 6104 and 6113.

(3) INCLUSION OF INCOME RECONCILIATION FORM FOR FAMILIES PROVIDED PREMIUM DISCOUNTS.—

(A) IN GENERAL.—A notice under this subsection shall include, in the case of a family that has been provided a premium discount under section 6103 (or section 6113) for the previous year, an income verification statement (described in section 1375) to be completed and returned to the regional alliance (along with any additional amounts owed) by the deadline specified in subsection (b). Such form shall require the submission of such information as Secretary specifies to establish or verify eligiblility for such premium discount.

(B) OTHER FAMILIES.—Any family which has not been provided such a discount but may be eligible for such a discount may submit such an income verification form and, if eligible, receive a rebate of the amount of excess family share paid for the previous year.

(C) ADDITIONAL INFORMATION.—The alliance shall permit a family to provide additional information relating to the amount of such reductions or the income of the family (insofar as it may relate to a premium discount or reduction in liability under section 6104 or 6113).

(4) TIMING OF NOTICE.—Notices under this subsection shall be mailed to each family at least 45 days before the deadline specified in subsection (b).

(b) DEADLINE FOR PAYMENT.—The deadline specified in this subsection for amounts owed for a year is such date as the Secretary may specify, taking into account the dates when the information specified in section 1343 becomes available to compute the amounts owed and the information required to file income reconcilation statements under section 1375. Amounts not paid by such deadline are subject to interest and penalty.

(c) CHANGE IN REGIONAL ALLIANCE.—In the case of a family that during a year changes the regional alliance through which the family obtains coverage under a regional alliance health plan, the Secretary shall establish rules which provide that the regional alliance in which the family last obtained such coverage in a year—

(1) is responsible for recovering amounts due under this subpart for the year (whether or not at-

tributable to periods of coverage obtained through that alliance);

(2) shall obtain such information, through the health information system implemented under section 5201, as the alliance may require in order to compute the amount of any liability owed under this subpart (taking into account any reduction in such amount under this section), and

(3) shall provide for the payment to other regional alliances of such amounts collected as may be attributable to amounts owed for periods of coverage obtained through such alliances.

(d) NO LOSS OF COVERAGE.—In no case shall the failure to pay amounts owed under this subsection result in an individual's or family's loss of coverage under this Act.

(e) DISPUTE RESOLUTION.—Each regional alliance shall establish a fair hearing mechanism for the resolution of disputes concerning amounts owed the alliance under this subpart.

**SEC. 1345. COLLECTIONS.**

(a) IN GENERAL.—Each regional alliance is responsible for the collection of all amounts owed the alliance (whether by individuals, employers, or others and whether on the basis of premiums owed, incorrect amounts of discounts or premium, cost sharing, or other reductions made, or otherwise), and no amounts are payable by the Federal Government under this Act (including section 9102) with respect to the failure to collect any such amounts. Each regional alliance shall use credit and collection procedures, including the imposition of interest charges and late fees for failure to make timely payment, as may be necessary to collect amounts owed to the alliance. States assist regional alliances in such collection process under section 1202(d).

(b) COLLECTION OF FAMILY SHARE.—

(1) WITHHOLDING.—

(A) IN GENERAL.—In the case of a family that includes a qualifying employee of an employer, the employer shall deduct from the wages of the qualifying employee (in a manner consistent with any rules of the Secretary of Labor) the amount of the family share of the premium for the plan in which the family is enrolled.

(B) MULTIPLE EMPLOYMENT.—In the case of a family that includes more than one qualifying employee, the family shall choose the employer to which subparagraph (A) will apply.

(C) PAYMENT.—Amounts withheld under this paragraph shall be maintained in a manner consistent with standards established by the Secretary of Labor and paid to the regional alliance involved in a manner consistent with the payment of employer premiums under subsection (c).

(D) SATISFACTION OF LIABILITY.—An amount deducted from wages of a qualifying employee by an employer is deemed to have been paid by the employee and to have satisfied the employee's obligation under subsection (a) to the extent of such amount.

(2) OTHER METHODS.—In the case of a family that does not include a qualifying employee, the regional alliance shall require payment to be made prospectively and such payment may be required to be made not less frequently than monthly. The Secretary may issue regulations in order to assure the timely and accurate collection of the family share due.

(c) TIMING AND METHOD OF PAYMENT OF EMPLOYER PREMIUMS.—

(1) FREQUENCY OF PAYMENT.—Payment of employer premiums under section 6121 for a month

shall be made not less frequently than monthly (or quarterly in the case of such payments made by virtue of section 6126). The Secretary of Labor may establish a method under which employers that pay wages on a weekly or biweekly basis are permitted to make such employer payments on such a weekly or biweekly basis.

(2) ELECTRONIC TRANSFER.—A regional alliance may require those employers that have the capacity to make payments by electronic transfer to make payments under this section by electronic transfer.

(d) ASSISTANCE.—

(1) EMPLOYER COLLECTIONS.—The Secretary of Labor shall provide regional alliances with such technical and other assistance as may promote the efficient collection of all amounts owed such alliances under this Act by employers. Such assistance may include the assessment of civil monetary penalties, not to exceed $5,000 or three times the amount of the liability owed, whichever is greater, in the case of repeated failure to pay (as specified in rules of the Secretary of Labor).

(2) FAMILY COLLECTIONS.—Except as provided in paragraph (1), the Secretary shall provide re-

gional alliances with such technical and other assistance as may promote the efficient collection of other amounts owed such alliances under this Act. Such assistance may include the assessment of civil monetary penalties, not to exceed $5,000 or three times the amount of the liability owed, whichever is greater, in the case of repeated failure to pay (as specified in rules of the Secretary).

(e) RECEIPT OF MISCELLANEOUS AMOUNTS.—For payments to regional alliances by—

(1) States, see subtitle A of title IX, and

(2) the Federal Government, see subtitle B of such title and section 1895 of the Social Security Act (as added by section 4003).

SEC. 1346. COORDINATION AMONG REGIONAL ALLIANCES.

(a) IN GENERAL.—The regional alliance which offers the regional alliance health plan in which a family is enrolled in December of each year (in this section referred to as the "final alliance") is responsible for the collection of any amounts owed under this subpart, without regard to whether the family resided in the alliance area during the entire year.

(b) PROVISION OF INFORMATION IN THE CASE OF CHANGE OF RESIDENCE.—In the case of a family that moves from one alliance area to another alliance area during a year, each regional alliance (other than the final alliance) is responsible for providing to the final alliance (through the national information system under section 5101 or otherwise) such information as the final alliance may require in order to determine the liability (and reductions in liability under section 6112) attributable to alliance credits provided by such regional alliance.

(c) DISTRIBUTION OF PROCEEDS.—In accordance with rules established by the Secretary, in consultation with the Secretary of Labor, the final alliance shall provide for the distribution of amounts collected under this subpart with respect to families in a year in an equitable manner among the regional alliances that provided health plan coverage to the families in the year.

(d) EXPEDITING PROCESS.—In order to reduce paperwork and promote efficiency in the collection of amounts owed regional alliances under this subpart, the Secretary may require or permit regional alliances to share such information (through the national information system under section 5101 or otherwise) as the Secretary determines to be cost-effective, subject to such confidentiality restrictions as may otherwise apply.

(e) STUDENTS.—In the case of a qualifying student who makes an election described in section 1012(e)(2)) (relating to certain full-time students who are covered under the plan of a parent but enrolled in a health plan offered by a different regional alliance from the one in which the parent is enrolled), the regional alliance that offered the plan to the parent shall provide for transfers of an appropriate portion of the premium (determined in accordance with procedures specified by the Board) to the other regional alliance in order to compensate that alliance for the provision of such coverage.

(f) PAYMENTS OF CERTAIN AMOUNTS TO CORPORATE ALLIANCES.—In the case of a married couple in which one spouse is a qualifying employee of a regional alliance employer and the other spouse is a qualifying employee of a corporate alliance employer, if the couple is enrolled with a corporate alliance health plan the regional alliance (which receives employer premium payments from such regional alliance employer with respect to such employee) shall pay to the corporate alliance the amounts so paid (or would be payable by the employer if section 6123 did not apply).

## Subpart B—Payments

### SEC. 1351. PAYMENT TO REGIONAL ALLIANCE HEALTH PLANS.

(a) COMPUTATION OF BLENDED PLAN PER CAPITA PAYMENT AMOUNT.—For purposes of making payments to plans under this section, each regional alliance shall compute, under section 6201(a), a blended plan per capita payment amount for each regional alliance health plan for enrollment in the alliance for a year.

(b) AMOUNT OF PAYMENT TO PLANS.—

(1) IN GENERAL.—Subject to subsection (e) and section 6121(b)(5)(B), each regional alliance shall provide for payment to each regional alliance health plan, in which an alliance eligible individual is enrolled, an amount equal to the net blended rate (described in paragraph (2)) adjusted (consistent with subsection (c)) to take into account the relative actuarial risk associated with the coverage with respect to the individual.

(2) NET BLENDED RATE.—The net blended rate described in this paragraph is the blended plan per capita payment amount (determined under section 6201(a)), reduced by—

(A) the consolidated set aside percentage specified under subsection (d), and

(B) any plan payment reduction imposed under section 6011 for the plan for the year.

(c) APPLICATION OF RISK ADJUSTMENT AND REINSURANCE METHODOLOGY.—Each regional alliance shall use the risk adjustment methodology developed under section 1541 in making payments to regional alliance health plans under this section, except as provided in section 1542.

(d) CONSOLIDATED SET ASIDE PERCENTAGE.—The consolidated set aside percentage, for a regional alliance for a year, is the sum of—

    (1) the administrative allowance percentage for the regional alliance, computed by the alliance under section 1352(b); and

    (2) 1.5 percentage points.

Amounts attributable to paragraph (2) are paid to the Federal Government (for academic health centers and graduate medical education) under section 1353.

(e) TREATMENT OF VETERANS, MILITARY, AND INDIAN HEALTH PLANS AND PROGRAMS.—

    (1) VETERANS HEALTH PLAN.—In applying this subtitle (and title VI) in the case of a regional alliance health plan that is a veterans health plan of the Department of Veterans Affairs, the following rules apply:

        (A) For purposes of applying subtitle A of title VI, families enrolled under the plan shall not be taken into account.

        (B) The provisions of subtitle A of title VI shall not apply to the plan, other than such provisions as require the plan to submit a per capita amount for each regional alliance area on a timely basis, which amount shall be treated as the final accepted bid of the plan for the area for purposes of subtitle B of such title and this section. This amount shall not be subject to negotiation and not subject to reduction under section 6011.

(C) For purposes of computing the blended plan per capita payment amount under this section, the AFDC and SSI proportions (under section 6202(a)) are deemed to be 0 percent.

(2) UNIFORMED SERVICES HEALTH PLAN.—In applying this subtitle (and title VI) in the case of a regional alliance health plan that is a Uniformed Services Health Plan of the Department of Defense, the following rules apply:

(A) For purposes of applying subtitle A of title VI, families enrolled under the plan shall not be taken into account.

(B) The provisions of subtitle A of title VI shall not apply to the plan, other than such provisions as require the plan to submit a per capita amount on a timely basis, which amount shall be treated as the final accepted bid of the plan for the area involved for purposes of subtitle B of such title and this section. This amount shall not be subject to negotiation and not subject to reduction under section 6011. The Board, in consultation with the Secretary of Defense, shall establish rules relating to the area (or areas) in which such a bid shall apply.

(C) For purposes of computing the blended plan per capita payment amount under this section, the AFDC and SSI proportions (under section 6202(a)) are deemed to be 0 percent.

(3) INDIAN HEALTH PROGRAMS.—In applying this subtitle (and title VI) in the case of a health program of the Indian Health Service, the following rules apply:

(A) Except as provided in this paragraph, the plan shall not be considered or treated to be a regional alliance health plan and for purposes of applying title VI, families enrolled under the program shall not be taken into account.

(B) In accordance with rules established by the Secretary, regional alliances shall act as agents for the collection of employer premium payments (including payments of corporate alliance employers) required under subtitle B of title VI with respect to qualifying employees who are enrolled under a health program of the Indian Health Service. The Secretary shall permit such alliances to retain a nominal fee to compensate them for such collection activities. In applying this subparagraph, the family share of premium for such employees is deemed to be zero for electing Indians (as defined in section 1012(d)(3)) and for other employees is the amount of the premium established under section 8306(b)(4)(A), employees are deemed to be residing in the area of residence (or area of employment), as specified under rules of the Secretary, and the class of enrollment shall be such class (or classes) as specified under rules of the Secretary.

## SEC. 1352. ALLIANCE ADMINISTRATIVE ALLOWANCE PERCENTAGE.

(a) SPECIFICATION BY ALLIANCE.—Before obtaining bids under 6004 from health plans for a year, each regional alliance shall establish the administrative allowance for the operation of regional alliance in the year.

(b) ADMINISTRATIVE ALLOWANCE PERCENTAGE.—Subject to subsection (c), the regional alliance shall compute an administrative allowance percentage for each year equal to—

(1) the administrative allowance determined under subsection (a) for the year, divided by

(2) the total of the amounts payable to regional alliance health plans under section 1343 (as estimated by the alliance and determined without regard to section 1343(d)).

(c) LIMITATION TO 2½ PERCENT.—In no case shall an administrative allowance percentage exceed 2.5 percent.

## SEC. 1353. PAYMENTS TO THE FEDERAL GOVERNMENT FOR ACADEMIC HEALTH CENTERS AND GRADUATE MEDICAL EDUCATION.

Each regional alliance shall make payment to the Secretary each year of an amount equal to the reduction in payments by the alliance to regional alliance health plans resulting from the consolidated set aside percentage under section 1351(d) including the 1.5 percentage points under paragraph (2) of such section.

### Subpart C—Financial Management

## SEC. 1361. MANAGEMENT OF FINANCES AND RECORDS.

(a) IN GENERAL.—Each regional alliance shall comply with standards established under section 1571(b) (relating to the management of finances, maintenance of records, accounting practices, auditing procedures, and financial reporting) and under section 1591(d) (relating to employer payments).

(b) SPECIFIC PROVISIONS.—In accordance with such standards—

    (1) FINANCIAL STATEMENTS.—

        (A) IN GENERAL.—Each regional alliance shall publish periodic audited financial statements.

        (B) ANNUAL FINANCIAL AUDIT.—

            (i) IN GENERAL.—Each regional alliance shall have an annual financial audit conducted by an independent auditor in accordance with generally accepted auditing standards.

            (ii) PUBLICATION.—A report on each such audit shall be made available to the public at nominal cost.

            (iii) REQUIRED ACTIONS FOR DEFICIENCIES.—If the report from such an audit does not bear an unqualified opinion, the alliance shall take such steps on a timely basis as may be necessary to correct any material deficiency identified in the report.

(C) ELIGIBILITY ERROR RATES.—Each regional alliance shall make eligibility determinations for premium discounts, liability reductions, and cost sharing reductions under sections 6104 and 6123, section 6113, and section 1371, respectively, in a manner that maintains the error rates below an applicable maximum permissible error rate specified by the Secretary (or the Secretary of Labor with respect to section 6123). In specifying such a rate, the Secretary shall take into account maximum permissible error rates recognized by the Federal Government under comparable State-administered programs.

(2) SAFEGUARDING OF FUNDS.—Each regional alliance shall safeguard family, employer, State, and Federal government payments to the alliance in accordance with fiduciary standards and shall hold such payments in financial institutions and instruments that meet standards recognized or established by the Secretary, in consultation with the Secretaries of Labor and the Treasury and taking into account current Federal laws and regulations relating to fiduciary responsibilities and financial management of public funds.

(3) CONTINGENCIES.—Each regional alliance shall provide that any surplus of funds resulting from an estimation discrepancy described in section 9201(b)(1)(D), up to a reasonable amount specified by the Secretary, shall be held in a contingency fund established by the alliance and used to fund any future shortfalls resulting from such a discrepancy.

(4) AUDITING OF EMPLOYER PAYMENTS.—

(A) IN GENERAL.—Each regional alliance is responsible for auditing the records of regional alliance employers to assure that employer payments (including the payment of amounts withheld) were made in the appropriate amount as provided under subpart A of part 2 of subtitle B of title VI.

(B) EMPLOYERS WITH EMPLOYEES RESIDING IN DIFFERENT ALLIANCE AREAS.—In the case of a regional alliance employer which has employees who reside in more than one alliance area, the Secretary of Labor, in consultation with the Secretary, shall establish a process for the coordination of regional alliance auditing activities among the regional alliances involved.

(C) APPEAL.—In the case of an audit conducted by a regional alliance on an employer under this paragraph, an employer or other regional alliance that is aggrieved by the determination in the audit is entitled to review of such audit by the Secretary of Labor in a manner to be provided by such Secretary.

**Subpart D—Reductions in Cost Sharing; Income Determinations**

**SEC. 1371. REDUCTION IN COST SHARING FOR LOW-INCOME FAMILIES.**

(a) REDUCTION.—

(1) IN GENERAL.—Subject to subsection (b), in the case of a family that is enrolled in a regional alliance health plan and that is either (A) an AFDC or SSI family or (B) is determined under this subpart to have family adjusted income below 150 percent of the applicable poverty level, the family is entitled to a reduction in cost sharing in accordance with this section.

(2) TIMING OF REDUCTION.—The reduction in cost sharing shall only apply to items and services furnished after the date the application for such reduction is approved under section 1372(c) and before the date of termination of the reduction under this subpart, or, in the case of an AFDC or SSI

family, during the period in which the family is such a family.

(3) INFORMATION TO PROVIDERS AND PLANS.—Each regional alliance shall provide, through electronic means and otherwise, health care providers and regional alliance health plans with access to such information as may be necessary in order to provide for the cost sharing reductions under this section.

(b) LIMITATION.—No reduction in cost sharing shall be available for families residing in an alliance area if the regional alliance for the area determines that there are sufficient low-cost plans (as defined in section 6104(b)(3)) that are lower or combination cost sharing plans available in the alliance area to enroll AFDC and SSI families and families with family adjusted income below 150 percent of the applicable poverty level.

(c) AMOUNT OF COST SHARING REDUCTION.—

(1) IN GENERAL.—Subject to paragraph (2), the reduction in cost sharing under this section shall be such reduction as will reduce cost sharing to the level of a lower or combination cost sharing plan.

(2) ADDITIONAL REDUCTION FOR AFDC AND SSI FAMILIES.—In the case of an AFDC or SSI family, in applying paragraph (1) (other than with respect

to hospital emergency room services for which there is no emergency medical condition, as defined in section 1867(e)(1) of the Social Security Act) there shall be substituted, for $5, $10, $20, and $25 in the table in section 1135(a), 20 percent of such respective amounts. The dollar amounts substituted by the previous sentence shall be subject to adjustment in the same manner under section 1136 as the dollar amounts otherwise specified in such section.

(d) ADMINISTRATION.—

(1) IN GENERAL.—In the case of an approved family (as defined in section 1372(b)(3)) enrolled in a regional alliance health plan, the regional alliance shall pay the plan for cost sharing reductions (other than cost sharing reductions under subsection (c)(2)) provided under this section and included in payments made by the plan to its providers.

(2) ESTIMATED PAYMENTS, SUBJECT TO RECONCILIATION.—Such payment shall be made initially on the basis of reasonable estimates of cost sharing reductions incurred by such a plan with respect to approved families and shall be reconciled not less often than quarterly based on actual claims for items and services provided.

(e) NO COST SHARING FOR INDIANS AND CERTAIN VETERANS AND MILITARY PERSONNEL.—The provisions of section 6104(a)(3) shall apply to cost sharing reductions under this section in the same manner as such provisions apply to premium discounts under section 6104.

### SEC. 1372. APPLICATION PROCESS FOR COST SHARING REDUCTIONS.

(a) APPLICATION.—

(1) IN GENERAL.—A regional alliance eligible family may apply for a determination of the family adjusted income of the family, for the purpose of establishing eligibility for cost sharing reductions under section 1371.

(2) FORM.—An application under this section shall include such information as may be determined by the regional alliance (consistent with rules developed by the Secretary) and shall include at least information about the family's employment status and income.

(b) TIMING.—

(1) IN GENERAL.—An application under this section may be filed at such times as the Secretary may provide, including during any open enrollment period, at the time of a move, or after a change in life circumstances (such as unemployment or di-

vorce) affecting class of enrollment or amount of family share or repayment amount.

(2) CONSIDERATION.—Each regional alliance shall approve or disapprove an application under this section, and notify the applicant of such decision, within such period (specified by the Secretary) after the date of the filing of the application.

(3) APPROVED FAMILY DEFINED.—In this section and section 1371, the term "approved family" means a family for which an application under this section is approved, until the date of termination of such approval under this section.

(c) APPROVAL OF APPLICATION.—

(1) IN GENERAL.—A regional alliance shall approve an application of a family under this section filed in a month if the application demonstrates that that family adjusted income of the family (as defined in subsection (d) and determined under paragraph (2)) is (or is expected to be) less than 150 percent of the applicable poverty level.

(2) USE OF CURRENT INCOME.—In making the determination under paragraph (1), a regional alliance shall take into account the income for the previous 3-month period and current wages from em-

ployment (if any), consistent with rules specified by the Secretary.

(d) FAMILY ADJUSTED INCOME.—

(1) IN GENERAL.—Except as provided in paragraph (4), in this Act the term "family adjusted income" means, with respect to a family, the sum of the adjusted incomes (as defined in paragraph (2)) for all members of the family (determined without regard to section 1012).

(2) ADJUSTED INCOME.—In paragraph (1), the term "adjusted income" means, with respect to an individual, adjusted gross income (as defined in section 62(a) of the Internal Revenue Code of 1986)—

    (A) determined without regard to sections 135, 162(l), 911, 931, and 933 of such Code, and

    (B) increased by the amount of interest received or accrued by the individual which is exempt from tax.

(3) PRESENCE OF ADDITIONAL DEPENDENTS.—At the option of an individual, a family may include (and not be required to separate out) the income of other individuals who are claimed as dependents of the family for income tax purposes, but such individ-

uals shall not be counted as part of the family for purposes of determining the size of the family.

(e) REQUIREMENT FOR PERIODIC CONFIRMATION AND VERIFICATION AND NOTICES.—

(1) CONFIRMATION AND VERIFICATION REQUIREMENT.—The continued eligibility of a family for cost sharing reductions under this section is conditioned upon the family's eligibility being—

(A) confirmed periodically by the regional alliance, and

(B) verified (through the filing of a new application under this section) by the regional alliance at the time income reconciliation statements are required to be filed under section 1375.

(2) RULES.—The Secretary shall issue rules related to the manner in which alliances confirm and verify eligibility under this section.

(3) NOTICES OF CHANGES IN INCOME AND EMPLOYMENT STATUS.—

(A) IN GENERAL.—Each approved family shall promptly notify the regional alliance of any material increase in the family adjusted income (as defined by the Secretary).

(B) RESPONSE.—If a regional alliance receives notice under subparagraph (A) (or from an employer under section 1602(b)(3)(A)(i)) or otherwise receives information indicating a potential significant change in the family's employment status or increase in adjusted family income, the regional alliance shall promptly take steps necessary to reconfirm the family's eligibility.

(f) TERMINATION OF COST SHARING REDUCTION.—The regional alliance shall, after notice to the family, terminate the reduction of cost sharing under this subpart for an approved family if the family fails to provide for confirmation or verification or notice required under subsection (c) on a timely basis or the alliance otherwise determines that the family is no longer eligible for such reduction. The previous sentence shall not prevent the family from subsequently reapplying for cost sharing reduction under this section.

(g) TREATMENT OF AFDC AND SSI RECIPIENTS.—

(1) NO APPLICATION REQUIRED.—AFDC and SSI families are not required to make an application under this section.

(2) NOTICE REQUIREMENT.—Each State (and the Secretary) shall notify each regional alliance, in

a manner specified by the Secretary, of the identity (and period of eligibility under the AFDC or SSI programs) of each AFDC and SSI recipient, unless such a recipient elects (in a manner specified by the Secretary) not to accept the reduction of cost sharing under this section.

### SEC. 1373. APPLICATION FOR PREMIUM REDUCTIONS AND REDUCTION IN LIABILITIES TO ALLIANCES.

(a) IN GENERAL.—Any regional alliance eligible family may apply for a determination of the family adjusted income of the family, for the purpose of establishing eligibility for a premium discount under section 6104 or a reduction in liability under section 6113.

(b) TIMING.—Such an application may be filed at such times as an application for a cost sharing reduction may be filed under section 1372(b) and also may be filed after the end of the year to obtain a rebate for excess premium payments made during a year.

(c) APPROVAL OF APPLICATION.—

(1) IN GENERAL.—A regional alliance shall approve an application of a family under this section filed in a month—

(A) for a premium discount under section 6104, if the application demonstrates that family adjusted income of the family (as determined under paragraph (2)) is (or is expected to be) less than 150 percent of the applicable poverty level, or

(B) for a reduction in liability under section 6113, if the application demonstrates that the wage-adjusted income (as defined in subsection 6113(d)) of the family (as determined under paragraph (2)) is (or is expected to be) less than 250 percent of the applicable poverty level.

(2) USE OF CURRENT INCOME.—In making the determination under paragraph (1), a regional alliance shall take into account the income for the previous 3-month period and current wages from employment (if any) and the statement of estimated income for the year (filed under section 1374(c)), consistent with rules specified by the Secretary.

(d) REQUIREMENT FOR PERIODIC CONFIRMATION AND VERIFICATION AND NOTICES.—The provisions of section (e) of section 1372 shall apply under this section in the same manner as it applies under such section, except that any reference to family adjusted income is deemed a reference to wage-adjusted income.

**Health Security Act**  *Title I, Subtitle D*

**SEC. 1374. GENERAL PROVISIONS RELATING TO APPLICATION PROCESS.**

(a) DISTRIBUTION OF APPLICATIONS.—Each regional alliance shall distribute applications under this subpart directly to consumers and through employers, banks, and designated public agencies.

(b) TO WHOM APPLICATION MADE.—Applications under this subpart shall be filed, by person or mail, with a regional alliance or an agency designated by the State for this purpose. The application may be submitted with an application to enroll with a health plan under this subtitle or separately.

(c) INCOME STATEMENT.—Each application shall include a declaration of estimated annual income for the year involved.

(d) FORM AND CONTENTS.—An application for a discount or reduction under this subpart shall be in a form and manner specified by the Secretary and shall require the provision of information necessary to make the determinations required under this subpart.

(e) FREQUENCY OF APPLICATIONS.—

(1) IN GENERAL.—An application under this subpart may be filed at any time during the year (including, in the case of section 1373, during the reconciliation process).

(2) CORRECTION OF INCOME.—Nothing in paragraph (1) shall be construed as preventing an individual or family from, at any time, submitting an application to reduce the amount of premium reduction or reduction of liability under this subpart based upon an increase in income from that stated in the previous application.

(e) TIMING OF REDUCTIONS AND DISCOUNTS.—

(1) IN GENERAL.—Subject to reconciliation under section 1375, premium discounts and cost sharing reductions under this subpart shall be applied to premium payments required (and for expenses incurred) after the date of approval of the application under this subpart.

(2) AFDC AND SSI RECIPIENTS.—In the case of an AFDC or SSI family, in applying paragraph (1), the date of approval of benefits under the AFDC or SSI program shall be considered the date of approval of an an application under this subpart.

(f) VERIFICATION.—The Secretary shall provide for verification, on a sample basis or other basis, of the information supplied in applications under this part. This verification shall be separate from the reconciliation provided under section 1375.

(g) HELP IN COMPLETING APPLICATIONS.—Each regional alliance shall assist individuals in the filing of applications and income reconciliation statements under this subpart.

(h) PENALTIES FOR INACCURATE INFORMATION.—

(1) INTEREST FOR UNDERSTATEMENTS.—Each individual who knowingly understates income reported in an application to a regional alliance under this subpart or otherwise makes a material misrepresentation of information in such an application shall be liable to the alliance for excess payments made based on such understatement or misrepresentation, and for interest on such excess payments at a rate specified by the Secretary.

(2) PENALTIES FOR MISREPRESENTATION.—In addition to the liability established under paragraph (1), each individual who knowingly misrepresents material information in an application under this subpart to a regional alliance shall be liable to the State in which the alliance is located for $2,000 or, if greater, three times the excess payments made based on such misrepresentation. The State shall provide for the transfer of a significant portion of such amount to the regional alliance involved.

## SEC. 1375. END-OF-YEAR RECONCILIATION FOR PREMIUM DISCOUNT AND REPAYMENT REDUCTION WITH ACTUAL INCOME.

(a) IN GENERAL.—In the case of a family whose application for a premium discount or reduction of liability for a year has been approved before the end of the year under this subpart, the family shall, subject to subsection (c) and by the deadline specified in section 1344(b) file with the regional alliance an income reconciliation statement to verify the family's adjusted income or wage-adjusted income, as the case may be, for the previous year. Such a statement shall contain such information as the Secretary may specify. Each regional alliance shall coordinate the submission of such statements with the notice and payment of family payments due under section 1344.

(b) RECONCILIATION OF PREMIUM PREMIUM DISCOUNT AND LIABILITY ASSISTANCE BASED ON ACTUAL INCOME.—Based on and using the income reported in the reconciliation statement filed under subsection (a) with respect to a family, the regional alliance shall compute the amount of premium discount or reduction in liability that should have been provided under section 6104 or section 6113 with respect for the family for the year involved. If the amount of such discount or liability reduction computed is—

(1) greater than the amount that has been provided, the family is liable to the regional alliance to pay (directly or through an increase in future family share of premiums or other payments) a total amount equal to the amount of the excess payment, or

(2) less than the amount that has been provided, the regional alliance shall pay to the family (directly or through a reduction in future family share of premiums or other payments) a total amount equal to the amount of the deficit.

(c) NO RECONCILIATION FOR AFDC AND SSI FAMILIES; NO RECONCILIATION FOR COST SHARING REDUCTIONS.—No reconciliation statement is required under this section—

(1) with respect to cost sharing reductions provided under section 1372, or

(2) for a family that only claims a premium discount or liability reduction under this subpart on the basis of being an AFDC or SSI family.

(d) DISQUALIFICATION FOR FAILURE TO FILE.—In the case of any family that is required to file a statement under this section in a year and that fails to file such a statement by the deadline specified, members of the family shall not be eligible for premium reductions under section

6104 or reductions in liability under section 6113 until such statement is filed. A regional alliance, using rules established by the Secretary, shall waive the application of this subsection if the family establishes, to the satisfaction of the alliance under such rules, good cause for the failure to file the statement on a timely basis.

(e) PENALTIES FOR FALSE INFORMATION.—Any individual that provides false information in a statement under subsection (a) is subject to the same liabilities as are provided under section 1374(h) for a misrepresentation of material fact described in such section.

(f) NOTICE OF REQUIREMENT.—Each regional alliance (directly or in coordination with other regional alliances) shall provide for written notice, at the end of each year, of the requirement of this section to each family which had received premium discount or reduction in liability under this subpart in any month during the preceding year and to which such requirement applies.

(g) TRANSMITTAL OF INFORMATION; VERIFICATION.—

(1) IN GENERAL.—Each participating State shall transmit annually to the Secretary such information relating to the income of families for the previous year as the Secretary may require to verify such income under this subpart.

(2) VERIFICATION.—Each participating State may use such information as it has available to it to assist regional alliances in verifying income of families with applications filed under this subpart. The Secretary of the Treasury may, consistent with section 6103 of the Internal Revenue Code of 1986, permit return information to be disclosed and used by a participating State in verifying such income but only in accordance with such section and only if the information is not directly disclosed to a regional alliance.

(h) CONSTRUCTION.—Nothing in this section shall be construed as authorizing reconciliation of any cost sharing reduction provided under this subpart.

## PART 4—RESPONSIBILITIES AND AUTHORITIES OF CORPORATE ALLIANCES

**SEC. 1381. CONTRACTS WITH HEALTH PLANS.**

(a) CONTRACTS WITH PLANS.—Subject to section 1382, each corporate alliance may—

(1) offer to individuals eligible to enroll under section 1311(c) coverage under an appropriate self-insured health plan (as defined in section 1400(b)), or

(2) negotiate with a State-certified health plan to enter into a contract with the plan for the enrollment of such individuals under the plan,

or do both.

(b) TERMS OF CONTRACTS WITH STATE-CERTIFIED HEALTH PLANS.—Contracts under this section between a corporate alliance and a State-certified health plan may contain such provisions (not inconsistent with the requirements of this title) as the alliance and plan may provide, except that in no case does such contract remove the obligation of the sponsor of the corporate alliance to provide for health benefits to corporate alliance eligible individuals consistent with this part.

## SEC. 1382. OFFERING CHOICE OF HEALTH PLANS FOR ENROLLMENT.

(a) IN GENERAL.—Each corporate alliance must provide to each eligible enrollee with respect to the alliance a choice of health plans among the plans which have contracts with the alliance under section 1381.

(b) OFFERING OF PLANS BY ALLIANCES.—A corporate alliance shall include among its health plan offerings for any eligible enrollee at least 3 health plans to enrollees, of which the alliance must offer—

(1) at least one fee-for-service plan (as defined in section 1322(b)(3)); and

(2) at least two health plans that are not fee-for-service plans.

SEC. 1383. ENROLLMENT; ISSUANCE OF HEALTH SECURITY CARD.

(a) IN GENERAL.—

(1) ENROLLMENT OF ALLIANCE ELIGIBLE INDIVIDUALS.—Each corporate alliance shall assure that each alliance eligible individual with respect to the alliance is enrolled in a corporate alliance health plan offered by the alliance, and shall establish and maintain methods and procedures consistent with this section sufficient to assure such enrollment. Such methods and procedures shall assure the enrollment of such individuals at the time they first become alliance eligible individuals with respect to the alliance.

(2) ISSUANCE OF HEALTH SECURITY CARDS.—A corporate alliance is responsible for the issuance of health security cards to corporate alliance eligible individuals under section 1001(b).

(b) RESPONSE TO POINT-OF-SERVICE NOTICES.—If a corporate alliance is notified under section 1323(b)(2) regarding an individual who has received services and appears to be an alliance eligible individual—

(1) the alliance shall promptly ascertain the individual's eligibility as an alliance eligible individual; and

(2) if the alliance determines that the individual is an alliance eligible individual—

(A) the alliance shall promptly provide for the enrollment of the individual in a health plan offered by the alliance (and notify the Secretary of Labor of such enrollment), and

(B) the alliance shall forward the claim for payment for the services to the health plan in which the individual is so enrolled and the plan shall make payment to the provider for such claim (in a manner consistent with requirements of the Secretary of Labor).

(c) ANNUAL OPEN ENROLLMENT; ENROLLMENT OF FAMILY MEMBERS; OVERSUBSCRIPTION OF PLANS.—The provisions of subsections (d) through (f) of section 1323 shall apply to a corporate alliance in the same manner as such provisions apply to a regional alliance.

(d) TERMINATION.—

(1) IN GENERAL.—The provisions of section 1323(g)(1) shall apply to a corporate alliance in the same manner as such provisions apply to a regional alliance.

(2) FAILURE TO PAY PREMIUMS.—If a corporate alliance fails to make premium payments to a health plan, the plan, after reasonable written notice to the alliance and the Secretary of Labor, may terminate coverage (and any contract with the alliance under this subpart). If such coverage is terminated the corporate alliance is responsible for the prompt enrollment of alliance eligible individuals whose coverage is terminated in another corporate alliance health plan.

(e) CORPORATE ALLIANCE TRANSITION.—Each corporate alliance must provide coverage—

(1) as of the first day of any month in which an individual first becomes a corporate alliance eligible individual, and

(2) through the end of the month in the case of a corporate alliance eligible individual who loses such eligibility during the month.

SEC. 1384. COMMUNITY-RATED PREMIUMS WITHIN PREMIUM AREAS.

(a) APPLICATION OF COMMUNITY-RATED PREMIUMS.—The premiums charged by a corporate alliance for enrollment in a corporate alliance health plan (not taking into account any employer premium payment required under section 6131) shall vary only by class of family enrollment (specified in section 1011(c)) and by premium area.

(b) DESIGNATION OF PREMIUM AREAS.—

(1) DESIGNATION.—Each corporate alliance shall designate premium areas to be used for the imposition of premiums (and calculation of employer premium payments) under this Act.

(2) CONDITIONS.—The boundaries of such areas shall reasonably reflect labor market areas or health care delivery areas and shall be consistent with rules the Secretary of Labor establishes (consistent with paragraph (3)) so that within such areas there are not substantial differences in average per capita health care expenditures.

(3) ANTI-REDLINING.—The provisions of paragraphs (4) and (5) of section 1202(b) (relating to redlining and metropolitan statistical areas) shall apply to the establishment of premium areas in the same manner as they apply to the establishment of the boundaries of regional alliance areas.

(c) APPLICATIONS OF CLASSES OF ENROLLMENT.—

(1) IN GENERAL.—The premiums shall be applied under this section based on class of family enrollment and shall vary based on such class in ac-

cordance with factors specified by the corporate alliance.

    (2) BASIS FOR FACTORS.—Such factors shall be the same in each premium and shall take into account such appropriate considerations (including the considerations the Board takes into account in the establishment of premium class factors under section 1531 and the costs of regional alliance health plans providing the comprehensive benefit package for families enrolled in the different classes) as the alliance considers appropriate, consistent with rules the Secretary of Labor establishes.

  (d) SPECIAL TREATMENT OF MULTIEMPLOYER ALLIANCES.—The Secretary of Labor shall provide for such exceptions to the requirements of this section in the case of a corporate alliance with a sponsor described in section 1311(b)(1)(B) as may be appropriate to reflect the unique and historical relationship between the employers and employees under such alliances.

## SEC. 1385. ASSISTANCE FOR LOW-WAGE FAMILIES.

  Each corporate alliance shall make an additional contribution towards the enrollment in health plans of the alliance by certain low-wage families in accordance with section 6131(b)(2).

## SEC. 1386. CONSUMER INFORMATION AND MARKETING; DATA COLLECTION AND QUALITY; ADDITIONAL DUTIES.

The provisions of sections 1325(a), 1327(a), 1328(a), and 1328(b) shall apply to a corporate alliance in the same manner as such provisions apply to a regional alliance.

## SEC. 1387. PLAN AND INFORMATION REQUIREMENTS.

(a) IN GENERAL.—A corporate alliance shall provide a written submission to the Secretary of Labor (in such form as the Secretary may require) detailing how the corporate alliance will carry out its activities under this part.

(b) ANNUAL INFORMATION.—A corporate alliance shall provide to the Secretary of Labor each year, in such form and manner as the Secretary may require, such information as the Secretary may require in order to monitor the compliance of the alliance with the requirements of this part.

(c) ANNUAL NOTICE OF EMPLOYEES OR PARTICIPANTS.—

(1) CORPORATE ALLIANCE.—Each corporate alliance shall submit to the Secretary of Labor, by not later than March 1 of each year, information on the number of full-time employees or participants obtaining coverage through the alliance as of January 1 of that year.

(2) EMPLOYERS THAT BECOME LARGE EMPLOYERS.—Each employer that is not a corporate alliance but employs 5,000 full-time employees as of January 1 of a year, shall submit to the Secretary of Labor, by not later than March 1 of the year, information on the number of such employees.

### SEC. 1388. MANAGEMENT OF FUNDS; RELATIONS WITH EMPLOYEES.

(a) MANAGEMENT OF FUNDS.—The management of funds by a corporate alliance shall be subject to the applicable fiduciary requirements of part 4 of subtitle B of title I of the Employee Retirement Income Security Act of 1974, together with the applicable enforcement provisions of part 5 of subtitle B of title I of such Act.

(b) MANAGEMENT OF FINANCES AND RECORDS; ACCOUNTING SYSTEM.—Each corporate alliance shall comply with standards relating to the management of finances and records and accounting systems as the Secretary of Labor shall specify.

### SEC. 1389. COST CONTROL.

Each corporate alliance shall control covered expenditures in a manner that meets the requirements of part 2 of subtitle A of title VI.

### SEC. 1390. PAYMENTS BY CORPORATE ALLIANCE EMPLOYERS TO CORPORATE ALLIANCES.

(a) LARGE EMPLOYER ALLIANCES.—In the case of a corporate alliance with a sponsor described in section 1311(b)(1)(A), the sponsor shall provide for the funding of benefits, through insurance or otherwise, consistent with section 6131, the applicable solvency requirements of sections 1395 and 1396, and any rules established by the Secretary of Labor.

(b) OTHER ALLIANCES.—In the case of a corporate alliance with a sponsor described in subparagraph (B) or (C) of section 1311(b)(1), a corporate alliance employer shall make payment of the employer premiums required under section 6131 under rules established by the corporate alliance, which rules shall be consistent with rules established by the Secretary of Labor.

### SEC. 1391. COORDINATION OF PAYMENTS.

(a) PAYMENTS OF CERTAIN AMOUNTS TO REGIONAL ALLIANCES.—In the case of a married couple in which one spouse is a qualifying employee of a regional alliance employer and the other spouse is a qualifying employee of a corporate alliance employer, if the couple is enrolled with a regional alliance health plan the corporate alliance (which receives employer premium payments from such corporate alliance employer with respect to such employee) shall pay to the regional alliance the amounts so paid.

(b) PAYMENTS OF CERTAIN AMOUNTS TO CORPORATE ALLIANCES.—In the case of a married couple in which one spouse is a qualifying employee of a corporate alliance employer and the other spouse is a qualifying employee of another corporate alliance employer, the corporate alliance of the corporate alliance health plan in which the couple is not enrolled shall pay to the corporate alliance of the plan in which the couple is enrolled any employer premium payments received from such corporate alliance employer with respect to such employee.

### SEC. 1392. APPLICABILITY OF ERISA ENFORCEMENT MECHANISMS FOR ENFORCEMENT OF CERTAIN REQUIREMENTS.

The provisions of sections 502 (relating to civil enforcement) and 504 (relating to investigative authority) of the Employee Retirement Income Security Act of 1974 shall apply to enforcement by the Secretary of Labor of this part in the same manner and to same extent as such provisions apply to enforcement of title I of such Act.

### SEC. 1393. APPLICABILITY OF CERTAIN ERISA PROTECTIONS TO ENROLLED INDIVIDUALS.

The provisions of sections 510 (relating to interference with rights protected under Act) and 511 (relating to coercive interference) of the Employee Retirement Income Security Act of 1974 shall apply, in relation to the provisions of this Act, with respect to individuals enrolled under corporate alliance health plans in the same manner and to the same extent as such provisions apply, in relation to the provisions of the Employee Retirement Income Security Act of 1974, with respect to participants and beneficiaries under employee welfare benefit plans covered by title I of such Act.

## SEC. 1394. DISCLOSURE AND RESERVE REQUIREMENTS.

(a) IN GENERAL.—The Secretary of Labor shall ensure that each corporate alliance health plan which is a self-insured plan maintains plan assets in trust as provided in section 403 of the Employee Retirement Income Security Act of 1974—

(1) without any exemption under section 403(b)(4) of such Act, and

(2) in amounts which the Secretary determines are sufficient to provide at any time for payment to health care providers of all outstanding balances owed by the plan at such time.

The requirements of the preceding sentence may be met through letters of credit, bonds, or other appropriate security to the extent provided in regulations of the Secretary.

(b) DISCLOSURE.—Each self-insured corporate alliance health plan shall notify the Secretary at such time as the financial reserve requirements of this section are not being met. The Secretary may assess a civil money penalty of not more than $100,000 against any corporate alliance for any failure to provide such notification in such form and manner and within such time periods as the Secretary may prescribe by regulation.

## SEC. 1395. TRUSTEESHIP BY THE SECRETARY OF INSOLVENT CORPORATE ALLIANCE HEALTH PLANS.

(d) APPOINTMENT OF SECRETARY AS TRUSTEE FOR INSOLVENT PLANS.—Whenever the Secretary of Labor determines that a corporate alliance health plan which is a self-insured plan will be unable to provide benefits when due or is otherwise in a financially hazardous condition as defined in regulations of the Secretary, the Secretary shall, upon notice to the plan, apply to the appropriate United States district court for appointment of the Secretary as trustee to administer the plan for the duration of the insolvency. The plan may appear as a party and other interested persons may intervene in the proceedings at the discretion of the court. The court shall appoint the Secretary trustee if the court determines that the trusteeship is necessary to protect the interests of the covered individuals or health care providers or to avoid any unreasonable deterioration of the financial condition of the plan or any unreasonable increase in the liability of the Corporate Alliance Insolvency Fund. The trusteeship of the

Secretary shall continue until the conditions described in the first sentence of this subsection are remedied or the plan is terminated.

(b) POWERS AS TRUSTEE.—The Secretary of Labor, upon appointment as trustee under subsection (a), shall have the power—

    (1) to do any act authorized by the plan, this Act, or other applicable provisions of law to be done by the plan administrator or any trustee of the plan,

    (2) to require the transfer of all (or any part) of the assets and records of the plan to the Secretary as trustee,

    (3) to invest any assets of the plan which the Secretary holds in accordance with the provisions of the plan, regulations of the Secretary, and applicable provisions of law,

    (4) to do such other acts as the Secretary deems necessary to continue operation of the plan without increasing the potential liability of the Corporate Alliance Insolvency Fund, if such acts may be done under the provisions of the plan,

    (5) to require the corporate alliance, the plan administrator, any contributing employer, and any employee organization representing covered individuals to furnish any information with respect to the

plan which the Secretary as trustee may reasonably need in order to administer the plan,

(6) to collect for the plan any amounts due the plan and to recover reasonable expenses of the trusteeship,

(7) to commence, prosecute, or defend on behalf of the plan any suit or proceeding involving the plan,

(8) to issue, publish, or file such notices, statements, and reports as may be required under regulations of the Secretary or by any order of the court,

(9) to terminate the plan and liquidate the plan assets in accordance with applicable provisions of this Act and other provisions of law, to restore the plan to the responsibility of the corporate alliance, or to continue the trusteeship,

(10) to provide for the enrollment of individuals covered under the plan in an appropriate regional alliance health plan, and

(11) to do such other acts as may be necessary to comply with this Act or any order of the court and to protect the interests of enrolled individuals and health care providers.

(b) NOTICE OF APPOINTMENT.—As soon as practicable after the Secretary's appointment as trustee, the Secretary shall give notice of such appointment to—

(1) the plan administrator,

(2) each enrolled individual,

(3) each employer who may be liable for contributions to the plan, and

(4) each employee organization which, for purposes of collective bargaining, represents enrolled individuals.

(d) ADDITIONAL DUTIES.—Except to the extent inconsistent with the provisions of this Act or part 4 of subtitle B of title I of the Employee Retirement Income Security Act of 1974, or as may be otherwise ordered by the court, the Secretary of Labor, upon appointment as trustee under this subsection, shall be subject to the same duties as those of a trustee under section 704 of title 11, United States Code, and shall have the duties of a fiduciary for purposes of such part 4.

(e) OTHER PROCEEDINGS.—An application by the Secretary of Labor under this subsection may be filed notwithstanding the pendency in the same or any other court of any bankruptcy, mortgage foreclosure, or equity receivership proceeding, or any proceeding to reorganize, conserve, or liquidate such plan or its property, or any proceeding to enforce a lien against property of the plan.

(f) JURISDICTION OF COURT.—

(1) IN GENERAL.—Upon the filing of an application for the appointment as trustee or the issuance of a decree under this subsection, the court to which the application is made shall have exclusive jurisdiction of the plan involved and its property wherever located with the powers, to the extent consistent with the purposes of this subsection, of a court of the United States having jurisdiction over cases under chapter 11 of title 11, United States Code. Pending an adjudication under paragraph (1) such court shall stay, and upon appointment by it of the Secretary of Labor as trustee, such court shall continue the stay of, any pending mortgage foreclosure, equity receivership, or other proceeding to reorganize, conserve, or liquidate the plan, the sponsoring alliance, or property of such plan or alliance, and any other suit against any receiver, conservator, or trustee of the plan, the sponsoring alliance, or property of the plan or alliance. Pending such adjudication and upon the appointment by it of the Secretary as trustee, the court may stay any proceeding to enforce a lien against property of the plan or the sponsoring alliance or any other suit against the plan or the alliance.

(2) VENUE.—An action under this subsection may be brought in the judicial district where the plan administrator resides or does business or where any asset of the plan is situated. A district court in which such action is brought may issue process with respect to such action in any other judicial district.

(g) PERSONNEL.—In accordance with regulations of the Secretary of Labor, the Secretary shall appoint, retain, and compensate accountants, actuaries, and other professional service personnel as may be necessary in connection with the Secretary's service as trustee under this subsection.

**SEC. 1396. GUARANTEED BENEFITS UNDER TRUSTEESHIP OF THE SECRETARY.**

(a) IN GENERAL.—Subject to subsection (b), the Secretary shall guarantee the payment of all benefits under a corporate alliance health plan which is a self-insured plan while such plan is under the Secretary's trusteeship under section 1396.

(b) LIMITATIONS.—Any increase in the amount of benefits under the plan resulting from a plan amendment which was made, or became effective, whichever is later, within 180 days (or such other reasonable time as may be prescribed in regulations of the Secretary of Labor) before the date of the Secretary's appointment as trustee of the plan shall be disregarded for purposes of determining the guarantee under this section.

(c) CORPORATE ALLIANCE HEALTH PLAN INSOLVENCY FUND.—

(1) ESTABLISHMENT.—The Secretary of Labor shall establish a Corporate Alliance Health Plan Insolvency Fund (hereinafter in this section referred to as the "Fund") from which the Secretary shall make payment of all guaranteed benefits under this section.

(2) RECEIPTS AND DISBURSEMENTS.—

(A) RECEIPTS.—The Fund shall be credited with—

(i) funds borrowed under paragraph (4),

(ii) assessments collected under section 1397, and

(iii) earnings on investment of the fund.

(B) DISBURSEMENTS.—The Fund shall be available—

(i) for making such payments as the Secretary determines are necessary to pay benefits guaranteed under this section,

(ii) to repay the Secretary of the Treasury such sums as may be borrowed (together with interest thereon) under paragraph (4), and

(iii) to pay the operational and administrative expenses of the Fund.

(3) BORROWING AUTHORITY.—At the direction of the Secretary of Labor, the Fund may, to the extent necessary to carry out the purposes of paragraph (1), issue to the Secretary of the Treasury notes or other obligations, in such forms and denominations, bearing such maturities, and subject to such terms and conditions as may be prescribed by the Secretary of the Treasury. Such notes or other obligations shall bear interest at a rate determined by the Secretary of the Treasury, taking into consideration the current average market yield on outstanding marketable obligations of the United States of comparable maturities during the month preceding the issuance of such notes or other obligations by the Fund. The Secretary of the Treasury shall purchase any notes or other obligations issued by the Fund under this paragraph, and for that purpose the Secretary of the Treasury may use as a public debt transaction the proceeds from the sale of

any securities issued under chapter 31 of title 31, United States Code and the purposes for which securities may be issued under such chapter are extended to include any purchase of such notes and obligations. The Secretary of the Treasury may at any time sell any of the notes or other obligations acquired by such Secretary under this paragraph. All redemptions, purchases, and sales by the Secretary of the Treasury of such notes or other obligations shall be treated as public debt transactions of the United States.

(4) INVESTMENT AUTHORITY.—Whenever the Secretary of Labor determines that the moneys of the Fund are in excess of current needs, the Secretary may request the investment of such amounts as the Secretary determines advisable by the Secretary of the Treasury in obligations issued or guaranteed by the United States, but, until all borrowings under paragraph (4) have been repaid, the obligations in which such excess moneys are invested may not yield a rate of return in excess of the rate of interest payable on such borrowings.

## SEC. 1397. IMPOSITION AND COLLECTION OF PERIODIC ASSESSMENTS ON SELF-INSURED CORPORATE ALLIANCE PLANS.

(a) IMPOSITION OF ASSESSMENTS.—Upon a determination that additional receipts to the Fund are necessary in order to enable the Fund to repay amounts borrowed by the Fund under section 1396(c)(3) while maintaining a balance sufficient to ensure the solvency of the Fund, the Secretary may impose assessments under this section. The Secretary shall prescribe from time to time such schedules of assessment rates and bases for the application of such rates as may be necessary to provide for such repayments.

(b) UNIFORMITY OF ASSESSMENTS.—The assessment rates prescribed by the Secretary for any period shall be uniform for all plans, except that the Secretary may vary the amount of such assessments by category, or waive the application of such assessments by category, taking into account differences in the financial solvency of, and financial reserves maintained by, plans in each category.

(c) LIMITATION ON AMOUNT OF ASSESSMENT.—The total amount assessed against a corporate alliance health plan under this section during a year may not exceed 2 percent of the total premiums paid to the plan with respect to corporate alliance eligible individuals enrolled with the plan during the year.

(d) PAYMENT OF ASSESSMENTS.—

(1) OBLIGATION TO PAY.—The designated payor of each plan shall pay the assessments imposed by the Secretary of Labor under this section with respect to that plan when they are due. Assessments under this section are payable at the time, and on an estimated, advance, or other basis, as determined by the Secretary. Assessments shall continue to accrue until the plan's assets are distributed pursuant to a termination procedure or the Secretary is appointed to serve as trustee of the plan under section 1395.

(2) LATE PAYMENT CHARGES AND INTEREST.—

(A) LATE PAYMENT CHARGES.—If any assessment is not paid when it is due, the Secretary may assess a late payment charge of not more than 100 percent of the assessment payment which was not timely paid.

(B) WAIVERS.—Subparagraph (A) shall not apply to any assessment payment made within 60 days after the date on which payment is due, if before such date, the designated payor obtains a waiver from the Secretary of Labor based upon a showing of substantial hardship arising from the timely payment of the assessment. The Secretary may grant a waiver under this subparagraph upon application made by the designated payor, but the Secretary may not grant a waiver if it appears that the designated payor will be unable to pay the assessment within 60 days after the date on which it is due.

(C) INTEREST.—If any assessment is not paid by the last date prescribed for a payment, interest on the amount of such assessment at the rate imposed under section 6601(a) of the Internal Revenue Code of 1986 shall be paid for the period from such last date to the date paid.

(e) CIVIL ACTION UPON NONPAYMENT.—If any designated payor fails to pay an assessment when due, the Secretary of Labor may bring a civil action in any district court of the United States within the jurisdiction of which the plan assets are located, the plan is administered, or in which a defendant resides or is found, for the recovery of the amount of the unpaid assessment, any late payment charge, and interest, and process may be served in any other district. The district courts of the United States shall have jurisdiction over actions brought under this subsection by the Secretary without regard to the amount in controversy.

(f) GUARANTEE HELD HARMLESS.—The Secretary of Labor shall not cease to guarantee benefits on account of the failure of a designated payor to pay any assessment when due.

(g) DESIGNATED PAYOR DEFINED.—

(1) IN GENERAL.—For purposes of this section, the term "designated payor" means—

(A) the employer or plan administrator in any case in which the eligible sponsor of the corporate alliance health plan is described in subparagraph (A) or (D) of section 1311(b)(1); and

(B) the contributing employers or the plan administrator in any case in which the eligible sponsor of the corporate alliance health plan is described in subparagraph (B) or (C) of section 1311(b)(1).

(2) CONTROLLED GROUPS.—If an employer is a member of a controlled group, each member of such group shall be jointly and severally liable for any assessments required to be paid by such employer. For purposes of the preceding sentence, the term "controlled group" means any group treated as a single

employer under subsection (b), (c), (m), or (o) of section 414 of the Internal Revenue Code of 1986.

## Subtitle E—Health Plans

**SEC. 1400. HEALTH PLAN DEFINED.**

(a) IN GENERAL.—In this Act, the term "health plan" means a plan that provides the comprehensive benefit package and meets the requirements of parts 1, 3, and 4.

(b) APPROPRIATE SELF-INSURED HEALTH PLAN.—In this Act, the term "appropriate self-insured health plan" means a group health plan (as defined in section 3(42) of the Employee Retirement Income Security Act of 1974) with respect to which the applicable requirements of title I of the Employee Retirement Income Security Act of 1974 are met and which is a self-insured plan.

(c) STATE-CERTIFIED HEALTH PLAN.—In this Act, the term "State-certified health plan" means a health plan that has been certified by a State under section 1203(a) (or, in the case in which the Board is exercising certification authority under section 1522(e), that has been certified by the Board).

(d) APPLICABLE REGULATORY AUTHORITY DEFINED.—In this subtitle, the term "applicable regulatory authority" means—

(1) with respect to a self-insured health plan, the Secretary of Labor, or

(2) with respect to a State-certified health plan, the State authority responsible for certification of the plan.

## PART 1—REQUIREMENTS RELATING TO COMPREHENSIVE BENEFIT PACKAGE

**SEC. 1401. APPLICATION OF REQUIREMENTS.**

No plan shall be treated under this Act as a health plan—

(1) unless the plan is a self-insured plan or a State-certified plan; or

(2) on and after the effective date of a finding by the applicable regulatory authority that the plan has failed to comply with such applicable requirements.

**SEC. 1402. REQUIREMENTS RELATING TO ENROLLMENT AND COVERAGE.**

(a) NO UNDERWRITING.—

(1) IN GENERAL.—Subject to paragraph (2), each health plan offered by a regional alliance or a corporate alliance must accept for enrollment every alliance eligible individual who seeks such enrollment. No plan may engage in any practice that has the effect of attracting or limiting enrollees on the

basis of personal characteristics, such as health status, anticipated need for health care, age, occupation, or affiliation with any person or entity.

(2) CAPACITY LIMITATIONS.—With the approval of the applicable regulatory authority, a health plan may limit enrollment because of the plan's capacity to deliver services or to maintain financial stability. If such a limitation is imposed, the limitation may not be imposed on a basis referred to in paragraph (1).

(b) NO LIMITS ON COVERAGE; NO PRE-EXISTING CONDITION LIMITS.—A health plan may not—

(1) terminate, restrict, or limit coverage for the comprehensive benefit package in any portion of the plan's service area for any reason, including nonpayment of premiums;

(2) cancel coverage for any alliance eligible individual until that individual is enrolled in another applicable health plan;

(3) exclude coverage of an alliance eligible individual because of existing medical conditions;

(4) impose waiting periods before coverage begins; or

(5) impose a rider that serves to exclude coverage of particular eligible individuals.

(c) ANTI-DISCRIMINATION.—

    (1) IN GENERAL.—No health plan may engage (directly or through contractual arrangements) in any activity, including the selection of a service area, that has the effect of discriminating against an individual on the basis of race, national origin, gender, income, health status, or anticipated need for health services.

    (2) SELECTION OF PROVIDERS FOR PLAN NETWORK.—In selecting among providers of health services for membership in a provider network, or in establishing the terms and conditions of such membership, a health plan may not engage in any practice that has the effect of discriminating against a provider—

        (A) based on the race, national origin, or gender of the provider; or

        (B) based on the income, health status, or anticipated need for health services of a patient of the provider.

    (3) NORMAL OPERATION OF HEALTH PLAN.—Except in the case of intentional discrimination, it shall not be a violation of this subsection, or of any regulation issued under this subsection, for any person to take any action otherwise prohibited under

this subsection, if the action is necessary to the normal operation of the health plan.

(4) REGULATIONS.—Not later than 1 year after the date of the enactment of this Act, the Secretary of Health and Human Services shall issue regulations in an accessible form to carry out this subsection.

(d) REQUIREMENTS FOR PLANS OFFERING LOWER COST SHARING.—Each health plan that offers enrollees the lower cost sharing schedule referred to in section 1131—

(1) shall apply such schedule to all items and services in the comprehensive benefit package;

(2) shall offer enrollees the opportunity to obtain coverage for out-of-network items and services (as described in subsection (f)(2)); and

(3) notwithstanding section 1403, in the case of an enrollee who obtains coverage for such items and services, may charge an alternative premium to take into account such coverage.

(e) TREATMENT OF COST SHARING.—Each health plan, in providing benefits in the comprehensive benefit package—

(1) shall include in its payments to providers, such additional reimbursement as may be necessary

to reflect cost sharing reductions to which individuals are entitled under section 1371, and

(2) shall maintain such claims or encounter records as may be necessary to audit the amount of such additional reimbursements and the individuals for which such reimbursement is provided.

(f) IN-NETWORK AND OUT-OF-NETWORK ITEMS AND SERVICES DEFINED.—

(1) IN-NETWORK ITEMS AND SERVICES.—For purposes of this Act, the term "in-network", when used with respect to items or services described in this subtitle, means items or services provided to an individual enrolled under a health plan by a health care provider who is a member of a provider network of the plan (as defined in paragraph (3)).

(2) OUT-OF-NETWORK ITEMS AND SERVICES.—For purposes of this Act, the term "out-of network", when used with respect to items or services described in this subtitle, means items or services provided to an individual enrolled under a health plan by a health care provider who is not a member of a provider network of the plan (as defined in paragraph (3)).

(3) PROVIDER NETWORK DEFINED.—A "provider network" means, with respect to a health plan,

providers who have entered into an agreement with the plan under which such providers are obligated to provide items and services in the comprehensive benefit package to individuals enrolled in the plan, or have an agreement to provide services on a fee-for-service basis.

(g) RELATION TO DETENTION.—A health plan is not required to provide any reimbursement to any detention facility for services performed in that facility for detainees in the facility.

## SEC. 1403. COMMUNITY RATING.

(a) REGIONAL ALLIANCE HEALTH PLANS.—Each regional alliance health plan may not vary the premium imposed with respect to residents of an alliance area, except as may be required under section 6102(a) with respect to different types of individual and family coverage under the plan.

(b) CORPORATE ALLIANCE HEALTH PLANS.—Each corporate alliance health plan may not vary the premium imposed with respect to individuals enrolled in the plan, except as may be required under section 1364 with respect to different types of individual and family coverage under the plan.

## SEC. 1404. MARKETING OF HEALTH PLANS; INFORMATION.

(a) REGIONAL ALLIANCE MARKETING RESTRICTIONS.—

(1) IN GENERAL.—The contract entered into between a regional alliance and a regional alliance health plan shall prohibit the distribution by the health plan of marketing materials within the regional alliance that contain false or materially misleading information and shall provide for prior approval by the regional alliance of any marketing materials to be distributed by the plan.

(2) ENTIRE MARKET.—A health plan offered by a health alliance may not distribute marketing materials to an area smaller than the entire area served by the plan.

(3) PROHIBITION OF TIE-INS.—A regional alliance health plan, and any agency of such a plan, may not seek to influence an individual's choice of plans in conjunction with the sale of any other insurance.

(b) INFORMATION AVAILABLE.—

(1) IN GENERAL.—Each regional alliance health plan must provide to the regional alliance and make available to alliance eligible individuals and health care professionals complete and timely information concerning the following:

(A) Costs.

(B) The identity, locations, qualifications, and availability of participating providers.

(C) Procedures used to control utilization of services and expenditures.

(D) Procedures for assuring and improving the quality of care.

(E) Rights and responsibilities of enrollees.

(F) Information on the number of plan members who disenroll from the plan.

(2) PROHIBITION AGAINST CERTIFICATION OF PLANS PROVIDING INACCURATE INFORMATION.—No regional alliance health plan may be a State-certified health plan under this title if the State determines that the plan submitted materially inaccurate information under paragraph (1).

(c) ADVANCE DIRECTIVES.—Each self-insured health plan and each State-certified health plan shall meet the requirement of section 1866(f) of the Social Security Act (relating to maintaining written policies and procedures respecting advance directives) in the same manner as such requirement relates to organizations with contracts under section 1876 of such Act.

SEC. 1405. GRIEVANCE PROCEDURE.

(a) IN GENERAL.—Each health plan must establish a grievance procedure for enrollees to use in pursuing complaints. Such procedure shall be consistent with subtitle C of title V.

(b) ADDITIONAL REMEDIES.—If the grievance procedure fails to resolve an enrollee's complaint—

> (1) in the case of an enrollee of a regional alliance health plan, the enrollee has the option of seeking assistance from the office of the ombudsman for the regional alliance established under section 1326(a), and
>
> (2) the enrollee may pursue additional legal remedies, including those provided under subtitle C of title V.

SEC. 1406. HEALTH PLAN ARRANGEMENTS WITH PROVIDERS.

(a) REQUIREMENT.—Each health plan must enter into such agreements with health care providers or have such other arrangements as may be necessary to assure the provision of all services covered by the comprehensive benefit package to eligible individuals enrolled with the plan.

(b) EMERGENCY AND URGENT CARE SERVICES.—

> (1) IN GENERAL.—Each health plan must cover emergency and urgent care services provided to en-

rollees, without regard to whether or not the provider furnishing such services has a contractual (or other) arrangement with the plan to provide items or services to enrollees of the plan.

(2) PAYMENT AMOUNTS.—In the case of emergency and urgent care provided to an enrollee outside of a health plan's service area, the payment amounts of the plan shall be based on the fee for service rate schedule established by the regional alliance for the alliance area where the services were provided.

(c) APPLICATION OF FEE SCHEDULE.—

(1) IN GENERAL.—Subject to paragraph (2), each regional alliance health plan or corporate alliance health plan that provides for payment for services on a fee-for-service basis shall make such payment in the amounts provided under the fee schedule established by the regional alliance under section 1322(c) (or, in the case of a plan offered in a State that has established a Statewide fee schedule under section 1322(c)(3), under such Statewide fee schedule).

(2) REDUCTION FOR PROVIDERS VOLUNTARILY REDUCING CHARGES.—If a provider under a health plan voluntarily agrees to reduce the amount

charged to an individual enrolled under the plan, the plan shall reduce the amount otherwise determined under the fee schedule applicable under paragraph (1) by the proportion of the reduction in such amount charged.

(3) REDUCTION FOR NONCOMPLYING PLAN.—Each regional alliance health plan that is a noncomplying plan shall provide for reductions in payments under the fee schedule to providers that are not participating providers in accordance with section 6012(b).

(d) PROHIBITION AGAINST BALANCE BILLING; REQUIREMENT OF DIRECT BILLING.—

(1) PROHIBITION OF BALANCE BILLING.—A provider may not charge or collect from an enrollee a fee in excess of the applicable payment amount under the applicable fee schedule under subsection (c), and the health plan and its enrollees are not legally responsible for payment of any amount in excess of such applicable payment amount for items and services covered under the comprehensive benefits package.

(2) DIRECT BILLING.—A provider may not charge or collect from an enrollee amounts that are payable by the health plan (including any cost shar-

ing reduction assistance payable by the plan) and shall submit charges to such plan in accordance with any applicable requirements of part 1 of subtitle B of title V (relating to health information systems).

(3) COVERAGE UNDER AGREEMENTS WITH PLANS.—The agreements or other arrangements entered into under subsection (a) between a health plan and the health care providers providing the comprehensive benefit package to individuals enrolled with the plan shall prohibit a provider from engaging in balance billing described in paragraph (1).

(e) IMPOSITION OF PARTICIPATING PROVIDER ASSESSMENT IN CASE OF A NONCOMPLYING PLAN.—Each health plan shall provide that if the plan is a noncomplying plan for a year under section 6012, payments to participating providers shall be reduced by the applicable network reduction percentage under such section.

## SEC. 1407. PREEMPTION OF CERTAIN STATE LAWS RELATING TO HEALTH PLANS.

(a) LAWS RESTRICTING PLANS OTHER THAN FEE-FOR-SERVICE PLANS.—Except as may otherwise be provided in this section, no State law shall apply to any services provided under a health plan that is not a fee-for-service plan (or a fee-for-service component of a plan) if such law has the effect of prohibiting or otherwise restricting plans from—

(1) except as provided in section 1203, limiting the number and type of health care providers who participate in the plan;

(2) requiring enrollees to obtain health services (other than emergency services) from participating providers or from providers authorized by the plan;

(3) requiring enrollees to obtain a referral for treatment by a specialized physician or health institution;

(4) establishing different payment rates for participating providers and providers outside the plan;

(5) creating incentives to encourage the use of participating providers; or

(6) requiring the use single-source suppliers for pharmacy, medical equipment, and other health products and services.

(b) PREEMPTION OF STATE CORPORATE PRACTICE ACTS.—Any State law related to the corporate practice of medicine and to provider ownership of health plans or other providers shall not apply to arrangements between health plans that are not fee-for-service plans and their participating providers.

(c) PARTICIPATING PROVIDER DEFINED.—In this title, a "participating provider" means, with respect to a health plan, a provider of health care services who is a member of a provider network of the plan (as described in section 1402(f)(3)).

**SEC. 1408. FINANCIAL SOLVENCY.**

Each regional alliance health plan must—

    (1) meet or exceed minimum capital requirements established by States under section 1204(a);

    (2) in the case of a plan operating in a State, must participate in the guaranty fund established by the State under section 1204(c); and

    (3) meet such other requirements relating to fiscal soundness as the State may establish (subject to the establishment of any alternative standards by the Board).

**SEC. 1409. REQUIREMENT FOR OFFERING COST SHARING POLICY.**

Each regional alliance health plan shall offer a cost sharing policy (as defined in section 1421(b)(2)) to each eligible family enrolled under the plan.

**SEC. 1410. QUALITY ASSURANCE.**

Each health plan shall comply with such quality assurance requirements as are imposed under subtitle A of title V with respect to such a plan.

## SEC. 1411. PROVIDER VERIFICATION.

Each health plan shall—

(1) verify the credentials of practitioners and facilities;

(2) ensure that all providers participating in the plan meet applicable State licensing and certification standards;

(3) oversee the quality and performance of participating providers, consistent with section 1410; and

(4) investigate and resolve consumer complaints against participating providers.

## SEC. 1412. CONSUMER DISCLOSURES OF UTILIZATION MANAGEMENT PROTOCOLS.

Each health plan shall disclose to enrollees (and prospective enrollees) the protocols used by the plan for controlling utilization and costs.

## SEC. 1413. CONFIDENTIALITY, DATA MANAGEMENT, AND REPORTING.

(a) IN GENERAL.—Each health plan shall comply with the confidentiality, data management, and reporting requirements imposed under subtitle B of title V.

(b) TREATMENT OF ELECTRONIC INFORMATION.—

(1) ACCURACY AND RELIABILITY.—Each health plan shall take such measures as may be necessary to ensure that health care information in electronic

form that the plan, or a member of a provider network of the plan, collects for or transmits to the Board under subtitle B of title V is accurate and reliable.

(2) PRIVACY AND SECURITY.—Each health plan shall take such measures as may be necessary to ensure that health care information described in paragraph (1) is not distributed to any individual or entity in violation of a standard promulgated by the Board under part 2 of subtitle B of title V.

## SEC. 1414. PARTICIPATION IN REINSURANCE SYSTEM.

Each regional alliance health plan of a State that has established a reinsurance system under section 1203(g) shall participate in the system in the manner specified by the State.

## PART 2—REQUIREMENTS RELATING TO SUPPLEMENTAL INSURANCE

## SEC. 1421. IMPOSITION OF REQUIREMENTS ON SUPPLEMENTAL INSURANCE.

(a) IN GENERAL.—An entity may offer a supplemental insurance policy but only if—

(1) in the case of a supplemental health benefit policy (as defined in subsection (b)(1)), the entity and the policy meet the requirements of section 1422; and

(2) in the case of a cost sharing policy (as defined in subsection (b)(2)), the entity and the policy meet the requirements of section 1423.

(b) POLICIES DEFINED.—

(1) SUPPLEMENTAL HEALTH BENEFIT POLICY.—

(A) IN GENERAL.—In this part, the term "supplemental health benefit policy" means a health insurance policy or health benefit plan offered to an alliance-eligible individual which provides—

(i) coverage for services and items not included in the comprehensive benefit package, or

(ii) coverage for items and services included in such package but not covered because of a limitation in amount, duration, or scope provided under such title,

or both.

(B) EXCLUSIONS.—Such term does not include the following:

(i) A cost sharing policy (as defined in paragraph (2)).

(ii) A long-term care insurance policy (as defined in section 2304(10)).

(iii) Insurance that limits benefits with respect to specific diseases (or conditions).

(iv) Hospital or nursing home indemnity insurance.

(v) A medicare supplemental policy (as defined in section 1882(g) of the Social Security Act).

(vi) Insurance with respect to accidents.

(2) COST SHARING POLICY.—In this part, the term "cost sharing policy" means a health insurance policy or health benefit plan offered to an alliance-eligible individual which provides coverage for deductibles, coinsurance, and copayments imposed as part of the comprehensive benefit package under title II, whether imposed under a higher cost sharing plan or with respect to out-of-network providers.

## SEC. 1422. STANDARDS FOR SUPPLEMENTAL HEALTH BENEFIT POLICIES.

(a) PROHIBITING DUPLICATION OF COVERAGE.—

(1) IN GENERAL.—No health plan, insurer, or any other person may offer—

(A) to any eligible individual a supplemental health benefit policy that duplicates any coverage provided in the comprehensive benefit package; or

>(B) to any medicare-eligible individual a supplemental health benefit policy that duplicates any coverage provided under part B of the medicare program.

(2) EXCEPTION FOR MEDICARE-ELIGIBLE INDIVIDUALS.—For purposes of this subsection, for the period in which an individual is a medicare-eligible individual and also is an alliance-eligible individual (and is enrolled under a regional alliance or corporate alliance health plan), paragraph (1)(A) (and not paragraph (1)(B)) shall apply.

(b) NO LIMITATION ON INDIVIDUALS OFFERED POLICY.—

(1) IN GENERAL.—Except as provided in paragraph (2), each entity offering a supplemental health benefit policy must accept for enrollment every individual who seeks such enrollment, subject to capacity and financial limits.

(2) EXCEPTION FOR CERTAIN OFFERORS.—Paragraph (1) shall not apply to any supplemental health benefit policy offered to an individual only on the basis of—

(A) the individual's employment (in the case of a policy offered by the individual's employer); or

(B) the individual's membership or enrollment in a fraternal, religious, professional, educational, or other similar organization.

(c) RESTRICTIONS ON MARKETING ABUSES.—Not later than January 1, 1996, the Board shall develop (in consultation with the States) minimum standards that prohibit marketing practices by entities offering supplemental health benefit policies that involve:

(1) Providing monetary incentives for or tying or otherwise conditioning the sale of the policy to enrollment in a regional alliance health plan of the entity.

(2) Using or disclosing to any party information about the health status or claims experience of participants in a regional alliance health plan for the purpose of marketing such a policy.

(d) CIVIL MONETARY PENALTY.—An entity that knowingly and willfully violates any provision of this section with respect to the offering of a supplemental health benefit policy to any individual shall be subject to a civil monetary penalty (not to exceed $10,000) for each such violation.

## SEC. 1423. STANDARDS FOR COST SHARING POLICIES.

(a) RULES FOR OFFERING OF POLICIES.—Subject to subsection (f), a cost sharing policy may be offered to an individual only if—

(1) the policy is offered by the regional alliance health plan in which the individual is enrolled;

(2) the regional alliance health plan offers the policy to all individuals enrolled in the plan;

(3) the plan offers each such individual a choice of a policy that provides standard coverage and a policy that provides maximum coverage (in accordance with standards established by the Board); and

(4) the policy is offered only during the annual open enrollment period for regional alliance health plans (described in section 1323(d)(1)).

(b) PROHIBITION OF COVERAGE OF COPAYMENTS.—Each cost sharing policy may not provide any benefits relating to any copayments established under the schedule of copayments and coinsurance under section 1135.

(c) EQUIVALENT COVERAGE FOR ALL SERVICES.—Each cost sharing policy must provide coverage for items and services in the comprehensive benefit package to the same extent as the policy provides coverage for all items and services in the package.

(d) REQUIREMENTS FOR PRICING.—

(1) IN GENERAL.—The price of any cost sharing policy shall—

(A) be the same for each individual to whom the policy is offered;

(B) take into account any expected increase in utilization resulting from the purchase of the policy by individuals enrolled in the regional alliance health plan; and

(C) not result in a loss-ratio of less than 90 percent.

(2) LOSS-RATIO DEFINED.—In paragraph (1)(C), a "loss-ratio" is the ratio of the premium returned to the consumer in payout relative to the total premium collected.

(e) LOSS OF STATE CERTIFICATION FOR REGIONAL ALLIANCE HEALTH PLANS FAILING TO MEET STANDARDS.—A State may not certify a regional alliance health plan that offers a cost sharing policy unless the plan and the policy meet the standards described in this section.

(f) SPECIAL RULES FOR FEHBP SUPPLEMENTAL PLANS.—Subsection (a) shall not apply to an FEHBP supplemental plan described in section 8203(f)(1), but only if the plan meets the following requirements:

(1) The plan must be offered to all individuals to whom such a plan is required to be offered under section 8204.

(2) The plan must offers each such individual a choice of a policy that provides standard coverage and a policy that provides maximum coverage (in accordance with standards established by the Board under subsection (a)(3)).

(3) The plan is offered only during the annual open enrollment period for regional alliance health plans (described in section 1323(d)(1)).

(4)(A) The price of the plan shall include an amount, established in accordance with rules established by the Board in consultation with the Office of Personnel Management, that takes into account any expected increase in utilization of the items and services in the comprehensive benefit package resulting from the purchase of the plan by individuals enrolled in a regional alliance health plan.

(B) The plan provides for payment, in a manner specified by the Board in the case of an individual enrolled in the plan and in a regional alliance health plan, to the regional alliance health plan of an amount equivalent to the additional amount described in subparagraph (A).

# PART 3—REQUIREMENTS RELATING TO ESSENTIAL COMMUNITY PROVIDERS

### SEC. 1431. HEALTH PLAN REQUIREMENT.

(a) IN GENERAL.—Subject to section 1432, each health plan shall, with respect to each electing essential community provider (as defined in subsection (d), other than a provider of school health services) located within the plan's service area, either—

    (1) enter into a written provider participation agreement (described in subsection (b)) with the provider, or

    (2) enter into a written agreement under which the plan shall make payment to the provider in accordance with subsection (c).

(b) PARTICIPATION AGREEMENT.—A participation agreement between a health plan and an electing essential community provider under this subsection shall provide that the health plan agrees to treat the provider in accordance with terms and conditions at least as favorable as those that are applicable to other providers participating in the health plan with respect to each of the following:

    (1) The scope of services for which payment is made by the plan to the provider.

    (2) The rate of payment for covered care and services.

(3) The availability of financial incentives to participating providers.

(4) Limitations on financial risk provided to other participating providers.

(5) Assignment of enrollees to participating providers.

(6) Access by the provider's patients to providers in medical specialties or subspecialties participating in the plan.

(c) PAYMENTS FOR PROVIDERS WITHOUT PARTICIPATION AGREEMENTS.—

(1) IN GENERAL.—Payment in accordance with this subsection is payment based, as elected by the electing essential community provider, either—

(A) on the fee schedule developed by the applicable health alliance (or the State) under section 1322(c), or

(B) on payment methodologies and rates used under the applicable Medicare payment methodology and rates (or the most closely applicable methodology under such program as the Secretary of Health and Human Services specifies in regulations).

(2) NO APPLICATION OF GATE-KEEPER LIMITATIONS.—Payment in accordance with this subsection

may be subject to utilization review, but may not be subject to otherwise applicable gate-keeper requirements under the plan.

(d) ELECTION.—

(1) IN GENERAL.—In this part, the term "electing essential community provider" means, with respect to a health plan, an essential community provider that elects this subpart to apply to the health plan.

(2) FORM OF ELECTION.—An election under this subsection shall be made in a form and manner specified by the Secretary, and shall include notice to the health plan involved. Such an election may be made annually with respect to a health plan, except that the plan and provider may agree to make such an election on a more frequent basis.

(e) SPECIAL RULE FOR PROVIDERS OF SCHOOL HEALTH SERVICES.—A health plan shall pay, to each provider of school health services located in the plan's service area an amount determined by the Secretary for such services furnished to enrollees of the plan.

## SEC. 1432. SUNSET OF REQUIREMENT.

(a) IN GENERAL.—Subject to subsection (d), the requirement of section 1431 shall only apply to health plans offered by a health alliance during the 5-year period beginning with the first year in which any regional alliance health plan is offered by the alliance.

(b) STUDIES.—In order to prepare recommendations under subsection (c), the Secretary shall conduct studies regarding essential community providers, including studies that assess—

> (1) the definition of essential community provider,
>
> (2) the sufficiency of the funding levels for providers, for both covered and uncovered benefits under this Act,
>
> (3) the effects of contracting requirements relating to such providers on such providers, health plans, and enrollees,
>
> (4) the impact of the payment rules for such providers, and
>
> (5) the impact of national health reform on such providers.

(c) RECOMMENDATIONS TO CONGRESS.—The Secretary shall submit to Congress, by not later than March 1, 2001, specific recommendations respecting whether, and to what extent, section 1431 should continue to apply to some or all essential community providers. Such recommendations may include a description of the particular types of such providers and circumstances under which such section should continue to apply.

(d) CONGRESSIONAL CONSIDERATION.—

(1) IN GENERAL.—Recommendations submitted under subsection (c) shall apply under this part (and may supersede the provisions of subsection (a)) unless a joint resolution (described in paragraph (2)) disapproving such recommendations is enacted, in accordance with the provisions of paragraph (3), before the end of the 60-day period beginning on the date on which such recommendations were submitted. For purposes of applying the preceding sentence and paragraphs (2) and (3), the days on which either House of Congress is not in session because of an adjournment of more than three days to a day certain shall be excluded in the computation of a period.

(2) JOINT RESOLUTION OF DISAPPROVAL.—A joint resolution described in this paragraph means only a joint resolution which is introduced within the 10-day period beginning on the date on which the Secretary submits recommendations under subsection (c) and—

(A) which does not have a preamble;

(B) the matter after the resolving clause of which is as follows: "That Congress disapproves the recommendations of the Secretary of Health and Human Services concerning the continued application of certain essential community provider requirements under section 1431 of the Health Security Act, as submitted by the Secretary on _____.", the blank space being filled in with the appropriate date; and

(C) the title of which is as follows: "Joint resolution disapproving recommendations of the Secretary of Health and Human Services concerning the continued application of certain essential community provider requirements under section 1431 of the Health Security Act, as submitted by the Secretary on _____.", the blank space being filled in with the appropriate date.

(3) PROCEDURES FOR CONSIDERATION OF RESOLUTION OF APPROVAL.—Subject to paragraph (4), the provisions of section 2908 (other than subsection (a)) of the Defense Base Closure and Realignment Act of 1990 shall apply to the consideration of a joint resolution described in paragraph (2) in the

same manner as such provisions apply to a joint resolution described in section 2908(a) of such Act.

(4) SPECIAL RULES.—For purposes of applying paragraph (3) with respect to such provisions—

(A) any reference to the Committee on Armed Services of the House of Representatives shall be deemed a reference to an appropriate Committee of the House of Representatives (specified by the Speaker of the House of Representatives at the time of submission of recommendations under subsection (c)) and any reference to the Committee on Armed Services of the Senate shall be deemed a reference to an appropriate Committee of the House of Representatives (specified by the Majority Leader of the Senate at the time of submission of recommendations under subsection (c)); and

(B) any reference to the date on which the President transmits a report shall be deemed a reference to the date on which the Secretary submits recommendations under subsection (c).

## PART 4—REQUIREMENTS RELATING TO WORKERS' COMPENSATION AND AUTOMOBILE MEDICAL LIABILITY COVERAGE

**SEC. 1441. REFERENCE TO REQUIREMENTS RELATING TO WORKERS COMPENSATION SERVICES.**

Each health plan shall meet the applicable requirements of part 2 of subtitle A of title VIII (relating to provision of workers compensation services to enrollees).

**SEC. 1442. REFERENCE TO REQUIREMENTS RELATING TO AUTOMOBILE MEDICAL LIABILITY SERVICES.**

Each health plan shall meet the applicable requirements of part 2 of subtitle B of title VIII (relating to provision of automobile medical liability services to enrollees).

# Subtitle F—Federal Responsibilities

## PART 1—NATIONAL HEALTH BOARD

### Subpart A—Establishment of National Health Board

**SEC. 1501. CREATION OF NATIONAL HEALTH BOARD; MEMBERSHIP.**

(a) IN GENERAL.—There is hereby created in the Executive Branch a National Health Board.

(b) COMPOSITION.—The Board is composed of 7 members appointed by the President, by and with the advice and consent of the Senate.

(c) CHAIR.—The President shall designate one of the members as chair. The chair serves a term concurrent with that of the President. The chair may serve a maximum of 3 terms. The chair shall serve as the chief executive officer of the Board.

(d) TERMS.—

(1) IN GENERAL.—Except as provided in paragraphs (2) and (4), the term of each member of the Board, except the chair, is 4 years and begins when the term of the predecessor of that member ends.

(2) INITIAL TERMS.—The initial terms of the members of the Board (other than the chair) first taking office after the date of the enactment of this Act, shall expire as designated by the President, two at the end of one year, two at the end of two years, and two at the end of three years.

(3) REAPPOINTMENT.—A member (other than the chair) may be reappointed for one additional term.

(4) CONTINUATION IN OFFICE.—Upon the expiration of a term of office, a member shall continue to serve until a successor is appointed and qualified.

(e) VACANCIES.—

(1) IN GENERAL.—Whenever a vacancy shall occur, other than by expiration of term, a successor shall be appointed by the President as provided above, by and with the consent of the Senate, to fill

such vacancy, and is appointed for the remainder of the term of the predecessor.

(2) NO IMPAIRMENT OF FUNCTION.—A vacancy in the membership of the Board does not impair the right of the remaining members to exercise all of the powers of the Board.

(3) ACTING CHAIR.—The Board may designate a Member to Act as chair during any period in which there is no chair designated by the President.

(f) MEETINGS; QUORUM.—

(1) MEETINGS.—At meetings of the Board the chair shall preside, and in the absence of the chair, the Board shall elect a member to act as chair pro tempore.

(2) QUORUM.—Four members of the Board shall constitute a quorum thereof.

## SEC. 1502. QUALIFICATIONS OF BOARD MEMBERS.

(a) CITIZENSHIP.—Each member of the Board shall be a citizen of the United States.

(b) BASIS OF SELECTION.—Board members will be selected on the basis of their experience and expertise in relevant subjects, including the practice of medicine, health care financing and delivery, state health systems, consumer protection, business, law, and delivery of care to vulnerable populations.

(c) EXCLUSIVE EMPLOYMENT.—During the term of appointment, Board members shall serve as employees of the Federal Government and shall hold no other employment.

(d) PROHIBITION OF CONFLICT OF INTEREST.—A member of the Board may not have a pecuniary interest in or hold an official relation to any health care plan, health care provider, insurance company, pharmaceutical company, medical equipment company, or other affected industry. Before entering upon the duties as a member of the Board, the member shall certify under oath compliance with this requirement.

(e) POST-EMPLOYMENT RESTRICTIONS.—After leaving the Board, former members are subject to post-employment restrictions applicable to comparable Federal employees.

(f) COMPENSATION OF BOARD MEMBERS.—Each member of the Board (other than the chair) shall receive an annual salary at the annual rate payable from time to time for level IV of the Executive Schedule. The chair of the Board, during the period of service as chair, shall receive an annual salary at the annual rate payable from time to time for level III of the Executive Schedule.

**SEC. 1503. GENERAL DUTIES AND RESPONSIBILITIES.**

(a) COMPREHENSIVE BENEFIT PACKAGE.—

(1) INTERPRETATION.—The Board shall interpret the comprehensive benefit package, adjust the delivery of preventive services under section 1153, and take such steps as may be necessary to assure that the comprehensive benefit package is available on a uniform national basis to all eligible individuals.

(2) RECOMMENDATIONS.—The Board may recommend to the President and the Congress appropriate revisions to such package. Such recommendations may reflect changes in technology, health care needs, health care costs, and methods of service delivery.

(b) ADMINISTRATION OF COST CONTAINMENT PROVISIONS.—The Board shall oversee the cost containment requirements of subtitle A of title VI and certify compliance with such requirements.

(c) COVERAGE AND FAMILIES.—The Board shall develop and implement standards relating to the eligibility of individuals for coverage in applicable health plans under subtitle A of title I and may provide such additional exceptions and special rules relating to the treatment of family members under section 1012 as the Board finds appropriate.

(d) QUALITY MANAGEMENT AND IMPROVEMENT.—The Board shall establish and have ultimate responsibility for a performance-based system of quality management and improvement as required by section 5001.

(e) INFORMATION STANDARDS.—The Board shall develop and implement standards to establish national health information system to measure quality as required by section 5101.

(f) PARTICIPATING STATE REQUIREMENTS.—Consistent with the provisions of subtitle C, the Board shall—

   (1) establish requirements for participating States,

   (2) monitor State compliance with those requirements,

   (3) provide technical assistance,

in a manner that ensures access to the comprehensive benefit package for all eligible individuals.

(g) DEVELOPMENT OF PREMIUM CLASS FACTORS.—The Board shall establish premium class factors under subpart D of this part.

(h) DEVELOPMENT OF RISK-ADJUSTMENT METHODOLOGY.—The Board shall develop a methodology for the risk-adjustment of premium payments to regional alliance health plans in accordance with part 3 of this subtitle.

(i) ENCOURAGING THE REASONABLE PRICING OF BREAKTHROUGH DRUGS.—The Board shall establish the

Breakthrough Drug Committee in accordance with subpart F of this part.

(j) FINANCIAL REQUIREMENTS.—The Board shall establish minimum capital requirements and requirements for guaranty funds under subpart G of this part.

(k) STANDARDS FOR HEALTH PLAN GRIEVANCE PROCEDURES.—The Board shall establish standards for health plan grievance procedures that are used by enrollees in pursuing complaints.

**SEC. 1504. ANNUAL REPORT.**

(a) IN GENERAL.—The Board shall prepare and send to the President and Congress an annual report addressing the overall implementation of the new health care system.

(b) MATTERS TO BE INCLUDED.—The Board shall include in each annual report under this section the following:

　　(1) Information on Federal and State implementation.

　　(2) Data related to quality improvement.

　　(3) Recommendations or changes in the administration, regulation and laws related to health care and coverage.

　　(4) A full account of all actions taken during the previous year.

**SEC. 1505. POWERS.**

(a) STAFF; CONTRACT AUTHORITY.—The Board shall have authority, subject to the provisions of the civil-service laws and chapter 51 and subchapter III of chapter 53 of title 5, United States Code, to appoint such officers and employees as are necessary to carry out its functions. To the extent provided in advance in appropriations Acts, the Board may contract with any person (including an agency of the Federal Government) for studies and analysis as required to execute its functions. Any employee of the Executive Branch may be detailed to the Board to assist the Board in carrying out its duties.

(b) ESTABLISHMENT OF ADVISORY COMMITTEES.—The Board may establish advisory committees.

(c) ACCESS TO INFORMATION.—The Board may secure directly from any department or agency of the United States information necessary to enable it to carry out its functions, to the extent such information is otherwise available to a department or agency of the United States. Upon request of the chair, the head of that department or agency shall furnish that information to the Board.

(d) DELEGATION OF AUTHORITY.—Except as otherwise provided in this Act, the Board may delegate any function to such officers and employees as the Board may designate and may authorize such successive redelegations of such functions with the Board as the Board deems to be necessary or appropriate. No delegation of functions by the Board shall relieve the Board of responsibility for the administration of such functions.

(e) RULEMAKING.—The National Health Board is authorized to establish such rules as may be necessary to carry out this Act.

SEC. 1506. FUNDING.

(a) AUTHORIZATION OF APPROPRIATIONS.—There are authorized to be appropriated to the Board such sums as may be necessary for fiscal years 1994, 1995, 1996, 1997, and 1998.

(b) SUBMISSION OF BUDGET.—Under the procedures of chapter 11 of title 31, United States Code, the budget for the Board for a fiscal year shall be reviewed by the Director of the Office of Management and Budget and submitted to the Congress as part of the President's submission of the Budget of the United States for the fiscal year.

## Subpart B—Responsibilities Relating to Review and Approval of State Systems

SEC. 1511. FEDERAL REVIEW AND ACTION ON STATE SYSTEMS.

(a) APPROVAL OF STATE SYSTEMS BY NATIONAL BOARD.—

(1) IN GENERAL.—The National Health Board shall approve a State health care system for which a document is submitted under section 1200(a) unless the Board finds that the system (as set forth in the document) does not (or will not) provide for the State meeting the responsibilities for participating States under this Act.

(2) REGULATIONS.—The Board shall issue regulations, not later than July 1, 1995, prescribing the requirements for State health care systems under parts 2 and 3 of subtitle C, except that in the case of a document submitted under section 1201(a) before the date of issuance of such regulations, the Board shall take action on such document notwithstanding the fact that such regulations have not been issued.

(3) NO APPROVAL PERMITTED FOR YEARS PRIOR TO 1996.—The Board may not approve a State health care system under this part for any year prior to 1996.

(b) REVIEW OF COMPLETENESS OF DOCUMENTS.—

(1) IN GENERAL.—If a State submits a document under subsection (a)(1), the Board shall notify the State, not later than 7 working days after the date of submission, whether or not the document is

complete and provides the Board with sufficient information to approve or disapprove the document.

(2) ADDITIONAL INFORMATION ON INCOMPLETE DOCUMENT.—If the Board notifies a State that the State's document is not complete, the State shall be provided such additional period (not to exceed 45 days) as the Board may by regulation establish in which to submit such additional information as the Board may require. Not later than 7 working days after the State submits the additional information, the Board shall notify the State respecting the completeness of the document.

(c) ACTION ON COMPLETED DOCUMENTS.—

(1) IN GENERAL.—The Board shall make a determination (and notify the State) on whether the State's document provides for implementation of a State system that meets the applicable requirements of subtitle C—

(A) in the case of a State that did not require the additional period described in subsection (b)(2) to file a complete document, not later than 90 days after notifying a State under subsection (b) that the State's document is complete, or

(B) in the case of a State that required the additional period described in subsection (b)(2) to file a complete document, not later than 90 days after notifying a State under subsection (b) that the State's document is complete.

(2) PLANS DEEMED APPROVED.—If the Board does not meet the applicable deadline for making a determination and providing notice established under paragraph (1) with respect to a State's document, the Board shall be deemed to have approved the State's document for purposes of this Act.

(d) OPPORTUNITY TO RESPOND TO REJECTED DOCUMENT.—

(1) IN GENERAL.—If (within the applicable deadline under subsection (c)(1)) the Board notifies a State that its document does not provide for implementation of a State system that meets the applicable requirements of subtitle C, the Board shall provide the State with a period of 30 days in which to submit such additional information and assurances as the Board may require.

(2) DEADLINE FOR RESPONSE.—Not later than 30 days after receiving such additional information and assurances, the Board shall make a determination (and notify the State) on whether the State's

document provides for implementation of a State system that meets the applicable requirements of subtitle C.

(3) PLAN DEEMED APPROVED.—If the Board does not meet the deadline established under paragraph (2) with respect to a State, the Board shall be deemed to have approved the State's document for purposes of this Act.

(e) APPROVAL OF PREVIOUSLY TERMINATED STATES.—If the Board has approved a State system under this part for a year but subsequently terminated the approval of the system under section 1513, the Board shall approve the system for a succeeding year if the State—

(1) demonstrates to the satisfaction of the Board that the failure that formed the basis for the termination no longer exists, and

(2) provides reasonable assurances that the types of actions (or inactions) which formed the basis for such termination will not recur.

(f) REVISIONS TO STATE SYSTEM.—

(1) SUBMISSION.—A State may revise a system approved for a year under this section, except that such revision shall not take effect unless the State has submitted to the Board a document describing

such revision and the Board has approved such revision.

(2) ACTIONS ON AMENDMENTS.—Not later than 60 days after a document is submitted under paragraph (1), the Board shall make a determination (and notify the State) on whether the implementation of the State system, as proposed to be revised, meets the applicable requirements of subtitle C. If the Board fails to meet the requirement of the preceding sentence, the Board shall be deemed to have approved the implementation of the State system as proposed to be revised.

(3) REJECTION OF AMENDMENTS.—Subsection (d) shall apply to an amendment submitted under this subsection in the same manner as it applies to a completed document submitted under subsection (b).

(g) NOTIFICATION OF NON-PARTICIPATING STATES.—If a State fails to submit a document for a State system by the deadline referred to in section 1200, or such a document is not approved under subsection (c), the Board shall immediately notify the Secretary of Health and Human Services and the Secretary of the Treasury of the State's failure for purposes of applying subpart B in that State.

## SEC. 1512. FAILURE OF PARTICIPATING STATES TO MEET CONDITIONS FOR COMPLIANCE.

(a) IN GENERAL.—In the case of a participating State, if the Board determines that the operation of the State system under subtitle C fails to meet the applicable requirements of this Act, sanctions shall apply against the State in accordance with subsection (b).

(b) TYPE OF SANCTION APPLICABLE.—The sanctions applicable under this part are as follows:

(1) If the Board determines that the State's failure does not substantially jeopardize the ability of eligible individuals in the State to obtain coverage for the comprehensive benefit package—

(A) the Board may order a regional alliance in the State to comply with applicable requirements of this Act and take such additional measures to assure compliance with such requirements as the Board may impose, if the Board determines that the State's failure relates to a requirement applicable to a regional alliance in the State, or

(B) if the Board does not take the action described in subparagraph (A) (or if the Board takes the action and determines that the action has not remedied the violation that led to the imposition of the sanction), the Board shall notify the Secretary of Health and Human Services, who shall reduce payments with respect to the State in accordance with section 1513.

(2) If the Board determines that the failure substantially jeopardizes the ability of eligible individuals in the State to obtain coverage for the comprehensive benefit package—

> (A) the Board shall terminate its approval of the State system; and
>
> (B) the Board shall notify the Secretary of Health and Human Services, who shall assume the responsibilities described in section 1522.

(c) TERMINATION OF SANCTION.—

(1) COMPLIANCE BY STATE.—A State against which a sanction is imposed may submit information at any time to the Board to demonstrate that the failure that led to the imposition of the sanction has been corrected.

(2) TERMINATION OF SANCTION.—If the Board determines that the failure that led to the imposition of a sanction has been corrected—

> (A) in the case of the sanction described in subsection (b)(1)(A), the Board shall notify the regional alliance against which the sanction is imposed; or

(B) in the case of any other sanction described in subsection (b), the Board shall notify the Secretary of Health and Human Services.

(d) PROTECTION OF ACCESS TO BENEFITS.—The Board and the Secretary of Health and Human Services shall exercise authority to take actions under this section with respect to a State only in a manner that assures the continuous coverage of eligible individuals under regional alliance health plans.

**SEC. 1513. REDUCTION IN PAYMENTS FOR HEALTH PROGRAMS BY SECRETARY OF HEALTH AND HUMAN SERVICES.**

(a) IN GENERAL.—Upon receiving notice from the Board under section 1512(b)(1)(B), the Secretary of Health and Human Services shall reduce the amount of any of the payments described in subsection (b) that would otherwise be made to individuals and entities in the State by such amount as the Secretary determines to be appropriate.

(b) PAYMENTS DESCRIBED.—The payments described in this subsection are as follows:

(1) Payments to academic health centers in the State under subtitle B of title III for medical education training programs funds.

(2) Payments to individuals and entities in the State for health research activities under section 301 and title IV of the Public Health Service Act.

(3) Payments to hospitals in the State under part 4 of subtitle E of title III (relating to payments to hospitals serving vulnerable populations)

### SEC. 1514. REVIEW OF FEDERAL DETERMINATIONS.

Any State or alliance affected by a determination by the Board under this subpart may appeal such determination in accordance with section 5231.

### SEC. 1515. FEDERAL SUPPORT FOR STATE IMPLEMENTATION.

(a) PLANNING GRANTS.—

(1) IN GENERAL.—Not later than 90 days after the date of the enactment of this Act, the Secretary shall make available to each State a planning grant to assist a State in the development of a health care system to become a participating State under subtitle C.

(2) FORMULA.—The Secretary shall establish a formula for the distribution of funds made available under this subsection.

(3) AUTHORIZATION OF APPROPRIATIONS.—There are authorized to be appropriated $50,000,000 in each of fiscal years 1995 and 1996.

(b) GRANTS FOR START-UP SUPPORT.—

(1) IN GENERAL.—The Secretary shall make available to States, upon their enacting of enabling legislation to become participating States, grants to assist in the establishment of regional alliances.

(2) FORMULA.—The Secretary shall establish a formula for the distribution of funds made available under this subsection.

(3) STATE MATCHING FUNDS REQUIRED.—Funds are payable to a State under this subsection only if the State provides assurances, satisfactory to the Secretary, that amounts of State funds (at least equal to the amount made available under this subsection) are expended for the purposes described in paragraph (1).

(4) AUTHORIZATION OF APPROPRIATIONS.—There are authorized to be appropriated $313,000,000 for fiscal year 1996, $625,000,000 for fiscal year 1997, and $313,000,000 for fiscal year 1998.

(c) FORMULA.—

(1) IN GENERAL.—The Board shall develop a formula for the distribution of

## Subpart C—Responsibilities in Absence of State Systems

### SEC. 1521. APPLICATION OF SUBPART.

(a) INITIAL APPLICATION.—This subpart shall apply with respect to a State as of January 1, 1998, unless—

(1) the State submits a document for a State system under section 1511(a)(1) by July 1, 1997, and

(2) the Board determines under section 1511 that such system meets the requirements of part 1 of subtitle C.

(b) TERMINATION OF APPROVAL OF SYSTEM OF PARTICIPATING STATE.—In the case of a participating State for which the Board terminates approval of the State system under section 1512(2), this subpart shall apply with respect to the State as of such date as is appropriate to assure the continuity of coverage for the comprehensive benefit package for eligible individuals in the State.

### SEC. 1522. FEDERAL ASSUMPTION OF RESPONSIBILITIES IN NON-PARTICIPATING STATES.

(a) NOTICE.—When the Board determines that this subpart will apply to a State for a calendar year, the Board shall notify the Secretary of Health and Human Services.

(b) ESTABLISHMENT OF REGIONAL ALLIANCE SYSTEM.—Upon receiving notice under subsection (a), the

Secretary shall take such steps, including the establishment of regional alliances, and compliance with other requirements applicable to participating States under subtitle C, as are necessary to ensure that the comprehensive benefit package is provided to eligible individuals in the State during the year.

(c) REQUIREMENTS FOR ALLIANCES.—Subject to section 1523, any regional alliance established by the Secretary pursuant to this section must meet all the requirements applicable under subtitle D to a regional alliance established and operated by a participating State, and the Secretary shall have the authority to fulfill all the functions of such an alliance.

(d) ESTABLISHMENT OF GUARANTY FUND.—

(1) ESTABLISHMENT.—The Secretary must ensure that there is a guaranty fund that meets the requirements established by the Board under section 1562, in order to provide financial protection to health care providers and others in the case of a failure of a regional alliance health plan under a regional alliance established and operated by the Secretary under this section.

(2) ASSESSMENTS TO PROVIDE GUARANTY FUNDS.—In the case of a failure of one or more regional alliance health plans under a regional alliance

established and operated by the Secretary under this section, the Secretary may require each regional alliance health plan under the alliance to pay an assessment to the Secretary in an amount not to exceed 2 percent of the premiums of such plans paid by or on behalf of regional alliance eligible individuals during a year for so long as necessary to generate sufficient revenue to cover any outstanding claims against the failed plan.

## SEC. 1523. IMPOSITION OF SURCHARGE ON PREMIUMS UNDER FEDERALLY-OPERATED SYSTEM.

(a) IN GENERAL.—If this subpart applies to a State for a calendar year, the premiums charged under the regional alliance established and operated by the Secretary in the State shall be equal to premiums that would otherwise be charged under a regional alliance established and operated by the State, increased by 15 percent. Such 15 percent increase shall be used to reimburse the Secretary for any administrative or other expenses incurred as a result of establishing and operating the system.

(b) TREATMENT OF SURCHARGE AS PART OF PREMIUM.—For purposes of determining the compliance of a State for which this subpart applies in a year with the requirements for budgeting under subtitle A of title VI for the year, the 15 percent increase described in subsection (a) shall be treated as part of the premium for payment to a regional alliance.

**SEC. 1524. RETURN TO STATE OPERATION.**

(a) APPLICATION PROCESS.—After the establishment and operation of an alliance system by the Secretary in a State under section 1522, the State may at any time apply to the Board for the approval of a State system in accordance with the procedures described in section 1511.

(b) TIMING.—If the Board approves the system of a State for which the Secretary has operated an alliance system during a year, the Secretary shall terminate the operation of the system, and the State shall establish and operate its approved system, as of January 1 of the first year beginning after the Board approves the State system. The termination of the Secretary's system and the operation of the State's system shall be conducted in a manner that assures the continuous coverage of eligible individuals in the State under regional alliance health plans.

**Subpart D—Establishment of Class Factors for Charging Premiums**

**SEC. 1531. PREMIUM CLASS FACTORS.**

(a) IN GENERAL.—For each of the classes of family enrollment (as specified in section 1011(c)), for purposes of title VI, the Board shall establish a premium class factor that reflects, subject to subsection (b), the relative actuarial value of the comprehensive benefit package of the class of family enrollment compared to such value of such package for individual enrollment.

(b) CONDITIONS.—In establishing such factors, the factor for the class of individual enrollment shall be 1 and the factor for the class of family enrollment of coverage of a married couple without children shall be 2.

## Subpart E—Risk Adjustment and Reinsurance Methodology for Payment of Plans

**SEC. 1541. DEVELOPMENT OF A RISK ADJUSTMENT AND REINSURANCE METHODOLOGY.**

(a) DEVELOPMENT.—

(1) INITIAL DEVELOPMENT.—Not later than April 1, 1995, the Board shall develop a risk adjustment and reinsurance methodology in accordance with this subpart.

(2) IMPROVEMENTS.—The Board shall make such improvements in such methodology as may be appropriate to achieve the purposes described in subsection (b)(1).

(b) METHODOLOGY.—

(1) PURPOSES.—Such methodology shall provide for the adjustment of payments to regional alliance health plans for the purposes of—

(A) assuring that payments to such plans reflect the expected relative utilization and expenditures for such services by each plan's enrollees compared to the average utilization and expenditures for regional alliance eligible individuals, and

(B) protecting health plans that enroll a disproportionate share of regional alliance eligible individuals with respect to whom expected utilization of health care services (included in the comprehensive benefit package) and expected health care expenditures for such services are greater than the average level of such utilization and expenditures for regional alliance eligible individuals.

(2) FACTORS TO BE CONSIDERED.—In developing such methodology, the Board shall take into account the following factors:

(A) Demographic characteristics.

(B) Health status.

(C) Geographic area of residence.

(D) Socio-economic status.

(E) Subject to paragraph (5), (i) the proportion of enrollees who are SSI recipients and

(ii) the proportion of enrollees who are AFDC recipients.

(F) Any other factors determined by the Board to be material to the purposes described in paragraph (1).

(3) ZERO SUM.—The methodology shall assure that the total payments to health plans by the regional alliance after application of the methodology are the same as the amount of payments that would have been made without application of the methodology.

(4) PROSPECTIVE ADJUSTMENT OF PAYMENTS.—The methodology, to the extent possible and except in the case of a mandatory reinsurance system described in subsection (b), shall be applied in manner that provides for the prospective adjustment of payments to health plans.

(5) TREATMENT OF SSI/AFDC ADJUSTMENT.—The Board is not required to apply the factor described in clause (i) or (ii) of paragraph (2)(E) if the Board determines that the application of the other risk adjustment factors described in paragraph (2) is sufficient to adjust premiums to take into account the enrollment in plans of AFDC recipients and SSI recipients.

(6) SPECIAL CONSIDERATION FOR MENTAL ILLNESS.—In developing the methodology under this section, the Board shall give consideration to the unique problems of adjusting payments to health plans with respect to individuals with mental illness.

(7) SPECIAL CONSIDERATION FOR VETERANS, MILITARY, AND INDIAN HEALTH PLANS.—In developing the methodology under this section, the Board shall give consideration to the special enrollment and funding provisions relating to plans described in section 1004(b).

(8) ADJUSTMENT TO ACCOUNT FOR USE OF ESTIMATES.—Subject to section 1346(b)(3) (relating to establishment of regional alliance reserve funds), if the total payments made by a regional alliance to all regional alliance health plans in a year under section 1324(c) exceeds, or is less than, the total of such payments estimated by the alliance in the application of the methodology under this subsection, because of a difference between—

> (A) the alliance's estimate of the distribution of enrolled families in different risk categories (assumed in the application of risk factors under this subsection in making payments to regional alliance health plans), and

(B) the actual distribution of such enrolled families in such categories,

the methodology under this subsection shall provide for an adjustment in the application of such methodology in the second succeeding year in a manner that would reduce, or increase, respectively, by the amount of such excess (or deficit) the total of such payments made by the alliance to all such plans.

(b) MANDATORY REINSURANCE.—

(1) IN GENERAL.—The methodology developed under this section may include a system of mandatory reinsurance, but may not include a system of voluntary reinsurance.

(2) REQUIREMENT IN CERTAIN CASES.—If the Board determines that an adequate system of prospective adjustment of payments to health plans to account for the health status of individuals enrolled by regional alliance health plans cannot be developed (and ready for implementation) by the date specified in subsection (a)(1), the Board shall include a mandatory reinsurance system as a component of the methodology. The Board may thereafter reduce or eliminate such a system at such time as the Board determines that an adequate prospective payment

adjustment for health status has been developed and is ready for implementation.

(3) REINSURANCE SYSTEM.—The Board, in developing the methodology for a mandatory reinsurance system under this subsection, shall—

(A) provide for health plans to make payments to state-established reinsurance programs for the purpose of reinsuring part or all of the health care expenses for items and services included in the comprehensive benefit package for specified classes of high-cost enrollees or specified high-cost treatments or diagnoses; and

(B) specify the manner of creation, structure, and operation of the system in each State, including—

(i) the manner (which may be prospective or retrospective) in which health plans make payments to the system, and

(ii) the type and level of reinsurance coverage provided by the system.

(c) CONFIDENTIALITY OF INFORMATION.—The methodology shall be developed in a manner consistent with privacy standards promulgated under section 5102(a). In developing such standards, the Board shall take into account any potential need of alliances for certain individually identifiable health information in order to carry out risk-adjustment and reinsurance activities under this Act, but only to the minimum extent necessary to carry out such activities and with protections provided to minimize the identification of the individuals to whom the information relates.

## SEC. 1542. INCENTIVES TO ENROLL DISADVANTAGED GROUPS.

The Board shall establish standards under which States may provide (under section 1203(e)(3)) for an adjustment in the risk-adjustment methodology developed under section 1541 in order to provide a financial incentive for regional alliance health plans to enroll individuals who are members of disadvantaged groups.

## SEC. 1543. ADVISORY COMMITTEE.

(a) IN GENERAL.—The Board shall establish an advisory committee to provide technical advice and recommendations regarding the development and modification of the risk adjustment and reinsurance methodology developed under this part.

(b) COMPOSITION.—Such advisory committee shall consist of 15 individuals and shall include individuals who are representative of health plans, regional alliances, consumers, experts, employers, and health providers.

## SEC. 1544. RESEARCH AND DEMONSTRATIONS.

The Secretary shall conduct and support research and demonstration projects to develop and improve, on a continuing basis, the risk adjustment and reinsurance methodology under this subpart.

## SEC. 1545. TECHNICAL ASSISTANCE TO STATES AND ALLIANCES.

The Board shall provide technical assistance to States and regional alliances in implementing the methodology developed under this subpart.

### Subpart F—Responsibilities for Financial Requirements

## SEC. 1551. CAPITAL STANDARDS FOR REGIONAL ALLIANCE HEALTH PLAN.

(a) IN GENERAL.—The Board shall establish, in consultation with the States, minimum capital requirements for regional alliance health plans, for purposes of section 1203(c).

(b) $500,000 MINIMUM.—Subject to paragraph (3), under such requirements there shall be not less than $500,000 of capital maintained for each plan offered in each alliance area, regardless of whether or not the same sponsor offered more than one of such plans.

(c) ADDITIONAL CAPITAL REQUIREMENTS.—The Board may require additional capital for factors likely to affect the financial stability of health plans, including the following:

>(1) Projected plan enrollment and number of providers participating in the plan.

>(2) Market share and strength of competition.

>(3) Extent and nature of risk-sharing with participating providers and the financial stability of risk-sharing providers.

>(4) Prior performance of the plan, risk history, and liquidity of assets.

(d) DEVELOPMENT OF STANDARDS BY NAIC.—The Board may request the National Association of Insurance Commissioners to develop model standards for the additional capital requirements described in subsection (c) and to present such standards to the Board not later than July 1, 1995. The Board may accept such standards as the standards to be applied under subsection (c) or modify the standards in any manner it finds appropriate.

### SEC. 1552. STANDARD FOR GUARANTY FUNDS.

(a) IN GENERAL.—In consultation with the States, the Board shall establish standards for guaranty funds established by States under section 1204(c).

(b) GUARANTY FUND STANDARDS.—The standards established under subsection (a) for a guaranty fund shall include the following:

(1) Each fund must have a method to generate sufficient resources to pay health providers and others in the case of a failure of a health plan (as described in section 1204(d)(4)) in order to meet obligations with respect to—

    (A) services rendered by the health plan for the comprehensive benefit package, including any supplemental coverage for cost sharing provided by the health plan, and

    (B) services rendered prior to health plan insolvency and services to patients after the insolvency but prior to their enrollment in other health plans.

(2) The fund is liable for all claims against the plan by health care providers with respect to their provision of items and services covered under the comprehensive benefit package to enrollees of the failed plan. Such claims, in full, shall take priority over all other claims. The fund also is liable, to the extent and in the manner provided in accordance with rules established by the Board, for other claims, including other claims of such providers and the claims of contractors, employees, governments, or any other claimants.

(3) The fund stands as a creditor for any payments owed the plan to the extent of the payments made by the fund for obligations of the plan.

(4) The fund has authority to borrow against future assessments (payable under section 1204(c)(2)) in order to meet the obligations of failed plans participating in the fund.

## PART 2—RESPONSIBILITIES OF DEPARTMENT OF HEALTH AND HUMAN SERVICES

### Subpart A—General Responsibilities

**SEC. 1571. GENERAL RESPONSIBILITIES OF SECRETARY OF HEALTH AND HUMAN SERVICES.**

(a) IN GENERAL.—Except as otherwise specifically provided under this Act (or with respect to administration of provisions in the Internal Revenue Code of 1986 or in the Employee Retirement Income Security Act of 1974), the Secretary of Health and Human Services shall administer and implement all of the provisions of this Act, except those duties delegated to the National Health Board, any other executive agency, or to any State.

(b) FINANCIAL MANAGEMENT STANDARDS.—The Secretary, in consultation with the Secretaries of Labor and the Treasury, shall establish, for purposes of section 1361, standards relating to the management of finances, maintenance of records, accounting practices, auditing procedures, and financial reporting for health alliances. Such standards shall take into account current Federal laws and regulations relating to fiduciary responsibilities and financial management of funds.

(c) AUDITING REGIONAL ALLIANCE PERFORMANCE.—The Secretary shall perform periodic financial and other audits of regional alliances to assure that such alliances are carrying out their responsibilities under this Act consistent with this Act. Such audits shall include audits of alliance performance in the areas of—

(1) assuring enrollment of all regional alliance eligible individuals in health plans,

(2) management of premium and cost sharing discounts and reductions provided; and

(3) financial management of the alliance, including allocation of collection shortfalls.

## SEC. 1572. ADVISORY COUNCIL ON BREAKTHROUGH DRUGS.

(a) IN GENERAL.—The Secretary shall appoint an Advisory Council on Breakthrough Drugs (in this section referred to as the "Council") that will examine the reasonableness of launch prices of new drugs that represent a breakthrough or significant advance over existing therapies.

(b) DUTIES.—(1) At the request of the Secretary, or a member of the Council, the Council shall make a determination regarding the reasonableness of launch prices of a breakthrough drug. Such a determination shall be based on:

 (A) prices of other drugs in the same therapeutic class;

 (B) cost information supplied by the manufacturer;

 (C) prices of the drug in countries specified in section 302(b)(4)(A) of the Federal Food, Drug, and Cosmetic Act; and

 (D) projected prescription volume, economies of scale, product stability, special manufacturing requirements and research costs.

(2) The Secretary shall review the determinations of the Council and publish the results of such review along with the Council's determination (including minority opinions) as a notice in the Federal Register.

(c) MEMBERSHIP.—The Council shall consist of a chair and 12 other persons, appointed without regard to the provisions of title 5, United States Code, governing appointments in the competitive service. The Council shall include a representative from the pharmaceutical industry, consumer organizations, physician organizations, the hospital industry, and the managed care industry. Other individuals appointed by the Secretary shall be recognized experts in the fields of health care economics, pharmacology, pharmacy and prescription drug reimbursement. Only one member of the Council may have direct or indirect financial ties to the pharmaceutical industry.

(d) TERM OF APPOINTMENTS.—Appointments shall be for a term of 3 years, except that the Secretary may provide initially for such shorter terms as will ensure that the terms of not more than 5 members expire in any one year.

(e) COMPENSATION.—Members of the Council shall be entitled to receive reimbursement of expenses and per diem in lieu of subsistence in the same manner as other members of advisory councils appointed by the Secretary are provided such reimbursements under the Social Security Act.

(f) NO TERMINATION.—Notwithstanding the provisions of the Federal Advisory Committee Act, the Council shall continue in existence until otherwise specified in law.

## Subpart B—Certification of Essential Community Providers

**SEC. 1581. CERTIFICATION.**

(a) IN GENERAL.—For purposes of this Act, the Secretary shall certify as an "essential community provider" any health care provider or organization that—

(1) is within any of the categories of providers and organizations specified in section 1582(a), or

(2) meets the standards for certification under section 1583(a).

(b) TIMELY ESTABLISHMENT OF PROCESS.—The Secretary shall take such actions as may be necessary to permit health care providers and organizations to be certified as essential community providers in a State before the beginning of the first year for the State.

**SEC. 1582. CATEGORIES OF PROVIDERS AUTOMATICALLY CERTIFIED.**

(a) IN GENERAL.—The categories of providers and organizations described in this subsection are as follows:

(1) MIGRANT HEALTH CENTERS.—A recipient or subrecipient of a grant under section 329 of the Public Health Service Act.

(2) COMMUNITY HEALTH CENTERS.—A recipient or subrecipient of a grant under section 330 of the Public Health Service Act.

(3) HOMELESS PROGRAM PROVIDERS.—A recipient or subrecipient of a grant under section 340 of the Public Health Service Act.

(4) PUBLIC HOUSING PROVIDERS.—A recipient or subrecipient of a grant under section 340A of the Public Health Service Act.

(5) FAMILY PLANNING CLINICS.—A recipient or subrecipient of a grant under title X of the Public Health Service Act.

(6) INDIAN HEALTH PROGRAMS.—A service unit of the Indian Health Service, a tribal organization, or an urban Indian program, as defined in the Indian Health Care Improvement Act.

(7) AIDS PROVIDERS UNDER RYAN WHITE ACT.—A public or private nonprofit health care provider that is a recipient or subrecipient of a grant under title XXIII of the Public Health Service Act.

(8) MATERNAL AND CHILD HEALTH PROVIDERS.—A public or private nonprofit entity that provides prenatal care, pediatric care, or ambulatory services to children, including children with special health care needs, and that receives funding for such care or services under title V of the Social Security Act.

(9) FEDERALLY QUALIFIED HEALTH CENTER; RURAL HEALTH CLINIC.—A Federally-qualified health center or a rural health clinic (as such terms are defined in section 1861(aa) of the Social Security Act.

(10) PROVIDER OF SCHOOL HEALTH SERVICES.—A provider of school health services that receives funding for such services under subtitle G of title III.

(11) COMMUNITY PRACTICE NETWORK.—A community practice networking receiving development funds under subtitle E of title III.

(b) SUBRECIPIENT DEFINED.—In this subpart, the term "subrecipient" means, with respect to a recipient of a grant under a particular authority, an entity that—

(1) is receiving funding from such a grant under a contract with the principal recipient of such a grant, and

(2) meets the requirements established to be a recipient of such a grant.

(c) HEALTH PROFESSIONAL DEFINED.—In this subpart, the term "health professional" means a physician, nurse, nurse practitioner, certified nurse midwife, physician assistant, psychologist, dentist, pharmacist, and other health care professional recognized by the Secretary.

## SEC. 1583. STANDARDS FOR ADDITIONAL PROVIDERS.

(a) STANDARDS.—The Secretary shall publish standards for the certification of additional categories of health care providers and organizations as essential community providers, including the categories described in subsection (b). Such a health care provider or organization shall not be certified unless the Secretary determines, under such standards, that health plans operating in the area served by the applicant would not be able to assure adequate access to items and services included in the comprehensive benefit package.

(b) CATEGORIES TO BE INCLUDED.—The categories described in this subsection are as follows:

(1) HEALTH PROFESSIONALS.—Health professionals—

(A) located in an area designated as a health professional shortage area (under section 332 of the Public Health Service Act), or

(B) providing a substantial amount of health services (as determined in accordance with standards established by the Secretary) to a medically underserved population (as designated under section 330 of such Act).

(2) INSTITUTIONAL PROVIDERS.—Public and private nonprofit hospitals and other institutional

health care providers located in such an area or providing health services to such a population.

(3) OTHER PROVIDERS.—Other public and private nonprofit agencies and organizations that—

    (A) are located in such an area or providing health services to such a population, and

    (B) provide health care and services essential to residents of such an area or such populations.

## SEC. 1584. CERTIFICATION PROCESS; REVIEW; TERMINATION OF CERTIFICATIONS.

(a) CERTIFICATION PROCESS.—

(1) PUBLICATION OF PROCEDURES.—The Secretary shall publish, not later than 6 months after the date of the enactment of this Act, the procedures to be used by health care professionals, providers, agencies, and organizations seeking certification under this subpart, including the form and manner in which an application for such certification is to be made.

(2) TIMELY DETERMINATION.—The Secretary shall make a determination upon such an application not later than 60 days (or 15 days in the case of a certification for an entity described in section 1582) after the date the complete application has

been submitted. The determination on an application for certification of an entity described in section 1582 shall only involve the verification that the entity is an entity described in such section.

(b) REVIEW OF CERTIFICATIONS.—The Secretary shall periodically review whether professionals, providers, agencies, and organizations certified under this subpart continue to meet the requirements for such certification.

(c) TERMINATION OR DENIAL OF CERTIFICATION.—

(1) PRELIMINARY FINDING.—If the Secretary preliminarily finds that an entity seeking certification under this section does not meet the requirements for such certification or such an entity certified under this subpart fails to continue to meet the requirements for such certification, the Secretary shall notify the entity of such preliminary finding and permit the entity an opportunity, under subtitle E of title V, to rebut such findings.

(2) FINAL DETERMINATION.—If, after such opportunity, the Secretary continues to find that such an entity continues to fail to meet such requirements, the Secretary shall terminate the certification and shall notify the entity, regional alliances, and corporate alliances of such termination and the effective date of the termination.

## SEC. 1585. NOTIFICATION OF HEALTH ALLIANCES AND PARTICIPATING STATES.

(a) IN GENERAL.—Not less often than annually the Secretary shall notify each participating State and each health alliance of essential community providers that have been certified under this subpart.

(b) CONTENTS.—Such notice shall include sufficient information to permit each health alliance to notify health plans of the identify of each entity certified as an essential community provider, including—

(1) the location of the provider within each plan's service area,

(2) the health services furnished by the provider, and

(3) other information necessary for health plans to carry out part 3 of subtitle E.

## PART 3—SPECIFIC RESPONSIBILITIES OF SECRETARY OF LABOR.

## SEC. 1591. RESPONSIBILITIES OF SECRETARY OF LABOR.

(a) IN GENERAL.—The Secretary of Labor is responsible—

(1) under subtitle D of title I, for the enforcement of requirements applicable to employers under regional health alliances (including requirements relating to payment of premiums) and the administration of corporate health alliances;

(2) under subtitle E of title I, with respect to elections by eligible sponsors to become corporate alliances and the termination of such elections;

(3) under section 1395, for the temporary assumption of the operation of self-insured corporate alliance health plans that are insolvent;

(4) under section 1396, for the establishment and administration of Corporate Alliance Health Plan Insolvency Fund;

(5) for carrying out any other responsibilities assigned to the Secretary under this Act; and

(6) for administering title I of the Employee Retirement Income Security Act of 1974 as it relates to group health plans maintained by corporate alliances.

(b) AGREEMENTS WITH STATES.—The Secretary of Labor may enter into agreements with States in order to enforce responsibilities of employers and corporate alliances, and requirements of corporate alliance health plans, under subtitle B of title I of the Employee Retirement Income Security Act of 1974.

(c) CONSULTATION WITH BOARD.—In carrying out activities under this Act with respect to corporate alliances, corporate alliance health plans, and employers, the

Secretary of Labor shall consult with the National Health Board.

(d) EMPLOYER-RELATED REQUIREMENTS.—

(1) IN GENERAL.—The Secretary of Labor, in consultation with the Secretary, shall be responsible for assuring that employers—

(A) make payments of any employer premiums (and withhold and make payment of the family share of premiums with respect to qualifying employees) as required under this Act, including auditing of regional alliance collection activities with respect to such payments,

(B) submit timely reports as required under this Act, and

(C) otherwise comply with requirements imposed on employers under this Act.

(2) AUDIT AND SIMILAR AUTHORITIES.—The Secretary of Labor—

(A) may carry out such audits (directly or through contract) and such investigations of employers and health alliances,

(B) may exercise such authorities under section 504 of Employee Retirement Income Security Act of 1974 (in relation to activities under this Act),

(C) may, with the permission of the Board, provide (through contract or otherwise) for such collection activities (in relation to amounts owed to regional alliances and for the benefit of such alliances), and

(D) may impose such civil penalties under section 1347(c),

as may be necessary to carry out such Secretary's responsibilities under this section.

(e) AUTHORITY.—The Secretary of Labor is authorized to issue such regulations as may be necessary to carry out responsibilities of the Secretary under this Act.

# Subtitle G—Employer Responsibilities

**SEC. 1601. PAYMENT REQUIREMENT.**

(a) IN GENERAL.—Each employer shall provide for payments required under section 6121 or 6131 in accordance with the applicable provisions of this Act.

(b) EMPLOYERS IN SINGLE-PAYER STATES.—In the case of an employer with respect to employees who reside in a single-payer State, the responsibilities of such employer under such system shall supersede the obligations of the employer under subsection (a), except as the Board may provide.

## SEC. 1602. REQUIREMENT FOR INFORMATION REPORTING.

(a) REPORTING OF END-OF-YEAR INFORMATION TO QUALIFYING EMPLOYEES.—

(1) IN GENERAL.—Each employer shall provide to each individual who was a qualifying employee of the employer during any month in the previous year information described in paragraph (2) with respect to the employee.

(2) INFORMATION TO BE SUPPLIED.—The information described in this paragraph, with respect to a qualifying employee, is the following (as specified by the Secretary):

(A) REGIONAL ALLIANCE INFORMATION.—With respect to each regional alliance through which the individual obtained health coverage:

(i) The total number of months of full-time equivalent employment (as determined for purposes of section 6121(d)) for each class of enrollment.

(ii) The amount of wages attributable to qualified employment and the amount of covered wages (as defined in paragraph (4)).

(iii) The total amount deducted from wages and paid for the family share of the premium.

(iv) Such other information as the Secretary of Labor may specify.

(B) CORPORATE ALLIANCE INFORMATION.—With respect to a qualifying employee who obtains coverage through a corporate alliance health plan:

(i) The total number of months of full-time equivalent employees (as determined under section 1901(b)(2)) for each class of enrollment.

(ii) Such other information as the Secretary of Labor may specify.

(3) ALLIANCE SPECIFIC INFORMATION.—In the case of a qualifying employee with respect to whom an employer made employer premium payments during the year to more than one regional alliance, the information under this subsection shall be reported separately with respect to each such alliance.

(4) COVERED WAGES DEFINED.—In this section, the term "covered wages" means wages paid an employee of an employer during a month in which the employee was a qualifying employee of the employer.

(b) REPORTING OF INFORMATION FOR USE OF REGIONAL ALLIANCES.—

(1) IN GENERAL.—Each employer (including corporate alliance employers) shall provide under subsection (f) on behalf of each regional alliance information described in paragraph (2) on an annual basis, information described in paragraph (3) on a monthly basis, and information described in paragraph (4) on a one-time basis, with respect to the employment of qualified employees in each year, month, or other time, respectively.

(2) INFORMATION TO BE SUPPLIED ON AN ANNUAL BASIS.—The information described in this paragraph, with respect to an employer, is the following (as specified by the Secretary of Labor).

(A) REGIONAL ALLIANCE INFORMATION.—With respect to each regional alliance to which employer premium payments were payable in the year:

(i) For each qualifying employee in the year—

(I) The total number of months of full-time equivalent employment (as determined for purposes of section 6121(d)) for the employee for each class of enrollment.

(II) The total amount deducted from wages and paid for the family share of the premium of the qualifying employee.

(ii) The total employer premium payment made under section 6121 for the year with respect to the employment of all qualifying employees residing in the alliance area and, in the case of an employer that has obtained (or seeks to obtain) a premium discount under section 6123, the total employer premium payment that would have been owed for such employment for the year but for such section.

(iii) The number of full-time equivalent employees (determined under section 6121(d)) for each class of family enrollment in the year (and for each month in the year in the case of an employer that has obtained or is seeking a premium discount under section 6123).

(iv) In the case of an employer to which section 6124 applies in a year, such additional information as the Secretary of

Labor may require for purposes of that section.

  (v) The amounts paid (and payable) pursuant to section 6125.

  (vi) The amount of covered wages for each qualified employee.

(3) INFORMATION ON A MONTHLY BASIS.—

 (A) IN GENERAL.—The information described in this paragraph for a month for an employer is such information as the Secretary of Labor may specify regarding—

  (i) the identity of each eligible individual who changed qualifying employee status with respect to the employer in the month; and

  (ii) in the case of such an individual described in subparagraph (B)(i)—

   (I) the regional alliance for the alliance area in which the individual resides, and

   (II) the individual's class of family enrollment.

 (B) CHANGES IN QUALIFYING EMPLOYEE STATUS DESCRIBED.—For purposes of subparagraph (A), an individual is considered to have changed qualifying employee status in a month if the individual either (i) is a qualifying employee of the employer in the month and was not a qualifying employee of the employer in the previous month, or (ii) is not a qualifying employee of the employer in the month but was a qualifying employee of the employer in the previous month.

(4) INITIAL INFORMATION.—Each employer, at such time before the first year in which qualifying employees of the employer are enrolled in regional alliance health plans as the Board may specify, shall provide for the reporting of such information relating to employment of eligible individuals as the Board may specify.

(c) RECONCILIATION OF EMPLOYER PREMIUM PAYMENTS.—

(1) PROVISION OF INFORMATION.—Each employer (whether or not the employer claimed (or claims) an employer premium discount under section 6123 for a year) that is liable for employer premium payments to a regional alliance for any month in a year shall provide the alliance with such information as the alliance may require (consistent with rules of the Secretary of Labor) to determine the appropriate

amount of employer premium payments that should have been made for all months in the year (taking into account any employer premium discount under section 6123 for the employer).

(2) DEADLINE.—Such information shall be provided not later than the beginning of February of the following year with the payment to be made for that month.

(3) RECONCILIATION.—

(A) CONTINUING EMPLOYERS.—Based on such information, the employer shall adjust the amount of employer premium payment made in the month in which the information is provided to reflect the amount by which the payments in the previous year were greater or less than the amount of payments that should have been made.

(B) DISCONTINUING EMPLOYERS.—In the case of a person that ceases to be an employer in a year, such adjustment shall be made in the form of a payment to, or from, the alliance involved.

(4) SPECIAL TREATMENT OF SELF-EMPLOYED INDIVIDUALS.—Except as the Secretary of Labor may provide, individuals who are employers only be

virtue of the operation of section 6126 shall have employer premium payments attributable to such section reconciled (in the manner previously described in this subsection) under the process for the collection of the family share of premiums under section 1344 rather than under this subsection.

(d) SPECIAL RULES FOR SELF-EMPLOYED.—

　　(1) IN GENERAL.—In the case of an individual who is treated as an employer under section 6126, the individual shall provide, under subsection (f) on behalf of each regional alliance, information described in paragraph (2) with respect to net earnings from self-employment income of the individual in each year.

　　(2) INFORMATION TO BE SUPPLIED.—The information described in this paragraph, with respect to an individual, is such information as may be necessary to compute the amount payable under section 6131 by virtue of section 6126.

(e) FORM.—Information shall be provided under this subsection in such electronic or other form as the Secretary specifies. Such specifications shall be done in a manner that, to the maximum extent practicable, simplifies administration for small employers.

(f) INFORMATION CLEARINGHOUSE FUNCTIONS.—

(1) DESIGNATION.—The Board shall provide for the use of the regional centers (which are part of the electronic data network under section 5103) to perform information clearinghouse functions under this section with respect to employers and regional and corporate alliances.

(2) FUNCTIONS.—The functions referred to in paragraph (1) shall include—

(A) receipt of information submitted by employers under subsection (b) on an annual (or one-time) basis,

(B) from the information received, transmittal of information required to regional alliances,

(C) such other functions as the Board specifies.

(g) DEADLINE.—Information required to be provided by an employer for a year under this section—

(1) to a qualifying employee shall be provided not later than the date the employer is required under law to provide for statements under section 6051 of the Internal Revenue Code of 1986 for that year, or

(2) to a health alliance (through a regional center) shall be provided not later than the date by

which information is required to be filed with the Secretary pursuant to agreements under section 232 of the Social Security Act for that year.

(h) NOTICE TO CERTAIN INDIVIDUALS WHO ARE NOT EMPLOYEES.—

(1) IN GENERAL.—A person that carries on a trade or business shall notify in writing each individual described in paragraph (2) that the person is not obligated to make any employer health care premium payment (under section 6121) in relation to the services performed by the individual for the person.

(2) INDIVIDUAL DESCRIBED.—An individual described in this paragraph, with respect to a person, is an individual who normally performs services for the person in the person's trade or business for more than 40 hours per month but who is not an employee of the person (within the meaning of section 1901(a)).

(3) TIMING; EFFECTIVE DATE.—Such notice shall be provided within a reasonable time after the individual begins performing services for the person, except that in no event is such a notice required to be provided with respect to services performed before January 1, 1998.

(4) EXCEPTIONS.—The Secretary shall issue regulations providing exceptions to the notice requirement of paragraph (1) with respect to individuals performing services on an irregular, incidental, or casual basis.

(5) MODEL NOTICE.—The Secretary shall publish a model notice that is easily understood by the average reader and that persons may use to satisfy the requirements of paragraph (1).

## SEC. 1603. REQUIREMENTS RELATING TO NEW EMPLOYEES.

(a) COMPLETION OF ENROLLMENT INFORMATION FORM.—At the time an individual is hired as a qualifying employee of a regional alliance employer, the employer shall obtain from the individual the following information (pursuant to rules established by the Secretary of Labor):

(1) The identity of the individual.

(2) The individual's alliance area of residence and whether the individual has moved from another alliance area.

(3) The class of family enrollment applicable to the individual.

(4) The health plan (and health alliance) in which the individual is enrolled at that time.

(5) If the individual has moved from another alliance area, whether the individual intends to enroll in a regional alliance health plan.

(b) TRANSMITTAL OF INFORMATION TO ALLIANCE.—

(1) IN GENERAL.—Each employer shall transmit the information obtained under subsection (a) to the regional alliance for the alliance area in which the qualifying employee resides (or will reside at the time of initial employment).

(2) DEADLINE.—Such information shall be transmitted within 30 days of the date of hiring of the employee.

(3) FORM.—Information under this section may be forwarded in electronic form to a regional alliance.

(c) PROVISION OF ENROLLMENT FORM AND INFORMATION.—In the case of an individual described in subsection (a)(5), the employer shall provide the individual, at the time of hiring, with—

(1) such information regarding the choice of, and enrollment in, regional alliance health plans, and

(2) such enrollment form,

as the regional alliance provides to the employer.

## SEC. 1604. AUDITING OF RECORDS.

Each regional alliance employer shall maintain such records, and provide the regional alliance for the area in which the employer maintains the principal place of employment (as specified by the Secretary of Labor) with access to such records, as may be necessary to verify and audit the information reported under this subtitle.

## SEC. 1605. PROHIBITION OF CERTAIN EMPLOYER DISCRIMINATION.

No employer may discriminate with respect to an employee on the basis of the family status of the employee or on the basis of the class of family enrollment selected with respect to the employee.

## SEC. 1606. PROHIBITION ON SELF-FUNDING OF COST SHARING BENEFITS BY REGIONAL ALLIANCE EMPLOYERS.

(a) PROHIBITION.—A regional alliance employer (and a corporate alliance employer with respect to employees who are regional alliance eligible individuals) may provide benefits to employees that consist of the benefits included in a cost sharing policy (as defined in section 1421(b)(2)) only through a contribution toward the purchase of a cost sharing policy which is funded primarily through insurance.

(b) INDIVIDUAL AND EMPLOYER RESPONSIBILITIES.—In the case of an individual who resides in a single-payer State and an employer with respect to employees who reside in such a State, the responsibilities of such individual and employer under such system shall supersede the obligations of the individual and employer under part 2 of this subtitle.

## SEC. 1607. EQUAL VOLUNTARY CONTRIBUTION REQUIREMENT.

(a) IN GENERAL.—An employer may not discriminate in the wages or compensation paid, or other terms or conditions of employment, with respect to an employee based on the health plan (or premium of such a plan) in which the employee is enrolled.

(b) REBATE REQUIRED IN CERTAIN CASES.—

(1) IN GENERAL.—Subject to paragraph (3), if—

(A) an employer makes available a voluntary premium payment on behalf of an employee towards the enrollment of the employee in a health plan, and

(B) the premium for the plan selected is less than the sum of the amounts of the employer premium payment (required under part 3) and the voluntary premium payment, the employer must rebate to the employee an amount equal to the difference described in subparagraph (B).

(2) REBATES.—

(A) IN GENERAL.—Any rebate provided under paragraph (1) shall be treated, for purposes of the Internal Revenue Code of 1986, as wages described in section 3121(a) of such Act.

(B) TREATMENT OF MULTIPLE FULL-TIME EMPLOYMENT IN A FAMILY.—In the case of—

(i) an individual who is an employee of more than one employer, or

(ii) a couple for which both spouses are employees,

if more than one employer provides for voluntary premium payments, the individual or couple may elect to have paragraph (1) applied with respect to all employment.

(c) EXCEPTION FOR COLLECTIVE BARGAINING AGREEMENT.—Subsections (a) and (b) shall not apply with respect to voluntary employer contributions made pursuant to a bona fide collective bargaining agreement.

(d) CONSTRUCTION.—

(1) Subsection (a) shall not be construed as preventing variations in net wages of an employee to

reflect the family share of premiums for the health plan selected, so long as any excess employer payments (as defined in paragraph (2)) are added to the pay of the employee involved.

(2) In paragraph (1), the term "excess employer payments" means, with respect to an employee, the amount by which the voluntary employer contribution toward health care expenses exceeds the family share of premium under section 6101(b) for such enrollment.

(e) VOLUNTARY EMPLOYER CONTRIBUTION DEFINED.—In this section, the term "voluntary employer contribution" means any payment designed to be used exclusively (or primarily) towards the cost of the family share of premiums for a health plan. Such term does not include any employer premiums required to be paid under part 3 of subtitle B of title VI.

### SEC. 1608. ENFORCEMENT.

In the case of a person that violates a requirement of this subtitle, the Secretary of Labor may impose a civil money penalty, in an amount not to exceed $10,000, for each violation with respect to each individual.

# [Subtitle H—Reserved]
# [Subtitle I—Reserved]
# Subtitle J—General Definitions; Miscellaneous Provisions

## PART 1—GENERAL DEFINITIONS

### SEC. 1901. DEFINITIONS RELATING TO EMPLOYMENT AND INCOME.

(a) IN GENERAL.—Except as otherwise specifically provided, in this Act the following definitions and rules apply:

　(1) EMPLOYER, EMPLOYEE, EMPLOYMENT, AND WAGES DEFINED.—Except as provided in this section—

　　(A) the terms "wages" and "employment" have the meanings given such terms under section 3121 of the Internal Revenue Code of 1986,

　　(B) the term "employee" hs the meaning given such term under subtitle C of such Code, and

　　(C) the term "employer" has the same meaning as the term "employer" as used in such section.

　(2) EXCEPTIONS.—For purposes of paragraph (1)—

(A) EMPLOYMENT.—

(i) EMPLOYMENT INCLUDED.—Paragraphs (1), (2), (5), (7) (other than clauses (i) through (iv) of subparagraph (C) and clauses (i) through (v) of subparagraph (F)), (8), (9), (10), (11), (13), (15), (18), and (19) of section 3121(b) of the Internal Revenue Code of 1986 shall not apply.

(ii) EXCLUSION OF INMATES AS EMPLOYEES.—Employment shall not include services performed in a penal institution by an inmate thereof or in a hospital or other health care institution by a patient thereof.

(B) WAGES.—

(i) IN GENERAL.—Paragraph (1) of section 3121(a) of the Internal Revenue Code of 1986 shall not apply.

(ii) TIPS NOT INCLUDED.—The term "wages" does not include cash tips.

(C) EXCLUSION OF EMPLOYEES OUTSIDE THE UNITED STATES.—The term "employee" does not include an individual who does not reside in the United States.

(D) EXCLUSION OF FOREIGN EMPLOYMENT.—The term "employee" does not include an individual—

(i) with respect to service, if the individual is not a citizen or resident of the United States and the service is performed outside the United States, or

(ii) with respect to service, if the individual is a citizen or resident of the United States and the service is performed outside the United States for an employer other than an American employer (as defined in section 3121(h) of the Internal Revenue Code of 1986).

(3) AGGREGATION RULES FOR EMPLOYERS.—For purposes of this Act—

(A) all employers treated as a single employer under subsection (a) or (b) of section 52 of the Internal Revenue Code of 1986 shall be treated as a single employer, and

(B) under regulations of the Secretary of Labor, all employees of organizations which are under common control with one or more organizations which are exempt from income tax under subtitle A of the Internal Revenue Code of 1986 shall be treated as employed by a single employer.

The regulations prescribed under subparagraph (B) shall be based on principles similar to the principles which apply to taxable organizations under subparagraph (A).

(4) EMPLOYER PREMIUM.—The term "employer premium" refers to the premium established and imposed under part 2 of subtitle B of title VI.

(b) QUALIFYING EMPLOYEE; FULL-TIME EMPLOYMENT.—

(1) QUALIFYING EMPLOYEE.—

(A) IN GENERAL.—In this Act, the term "qualifying employee" means, with respect to an employer for a month, an employee (other than a covered child, as defined in subparagraph (C)) who is employed by the employer for at least 40 hours (as determined under paragraph (3)) in the month.

(B) NO SPECIAL TREATMENT OF MEDICARE BENEFICIARIES, SSI RECIPIENTS, AFDC RECIPIENTS, AND OTHERS.—Subparagraph (A) shall apply regardless of whether or not the qualifying employee is a medicare-eligible individual, an SSI recipient, an AFDC recipient, an individual described in section 1004(b), an eligible individual or is authorized to be so employed.

(C) COVERED CHILD DEFINED.—In subparagraph (A), the term "covered child" means an eligible individual who is a child and is enrolled under a health plan as a family member described in section 1011(b)(2)(B).

(2) FULL-TIME EQUIVALENT EMPLOYEES; PART-TIME EMPLOYEES.—

(A) IN GENERAL.—For purposes of this Act, a qualifying employee who is employed by an employer—

(i) for at least 120 hours in a month, is counted as 1 full-time equivalent employee for the month and shall be deemed to be employed on a full-time basis, or

(ii) for at least 40 hours, but less than 120 hours, in a month, is counted as a fraction of a full-time equivalent employee in the month equal to the full-time employment ratio (as defined in subparagraph (B)) for the employee and shall be deemed to be employed on a part-time basis.

(B) FULL-TIME EMPLOYMENT RATIO DEFINED.—For purposes of this Act, the term "full-time employment ratio" means, with respect to a qualifying employee of an employer in a month, the lesser of 1 or the ratio of—

(i) the number of hours of employment such employee is employed by such employer for the month (as determined under paragraph (3)), to

(ii) 120 hours.

(C) FULL-TIME EMPLOYEE.—For purposes of this Act, the term "full-time employee" means, with respect to an employer, an employee who is employed on a full-time basis (as specified in subparagraph (A)) by the employer.

(3) HOURS OF EMPLOYMENT.—

(A) IN GENERAL.—For purposes of this Act, the Board shall specify the method for computing hours of employment for employees of an employer consistent with this paragraph. The Board shall take into account rules used for purposes of applying the Fair Labor Standards Act.

(B) HOURLY WAGE EARNERS.—In the case of an individual who receives compensation (in the form of hourly wages or compensation) for the performance of services, the individual is considered to be "employed" by an employer for an hour if compensation is payable with respect to that hour of employment, without regard to whether or not the employee is actually performing services during such hours.

(4) TREATMENT OF SALARIED EMPLOYEES AND EMPLOYEE PAID ON CONTINGENT OR BONUS ARRANGEMENTS.—In the case of an employee who receives compensation on a salaried basis or on the basis of a commission (or other contigent or bonus basis), rather than an hourly, the Board shall establish rules for the conversion of the compensation to hours of employment, taking into account the minimum monthly compensation levels for workers employed on a full-time basis under the Fair Labor Standards Act and other factors the Board considers relevant.

(c) DEFINITIONS RELATING TO SELF-EMPLOYMENT.—In this Act:

(1) NET EARNINGS FROM SELF-EMPLOYMENT.—The term "net earnings from self-employ-

ment" has the meaning given such term under section 1402(a) of the Internal Revenue Code of 1986.

(2) SELF-EMPLOYED INDIVIDUAL.—The term "self-employed individual" means, for a year, an individual who has net earnings from self-employment for the year.

**SEC. 1902. OTHER GENERAL DEFINITIONS.**

Except as otherwise specifically provided, in this Act the following definitions apply:

(1) ALIEN PERMANENTLY RESIDING IN THE UNITED STATES UNDER COLOR OF LAW.—The term "alien permanently residing in the United States under color of law" means an alien lawfully admitted for permanent residence (within the meaning of section 101(a)(19) of the Immigration and Nationality Act), and includes any of the following:

(A) An alien who is admitted as a refugee under section 207 of the Immigration and Nationality Act.

(B) An alien who is granted asylum under section 208 of such Act.

(C) An alien whose deportation is withheld under section 243(h) of such Act.

(D) An alien who is admitted for temporary residence under section 210, 210A, or 245A of such Act.

(E) An alien who has been paroled into the United States under section 212(d)(5) of such Act for an indefinite period or who has been granted extended voluntary departure as a member of a nationality group.

(F) An alien who is the spouse or unmarried child under 21 years of age of a citizen of the United States, or the parent of such a citizen if the citizen is over 21 years of age, and with respect to whom an application for adjustment to lawful permanent residence is pending.

(G) An alien within such other classification of permanent resident aliens as the National Health Board may establish by regulation.

(2) AFDC FAMILY.—The term "AFDC family" means a family composed entirely of one or more AFDC recipients.

(3) AFDC RECIPIENT.—The term "AFDC recipient" means an individual who is receiving aid or assistance under any plan of the State approved

under title I, X, XIV, or XVI, or part A or part E of title IV, of the Social Security Act.

(4) ALLIANCE AREA.—The term "alliance area" means the area served by a regional alliance and specified under section 1202(b).

(5) ALLIANCE ELIGIBLE INDIVIDUAL.—The term "alliance eligible individual" means, with respect to a health alliance, an eligible individual with respect to whom the applicable health plan is a health plan offered by or through such alliance and does not include a prisoner.

(6) APPLICABLE HEALTH PLAN.—The term "applicable health plan" means, with respect to an eligible individual, the health plan specified pursuant to section 1004 and part 2 of subtitle A.

(7) COMBINATION COST SHARING PLAN.—The term "combination cost sharing plan" means a health plan that provides combination cost sharing schedule (consistent with section 1134).

(8) COMPREHENSIVE BENEFIT PACKAGE.—The term "comprehensive benefit package" means the package of health benefits provided under subtitle B of title II.

(9) CONSUMER PRICE INDEX; CPI.—The terms consumer price index" and "CPI" mean the

Consumer Price Index for all urban consumers (U.S. city average), as published by the Bureau of Labor Statistics.

(10) CORPORATE ALLIANCE ELIGIBLE INDIVIDUAL.—The term "corporate alliance eligible individual" means, with respect to a corporate alliance, an eligible individual with respect to whom the corporate alliance is the applicable health plan.

(11) CORPORATE ALLIANCE EMPLOYER.—The term "corporate alliance employer" means, with respect to a corporate alliance, an employer of an individual who is a participant in a corporate alliance health plan of that alliance.

(12) CORPORATE ALLIANCE HEALTH PLAN.—The term "corporate alliance health plan" means a health plan offered by a corporate alliance under part 2 of subtitle E.

(13) DISABLED SSI RECIPIENT.—The term "disabled SSI recipient" means an individual who—

(A) is an SSI recipient, and

(B) has been determined to be disabled for purposes of the supplemental security income program (under title XVI of the Social Security Act).

(14) ELIGIBLE ENROLLEE.—The term "eligible enrollee" means, with respect to an health plan offered by a health alliance, an alliance eligible individual, but does not include such an individual if the individual is enrolled under such a plan as the family member of another alliance eligible individual.

(15) ESSENTIAL COMMUNITY PROVIDER.—The term "essential community provider" means an entity certified as such a provider under subpart B of part 2 of subtitle F.

(16) FEE-FOR-SERVICE PLAN.—The term "fee-for-service plan" means a health plan described in section 1322(b)(2)(A).

(17) FIRST YEAR.—The term "first year" means, with respect to—

(A) a State that is a participating State in a year before 1998, the year in which the State first is a participating State, or

(B) any other State, 1998.

(18) HIGHER COST SHARING PLAN.—The term "higher cost sharing plan" means a health plan that provides a high cost sharing schedule (consistent with section 1133).

(19) LONG-TERM NONIMMIGRANT.—The term "long-term nonimmigrant" means a nonimmigrant

described in subparagraph (E), (H), (I), (J), (K), (L), (M), (N), (O), (Q), or (R) of section 101(a)(15) of the Immigration and Nationality Act or an alien within such other classification of nonimmigrant as the National Health Board may establish by regulation.

(20) LOWER COST SHARING PLAN.—The term "lower cost sharing plan" means a health plan that provides a lower cost sharing schedule (consistent with section 1132).

(21) MEDICARE PROGRAM.—The term "medicare program" means the health insurance program under title XVIII of the Social Security Act.

(22) MEDICARE-ELIGIBLE INDIVIDUAL.—The term "medicare-eligible individual" means, subject to section 1012(a), an individual who is entitled to benefits under part A of the medicare program.

(23) MOVE.—The term "move" means, respect to an individual, a change of residence of the individual from one alliance area to another alliance area.

(24) NATIONAL HEALTH BOARD; BOARD.—The terms "National Health Board" and "Board" mean the National Health Board established under part 1 of subtitle F of title I.

(25) POVERTY LEVEL.—

    (A) IN GENERAL.—The term "applicable poverty level" means, for a family for a year, the official poverty line (as defined by the Office of Management and Budget, and revised annually in accordance with section 673(2) of the Omnibus Budget Reconciliation Act of 1981) applicable to a family of the size involved (as determined under subparagraph (B)) for 1994 adjusted by the percentage increase or decrease described in subparagraph (C) for the year involved.

    (B) FAMILY SIZE.—In applying the applicable poverty level to—

        (i) an individual enrollment, the family size is deemed to be one person;

        (ii) a couple-only enrollment, the family size is deemed to be two persons;

        (iii) a single parent enrollment, the family size is deemed to be three persons; or

        (iv) a dual parent, the family size is deemed to be four persons.

    (C) PERCENTAGE ADJUSTMENT.—The percentage increase or decrease described in this subparagraph for a year is the percentage increase or decrease by which the average CPI for the 12-month-period ending with August 31 of the preceding year exceeds such average for the 12-month period ending with August 31, 1993.

(D) ROUNDING.—Any adjustment made under subparagraph (A) for a year shall be rounded to the nearest multiple of $100.

(26) PRISONER.—The term "prisoner" means, as specified by the Board, an eligible individual during a period of imprisonment under Federal, State, or local authority after conviction as an adult.

(27) REGIONAL ALLIANCE ELIGIBLE INDIVIDUAL.—The term "regional alliance eligible individual" means an eligible individual with respect to whom a regional alliance health plan is an applicable health plan.

(28) REGIONAL ALLIANCE EMPLOYER.—The term "regional alliance employer" means an employer that is meeting the requirement of section 1003 other than through an agreement with one or more health alliances.

(29) REGIONAL ALLIANCE HEALTH PLAN.—The term "regional alliance health plan" means a health

plan offered by a regional alliance under part 1 of subtitle E of title I.

(30) RESIDE.—

(A) An individual is considered to reside in the location in which the individual maintains a primary residence (as established under rules of the National Health Board).

(B) Under such rules and subject to section 1323(c), in the case of an individual who maintains more than one residence, the primary residence of the individual shall be determined taking into account the proportion of time spent at each residence.

(C) In the case of a couple only one spouse of which is a qualifying employee, except as the Board may provide, the residence of the employee shall be the residence of the couple.

(31) SECRETARY.—The term "Secretary" means the Secretary of Health and Human Services.

(32) SSI FAMILY.—The term "SSI family" means a family composed entirely of one or more SSI recipients.

(33) SSI RECIPIENT.—The term "SSI recipient" means an individual—

(A) with respect to whom supplemental security income benefits are being paid under title XVI of the Social Security Act,

(B) who receiving a supplementary payment under section 1616 of such Act or under section 212 of Public Law 93–66, or

(C) who receiving monthly benefits under section 1619(a) of such Act (whether or not pursuant to section 1616(c)(3) of such Act).

(34) STATE.—The term "State" includes the District of Columbia, Puerto Rico, the Virgin Islands, Guam, American Samoa, and the Northern Mariana Islands.

(35) STATE MEDICAID PLAN.—The term "State medicaid plan" means a plan of medical assistance of a State approved under title XIX of the Social Security Act.

(36) UNDOCUMENTED ALIEN.—The term "undocumented alien" means an alien who is not a long-term nonimmigrant, a diplomat, or described in section 1004(c).

(37) UNITED STATES.—The term "United States" means the 50 States, the District of Columbia, Puerto Rico, the Virgin Islands, Guam, American Samoa, and Northern Mariana Islands.

# PART 2—MISCELLANEOUS PROVISIONS

## SEC. 1911. USE OF INTERIM, FINAL REGULATIONS.

In order to permit the timely implementation of the provisions of this Act, the National Health Board, the Secretary of Health and Human Services, the Secretary of Labor are each authorized to issue regulations under this Act on an interim basis that become final on the date of publication, subject to change based on subsequent public comment.

## SEC. 1912. SOCIAL SECURITY ACT REFERENCES.

Except as may otherwise be provided, any reference in this title, or in title V or VI, to the Social Security Act shall be to the Social Security Act as in effect on the date of the enactment of this Act.

# TITLE II—NEW BENEFITS

TABLE OF CONTENTS OF TITLE

## Subtitle A—Medicare Outpatient Prescription Drug Benefit

Sec. 2001. Coverage of outpatient prescription drugs.
Sec. 2002. Payment rules and related requirements for outpatient drugs.
Sec. 2003. Medicare rebates for covered outpatient drugs.
Sec. 2004. Counseling by participating pharmacies.
Sec. 2005. Extension of 25 percent rule for portion of premium attributable to covered outpatient drugs.
Sec. 2006. Coverage of home infusion drug therapy services.
Sec. 2007. Civil money penalties for excessive charges.
Sec. 2008. Conforming amendments to medicaid program.
Sec. 2009. Effective date.

## Subtitle B—Long-Term Care

### PART 1—STATE PROGRAMS FOR HOME AND COMMUNITY-BASED SERVICES FOR INDIVIDUALS WITH DISABILITIES

Sec. 2101. State programs for home and community-based services for individuals with disabilities.
Sec. 2102. State plans.
Sec. 2103. Individuals with disabilities defined.
Sec. 2104. Home and community-based services covered under State plan.
Sec. 2105. Cost sharing.
Sec. 2106. Quality assurance and safeguards.
Sec. 2107. Advisory groups.
Sec. 2108. Payments to States.
Sec. 2109. Total Federal budget; allotments to States.

### PART 2—MEDICAID NURSING HOME IMPROVEMENTS

Sec. 2201. Reference to amendments.

### PART 3—PRIVATE LONG-TERM CARE INSURANCE

#### SUBPART A—GENERAL PROVISIONS

Sec. 2301. Federal regulations; prior application or certain requirements.
Sec. 2302. National Long-term Care Insurance Advisory Council.
Sec. 2303. Relation to State law.
Sec. 2304. Definitions.

#### SUBPART B—FEDERAL STANDARDS AND REQUIREMENTS

Sec. 2321. Requirements to facilitate understanding and comparison of benefits.
Sec. 2322. Requirements relating to coverage.
Sec. 2323. Requirements relating to premiums.
Sec. 2324. Requirements relating to sales practices.
Sec. 2325. Continuation, renewal, replacement, conversion, and cancellation of policies.
Sec. 2326. Requirements relating to payment of benefits.

SUBPART C—ENFORCEMENT

Sec. 2342. State programs for enforcement of standards.
Sec. 2342. Authorization of appropriations for State programs.
Sec. 2343. Allotments to States.
Sec. 2344. Payments to States.
Sec. 2345. Federal oversight of State enforcement.
Sec. 2346. Effect of failure to have approved State program.

SUBPART D—CONSUMER EDUCATION GRANTS

Sec. 2361. Grants for consumer education.

PART 4—TAX TREATMENT OF LONG-TERM CARE INSURANCE AND SERVICES

Sec. 2401. Reference to tax provisions.

PART 5—TAX INCENTIVES FOR INDIVIDUALS WITH DISABILITIES WHO WORK

Sec. 2501. Reference to tax provision.

PART 6—DEMONSTRATION AND EVALUATION

Sec. 2601. Demonstration on acute and long-term care integration.
Sec. 2602. Performance review of the long-term care programs.

# Subtitle A—Medicare Outpatient Prescription Drug Benefit

**SEC. 2001. COVERAGE OF OUTPATIENT PRESCRIPTION DRUGS.**

(a) COVERED OUTPATIENT DRUGS AS MEDICAL AND OTHER HEALTH SERVICES.—Section 1861(s)(2)(J) of the Social Security Act (42 U.S.C. 1395x(s)(2)(J)) is amended to read as follows:

"(J) covered outpatient drugs;".

(b) DEFINITION OF COVERED OUTPATIENT DRUG.—Section 1861(t) of such Act (42 U.S.C. 1395x(t)), as amended by section 13553(b) of the Omnibus Budget Reconciliation Act of 1993 (hereafter in this subtitle referred to as "OBRA–1993"), is amended—

(1) in the heading, by adding at the end the following: "; Covered Outpatient Drugs";

(2) in paragraph (1), by striking "paragraph (2)" and inserting "the succeeding paragraphs of this subsection"; and

(3) by striking paragraph (2) and inserting the following:

"(2) Except as otherwise provided in paragraph (3), the term 'covered outpatient drug' means any of the following products used for a medically accepted indication (as described in paragraph (4)):

"(A) A drug which may be dispensed only upon prescription and—

"(i) which is approved for safety and effectiveness as a prescription drug under section 505 or 507 of the Federal Food, Drug, and Cosmetic Act or which is approved under section 505(j) of such Act;

"(ii)(I) which was commercially used or sold in the United States before the date of the enactment of the Drug Amendments of 1962 or which is identical, similar, or related (within the meaning of section 310.6(b)(1) of title 21 of the Code of Federal Regulations) to such a drug, and (II) which has not been the subject of a final determination by the Secretary that it is a 'new drug' (within the meaning of section 201(p) of the Federal Food, Drug, and Cosmetic Act) or an action brought by the Secretary under section 301, 302(a), or 304(a) of such Act to enforce section 502(f) or 505(a) of such Act; or

"(iii)(I) which is described in section 107(c)(3) of the Drug Amendments of 1962 and for which the Secretary has determined there is a compelling justification for its medical need, or is identical, similar, or related (within the meaning of section 310.6(b)(1) of title 21 of the Code of Federal Regulations) to such a drug, and (II) for which the Secretary has not issued a notice of an opportunity for a hearing under section 505(e) of the Federal Food, Drug, and Cosmetic Act on a proposed order of the Secretary to withdraw approval of an application for such drug under such section because the Secretary has determined that the drug is less than effective for all conditions of use prescribed, recommended, or suggested in its labeling;

"(B) A biological product which—

"(i) may only be dispensed upon prescription,

"(ii) is licensed under section 351 of the Public Health Service Act, and

"(iii) is produced at an establishment licensed under such section to produce such product; and

"(C) Insulin certified under section 506 of the Federal Food, Drug, and Cosmetic Act.

"(3) The term 'covered outpatient drug' does not include any product which is intravenously administered in a home setting unless it is a covered home infusion drug (as described in paragraph (5)).

"(4) For purposes of paragraph (2), the term 'medically accepted indication', with respect to the use of an outpatient drug, includes any use which has been approved by the Food and Drug Administration for the drug, and includes another use of the drug if—

"(A) the drug has been approved by the Food and Drug Administration; and

"(B)(i) such use is supported by one or more citations which are included (or approved for inclusion) in one or more of the following compendia: the American Hospital Formulary Service-Drug Information, the American Medical Association Drug

Evaluations, the United States Pharmacopoeia-Drug Information, and other authoritative compendia as identified by the Secretary, unless the Secretary has determined that the use is not medically appropriate or the use is identified as not indicated in one or more such compendia, or

"(ii) the carrier involved determines, based upon guidance provided by the Secretary to carriers for determining accepted uses of drugs, that such use is medically accepted based on supportive clinical evidence in peer reviewed medical literature appearing in publications which have been identified for purposes of this clause by the Secretary.

The Secretary may revise the list of compendia in paragraph (B)(i) designated as appropriate for identifying medically accepted indications for drugs.

"(5)(A) For purposes of paragraph (3), the term 'covered home infusion drug' means a covered outpatient drug dispensed to an individual that—

"(i) is administered intravenously, subcutaneously, epidurally, or through other means determined by the Secretary, using an access device that is inserted in to the body and an infusion device to control the rate of flow of the drug, "(ii) is administered in the individual's home (including an institution used as his home, other than a hospital under subsection (e) or a skilled nursing facility that meets the requirements of section 1819(a)), and

"(iii)(I) is an antibiotic drug and the Secretary has not determined, for the specific drug or the indication to which the drug is applied, that the drug cannot generally be administered safely and effectively in a home setting, or

"(II) is not an antibiotic drug and the Secretary has determined, for the specific drug or the indication to which the drug is applied, that the drug can generally be administered safely and effectively in a home setting.

"(B) Not later than January 1, 1996, (and periodically thereafter), the Secretary shall publish a list of the drugs, and indications for such drugs, that are covered home infusion drugs, with respect to which home infusion drug therapy may be provided under this title.".

(c) EXCEPTIONS; EXCLUSIONS FROM COVERAGE.—Section 1862(a) of such Act (42 U.S.C. 1395y(a)), as amended by sections 4034(b)(4) and 4118(b), is amended—

(1) by striking "and" at the end of paragraph (15),

(2) by striking the period at the end of paragraph (16) and inserting "; or", and

(3) by inserting after paragraph (16) the following new paragraph:

"(17) A covered outpatient drug (as described in section 1861(t))—

"(A) when furnished as part of, or as incident to, any other item or service for which payment may be made under this title, or

"(B) which is listed under paragraph (2) of section 1927(d) (other than subparagraph (I) or (J) of such paragraph) as a drug which may be excluded from coverage under a State plan under title XIX and which the Secretary elects to exclude from coverage under this part.

(d) OTHER CONFORMING AMENDMENTS.—(1) Section 1861 of such Act (42 U.S.C. 1395x) is amended—

(A) in subsection (s)(2), as amended by section 13553 of OBRA–1993—

(i) by striking subparagraphs (O) and (Q),

(ii) by adding "and" at the end of subparagraph (N),

(iii) by striking "; and" at the end of subparagraph (P) and inserting a period, and

(iv) by redesignating subparagraph (P) as subparagraph (O); and

(B) by striking the subsection (jj) added by section 4156(a)(2) of the Omnibus Budget Reconciliation Act of 1990.

(2) Section 1881(b)(1)(C) of such Act (42 U.S.C. 1395rr(b)(1)(C)), as amended by section 13566(a) of OBRA–1993, is amended by striking "section 1861(s)(2)(P)" and inserting "section 1861(s)(2)(O)".

### SEC. 2002. PAYMENT RULES AND RELATED REQUIREMENTS FOR COVERED OUTPATIENT DRUGS.

(a) IN GENERAL.—Section 1834 of the Social Security Act (42 U.S.C. 1395m) is amended by inserting after subsection (c) the following new subsection:

"(d) PAYMENT FOR AND CERTAIN REQUIREMENTS CONCERNING COVERED OUTPATIENT DRUGS.—

"(1) DEDUCTIBLE.—

"(A) IN GENERAL.—Payment shall be made under paragraph (2) only for expenses incurred by an individual for a covered outpatient drug during a calendar year after the individual has incurred expenses in the year for such drugs (during a period in which the individual is entitled to benefits under this part) equal to the deductible amount for that year.

"(B) DEDUCTIBLE AMOUNT.—

"(i) For purposes of subparagraph (A), the deductible amount is—

"(I) for 1996, $250, and

"(II) for any succeeding year, the amount (rounded to the nearest dollar) that the Secretary estimates will ensure that the percentage of the average number of individuals covered under this part (other than individuals enrolled with an eligible organization under section 1876 or an organization described in section 1833(a)(1)(A)) during the year who will incur expenses for covered outpatient drugs equal to or greater than such amount will be the same as the percentage for the previous year.

"(ii) The Secretary shall promulgate the deductible amount for 1997 and each succeeding year during September of the previous year.

"(C) SPECIAL RULE FOR DETERMINATION OF EXPENSES INCURRED.—In determining the amount of expenses incurred by an individual for covered outpatient drugs during a year for purposes of subparagraph (A), there shall not be included any expenses incurred with respect to a drug to the extent such expenses exceed the payment basis for such drug under paragraph (3).

"(2) PAYMENT AMOUNT.—

"(A) IN GENERAL.—Subject to the deductible established under paragraph (1), the amount payable under this part for a covered outpatient drug furnished to an individual during a calendar year shall be equal to—

"(i) 80 percent of the payment basis described in paragraph (3), in the case of an individual who has not incurred expenses for covered outpatient drugs during the year (including the deductible imposed under paragraph (1)) in excess of the out-of-pocket limit for the year under subparagraph (B); and "(ii) 100 percent of the payment basis described in paragraph (3), in the case of any other individual.

"(B) OUT-OF-POCKET LIMIT DESCRIBED.—

"(i) For purposes of subparagraph (A), the out-of-pocket limit for a year is equal to—

"(I) for 1996, $1000, and

"(II) for any succeeding year, the amount (rounded to the nearest dollar) that the Secretary estimates will ensure that the percentage of the average number of individuals covered under this part (other than individuals enrolled with an eligible organization under section 1876 or an organization described in section 1833(a)(1)(A)) during the year who will incur expenses for covered outpatient drugs equal to or greater than such amount will be the same as the percentage for the previous year.

"(ii) The Secretary shall promulgate the out-of-pocket limit for 1997 and each succeeding year during September of the previous year.

"(C) SPECIAL RULE FOR DETERMINATION OF EXPENSES INCURRED.—In determining the amount of expenses incurred by an individual for covered outpatient drugs during a year for purposes of subparagraph (A), there shall not be included any expenses incurred with respect to a drug to the extent such expenses exceed the payment basis for such drug under paragraph (3).

"(3) PAYMENT BASIS.—For purposes of paragraph (2), the payment basis is the lesser of—

"(A) the actual charge for a covered outpatient drug, or

"(B) the applicable payment limit established under paragraph (4).

"(4) PAYMENT LIMITS.—

"(A) PAYMENT LIMIT FOR SINGLE SOURCE DRUGS AND MULTIPLE SOURCE DRUGS WITH RESTRICTIVE PRESCRIPTIONS.—In the case of a covered outpatient drug that is a multiple source drug which has a restrictive prescription, or that is single source drug, the payment limit for a payment calculation period is equal to—

"(i) for drugs furnished after 1996, the 90th percentile of the actual charges (computed on the geographic basis specified by the Secretary) for the drug product for the second previous payment calculation period, or

"(ii) the amount of the administrative allowance (established under paragraph (5)) plus the product of the number of dosage units dispensed and the per unit estimated acquisition cost for the drug product (determined under subparagraph (C)) for the period,

whichever is less.

"(B) PAYMENT LIMIT FOR MULTIPLE SOURCE DRUGS WITHOUT RESTRICTIVE PRESCRIPTIONS.—In the case of a drug that is a multiple source drug which does not have a restrictive prescription, the payment limit for a payment calculation period is equal to the amount of the administrative allowance (established under paragraph (5)) plus the product of the number of dosage units dispensed and the unweighted median of the unit estimated acquisition cost (determined under subparagraph (C)) for the drug products for the period.

"(C) DETERMINATION OF UNIT PRICE.—

"(i) IN GENERAL.—The Secretary shall determine, for the dispensing of a covered outpatient drug product in a payment calculation period, the estimated acquisition cost for the drug product. With respect to any covered outpatient drug product, such cost may not exceed 93 percent of the average manufacturer non-retail price for the drug (as defined in section 1850(f)(2)) during the period.

"(ii) COMPLIANCE WITH REQUEST FOR INFORMATION.—If a wholesaler or direct seller of a covered outpatient drug refuses, after being requested by the Secretary, to provide price information requested to carry out clause (i), or deliberately provides information that is false, the Secretary may impose a civil money penalty of not to exceed $10,000 for each such refusal or provision of false information. The provisions of section 1128A (other than subsections (a) and (b)) shall apply to civil money penalties under the previous sentence in the same manner as they apply to a penalty or proceeding under section 1128A(a). Information gathered pursuant to clause (i) shall not be disclosed except as the Secretary determines to be necessary to carry out the purposes of this part.

"(5) ADMINISTRATIVE ALLOWANCE FOR PURPOSES OF PAYMENT LIMIT.—

"(A) IN GENERAL.—Except as provided in subparagraph (B), the administrative allowance under paragraph (4) is—

"(i) for 1996, $5, and

"(ii) for each succeeding year, the amount for the previous year adjusted by the percentage change in the consumer price index for all urban consumers (U.S. city average) for the 12-month period ending with June of that previous year.

"(B) REDUCTION FOR MAIL ORDER PHARMACIES.—The Secretary may, after consulting with representatives of pharmacists, individuals enrolled under this part, and of private insurers, reduce the administrative allowances established under subparagraph (A) for any covered outpatient drug dispensed by a mail order pharmacy, based on differences between such pharmacies and other pharmacies with respect to operating costs and other economies.

"(6) ASSURING APPROPRIATE PRESCRIBING AND DISPENSING PRACTICES.—

"(A) IN GENERAL.—The Secretary shall establish a program to identify (and to educate physicians and pharmacists concerning)—

"(i) instances or patterns of unnecessary or inappropriate prescribing or dispensing practices for covered outpatient drugs,

"(ii) instances or patterns of substandard care with respect to such drugs,

"(iii) potential adverse reactions, and

"(iv) appropriate use of generic products.

"(B) STANDARDS.—In carrying out the program under subparagraph (A), the Secretary shall establish for each covered outpatient drug standards for the prescribing of the drug which are based on accepted medical practice. In establishing such standards, the Secretary shall incorporate standards from such current authoritative compendia as the Secretary may select, except that the Secretary may modify such a standard by regulation on the basis of scientific and medical information that such standard is not consistent with the safe and effective use of the drug.

"(C) DRUG USE REVIEW.—The Secretary may provide for a drug use review program with respect to covered outpatient drugs dispensed to individuals eligible for benefits under this part. Such program may include such elements as the Secretary determines to be necessary to assure that prescriptions (i) are appropriate, (ii) are medically necessary, and (iii) are not likely to result in adverse medical results, including any elements of the State drug use review programs required under section 1927(g) that the Secretary determines to be appropriate.

"(7) ADMINISTRATIVE IMPROVEMENTS.—The Secretary shall develop, in consultation with representatives of pharmacies and of other interested persons, a standard claims form for covered outpatient drugs in accordance with title V of the Health Security Act.

"(8) DEFINITIONS.—In this subsection:

"(A) MULTIPLE AND SINGLE SOURCE DRUGS.—The terms 'multiple source drug' and 'single source drug' have the meanings of those terms under section 1927(k)(7).

"(B) RESTRICTIVE PRESCRIPTION.—A drug has a 'restrictive prescription' only if—

"(i) in the case of a written prescription, the prescription for the drug indicates, in the handwriting of the physician or other person prescribing the drug and with an appropriate phrase (such as 'brand medically necessary') recognized by the Secretary, that a particular drug product must be dispensed, or

"(ii) in the case of a prescription issued by telephone—

"(I) the physician or other person prescribing the drug (through use of such an appropriate phrase) states that a particular drug product must be dispensed, and

"(II) the physician or other person submits to the pharmacy involved, within 30 days after the date of the telephone prescription, a written confirmation which is in the handwriting of the physician or other person prescribing the drug and which indicates with such appropriate phrase that the particular drug product was required to have been dispensed.

"(C) PAYMENT CALCULATION PERIOD.—The term 'payment calculation period' means the 6-month period beginning with January of each year and the 6-month period beginning with July of each year.".

(b) SUBMISSION OF CLAIMS BY PHARMACIES.—Section 1848(g)(4) of such Act (42 U.S.C. 1395w–4(g)(4)) is amended—

 (1) in the heading—

  (A) by striking "PHYSICIAN", and

  (B) by inserting "BY PHYSICIANS AND SUPPLIERS" after "CLAIMS",

 (2) in the matter in subparagraph (A) preceding clause (i)—

(A) by striking "For services furnished on or after September 1, 1990, within 1 year" and inserting "Within 1 year (90 days in the case of covered outpatient drugs)",

(B) by striking "a service" and inserting "an item or service", and

(C) by inserting "or of providing a covered outpatient drug," after "basis," and

(3) in subparagraph (A)(i), by inserting "item or" before "service.

(c) SPECIAL RULES FOR CARRIERS.—

(1) USE OF REGIONAL CARRIERS.—Section 1842(b)(2) of such Act (42 U.S.C. 1395u(b)(2)) is amended by adding at the end the following:

"(D) With respect to activities related to covered outpatient drugs, the Secretary may enter into contracts with carriers under this section to perform the activities on a regional basis.".

(2) PAYMENT ON OTHER THAN A COST BASIS.—Section 1842(c)(1)(A) of such Act (42 U.S.C. 1395u(c)(1)(A)) is amended—

(A) by inserting "(i)" after "(c)(1)(A)",

(B) in the first sentence, by inserting ", except as otherwise provided in clause (ii)," after "under this part, and", and

(C) by adding at the end the following:

"(ii) To the extent that a contract under this section provides for activities related to covered outpatient drugs, the Secretary may provide for payment for those activities based on any method of payment determined by the Secretary to be appropriate.".

(3) USE OF OTHER ENTITIES FOR COVERED OUTPATIENT DRUGS.—Section 1842(f) of such Act (42 U.S.C. 1395u(f)) is amended—

(A) by striking "and" at the end of paragraph (1),

(B) by substituting "; and" for the period at the end of paragraph (2), and,

(C) by adding at the end the following:

"(3) with respect to activities related to covered outpatient drugs, any other private entity which the Secretary determines is qualified to conduct such activities.".

(4) DESIGNATED CARRIERS TO PROCESS CLAIMS OF RAILROAD RETIREES.—Section 1842(g) of such Act (42 U.S.C. 1395u(g)) is amended by inserting "(other than functions related to covered outpatient drugs)" after "functions".

(d) CONTRACTS FOR AUTOMATIC DATA PROCESSING EQUIPMENT.—Actions taken before 1995 that affect contracts related to the processing of claims for covered outpatient drugs (as defined in section 1861(t) of the Social Security Act) shall not be subject to section 111 of the Federal Property and Administrative Services Act of 1949, and shall not be subject to administrative or judicial review.

(e) CONFORMING AMENDMENTS.—

(1)(A) Section 1833(a)(1) of such Act (42 U.S.C. 1395l(a)(1)), as amended by section 13544(b)(2) of OBRA–1993, is amended—

(i) by striking "and" at the end of clause (O), and

(ii) by inserting before the semicolon at the end the following: ", and (Q) with respect to covered outpatient drugs, the amounts paid shall be as prescribed by section 1834(d)".

(B) Section 1833(a)(2) of such Act (42 U.S.C. 1395l(a)(2)) is amended in the matter preceding subparagraph (A) by inserting ", except for covered outpatient drugs," after "and (I) of such section".

(2) Section 1833(b)(2) of such Act (42 U.S.C. 1395l(b)(2)) is amended by inserting "or with respect to covered outpatient drugs" before the comma.

(3) The first sentence of section 1842(h)(2) of such Act (42 U.S.C. 1395u(h)(2)) is amended by inserting "(other than a carrier described in subsection (f)(3))" after "Each carrier".

(4) The first sentence of section 1866(a)(2)(A) of such Act (42 U.S.C. 1395cc(a)(2)(A)) is amended—

(A) in clause (i), by inserting "section 1834(d), after "section 1833(b),", and

(B) in clause (ii), by inserting ", other than for covered outpatient drugs," after "provider)".

### SEC. 2003. MEDICARE REBATES FOR COVERED OUTPATIENT DRUGS.

(a) IN GENERAL.—Part B of title XVIII of the Social Security Act is amended by adding at the end the following new section:

"REBATES FOR COVERED OUTPATIENT DRUGS

"Sec. 1850. (a) REQUIREMENT FOR REBATE AGREEMENT.—In order for payment to be available under this part for covered outpatient drugs of a manufacturer dispensed on or after January 1, 1996, the manufacturer must have entered into and have in effect a rebate agreement with the Secretary meeting the requirements of subsection (b), and an agreement to give equal access to discounts in accordance with subsection (e).

"(b) TERMS, IMPLEMENTATION, AND ENFORCEMENT OF REBATE AGREEMENT.—

"(1) PERIODIC REBATES.—

"(A) IN GENERAL.—A rebate agreement under this section shall require the manufacturer to pay to the Secretary for each calendar quarter, not later than 30 days after the date of receipt of the information described in paragraph (2) for such quarter, a rebate in an amount determined under subsection (c) for all covered outpatient drugs of the manufacturer described in subparagraph (B).

"(B) DRUGS INCLUDED IN QUARTERLY REBATE CALCULATION.—Drugs subject to rebate with respect to a calendar quarter are drugs which are either—

"(i) dispensed by participating pharmacies during such quarter to individuals (other than individuals enrolled with an eligible organization with a contract under section 1876) eligible for benefits under this part, as reported by such pharmacies to the Secretary, or

"(ii) dispensed by nonparticipating pharmacies to such individuals and included in claims for payment of benefits received by the Secretary during such quarter.

"(2) INFORMATION FURNISHED TO MANUFACTURERS.—

"(A) IN GENERAL.—The Secretary shall report to each manufacturer, not later than 60 days after the end of each calendar quarter, information on the total number, for each covered outpatient drug, of units of each dosage form, strength, and package size dispensed under the plan during the quarter, on the basis of the data reported to the Secretary described in paragraph (1)(B).

"(B) AUDIT.—The Comptroller General may audit the records of the Secretary to the extent necessary to determine the accuracy of reports by the Secretary pursuant to subparagraph (A). Adjustments to rebates shall be made to the extent determined necessary by the audit to reflect actual units of drugs dispensed.

"(3) PROVISION OF PRICE INFORMATION BY MANUFACTURER.—

"(A) QUARTERLY PRICING INFORMATION.—Each manufacturer with an agreement in effect under this section shall report to the Secretary, not later than 30 days after the last day of each calendar quarter, on the average manufacturer retail price and the average manufacturer non-retail price for each dosage form and strength of each covered outpatient drug for the quarter.

"(B) BASE QUARTER PRICES.—Each manufacturer of a covered outpatient drug with an agreement under this section shall report to the Secretary, by not later than 30 days after the effective date of such agreement (or, if later, 30 days after the end of the base quarter), the average manufacturer retail price, for such base quarter, for each dosage form and strength of each such covered drug.

"(C) VERIFICATION OF AVERAGE MANUFACTURER PRICE.—The Secretary may inspect the records of manufacturers, and survey wholesalers, pharmacies, and institutional purchasers of drugs, as necessary to verify prices reported under subparagraph (A).

"(D) PENALTIES.—

"(i) CIVIL MONEY PENALTIES.—The Secretary may impose a civil money penalty on a manufacturer with an agreement under this section—

"(I) for failure to provide information required under subparagraph (A) on a timely basis, in an amount up to $10,000 per day of delay;

"(II) for refusal to provide information about charges or prices requested by the Secretary for purposes of verification pursuant to subparagraph (C), in an amount up to $100,000; and

"(III) for provision, pursuant to subparagraph (A) or (B), of information that the manufacturer knows or should know is false, in an amount up to $100,000 per item of information. Such civil money penalties are in addition to any other penalties prescribed by law. The provisions of section 1128A (other than subsections (a) (with respect to amounts of penalties or additional assessments) and (b)) shall apply to a civil money penalty under this subparagraph in the same manner as such provisions apply to a penalty or proceeding under section 1128A(a).

"(ii) TERMINATION OF AGREEMENT.—If a manufacturer with an agreement under this section has not provided information required under subparagraph (A) or (B) within 90 days of the deadline imposed, the Secretary may suspend the agreement with respect to covered outpatient drugs dispensed after the end of such 90-day period and until the date such information is reported (but in no case shall a suspension be for less than 30 days).

"(4) LENGTH OF AGREEMENT.—

"(A) IN GENERAL.—A rebate agreement shall be effective for an initial period of not less than one year and shall be automatically renewed for a period of not less than one year unless terminated under subparagraph (B).

"(B) TERMINATION.—

"(i) BY THE SECRETARY.—The Secretary may provide for termination of a rebate agreement for violation of the requirements of the agreement or other good cause shown. Such termination shall not be effective earlier than 60 days after the date of notice of such termination. The Secretary shall afford a manufacturer an opportunity for a hearing concerning such termination, but such hearing shall not delay the effective date of the termination.

"(ii) BY A MANUFACTURER.—A manufacturer may terminate a rebate agreement under this section for any reason. Any such termination shall not be effective until the calendar quarter beginning at least 60 days after the date the manufacturer provides notice to the Secretary.

"(iii) EFFECTIVE DATE OF TERMINATION.—Any termination under this subparagraph shall not affect rebates due under the agreement before the effective date of its termination.

"(iv) NOTICE TO PHARMACIES.—In the case of a termination under this subparagraph, the Secretary shall notify pharmacies that are participating suppliers under this part and physician organizations not less than 30 days before the effective date of such termination.

"(c) AMOUNT OF REBATE.—

"(1) BASIC REBATE.—Each manufacturer shall remit a basic rebate to the Secretary for each calendar quarter in an amount, with respect to each dosage form and strength of a covered drug (except as provided under paragraph (4)), equal to the product of—

"(A) the total number of units subject to rebate for such quarter, as described in subsection (b)(1)(B); and

"(B) the greater of—

"(i) the difference between the average manufacturer retail price and the average manufacturer non-retail price,

"(ii) 17 percent of the average manufacturer retail price, or

"(iii) the amount determined pursuant to paragraph (4).

"(2) ADDITIONAL REBATE.—Each manufacturer shall remit to the Secretary, for each calendar quarter, an additional rebate for each dosage form and strength of a covered drug (except as provided under paragraph (4)), in an amount equal to—

"(A) the total number of units subject to rebate for such quarter, as described in subsection (b)(1)(B), multiplied by

"(B) the amount, if any, by which the average manufacturer retail price for covered drugs of the manufacturer exceeds the average manufacturer retail price for the base quarter, increased by the percentage increase in the Consumer Price Index for all urban consumers (U.S. average) from the end of such base quarter to the month before the beginning of such calendar quarter.

"(3) NEGOTIATED REBATE AMOUNT FOR NEW DRUGS.—

"(A) IN GENERAL.—The Secretary may negotiate with the manufacturer a per-unit rebate amount, in accordance with this paragraph, for any covered outpatient drug (except as provided under paragraph (4)) first marketed after June 30, 1993—

"(i) which is not marketed in any country specified in section 802(b)(4)(A) of the Federal Food, Drug, and Cosmetic Act and for which the Secretary believes the average manufacturer's retail price may be excessive, or

"(ii) which is marketed in one or more of such countries, at prices significantly lower than the average manufacturer retail price.

"(B) MAXIMUM REBATE AMOUNT FOR DRUGS MARKETED IN CERTAIN COUNTRIES.—The rebate negotiated pursuant to this paragraph for a drug described in subparagraph (A)(ii) may be an amount up to the difference between the average manufacturer retail price and any price at which the drug is available to wholesalers in a country specified in such section 802(b)(4)(A).

"(C) FACTORS TO BE CONSIDERED.—In making determinations with respect to the prices of a covered drug described in subparagraph (A) and in negotiating a rebate amount pursuant to this paragraph, the Secretary shall take into consideration, as applicable and appropriate, the prices of other drugs in the same therapeutic class, cost information requested by the Secretary and supplied by the manufacturer or estimated by the Secretary, prescription volumes, economies of scale, product stability, special manufacturing requirements, prices of the drug in countries specified in subparagraph (A)(i) (in the case of a drug described in such subparagraph), and other relevant factors.

"(D) OPTION TO EXCLUDE COVERAGE.—If the Secretary is unable to negotiate with the manufacturer an acceptable rebate amount with respect to a covered outpatient drug pursuant to this paragraph, the Secretary may exclude such drug from coverage under this part.

"(E) EFFECTIVE DATE OF EXCLUSION FROM COVERAGE.—An exclusion of a drug from coverage pursuant to subparagraph (D) shall be effective on and after—

"(i) the date 6 months after the effective date of marketing approval of such drug by the Food and Drug Administration, or

"(ii) (if earlier) the date the manufacturer terminates negotiations with the Secretary concerning the rebate amount.

"(4) NO REBATE REQUIRED FOR GENERIC DRUGS.—Paragraphs (1) through (3) shall not apply with respect to a covered outpatient drug that is not a single source drug or an innovator multiple source drug (as such terms are defined in section 1927(k)).

"(5) DEPOSIT OF REBATES.—The Secretary shall deposit rebates under this section in the Federal Supplementary Medical Insurance Trust Fund established under section 1841.

"(d) CONFIDENTIALITY OF INFORMATION.—Notwithstanding any other provision of law, information disclosed by a manufacturer under this section is confidential and shall not be disclosed by the Secretary, except—

"(A) as the Secretary determines to be necessary to carry out this section,

"(B) to permit the Comptroller General to review the information provided, and

"(C) to permit the Director of the Congressional Budget Office to review the information provided.

"(e) AGREEMENT TO GIVE EQUAL ACCESS TO DISCOUNTS.—An agreement under this subsection by a manufacturer of covered outpatient drugs shall guarantee that the manufacturer will offer, to each wholesaler or retailer (or other purchaser representing a group of such wholesalers or retailers) that purchases such drugs on substantially the same terms (including such terms as prompt payment, cash payment, volume purchase, single-site delivery, the use of formularies by purchasers, and any other terms effectively reducing the manufacturer's costs) as any other purchaser (including any institutional purchaser) the same price for such drugs as is offered to such other purchaser. In determining a manufacturer's compliance with the previous sentence, there shall not be taken into account terms offered to the Department of Veterans Affairs, the Department of Defense, or any public program.

"(f) DEFINITIONS.—For purposes of this section—

"(1) AVERAGE MANUFACTURER RETAIL PRICE.—The term 'average manufacturer retail price' means, with respect to a covered outpatient drug of a manufacturer for a calendar quarter, the average price (inclusive of discounts for cash payment, prompt payment, volume purchases, and rebates (other than rebates under this section), but exclusive of nominal prices) paid to the manufacturer for the drug in the United States for drugs distributed to the retail pharmacy class of trade.

"(2) AVERAGE MANUFACTURER NON-RETAIL PRICE.—The term 'average manufacturer non-retail price' means, with respect to a covered outpatient drug of a manufacturer for a calendar quarter, the weighted average price (inclusive of discounts for cash payment, prompt payment, volume purchases, and rebates (other than rebates under this section), but exclusive of nominal prices) paid to the manufacturer for the drug in the United States by hospitals and other institutional purchasers that purchase drugs for institutional use and not for resale.

"(3) BASE QUARTER.—The term 'base quarter' means, with respect to a covered outpatient drug of a manufacturer, the calendar quarter beginning April 1, 1993, or (if later) the first full calendar quarter during which the drug was marketed in the United States.

"(4) COVERED DRUG.—The term 'covered drug' includes each innovator multiple source drug and single source drug, as those terms are defined in section 1927(k)(7).

"(5) MANUFACTURER.—The term 'manufacturer' means, with respect to a covered outpatient drug—

"(A) the entity whose National Drug Code number (as issued pursuant to section 510(e) of the Federal Food, Drug, and Cosmetic Act) appears on the labeling of the drug; or

"(B) if the number described in subparagraph (A) does not appear on the labeling of the drug, the person named as the applicant in a human drug application (in the case of a new drug) or the product license application (in the case of a biological product) for such drug approved by the Food and Drug Administration.".

(b) CONFORMING AMENDMENT RELATING TO EXCLUSIONS FROM COVERAGE.—Section 1862(a)(18) of such Act (42 U.S.C. 1395y(a)), as added by section 2001(c), is amended—

(A) by striking "or" at the end of subparagraph (A),

(B) by striking the period at the end of subparagraph (B) and inserting ", or", and

(C) by adding at the end the following new subparagraphs:

"(C) furnished during a year for which the drug's manufacturer does not have in effect a rebate agreement with the Secretary that meets the requirements of section 1850 for the year, or

"(D) excluded from coverage during the year by the Secretary pursuant to section 1850(c)(3)(D) (relating to negotiated rebate amounts for certain new drugs).".

### SEC. 2004. COUNSELING BY PARTICIPATING PHARMACIES.

Section 1842(h) of the Social Security Act (42 U.S.C. 1395u(h)) is amended by adding at the end the following:

"(8) A pharmacy that is a participating supplier under this part shall agree to answer questions of individuals enrolled under this part who receive a covered outpatient drug from the pharmacy regarding the appropriate use of the drug, potential interactions between the drug and other drugs dispensed to the individual, and other matters relating to the dispensing of such drugs.".

### SEC. 2005. EXTENSION OF 25 PERCENT RULE FOR PORTION OF PREMIUM ATTRIBUTABLE TO COVERED OUTPATIENT DRUGS.

Section 1839(e) of the Social Security Act (42 U.S.C. 1395r(e)) is amended by adding at the end the following:

"(3) Notwithstanding the provisions of subsection (a), the portion of the monthly premium for each individual enrolled under this part for each month after December 1998 that is attributable to covered outpatient drugs shall be an amount equal to 50 percent of the portion of the monthly actuarial rate for enrollees age 65 and over, as determined under subsection (a)(1) and applicable to such month, that is attributable to covered outpatient drugs.".

**SEC. 2006. COVERAGE OF HOME INFUSION DRUG THERAPY SERVICES.**

(a) IN GENERAL.—Section 1832(a)(2)(A) of the Social Security Act (42 U.S.C. 1395k(a)(2)(A)) is amended by inserting "and home infusion drug therapy services" before the semicolon.

(b) HOME INFUSION DRUG THERAPY SERVICES DEFINED.—Section 1861 of such Act (42 U.S.C. 1395x) is amended—

    (1) by redesignating the subsection (jj) inserted by section 4156(a)(2) of the Omnibus Budget Reconciliation Act of 1990 as subsection (kk); and

    (2) by inserting after such subsection the following new subsection:

    "Home Infusion Drug Therapy Services

    "(ll)(1) The term 'home infusion drug therapy services' means the items and services described in paragraph (2) furnished to an individual who is under the care of a physician—

        "(A) in a place of residence used as the individual's home,

        "(B) by a qualified home infusion drug therapy provider (as defined in paragraph (3)) or by others under arrangements with them made by that provider, and

"(C) under a plan established and periodically reviewed by a physician.

"(2) The items and services described in this paragraph are such nursing, pharmacy, and related services (including medical supplies, intravenous fluids, delivery, and equipment) as are necessary to conduct safely and effectively a drug regimen through use of a covered home infusion drug (as defined in subsection (t)(5)), but do not include such covered outpatient drugs.

"(3) The term 'qualified home infusion drug therapy provider' means any entity that the secretary determines meets the following requirements:

"(A) The entity is capable of providing or arranging for the items and services described in paragraph (2) and covered home infusion drugs.

"(B) The entity maintains clinical records on all patients.

"(C) The entity adheres to written protocols and policies with respect to the provision of items and services.

"(D) The entity makes services available (as needed) seven days a week on a 24-hour basis.

"(E) The entity coordinates all service with the patient's physician.

"(F) The entity conducts a quality assessment and assurance program, including drug regimen review and coordination of patient care.

"(G) The entity assures that only trained personnel provide covered home infusion drugs (and any other service for which training is required to provide the service safely).

"(H) The entity assumes responsibility for the quality of services provided by others under arrangements with the entity.

"(I) In the case of an entity in any State in which State or applicable local law provides for the licensing of entities of this nature, (A) is licensed pursuant to such law, or (B) is approved, by the agency of such State or locality responsible for licensing entities of this nature, as meeting the standards established for such licensing.

"(J) The entity meets such other requirements as the Secretary may determine are necessary to assure the safe and effective provision of home infusion drug therapy services and the efficient administration of the home infusion drug therapy benefit.".

(c) PAYMENT.—

(1) IN GENERAL.—Section 1833 of such Act (42 U.S.C. 1395l) is amended—

(A) in subsection (a)(2)(B), by striking "or (E)" and inserting "(E), or (F)",

(B) in subsection (a)(2)(D), by striking "and" at the end,

(C) in subsection (a)(2)(E), by striking the semicolon and inserting "; and",

(D) by inserting after subsection (a)(2)(E) the following new subparagraph:

"(F) with resect to home infusion drug therapy services, the amounts described in section 1834(j);",

(E) in the first sentence of subsection (b), by striking "services, (3)" and inserting "services and home infusion drug therapy services, (3)".

(2) AMOUNT DESCRIBED.—Section 1834 of such Act, as amended by section 13544(b)(i) of OBRA–1993, is amended by adding at the end the following new subsection:

"(j) HOME INFUSION DRUG THERAPY SERVICES.—

"(1) IN GENERAL.—With respect to home infusion drug therapy services, payment under this part shall be made in an amount equal to the lesser of the actual charges for such services or the fee schedule established under paragraph (2).

"(2) ESTABLISHMENT OF FEE SCHEDULE.—
The Secretary shall establish by regulation before the beginning of 1996 and each succeeding year a fee schedule for home infusion drug therapy services for which payment is made under this part. A fee schedule established under this subsection shall be on a per diem basis.".

(3) PROHIBITION ON CERTAIN REFERRALS.—Section 1877(h)(6) of such Act (42 U.S.C. 1395nn(h)(6)), as amended by section 13562(a) of OBRA–1993, is amended by adding at the end the following:

"(L) Home infusion drug therapy services.".

(d) CERTIFICATION.—Section 1835(a)(2) of such Act (42 U.S.C. 1395n(a)(2)) is amended—

(1) by striking "and" at the end of subparagraph (E),

(2) by striking the period at the end of subparagraph (F) and inserting "; and", and

(3) by inserting after subparagraph (F) the following:

"(G) in the case of home infusion drug therapy services, (i) such services are or were required because the individual needed such services for the administration of a covered home infusion drug, (ii) a plan for furnishing such services has been established and is reviewed periodically by a physician, and (iii) such services are or were furnished while the individual is or was under the care of a physician.".

(e) CERTIFICATION OF HOME INFUSION DRUG THERAPY PROVIDERS; INTERMEDIATE SANCTIONS FOR NONCOMPLIANCE.—

(1) TREATMENT AS PROVIDER OF SERVICES.—Section 1861(u) of such Act (42 U.S.C. 1395x(u)) is amended by inserting "home infusion drug therapy provider," after "hospice program,".

(2) CONSULTATION WITH STATE AGENCIES AND OTHER ORGANIZATIONS.—Section 1863 of such Act (42 U.S.C. 1395z) is amended by striking "and (dd)(2)" and inserting "(dd)(2), and (ll)(3)".

(3) USE OF STATE AGENCIES IN DETERMINING COMPLIANCE.—Section 1864(a) of such Act (42 U.S.C. 1395aa(a)) is amended—

(A) in the first sentence, by striking "an agency is a hospice program" and inserting "an agency or entity is a hospice program or a home infusion drug therapy provider," after "home health agency, or whether"; and

(B) in the second sentence—

(i) by striking "institution or agency" and inserting "institution, agency, or entity", and

(ii) by striking "or hospice program" and inserting "hospice program, or home infusion drug therapy provider".

(4) APPLICATION OF INTERMEDIATE SANCTIONS.—Section 1846 of such Act (42 U.S.C. 1395w–2) is amended—

(A) in the heading, by adding "AND FOR QUALIFIED HOME INFUSION DRUG THERAPY PROVIDERS" at the end,

(B) in subsection (a), by inserting "or that a qualified home infusion drug therapy provider that is certified for participation under this title no longer substantially meets the requirements of section 1861(ll)(3)" after "under this part", and

(C) in subsection (b)(2)(A)(iv), by inserting "or home infusion drug therapy services" after "clinical diagnostic laboratory tests".

(f) USE OF REGIONAL INTERMEDIARIES IN ADMINISTRATION OF BENEFIT.—Section 1816 of such Act (42 U.S.C. 1395h) is amended by adding at the end the following new subsection:

"(k) With respect to carrying out functions relating to payment for home infusion drug therapy services and covered home infusion drugs, the Secretary may enter into contracts with agencies or organizations under this section to perform such functions on a regional basis.".

## SEC. 2007. CIVIL MONEY PENALTIES FOR EXCESSIVE CHARGES.

Section 1128A(a) of the Social Security Act (42 U.S.C. 1320a–7a(a)), as amended by sections 4041(a)(1), 4043(a)(1), and 4043(c), is amended—

(1) by striking ",or" at the end of paragraph (5) and adding a semicolon,

(3) by adding "or" at the end of paragraph (6), and

(4) by inserting after paragraph (6) the following:

"(7) in the case of a pharmacy, presents or causes to be presented to any person a request for payment for covered outpatient drugs (as defined in section 1861(t)) dispensed to an individual enrolled under part B of title XVIII and for which the amount charged by the pharmacy is greater than the amount the pharmacy charges the general public (as determined by the Secretary);".

## SEC. 2008. CONFORMING AMENDMENTS TO MEDICAID PROGRAM.

(a) IN GENERAL.—

(1) REQUIRING MEDICARE REBATE AS CONDITION OF COVERAGE.—The first sentence of section 1927(a)(1) of the Social Security Act (42 U.S.C. 1396r–8(a)(1)) is amended—

(A) in the first sentence of paragraph (1), by striking "and paragraph (6)" and inserting ", paragraph (6), and (for calendar quarters beginning on or after January 1, 1996) paragraph (7)"; and

(B) by adding at the end the following new paragraph:

"(7) REQUIREMENT RELATING TO REBATE AGREEMENTS FOR COVERED OUTPATIENT DRUGS UNDER MEDICARE PROGRAM.—A manufacturer meets the requirements of this paragraph for quarters in a year if the manufacturer has in effect an agreement with the Secretary under section 1850 for providing rebates for covered outpatient drugs furnished to individuals under title XVIII during the year.".

(2) NON-DUPLICATION OF REBATES.—Section 1927(b)(1) of the Social Security Act (42 U.S.C. 1396r–8(b)(1)) is amended—

(A) by redesignating subparagraph (B) as subparagraph (C), and

(B) by inserting after subparagraph (A) the following new subparagraph:

"(B) NON-DUPLICATION OF MEDICARE REBATE.—Covered drugs furnished to an individual eligible for benefits under both part B of title XVIII and a State plan under this title shall not be included in the determination of units of covered outpatient drugs subject to rebate under this section.".

(b) EFFECTIVE DATE.—The amendments made by subsection (a) shall apply to quarters beginning on or after January 1, 1996.

## SEC. 2009. EFFECTIVE DATE.

The amendments made by this subtitle shall apply to items and services furnished on or after January 1, 1996.

# Subtitle B—Long-Term Care

## PART 1—STATE PROGRAMS FOR HOME AND COMMUNITY-BASED SERVICES FOR INDIVIDUALS WITH DISABILITIES

### SEC. 2101. STATE PROGRAMS FOR HOME AND COMMUNITY-BASED SERVICES FOR INDIVIDUALS WITH DISABILITIES.

(a) IN GENERAL.—Each State that has a plan for the home and community-based services to individuals with disabilities submitted to and approved by the Secretary under section 2102(b) is entitled to payment in accordance with section 2108.

(b) NO INDIVIDUAL ENTITLEMENT ESTABLISHED.—Nothing in this part shall be construed to create an entitlement in individuals or a requirement that a State with such an approved plan expend the entire amount of funds to which it is entitled in any year.

(c) STATE DEFINED.—In this subpart, the term "State" includes the District of Columbia, Puerto Rico, the Virgin Islands, Guam, American Samoa, and the Northern Mariana Islands.

### SEC. 2102. STATE PLANS.

(a) PLAN REQUIREMENTS.—In order to be approved under subsection (b), a State plan for home and community-based services for individuals with disabilities must meet the following requirements (except to the extent provided in subsection (b)(2), relating to phase-in period):

(1) ELIGIBILITY.—

(A) IN GENERAL.—Within the amounts provided by the State (and under section 2108) for such program, the plan shall provide that services under the plan will be available to individuals with disabilities (as defined in section 2103(a)) in the State.

(B) INITIAL SCREENING.—The plan shall provide a process for the initial screening of individuals who appear to have some reasonable likelihood of being an individual with disabilities.

(C) RESTRICTIONS.—The plan may not limit the eligibility of individuals with disabilities based on—

(i) income,

(ii) age,

(iii) geography,

(iv) nature, severity, or category of disability,

(v) residential setting (other than an institutional setting), or

(vi) other grounds specified by the Secretary.

(D) MAINTENANCE OF EFFORT.—The plan must provide assurances that, in the case of an individual receiving medical assistance for home and community-based services under the State medicaid plan as of the date of the enactment of this Act, the State will continue to make available (either under this plan, under the State medicaid plan, or otherwise) to such individual an appropriate level of assistance for home and community-based services, taking into account the level of assistance provided as of such date and the individual's need for home and community-based services.

(2) SERVICES.—

(A) SPECIFICATION.—Consistent with section 2104, the plan shall specify—

(i) the services made available under the State plan,

(ii) the extent and manner in which such services are allocated and made available to individuals with disabilities, and

(iii) the manner in which services under the State plan are coordinated with each other and with health and long-term care services available outside the plan for individuals with disabilities.

Subject to section 2104(e)(1)(B), such services may be delivered in an individual's home, a range of community residential arrangements, or outside the home.

(B) ALLOCATION.—The State plan—

(i) shall specify how it will allocate services under the plan, during and after the 7-fiscal-year phase-in period beginning with fiscal year 1996, among covered individuals with disabilities, and

(ii) may not allocate such services based on the income or other financial resources of such individuals.

(C) LIMITATION ON LICENSURE OR CERTIFICATION.—The State may not subject consumer-directed providers of personal assistance services to licensure, certification, or other requirements which the Secretary finds not to be necessary for the health and safety of individuals with disabilities.

(D) CONSUMER CHOICE.—To the extent possible, the choice of an individual with disabilities (and that individual's family) regarding which covered services to receive and the providers who will provide such services shall be followed.

(E) REQUIREMENT TO SERVE LOW-INCOME INDIVIDUALS.—The State plan shall assure that—

(i) the proportion of the population of low-income individuals with disabilities in the State that represents individuals with disabilities who are provided home and community-based services either under the plan, under the State medicaid plan, or under both, is not less than

(ii) the proportion of the population of the State that represents individuals who are low-income individuals.

(3) COST SHARING.—The plan shall impose cost sharing with respect to covered services only in accordance with section 2105.

(4) TYPES OF PROVIDERS AND REQUIREMENTS FOR PARTICIPATION.—The plan shall specify—

(A) the types of service providers eligible to participate in the program under the plan, which shall include consumer-directed providers, and

  (B) any requirements for participation applicable to each type of service provider.

(5) BUDGET.—The plan shall specify how the State will manage Federal and State funds available under the plan during each 5-fiscal-year period (with the first such period beginning with fiscal year 1996) to serve all categories of individuals with disabilities and meet the requirements of this subsection.

(6) PROVIDER REIMBURSEMENT.—

  (A) PAYMENT METHODS.—The plan shall specify the payment methods to be used to reimburse providers for services furnished under the plan. Such methods may include retrospective reimbursement on a fee-for-service basis, prepayment on a capitation basis, payment by cash or vouchers to individuals with disabilities, or any combination of these methods. In the case of the use of cash or vouchers, the plan shall specify how the plan will assure compliance with applicable employment tax provisions.

  (B) PAYMENT RATES.—The plan shall specify the methods and criteria to be used to set payment rates for services furnished under the plan (including rates for cash payments or vouchers to individuals with disabilities).

(C) PLAN PAYMENT AS PAYMENT IN FULL.—The plan shall restrict payment under the plan for covered services to those providers that agree to accept the payment under the plan (at the rates established pursuant to subparagraph (B)) and any cost sharing permitted or provided for under section 2105 as payment in full for services furnished under the plan.

(7) QUALITY ASSURANCE AND SAFEGUARDS.—The State plan shall provide for quality assurance and safeguards for applicants and beneficiaries in accordance with section 2106.

(8) ADVISORY GROUP.—The State plan shall—

(A) assure the establishment and maintenance of an advisory group under section 2107(b), and

(B) include the documentation prepared by the group under section 2107(b)(4)..

(9) ADMINISTRATION.—

(A) STATE AGENCY.—The plan shall designate a State agency or agencies to administer (or to supervise the administration of) the plan.

(B) ADMINISTRATIVE EXPENDITURES.—Effective beginning with fiscal year 2003, the plan shall contain assurances that not more than 10 percent of expenditures under the plan for all quarters in any fiscal year shall be for administrative costs.

(C) COORDINATION.—The plan shall specify how the plan—

(i) will be integrated with the State medicaid plan, titles V and XX of the Social Security Act, programs under the Older Americans Act of 1965, programs under the Developmental Disabilities Assistance and Bill of Rights Act, the Individuals with Disabilities Education Act, and any other Federal or State programs that provide services or assistance targeted to individuals with disabilities, and

(ii) will be coordinated with health plans.

(10) REPORTS AND INFORMATION TO SECRETARY; AUDITS.—The plan shall provide that the State will furnish to the Secretary—

(A) such reports, and will cooperate with such audits, as the Secretary determines are needed concerning the State's administration of its plan under this subpart, including the processing of claims under the plan, and

 (B) such data and information as the Secretary may require in order to carry out the Secretary's responsibilities.

 (11) USE OF STATE FUNDS FOR MATCHING.—

  (A) IN GENERAL.—The plan shall provide assurances that Federal funds will not be used to provide for the State share of expenditures under this subpart.

  (B) INCORPORATION OF DISQUALIFICATION FOR CERTAIN PROVIDER-RELATED DONATIONS AND HEALTH RELATED TAXES.—The Secretary shall apply the provisions of section 1903(w) of the Social Security Act to plans and payment under this title in a manner similar to the manner in which such section applies to plans and payment under title XIX of such Act.

(b) APPROVAL OF PLANS.—The Secretary shall approve a plan submitted by a State if the Secretary determines that the plan—

 (1) was developed by the State after consultation with individuals with disabilities and representatives of groups of such individuals, and

(2) meets the requirements of subsection (a).

(c) MONITORING.—The Secretary shall monitor the compliance of State plans with the eligibility requirements of section 2103 and may monitor the compliance of such plans with other requirements of this subpart.

(d) REGULATIONS.—The Secretary shall issue such regulations as may be appropriate to carry out this subpart on a timely basis.

## SEC. 2103. INDIVIDUALS WITH DISABILITIES DEFINED.

(a) IN GENERAL.—In this subpart, the term "individual with disabilities" means any individual within one or more of the following 4 categories of individuals:

(1) INDIVIDUALS REQUIRING HELP WITH ACTIVITIES OF DAILY LIVING.—An individual of any age who—

(A) requires hands-on or standby assistance, supervision, or cueing (as defined in regulations) to perform three or more activities of daily living (as defined in subsection (c)), and

(B) is expected to require such assistance, supervision, or cueing over a period of at least 100 days.

(2) INDIVIDUALS WITH SEVERE COGNITIVE OR MENTAL IMPAIRMENT.—An individual of any age—

(A) whose score, on a standard mental status protocol (or protocols) appropriate for measuring the individual's particular condition specified by the Secretary, indicates either severe cognitive impairment or severe mental impairment, or both;

(B) who—

(i) requires hands-on or standby assistance, supervision, or cueing with one or more activities of daily living,

(ii) requires hands-on or standby assistance, supervision, or cueing with at least such instrumental activity (or activities) of daily living related to cognitive or mental impairment as the Secretary specifies, or

(iii) displays symptoms of one or more serious behavioral problems (that is on a list of such problems specified by the Secretary) which create a need for supervision to prevent harm to self or others, and

(C) whose is expected to meet the requirements of subparagraphs (A) and (B) over a period of at least 100 days.

(3) INDIVIDUALS WITH SEVERE OR PROFOUND MENTAL RETARDATION.—An individual of any age who has severe or profound mental retardation (as determined according to a protocol specified by the Secretary).

(4) SEVERELY DISABLED CHILDREN.—An individual under 6 years of age who—

 (A) has a severe disability or chronic medical condition,

 (B) but for receiving personal assistance services or any of the services described in section 2104(d)(1), would require institutionalization in a hospital, nursing facility, or intermediate care facility for the mentally retarded, and

 (C) is expected to have such disability or condition and require such services over a period of at least 100 days.

(b) DETERMINATION.—

(1) IN GENERAL.—The determination of whether an individual is an individual with disabilities shall be made, by persons or entities specified under the State plan, using a uniform protocol consisting of an initial screening and assessment specified by the Secretary. A State may collect additional information, at the time of obtaining information to

make such determination, in order to provide for the assessment and plan described in section 2104(b) or for other purposes. The State shall establish a fair hearing process for appeals of such determinations.

(2) PERIODIC REASSESSMENT.—The determination that an individual is an individual with disabilities shall be considered to be effective under the State plan for a period of not more than 12 months (or for such longer period in such cases as a significant change in an individual's condition that may affect such determination is unlikely). A reassessment shall be made if there is a significant change in an individual's condition that may affect such determination.

(c) ACTIVITY OF DAILY LIVING DEFINED.—In this subpart, the term "activity of daily living" means any of the following: eating, toileting, dressing, bathing, and transferring in and out of bed.

SEC. 2104. HOME AND COMMUNITY-BASED SERVICES COVERED UNDER STATE PLAN.

(a) SPECIFICATION.—

(1) IN GENERAL.—Subject to the succeeding provisions of this section, the State plan under this subpart shall specify—

(A) the home and community-based services available under the plan to individuals with disabilities (or to such categories of such individuals), and

(B) any limits with respect to such services.

(2) FLEXIBILITY IN MEETING INDIVIDUAL NEEDS.—The services shall be specified in a manner that permits sufficient flexibility for providers to meet the needs of individuals with disabilities in a cost effective manner. Subject to subsection (e)(1)(B), such services may be delivered in an individual's home, a range of community residential arrangements, or outside the home.

(b) REQUIREMENT FOR NEEDS ASSESSMENT AND PLAN OF CARE.—

(1) IN GENERAL.—The State plan shall provide for home and community-based services to an individual with disabilities only if—

(A) a comprehensive assessment of the individual's need for home and community-based services (regardless of whether all needed services are available under the plan) has been made,

(B) an individualized plan of care based on such assessment is developed, and

(C) such services are provided consistent with such plan of care.

(2) INVOLVEMENT OF INDIVIDUALS.—The individualized plan of care under paragraph (1)(B) for an individual with disabilities shall—

(A) be developed by qualified individuals (specified under the State plan),

(B) be developed and implemented in close consultation with the individual and the individual's family,

(C) be approved by the individual (or the individual's representative), and

(D) be reviewed and updated not less often than every 6 months.

(3) PLAN OF CARE.—The plan of care under paragraph (1)(B) shall—

(A) specify which services specified under the individual plan will be provided under the State plan under this subpart,

(B) identify (to the extent possible) how the individual will be provided any services specified under the plan of care and not provided under the State plan, and

(C) specify how the provision of services to the individual under the plan will be coordinated with the provision of other health care services to the individual.

The State shall make reasonable efforts to identify and arrange for services described in subparagraph (B). Nothing in this subsection shall be construed as requiring a State (under the State plan or otherwise) to provide all the services specified in such a plan.

(c) MANDATORY COVERAGE OF PERSONAL ASSISTANCE SERVICES.—The State plan shall include, in the array of services made available to each category of individuals with disabilities, both agency-administered and consumer-directed personal assistance services (as defined in subsection (g)).

(d) ADDITIONAL SERVICES.—

(1) TYPES OF SERVICES.—Subject to subsection (e), services available under a State plan under this subpart shall include any (or all) of the following:

(A) Case management.

(B) Homemaker and chore assistance.

(C) Home modifications.

(D) Respite services.

(E) Assistive devices.

(F) Adult day services.

(G) Habilitation and rehabilitation.

(H) Supported employment.

(I) Home health services.

(J) Any other care or assistive services (approved by the Secretary) that the State determines will help individuals with disabilities to remain in their homes and communities.

(2) CRITERIA FOR SELECTION OF SERVICES.—The State plan shall specify—

(A) the methods and standards used to select the types, and the amount, duration, and scope, of services to be covered under the plan and to be available to each category of individuals with disabilities, and

(B) how the types, and the amount, duration, and scope, of services specified meet the needs of individuals within each of the 4 categories of individuals with disabilities.

(e) EXCLUSIONS AND LIMITATIONS.—

(1) IN GENERAL.—A State plan may not provide for coverage of—

(A) room and board,

(B) services furnished in a hospital, nursing facility, intermediate care facility for the mentally retarded, or other institutional setting specified by the Secretary,

   (C) items and services to the extent coverage is provided for the individual under a health plan or the medicare program.

  (2) TAKING INTO ACCOUNT INFORMAL CARE.—A State plan may take into account, in determining the amount and array of services made available to covered individuals with disability, the availability of informal care.

 (f) PAYMENT FOR SERVICES.—A State plan may provide for the use of—

  (1) vouchers,

  (2) cash payments directly to individuals with disabilities,

  (3) capitation payments to health plans, and

  (4) payment to providers,

to pay for covered services.

 (g) PERSONAL ASSISTANCE SERVICES.—

  (1) IN GENERAL.—In this section, the term "personal assistance services" means those services specified under the State plan as personal assistance services and shall include at least hands-on and standby assistance, supervision, and cueing with ac-

tivities of daily living, whether agency-administered or consumer-directed (as defined in paragraph (2)).

(2) CONSUMER-DIRECTED; AGENCY-ADMINISTERED.—In this part:

(A) The term "consumer-directed" means, with reference to personal assistance services or the provider of such services, services that are provided by an individual who is selected and managed (and, at the individual's option, trained) by the individual receiving the services.

(B) The term "agency-administered" means, with respect to such services, services that are not consumer-directed.

### SEC. 2105. COST SHARING.

(a) NO OR NOMINAL COST SHARING FOR POOREST.—The State plan may not impose any cost sharing (other than nominal cost sharing) for individuals with income (as determined under subsection (c)) less than 150 percent of the poverty level (as defined in section 1902(25)) applicable to a family of the size involved.

(b) SLIDING SCALE FOR REMAINDER.—The State plan shall impose cost sharing in the form of coinsurance (based on the amount paid under the State plan for a service)—

(1) at a rate of 10 percent for individuals with disabilities with income not less than 150 percent, and less than 250 percent, of the poverty level applicable to a family of the size involved;

(2) at a rate of 25 percent for such individuals with income not less than 250 percent, and less than 400 percent, of the poverty level applicable to a family of the size involved; and

(3) at a rate of 40 percent for such individuals with income equal to at least 400 percent of the poverty level applicable to a family of the size involved.

(c) DETERMINATION OF INCOME FOR PURPOSES OF COST SHARING.—The State plan shall specify the process to be used to determine the income of an individual with disabilities for purposes of this section. Such process shall be consistent with standards specified by the Secretary.

**SEC. 2106. QUALITY ASSURANCE AND SAFEGUARDS.**

(a) QUALITY ASSURANCE.—The State plan shall specify how the State will ensure and monitor the quality of services, including—

(1) safeguarding the health and safety of individuals with disabilities,

(2) the minimum standards for agency providers and how such standards will be enforced,

(3) the minimum competency requirements for agency provider employees who provide direct services under this subpart and how the competency of such employees will be enforced,

(4) obtaining meaningful consumer input, including consumer surveys that measure the extent to which participants receive the services described in the plan of care and participant satisfaction with such services,

(5) participation in quality assurance activities, and

(6) specifying the role of the long-term care ombudsman (under the Older Americans Act of 1965) and the Protection and Advocacy Agency (under the Developmental Disabilities Assistance and Bill of Rights Act) in assuring quality of services and protecting the rights of individuals with disabilities.

(b) SAFEGUARDS.—

(1) CONFIDENTIALITY.—The State plan shall provide safeguards which restrict the use or disclosure of information concerning applicants and beneficiaries to purposes directly connected with the administration of the plan (including performance reviews under section 2602).

(2) SAFEGUARDS AGAINST ABUSE.—The State plans shall provide safeguards against physical, emotional, or financial abuse or exploitation (specifically including appropriate safeguards in cases where payment for program benefits is made by cash payments or vouchers given directly to individuals with disabilities).

## SEC. 2107. ADVISORY GROUPS.

(a) FEDERAL ADVISORY GROUP.—

(1) ESTABLISHMENT.—The Secretary shall establish an advisory group, to advise the Secretary and States on all aspects of the program under this subpart.

(2) COMPOSITION.—The group shall be composed of individuals with disabilities and their representatives, providers, Federal and State officials, and local community implementing agencies and a majority of its members shall be individuals with disabilities and their representatives.

(b) STATE ADVISORY GROUPS.—

(1) IN GENERAL.—Each State plan shall provide for the establishment and maintenance of an advisory group to advise the State on all aspects of the State plan under this subpart.

(2) COMPOSITION.—Members of each advisory group shall be appointed by the Governor (or other chief executive officer of the State) and shall include individuals with disabilities and their representatives, providers, State officials, and local community implementing agencies and a majority of its members shall be individuals with disabilities and their representatives.

(3) SELECTION OF MEMBERS.—Each State shall establish a process whereby all residents of the State, including individuals with disabilities and their representatives, shall be given the opportunity to nominate members to the advisory group.

(4) PARTICULAR CONCERNS.—Each advisory group shall—

(A) before the State plan is developed, advise the State on guiding principles and values, policy directions, and specific components of the plan,

(B) meet regularly with State officials involved in developing the plan, during the development phase, to review and comment on all aspects of the plan,

(C) participate in the public hearings to help assure that public comments are addressed to the extent practicable,

(D) document any differences between the group's recommendations and the plan,

(E) document specifically the degree to which the plan is consumer-directed, and

(F) meet regularly with officials of the designated State agency (or agencies) to provide advice on all aspects of implementation and evaluation of the plan.

**SEC. 2108. PAYMENTS TO STATES.**

(a) IN GENERAL.—Subject to section 2102(a)(9)(B) (relating to limitation on payment for administrative costs), the Secretary shall pay to each State with a plan approved under this subpart, for each quarter, from its allotment under section 2109(b), an amount equal to—

(1) the Federal matching percentage (as defined in subsection (b)) of amount demonstrated by State claims to have been expended during the quarter for home and community-based services under the plan for individuals with disabilities; plus

(2) an amount equal to 90 percent of amount expended during the quarter under the plan for activities (including preliminary screening) relating to

determination of eligibility and performance of needs assessment; plus

(3) an amount equal to 90 percent (or, beginning with quarters in fiscal year 2003, 75 percent) of the amount expended during the quarter for the design, development, and installation of mechanical claims processing systems and for information retrieval; plus

(4) an amount equal to 50 percent of the remainder of the amounts expended during the quarter as found necessary by the Secretary for the proper and efficient administration of the State plan.

(b) FEDERAL MATCHING PERCENTAGE.—

(1) IN GENERAL.—In subsection (a), the term "Federal matching percentage" means, with respect to a State, the reference percentage specified in paragraph (2) increased by 28 percentage points, except that the Federal matching percentage shall in no case be less than 75 percent or more than 95 percent.

(2) REFERENCE PERCENTAGE.—

(A) IN GENERAL.—The reference percentage specified in this paragraph is 100 percent less the State percentage specified in subparagraph (B), except that—

(i) the percentage under this paragraph shall in no case be less than 50 percent or more than 83 percent, and

(ii) the percentage for Puerto Rico, the Virgin Islands, Guam, the Northern Mariana Islands, and American Samoa shall be 50 percent.

(B) STATE PERCENTAGE.—The State percentage specified in this subparagraph is that percentage which bears the same ratio to 45 percent as the square of the per capita income of such State bears to the square of the per capita income of the continental United States (including Alaska) and Hawaii.

(c) PAYMENTS ON ESTIMATES WITH RETROSPECTIVE ADJUSTMENTS.—The method of computing and making payments under this section shall be as follows:

(1) The Secretary shall, prior to the beginning of each quarter, estimate the amount to be paid to the State under subsection (a) for such quarter, based on a report filed by the State containing its estimate of the total sum to be expended in such quarter, and such other information as the Secretary may find necessary.

(2) From the allotment available therefore, the Secretary shall pay the amount so estimated, reduced or increased, as the case may be, by any sum (not previously adjusted under this section) by which the Secretary finds that the estimate of the amount to be paid the State for any prior period under this section was greater or less than the amount which should have been paid.

(d) APPLICATION OF RULES REGARDING LIMITATIONS ON PROVIDER-RELATED DONATIONS AND HEALTH CARE RELATED TAXES.—The provisions of section 1903(w) of the Social Security Act shall apply to payments to States under this section in the same manner as they apply to payments to States under section 1903(a) of such Act.

## SEC. 2109. TOTAL FEDERAL BUDGET; ALLOTMENTS TO STATES.

(a) TOTAL FEDERAL BUDGET.—

(1) FISCAL YEARS 1996 through 2003.—For purposes of this subpart, the total Federal budget for State plans under this subpart for each of fiscal years 1996 through 2003 is the following:

(A) For fiscal year 1996, 4.5 billion.

(B) For fiscal year 1997, 7.8 billion.

(C) For fiscal year 1998, 11.0 billion.

(D) For fiscal year 1999, 14.7 billion.

(E) For fiscal year 2000, 18.7 billion. [$56 to 2000}

(F) For fiscal year 2001, 26.7 billion. [48-56 for out years]

(G) For fiscal year 2002, 35.5 billion.

(H) For fiscal year 2003, 38.3 billion.

(2) SUBSEQUENT FISCAL YEARS.—For purposes of this subpart, the total Federal budget for State plans under this subpart for each fiscal year after fiscal year 2003 is the total Federal budget under this subsection for the preceding fiscal year multiplied by—

(A) a factor (described in paragraph (3)) reflecting the change in the CPI for the fiscal year, and

(B) a factor (described in paragraph (4)) reflecting the change in the number of individuals with disabilities for the fiscal year.

(3) CPI INCREASE FACTOR.—For purposes of paragraph (2)(A), the factor described in this paragraph for a fiscal year is the ratio of—

(A) the annual average index of the consumer price index for the preceding fiscal year, to—

(B) such index, as so measured, for the second preceding fiscal year.

(4) DISABLED POPULATION FACTOR.—For purposes of paragraph (2)(B), the factor described in this paragraph for a fiscal year is 100 percent plus (or minus) the percentage increase (or decrease) change in the disabled population of the United States (as determined for purposes of the most recent update under subsection (b)(3)(D).

[review:] (5) ADDITIONAL FUNDS DUE TO MEDICAID OFFSETS.—

(A) IN GENERAL.—Each participating State must provide the Secretary with information concerning offsets and reductions in the medicaid program resulting from home and community-based services provided under this title, that would have been paid for under the State medicaid plan but for the provision of similar services under the program under this title.

(B) REPORTS.—Each State with a program under this title shall submit such reports to the Secretary as the Secretary may require in order to monitor compliance with subparagraph (A).

(C) COMPLIANCE.—The Secretary shall review such reports. The Secretary shall increase the total Federal budget for State plans under subsection (a)(1) by the amount of any reduction in Federal expenditures for medical assistance under the State medicaid plan for home and community based services.

(D) NO DUPLICATE PAYMENT.—No paymet may be made to a State under this section for any services to the extent that the State received payment for such services under section 1903(a) of the Social Security Act.

(b) ALLOTMENTS TO STATES.—

(1) IN GENERAL.—The Secretary shall allot to each State for each fiscal year an amount that bears the same ratio to the total Federal budget for the fiscal year (specified under paragraph (1) or (2) of subsection (a)) as the State allotment factor (under paragraph (2) for the State for the fiscal year) bears to the sum of such factors for all States for that fiscal year.

(2) STATE ALLOTMENT FACTOR.—

(A) IN GENERAL.—For each State for each fiscal year, the Secretary shall compute a State allotment factor equal to the sum of—

(i) the base allotment factor (specified in subparagraph (B)), and

(ii) the low income allotment factor (specified in subparagraph (C)),

for the State for the fiscal year.

(B) BASE ALLOTMENT FACTOR.—The base allotment factor, specified in this subparagraph, for a State for a fiscal year is equal to the product of the following:

(i) NUMBER OF INDIVIDUALS WITH DISABILITIES.—The number of individuals with disabilities in the State (determined under paragraph (3)) for the fiscal year.

(ii) 80 PERCENT OF THE NATIONAL PER CAPITA BUDGET.—80 percent of the national average per capita budget amount (determined under paragraph (4)) for the fiscal year.

(iii) WAGE ADJUSTMENT FACTOR.—The wage adjustment factor (determined under paragraph (5)) for the State for the fiscal year.

(iv) FEDERAL MATCHING RATE.—The Federal matching rate (determined under section 2108(b)) for the fiscal year.

(C) LOW INCOME ALLOTMENT FACTOR.—
The low income allotment factor, specified in this subparagraph, for a State for a fiscal year is equal to the product of the following:

(i) NUMBER OF INDIVIDUALS WITH DISABILITIES.—The number of individuals with disabilities in the State (determined under paragraph (3)) for the fiscal year.

(ii) 10 PERCENT OF THE NATIONAL PER CAPITA BUDGET.—10 percent of the national average per capita budget amount (determined under paragraph (4)) for the fiscal year.

(iii) WAGE ADJUSTMENT FACTOR.—The wage adjustment factor (determined under paragraph (5)) for the State for the fiscal year.

(iv) FEDERAL MATCHING RATE.—The Federal matching rate (determined under section 2108(b)) for the fiscal year.

(v) LOW INCOME INDEX.—The low income index (determined under paragraph (6)) for the State for the preceding fiscal year.

(3) NUMBER OF INDIVIDUALS WITH DISABILITIES.—The number of individuals with disabilities in a State for a fiscal year shall be determined as follows:

    (A) BASE.—The Secretary shall determine the number of individuals in the State by age, sex, and income category, based on the 1990 decennial census, adjusted (as appropriate) by the March 1994 current population survey.

    (B) DISABILITY PREVALENCE LEVEL BY POPULATION CATEGORY.—The Secretary shall determine, for each such age, sex, and income category, the national average proportion of the population of such category that represents individuals with disabilities. The Secretary may conduct periodic surveys in order to determine such proportions.

    (C) BASE DISABLED POPULATION IN A STATE.—The number of individuals with disabilities in a State in 1994 is equal to the sum of the products, for such each age, sex, and income category, of—

        (i) the population of individuals in the State in the category (determined under subparagraph (A)), and

(ii) the national average proportion for such category (determined under subparagraph (B)).

(D) UPDATE.—The Secretary shall determine the number of individuals with disabilities in a State in a fiscal year equal to the number determined under subparagraph (C) for the State increased (or decreased) by the percentage increase (or decrease) in the disabled population of the State as determined under the current population survey from 1994 to the year before the fiscal year involved.

(4) NATIONAL PER CAPITA BUDGET AMOUNT.—The national average per capita budget amount, for a fiscal year, is—

(A) the total Federal budget specified under subsection (a) for the fiscal year; divided by

(B) the sum, for the fiscal year, of the numbers of individuals with disabilities (determined under paragraph (3)) for all the States for the fiscal year.

(5) WAGE ADJUSTMENT FACTOR.—The wage adjustment factor, for a State for a fiscal year, is equal to the ratio of—

(A) the average hourly wages for service workers (other than household or protective services) in the State, to

(B) the national average hourly wages for service workers (other than household or protective services).

The hourly wages shall be determined under this paragraph based on data from the most recent decennial census for which such data are available.

(6) LOW INCOME INDEX.—The low income index for each State for a fiscal year is the ratio, determined for the preceding fiscal year, of—

(A) the percentage of the State's population that has income below 150 percent of the poverty level, to

(B) the percentage of the population of the United States that has income below 150 percent of the poverty level.

Such percentages shall be based on data from the most recent decennial census for which such data are available, adjusted by data from the most recent current population survey as determined appropriate by the Secretary.

(c) STATE ENTITLEMENT.—This subpart constitutes budget authority in advance of appropriations Acts, and represents the obligation of the Federal Government to provide for the payment to States of amounts described in section 2109(a).

## PART 2—MEDICAID NURSING HOME IMPROVEMENTS

### SEC. 2201. REFERENCE TO AMENDMENTS.

For amendments to the medicaid program under title XIX of the Social Security Act to improvement nursing home benefits under such program, see part 2 of subtitle C of title IV.

## PART 3—PRIVATE LONG-TERM CARE INSURANCE

### Subpart A—General Provisions

### SEC. 2301. FEDERAL REGULATIONS; PRIOR APPLICATION OR CERTAIN REQUIREMENTS.

(a) IN GENERAL.—The Secretary, with the advice and assistance of the Advisory Council, as appropriate, shall promulgate regulations as necessary to implement the provisions of this part, in accordance with the timetable specified in subsection (b).

(b) TIMETABLE FOR PUBLICATION OF REGULATIONS.—

(1) FEDERAL REGISTER NOTICE.—Within 120 days after the date a majority of the members are first appointed to the Advisory Council pursuant to section 2302, the Secretary shall publish in the Fed-

eral Register a notice setting forth the projected timetable for promulgation of regulations required under this part. Such timetable shall indicate which regulations are proposed to be published by the end of the first, second, and third years after appointment of the Advisory Council.

(2) FINAL DEADLINE.—All regulations required under this part shall be published by the end of the third year after appointment of the Advisory Council.

(c) PROVISIONS EFFECTIVE WITHOUT REGARD TO PROMULGATION OF REGULATIONS.—

(1) IN GENERAL.—Notwithstanding any other provision of this part, insurers shall be required, not later than 6 months after the enactment of this Act, regardless of whether final implementing regulations have been promulgated by the Secretary, to comply with the following provisions of this part:

(A) Section 2321(c) (standard outline of coverage);

(B) Section 2321(d) (reporting to State insurance commissioners);

(C) Section 2322(b) (preexisting condition exclusions);

(D) Section 2322(c) (limiting conditions on benefits);

(E) Section 2322(d) (inflation protection);

(F) Section 2324 (sales practices);

(G) Section 2325 (continuation, renewal, replacement, conversion, and cancellation of policies); and

(H) Section 2326 (payment of benefits).

(2) INTERIM REQUIREMENTS.—Before the effective date of applicable regulations promulgated by the Secretary implementing requirements of this part as specified below, such requirements will be considered to be met—

(A) in the case of section 2321(c) (requiring a standard outline of coverage), if the long-term care insurance policy meets the requirements of section 6.G.(2) of the NAIC Model Act and of section 24 of the NAIC Model Regulation;

(B) in the case of section 2321(d) (requiring reporting to the State insurance commissioner), if the insurer meets the requirements of section 14 of the NAIC Model Regulation;

(C) in the case of section 2322(c)(1) (general requirements concerning limiting conditions on benefits), if such policy meets the requirements of section 6.D. of the NAIC Model Act;

(D) in the case of section 2322(c)(2) (limiting conditions on home health care or community-based services) if such policy meets the requirements of section 11 of the NAIC Model Regulations;

(E) in the case of section 2322(d) (concerning inflation protection), if the insurer meets the requirements of section 12 of the NAIC Model Regulation;

(F) in the case of section 2324(b) (concerning applications for the purchase of insurance), if the insurer meets the requirements of section 10 of the NAIC Model Regulation;

(G) in the case of section 2324(d) (concerning compensation for the sale of policies), if the insurer meets the requirements of the optional regulation entitled "Permitted Compensation Arrangements" included in the NAIC Model Regulation;

(H) in the case of section 2324(g) (concerning sales through employers or membership organizations), if the insurer and the membership organization meet the requirements of section 21.C. of the NAIC Model Regulation;

(I) in the case of section 2324(h) (concerning interstate sales of group policies), if the insurer and the policy meet the requirements of section 5 of the NAIC Model Act; and

(J) in the case of section 2325(f) (concerning continuation, renewal, replacement, and conversion of policies), if the insurer and the policy meet the requirements of section 7 of the NAIC Model Regulation.

## SEC. 2302. NATIONAL LONG-TERM CARE INSURANCE ADVISORY COUNCIL.

(a) APPOINTMENT.—The Secretary shall appoint an advisory board to be known as the National Long-Term Care Insurance Advisory Council.

(b) COMPOSITION.—

(1) NUMBER AND QUALIFICATIONS OF MEMBERS.—The Advisory Council shall consist of 5 members, each of whom has substantial expertise in matters relating to the provision and regulation of long-term care insurance. At least one member shall have experience as a State insurance commissioner or legislator with expertise in policy development

with respect to, and regulation of, long-term care insurance.

(2) TERMS OF OFFICE.—

(A) IN GENERAL.—Except as otherwise provided in this subsection, members shall be appointed for terms of office of 5 years.

(B) INITIAL MEMBERS.—Of the initial members of the Council, one shall be appointed for a term of 5 years, one for 4 years, one for 3 years, one for 2 years, and one for 1 year.

(C) TWO-TERM LIMIT.—No member shall be eligible to serve in excess of two consecutive terms, but may continue to serve until such member's successor is appointed.

(3) VACANCIES.—Any member appointed to fill a vacancy occurring before the expiration of the term of such member's predecessor shall be appointed for the remainder of such term.

(4) REMOVAL.—No member may be removed during the member's term of office except for just and sufficient cause.

(c) CHAIRPERSON.—The Secretary shall appoint a Chairperson from among the members.

(d) COMPENSATION.—

(1) IN GENERAL.—Except as provided in paragraph (3), members of the Advisory Council, while serving on business of the Advisory Council, shall be entitled to receive compensation at a rate not to exceed the daily equivalent of the rate specified for level V of the Executive Schedule under section 5316 of title 5, United States Code.

(2) TRAVEL.—Except as provided in paragraph (3), members of the Advisory Council, while serving on business of the Advisory Council away from their homes or regular places of business, may be allowed travel expenses (including per diem in lieu of subsistence) as authorized by section 5703(b) of title 5, United States Code, for persons in the Government service employed intermittently.

(3) RESTRICTION.—A member of the Advisory Council may not be compensated under this section if the member is receiving compensation or travel expenses from another source while serving on business of the Advisory Council.

(e) MEETINGS.—The Advisory Council shall meet not less often than 2 times a year at the direction of the Chairperson.

(f) STAFF AND SUPPORT.—

(1) IN GENERAL.—The Advisory Council shall have a salaried executive director appointed by the Chairperson, and staff appointed by the executive director with the approval of the Chairperson.

(2) FEDERAL ENTITIES.—The head of each Federal department and agency shall make available to the Advisory Council such information and other assistance as it may require to carry out its responsibilities.

(g) GENERAL RESPONSIBILITIES.—The Advisory Council shall—

(1) provide advice, recommendations, and assistance to the Secretary on matters relating to long-term care insurance as specified in this part and as otherwise required by the Secretary;

(2) collect, analyze, and disseminate information relating to long-term care insurance in order to increase the understanding of insurers, providers, consumers, and regulatory bodies of the issues relating to, and to facilitate improvements in, such insurance;

(3) develop for the Secretary's consideration proposed models, standards, requirements, and procedures relating to long-term care insurance, as appropriate, with respect to the content and format of

insurance policies, agent and insurer practices concerning the sale and servicing of such policies, and regulatory activities; and

(4) monitor the development of the long-term care insurance market (including policies, marketing practices, pricing, eligibility and benefit preconditions, and claims payment procedures) and advise the Secretary concerning the need for regulatory changes.

(h) SPECIFIC MATTERS FOR CONSIDERATION.—The Advisory Council shall consider, and provide views and recommendations to the Secretary concerning, the following matters relating to long-term care insurance:

(1) UNIFORM TERMS, DEFINITIONS, AND FORMATS.—The Advisory Council shall develop and propose to the Secretary uniform terminology, definitions, and formats for use in long-term care insurance policies.

(2) STANDARD OUTLINE OF COVERAGE.—The Advisory Council shall develop and propose to the Secretary a standard format for use by all insurers offering long-term care policies for the outline of coverage required pursuant to section 2321(c).

(3) PREMIUMS.—

(A) CONSIDERATION OF FEDERAL REQUIREMENTS.—The Advisory Council shall consider, and make recommendations to the Secretary concerning—

(i) whether Federal standards should be established governing the amounts of and rates of increase in premiums in long-term care policies, and

(ii) if so, what factors should be taken into account (and whether such factors should include the age of the insured, actuarial information, cost of care, lapse rates, financial reserve requirements, insurer solvency, and tax treatment of premiums, and benefits.

(4) UPGRADES OF COVERAGE.—The Advisory Council shall consider, and make recommendations to the Secretary concerning, whether Federal standards are needed governing the terms and conditions insurers may place on insured individuals' eligibility to obtain improved coverage (including any restrictions considered advisable with respect to premium increases, agent commissions, medical underwriting, and age rating).

(5) THRESHOLD CONDITIONS FOR PAYMENT OF BENEFITS.—The Advisory Council shall—

    (A) consider, and make recommendations to the Secretary concerning, the advisability of establishing standardized sets of threshold conditions (based on degrees of functional or cognitive impairment or on other conditions) for payment of covered benefits;

    (B) to the extent found appropriate, recommend to the Secretary specific sets of threshold conditions to be used for such purpose;

    (C) develop and propose to the Secretary, with respect to assessments of insured individuals' levels of need for purposes of receipt of covered benefits—

        (i) professional qualification standards applicable to individuals making such determinations; and

        (ii) uniform procedures and formats for use in performing and documenting such assessments.

(6) DISPUTE RESOLUTION.—The Advisory Council shall consider, and make recommendations to the Secretary concerning, procedures that insurers and States should be required to implement to

afford insured individuals a reasonable opportunity to dispute denial of benefits under a long-term care insurance policy.

(7) SALES AND SERVICING OF POLICIES.—The Advisory Council shall consider, and make recommendations to the Secretary concerning—

(A) training and certification to be required of agents involved in selling or servicing long-term care insurance policies;

(B) appropriate limits on commissions or other compensation paid to agents for the sale or servicing of such policies;

(C) sales practices that should be prohibited or limited with respect to such policies (including any financial limits that should be applied concerning the individuals to whom such policies may be sold); and

(D) appropriate standards and requirements with respect to sales of such policies by or through employers and other entities, to employees, members, or affiliates of such entities.

(8) CONTINUING CARE RETIREMENT COMMUNITIES.—The Advisory Council shall consider, and make recommendations to the Secretary concerning, the extent to which the long-term care insurance as-

pects of continuing care retirement community arrangements should be subject to regulation under this part (and the Secretary, in consultation with the Secretary of the Treasury, shall consider such recommendations and promulgate appropriate regulations).

(i) ACTIVITIES.—In order to carry out its responsibilities under this part, the Advisory Council is authorized to—

　　(1) consult individuals and public and private entities with experience and expertise in matters relating to long-term care insurance (and shall consult the National Association of Insurance Commissioners);

　　(2) conduct meetings and hold hearings;

　　(3) conduct research (either directly or under grant or contract);

　　(4) collect, analyze, publish, and disseminate data and information (either directly or under grant or contract); and

　　(5) develop model formats and procedures for insurance policies and marketing materials; and develop proposed standards, rules, and procedures for regulatory programs.

(j) AUTHORIZATION OF APPROPRIATIONS.—There are authorized to be appropriated, for activities of the Advisory Council, $1,500,000 for fiscal year 1995, and $2,000,000 for each succeeding fiscal year.

**SEC. 2303. RELATION TO STATE LAW.**

Nothing in this part shall be construed as preventing a State from applying standards that provide greater protection to insured individuals under long-term care insurance policies than the standards promulgated under this part, except that such State standards may not be inconsistent with any of the requirements of this part or of regulations hereunder.

**SEC. 2304. DEFINITIONS.**

For purposes of this part:

(1) ACTIVITY OF DAILY LIVING.—The term "activity of daily living" means any of the following: eating, toileting, dressing, bathing, and transferring in and out of bed.

(2) ADULT DAY CARE.—The term "adult day care" means a program providing social and health-related services during the day to six or more adults with disabilities (or such smaller number as the Secretary may specify in regulations) in a community group setting outside the home.

(3) ADVISORY COUNCIL.—The term "Advisory Council" means the National Long-Term Care Insurance Advisory Council established pursuant to section 2302.

(4) CERTIFICATE.—The term "certificate" means a document issued to an individual as evidence of such individual's coverage under a group insurance policy.

(5) CONTINUING CARE RETIREMENT COMMUNITY.—The term "continuing care retirement community" means a residential community operated by a private entity that enters into contractual agreements with residents under which such entity guarantees, in consideration for residents' purchase of or periodic payment for membership in the community, to provide for such residents' future long-term care needs.

(6) DESIGNATED REPRESENTATIVE.—The term "designated representative" means the person designated by an insured individual (or, if such individual is incapacitated, pursuant to an appropriate administrative or judicial procedure) to communicate with the insurer on behalf of such individual in the event of such individual's incapacitation.

(7) HOME HEALTH CARE.—The term "home health care" means medical and nonmedical services including such services as homemaker services, assistance with activities of daily living, and respite care provided to individuals in their residences.

(8) INSURED INDIVIDUAL.—The term "insured individual" means, with respect to a long-term care insurance policy, any individual who has coverage of benefits under such policy.

(9) INSURER.—The term "insurer" means any person that offers or sells an individual or group long-term care insurance policy under which such person is at risk for all or part of the cost of benefits under the policy, and includes any agent of such person.

(10) LONG-TERM CARE INSURANCE POLICY.—The term "long-term care insurance policy" has the meaning given that term in section 4 of the NAIC Model Act, except that the last sentence of such section shall not apply.

(11) NAIC MODEL ACT.—The term "NAIC Model Act" means the Long-Term Care Insurance Model Act published by the NAIC, as amended through January 1993.

(12) NAIC MODEL REGULATION.—The term "NAIC Model Regulation" means the Long-Term Care Insurance Model Regulation published by the NAIC, as amended through January 1993.

(13) NURSING FACILITY.—The term "nursing facility" means a facility licensed by the State to provide to residents—

> (A) skilled nursing care and related services for residents who require medical or nursing care;
>
> (B) rehabilitation services for the rehabilitation of injured, disabled, or sick individuals, or
>
> (C) on a regular basis, health-related care and services to individuals who because of their mental or physical condition require care and services (above the level of room and board) which can be made available to them only through institutional facilities.

(14) POLICYHOLDER.—The term "policyholder" means the entity which is the holder of record of a group long-term care insurance policy.

(15) RESIDENTIAL CARE FACILITY.—The term "residential care facility" means a facility (including a nursing facility) that—

(A) provides to residents medical or personal care services (including at a minimum assistance with activities of daily living) in a setting other than an individual or single-family home, and

(B) does not provide services of a higher level than can be provided by a nursing facility.

(16) RESPITE CARE.—The term "respite care" means the temporary provision of care (including assistance with activities of daily living) to an individual, in the individual's home or another setting in the community, for the purpose of affording such individual's unpaid caregiver a respite from the responsibilities of such care.

(17) STATE INSURANCE COMMISSIONER.—The term "State insurance commissioner" means the State official bearing such title, or, in the case of a jurisdiction where such title is not used, the State official with primary responsibility for the regulation of insurance.

**Subpart B—Federal Standards and Requirements**

**SEC. 2321. REQUIREMENTS TO FACILITATE UNDERSTANDING AND COMPARISON OF BENEFITS.**

(a) IN GENERAL.—The Secretary, after considering (where appropriate) recommendations of the Advisory

Council, shall promulgate regulations designed to standardize formats and terminology used in long-term care insurance policies, to require insurers to provide to customers and beneficiaries information on the range of public and private long-term care coverage available, and to establish such other requirements as may be appropriate to promote consumer understanding and facilitate comparison of benefits, which shall include at a minimum the requirements specified in this section.

(b) UNIFORM TERMS, DEFINITIONS, AND FORMATS.—Insurers shall be required to use, in long-term care insurance policies, uniform terminology, definitions of terms, and formats, in accordance with regulations promulgated by the Secretary, after considering recommendations of the Advisory Council.

(c) STANDARD OUTLINE OF COVERAGE.—

(1) IN GENERAL.—Insurers shall be required to develop for each long-term care insurance policy offered or sold, to include as a part of each such policy, and to make available to each potential purchaser and furnish to each insured individual and policyholder, an outline of coverage under such policy that—

(A) includes the elements specified in paragraph (2),

(B) is in a uniform format (as prescribed by Secretary on the basis of recommendations by the Advisory Council),

(C) accurately and clearly reflects the contents of the policy, and

(D) is updated periodically on such timetable as may be required by the Secretary (or more frequently as necessary to reflect significant changes in outlined information).

(2) CONTENTS OF OUTLINE.—The outline of coverage for each long-term care insurance policy shall include at least the following:

(A) BENEFITS.—A description of—

(i) the principal benefits covered, including the extent of—

(I) benefits for services furnished in residential care facilities, and

(II) other benefits,

(ii) the principal exclusions from and limitations on coverage,

(iii) the terms and conditions, if any, upon which the insured individual may obtain upgraded benefits, and

(iv) the threshold conditions for entitlement to receive benefits.

(B) CONTINUATION, RENEWAL, AND CONVERSION.—A statement of the terms under which a policy may be—

(i) returned (and premium refunded) during an initial examination period,

(ii) continued in force or renewed,

(iii) converted to an individual policy (in the case of coverage under a group policy),

(C) CANCELLATION.—A statement of the circumstances in which a policy may be terminated, and the refund or nonforfeitures benefits (if any) applicable in each such circumstance, including—

(i) death of the insured individual,

(ii) nonpayment of premiums,

(iii) election by the insured individual not to renew,

(iv) any other circumstance.

(D) PREMIUM.—A statement of—

(i) the total annual premium, and the portion of such premium attributable to each covered benefit,

(ii) any reservation by the insurer of a right to change premiums,

(iii) any limit on annual premium increases,

(iv) any expected premium increases associated with automatic or optional benefit increases (including inflation protection), and

(v) any circumstances under which payment of premium is waived.

(E) DECLARATION CONCERNING SUMMARY.—A statement, in bold face type on the face of the document in language understandable to the average individual, that the outline of coverage is a summary only, not a contract of insurance, and that the policy contains the contractual provisions that govern.

(F) COST/VALUE COMPARISON.—

(i) Information on average costs (and variation in such costs) for nursing facility care (and such other care as the Secretary may specify) and information on the value of benefits relative to such costs.

(ii) A comparison of benefits, over a period of at least 20 years, for policies with and without inflation protection.

(iii) A declaration as to whether the amount of benefits will increase over time, and, if so, a statement of the type and amount of, any limitations on, and any premium increases for, such benefit increases.

(G) TAX TREATMENT.—A statement of the Federal income tax treatment of premiums and benefits under the policy, as determined by the Secretary of the Treasury.

(H) OTHER.—Such other information as the Secretary may require.

(d) REPORTING TO STATE INSURANCE COMMISSIONER.—Each insurer shall be required to report at least annually, to the State insurance commissioner of each State in which any long-term care insurance policy of the insurer is sold, such information, in such format, as the Secretary may specify with respect to each such policy, including—

(1) the standard outline of coverage required pursuant to subsection (c);

(2) lapse rates and replacement rates for such policies;

(3) the ratio of premiums collected to benefits paid;

(4) reserves;

(5) written materials used in sale or promotion of such policy; and

(6) any other information the Secretary may require.

(e) COMPARISON OF LONG-TERM CARE COVERAGE ALTERNATIVES.—Each insurer shall be required to furnish to each individual before a long-term care insurance policy of the insurer is sold to the individual information on the conditions of eligibility for, and benefits under, each of the following:

> (1) POLICIES OFFERED BY THE INSURER.—The standard outline of coverage, and such other information as the Secretary may specify, with respect to each long-term care insurance policy offered by the insurer.
>
> (2) COMPARISON TO OTHER AVAILABLE PRIVATE INSURANCE.—Information, in such format as may be required under this part, on—
>
>> (A) benefits offered under long-term care insurance policies of the insurer (and the threshold conditions for receipt by an insured individual of each such benefit); and
>>
>> (B) additional benefits available under policies offered by other private insurers (to the

extent such information is made available by the State insurance commissioner).

(3) PUBLIC PROGRAMS; REGIONAL ALLIANCES.—Information furnished to the insurer, pursuant to section 2342(b)(2), by the State in which such individual resides, on conditions of eligibility for, and long-term care benefits (or the lack of such benefits) under—

    (A) each public long-term care program administered by the State,

    (B) the Medicare programs under title XVIII of the Social Security Act; and

    (C) each regional alliance operating in the State.

## SEC. 2322. REQUIREMENTS RELATING TO COVERAGE.

(a) IN GENERAL.—The Secretary, after considering (where appropriate) recommendations of the Advisory Council, shall promulgate regulations establishing requirements with respect to the terms of and benefits under long-term care insurance policies, which shall include at a minimum the requirements specified in this section.

(b) LIMITATIONS ON PREEXISTING CONDITION EXCLUSIONS.—

    (1) INITIAL POLICIES.—A long-term care insurance policy may not exclude or limit coverage for

any service or benefit, the need for which is the result of a medical condition or disability because an insured individual received medical treatment for, or was diagnosed as having, such condition before the issuance of the policy, unless—

>(A) the insurer, prior to issuance of the policy, determines and documents (with evidence including written evidence that such condition has been treated or diagnosed by a qualified health care professional) that the insured individual had such condition during the 6-month period (or such longer period as the Secretary may specify) ending on the effective date of the policy; and

>(B) the need or such service or benefit begins within 6 months (or such longer period as the Secretary may specify) following the effective date of the policy.

(2) REPLACEMENT POLICIES.—Solely for purposes of the requirements of paragraph (1), with respect to an insured individual, the effective date of a long-term care insurance policy issued to replace a previous policy, with respect to benefits which are the same as or substantially equivalent to benefits under such previous policy, shall be considered to be

the effective date of such previous policy with respect to such individual.

(c) LIMITING CONDITIONS ON BENEFITS.—

(1) IN GENERAL.—A long-term care insurance policy may not—

(A) condition eligibility for benefits for a type of service on the need for or receipt of any other type of service (such as prior hospitalization or institutionalization, or a higher level of care than the care for which benefits are covered);

(B) condition eligibility for any benefit (where the need for such benefit has been established by an independent assessment of impairment) on any particular medical diagnosis (including any acute condition) or on one of a group of diagnoses;

(C) condition eligibility for benefits furnished by licensed or certified providers on compliance by such providers with conditions not required under Federal or State law; or

(D) condition coverage of any service on provision of such service by a provider, or in a setting, providing a higher level of care than that required by an insured individual.

(2) HOME CARE OR COMMUNITY-BASED SERVICES.—A long-term care insurance policy that provides benefits for any home care or community-based services provided in a setting other than a residential care facility—

(A) may not limit such benefits to services provided by registered nurses or licensed practical nurses;

(B) may not limit such benefits to services furnished by persons or entities participating in programs under titles XVIII and XIX of the Social Security Act and in part 1 of this subtitle; and

(C) must provide, at a minimum, benefits for personal assistance with activities of daily living, home health care, adult day care, and respite care.

(3) NURSING FACILITY SERVICES.—A long-term care insurance policy that provides benefits for any nursing facility services—

(A) must provide benefits for such services provided by all types of nursing facilities licensed by the State, and

(B) may provide benefits for care in other residential facilities.

(4) PROHIBITION ON DISCRIMINATION BY DIAGNOSIS.—A long-term care insurance policy may not provide for treatment of—

(A) Alzheimer's disease or any other progressive degenerative dementia of an organic origin,

(B) any organic or inorganic mental illness,

(C) mental retardation or any other cognitive or mental impairment, or

(D) HIV infection or AIDS,

different from the treatment of any other medical condition for purposes of determining whether threshold conditions for the receipt of benefits have been met, or the amount of benefits under the policy.

(d) INFLATION PROTECTION.—

(1) REQUIREMENT TO OFFER.—An insurer offering for sale any long-term care insurance policy shall be required to afford the purchaser the option to obtain coverage under such policy (upon payment of increased premiums) of annual increases in benefits at rates in accordance with paragraph (2).

(2) RATE INCREASE IN BENEFITS.—For purposes of paragraph (1), the benefits under a policy

for each year shall be increased by a percentage of the full value of benefits under the policy for the previous year, which shall be not less than 5 percent of such value (or such other rate of increase as may be determined by the Secretary to be adequate to offset increases in the costs of long-term care services for which coverage is provided under the policy).

(3) REQUIREMENT OF WRITTEN REJECTION.—Inflation protection in accordance with paragraph (1) may be excluded from the coverage under a policy only if the insured individual (or, if different, the person responsible for payment of premiums has rejected in writing the option to obtain such coverage.

### SEC. 2323. REQUIREMENTS RELATING TO PREMIUMS.

(a) IN GENERAL.—The Secretary, after considering (where appropriate) recommendations of the Advisory Council, shall promulgate regulations establishing requirements applicable to premiums for long-term care insurance policies, which shall include at a minimum the requirements specified in this section.

(b) LIMITATIONS ON RATES AND INCREASES.—The Secretary, after considering recommendations of the Advisory Council, may establish by regulation such standards and requirements as may be determined appropriate with respect to—

(1) mandatory or optional State procedures for review and approval of premium rates and rate increases or decreases;

(2) limitations on the amount of initial premiums, or on the rate or amount of premium increases;

(3) the factors to be taken into consideration by an insurer in proposing, and by a State in approving or disapproving, premium rates and increases; and

(4) the extent to which consumers should be entitled to participate or be represented in the rate-setting process and to have access to actuarial and other information relied on in setting rates.

## SEC. 2324. REQUIREMENTS RELATING TO SALES PRACTICES.

(a) IN GENERAL.—The Secretary, after considering (where appropriate) recommendations of the Advisory Council, shall promulgate regulations establishing requirements applicable to the sale or offering for sale of long-term care insurance policies, which shall include at a minimum the requirements specified in this section.

(b) APPLICATIONS.—Any insurer that offers any long-term care insurance policy (including any group policy) shall be required to meet such requirements with respect to the content, format, and use of application forms for long-term care insurance as the Secretary may require by regulation.

(c) AGENT TRAINING AND CERTIFICATION.—An insurer may not sell or offer for sale a long-term care insurance policy through an agent who does not comply with minimum standards with respect to training and certification established by the Secretary after consideration of recommendations by the Advisory Council.

(d) COMPENSATION FOR SALE OF POLICIES.—Compensation by an insurer to an agent or agents for the sale of an original long-term care insurance policy, or for servicing or renewing such a policy, may not exceed amounts (or percentage shares of premiums or other reference amounts) specified by the Secretary in regulations, after considering recommendations of the Advisory Council.

(e) PROHIBITED SALES PRACTICES.—The following practices by insurers shall be prohibited with respect to the sale or offer for sale of long-term care insurance policies:

   (1) FALSE AND MISLEADING REPRESENTATIONS.—Making any statement or representation—

      (A) which the insurer knows or should know is false or misleading (including the inaccurate, incomplete, or misleading comparison of long-term care insurance policies or insurers), and

(B) which is intended, or would be likely, to induce any person to purchase, retain, terminate, forfeit, permit to lapse, pledge, assign, borrow against, convert, or effect a change with respect to, any long-term care insurance policy.

(2) INACCURATE COMPLETION OF MEDICAL HISTORY.—Making or causing to be made (by any means including failure to inquire about or to record information relating to preexisting conditions) statements or omissions, in records detailing the medical history of an applicant for insurance, which the insurer knows or should know render such records false, incomplete, or misleading in any way material to such applicant's eligibility for or coverage under a long-term care insurance policy.

(3) UNDUE PRESSURE.—Employing force, fright, threat, or other undue pressure, whether explicit or implicit, which is intended, or would be likely, to induce the purchase of a long-term care insurance policy.

(4) COLD LEAD ADVERTISING.—Using, directly or indirectly, any method of contacting consumers (including any method designed to induce consumers

to contact the insurer or agent) for the purpose of inducing the purchase of long-term care insurance (regardless of whether such purpose is the sole or primary purpose of the contact) without conspicuously disclosing such purpose.

(f) PROHIBITION ON SALE OF DUPLICATE BENEFITS.—An insurer or agent may not sell or issue to an individual a long-term care insurance policy that the insurer or agent knows or should know provides for coverage that duplicates coverage already provided in another long-term care insurance policy held by such individual (unless the policy is intended to replace such other policy).

(g) SALES THROUGH EMPLOYERS OR MEMBERSHIP ORGANIZATIONS.—

(1) REQUIREMENTS CONCERNING SUCH ARRANGEMENTS.—In any case where an employer, organization, association, or other entity (referred to as a "membership entity") endorses a long-term care insurance policy to, or such policy is marketed or sold through such membership entity to, employees, members, or other individuals affiliated with such membership entity—

(A) the insurer offering such policy shall not permit its marketing or sale through such entity unless the requirements of this subsection are met; and

(B) a membership entity that receives any compensation for such sale, marketing, or endorsement of such policy shall be considered the agent of the insurer for purposes of this part.

(2) DISCLOSURE AND INFORMATION REQUIREMENTS.—A membership entity that endorses a long-term care insurance policy, or through which such policy is sold, to individuals affiliated with such entity, shall—

(A) disclose prominently, in a form and manner designed to ensure that each such individual who receives information concerning any such policy through such entity is aware of and understands such disclosure—

(i) the manner in which the insurer and policy were selected;

(ii) the extent (if any) to which a person independent of the insurer with expertise in long-term care insurance analyzed the advantages and disadvantages of such policy from the standpoint of such individuals (including such matters as the merits of the policy compared to other available benefit packages, and the financial stability of the insurer), and the results of any such analysis;

(iii) any organizational or financial ties between the entity (or a related entity) and the insurer (or a related entity);

(iv) the nature of compensation arrangements (if any) and the amount of compensation (including all fees, commissions, and other forms of financial support) for the endorsement or sale of such policy; and

(B) make available to such individuals, either directly or through referrals, appropriate counseling to assist such individuals to make educated and informed decisions concerning the purchase of such policies.

### SEC. 2325. CONTINUATION, RENEWAL, REPLACEMENT, CONVERSION, AND CANCELLATION OF POLICIES.

(a) IN GENERAL.—The Secretary, after considering (where appropriate) recommendations of the Advisory Council, shall promulgate regulations establishing requirements applicable to the renewal, replacement, conversion, and cancellation of long-term care insurance policies, which shall include at a minimum the requirements specified in this section.

(b) INSURED'S RIGHT TO CANCEL DURING EXAMINATION PERIOD.—Each individual insured (or, if different, each individual liable for payment of premiums) under a long-term care insurance policy shall have the unconditional right to return the policy within 30 days after the date of its issuance and delivery, and to obtain a full refund of any premium paid.

(c) INSURER'S RIGHT TO CANCEL (OR DENY BENEFITS) BASED ON FRAUD OR NONDISCLOSURE.—An insurer shall have the right to cancel a long-term care insurance policy, or to refuse to pay a claim for benefits, based on evidence that the insured falsely represented or failed to disclose information material to the determination of eligibility to purchase such insurance, but only if—

(1) the insurer presents written documentation, developed at the time the insured applied for such insurance, of the insurer's request for the information thus withheld or misrepresented, and the insured individual's response to such request;

(2) the insurer presents medical records or other evidence showing that the insured individual knew or should have known that such response was false, incomplete, or misleading;

(3) notice of cancellation is furnished to the insured individual before the date 3 years after the effective date of the policy (or such earlier date as the Secretary may specify in regulations); and

(4) the insured individual is afforded the opportunity to review and refute the evidence presented by the insurer pursuant to paragraphs (1) and (2).

(d) INSURER'S RIGHT TO CANCEL FOR NONPAYMENT OF PREMIUMS.—

(1) IN GENERAL.—Insurers shall have the right to cancel long-term care insurance policies for nonpayment of premiums, subject to the provisions of this subsection and subsection (e) (relating to nonforfeiture).

(2) NOTICE AND ACKNOWLEDGEMENT.—

(A) IN GENERAL.—The insurer may not cancel coverage of an insured individual until—

(i) the insurer, not earlier than the date when such payment is 30 days past due, has given written notice to the insured individual (by registered letter or the equivalent) of such intent, and

(ii) 30 days have elapsed since the insurer obtained written acknowledgment of receipt of such notice from the insured individual (or the designated representative, at the insured individual's option or in the case of an insured individual determined to be incapacitated in accordance with paragraph (4)).

(B) ADDITIONAL REQUIREMENT FOR GROUP POLICIES.—In the case of a group long-term care insurance policy, the notice and acknowledgement requirements of subparagraph (A) apply with respect to the policyholder and to each insured individual.

(3) REINSTATEMENT OF COVERAGE OF INCAPACITATED INDIVIDUALS.—In any case where the coverage of an individual under a long-term care insurance policy has been canceled pursuant to paragraph (2), the insurer shall be required to reinstate full coverage of such individual under such policy, retroactive to the effective date of cancellation, if the insurer receives from such individual (or the designated representative of such individual), within 5 months after such date—

(A) evidence of a determination of such individual's incapacitation in accordance with paragraph (4) (whether made before or after such date), and

(B) payment of all premiums due and past due, and all charges for late payment.

(4) DETERMINATION OF INCAPACITATION.—For purposes of this subsection, the term "determination of incapacitation" means a determination by a qualified health professional (in accordance with such requirements as the Secretary may specify), that an insured individual has suffered a cognitive impairment or loss of functional capacity which could reasonably be expected to render the individual permanently or temporarily unable to deal with business or financial matters. The standard used to make such determination shall not be more stringent than the threshold conditions for the receipt of covered benefits.

(5) DESIGNATION OF REPRESENTATIVE.—The insurer shall be required—

(A) to require the insured individual, at the time of sale or issuance of a long-term care insurance policy—

(i) to designate a representative for purposes of communication with the insurer concerning premium payments in the event the insured individual cannot be located or is incapacitated, or

                    (ii) to complete a signed and dated statement declining to designate a representative, and

            (B) to obtain from the insured individual, at the time of each premium payment (but in no event less often than once in each 12-month period) reconfirmation or revision of such designation or declination.

(e) NONFORFEITURE.—

    (1) IN GENERAL.—The Secretary, after consideration of recommendations by the Advisory Council, shall by regulation require appropriate nonforfeiture benefits with respect to each long-term care insurance policy that lapses for any reason (including nonpayment of premiums, cancellation, or failure to renew, but excluding lapses due to death) after remaining in effect beyond a specified minimum period.

    (2) NONFORFEITURE BENEFITS.—The standards established under this subsection shall require that the amount or percentage of nonforfeiture benefits shall increase proportionally with the amount of premiums paid by a policyholder.

(f) CONTINUATION, RENEWAL, REPLACEMENT, AND CONVERSION OF POLICIES.—

(1) IN GENERAL.—Insurers shall not be permitted to cancel, or refuse to renew (or replace with a substantial equivalent), any long-term care insurance policy for any reason other than for fraud or material misrepresentation (as provided in subsection (c)) or for nonpayment of premium (as provided in subsection (d)).

(2) DURATION AND RENEWAL OF POLICIES.—Each long-term care insurance policy shall contain a provision that clearly states—

(A) the duration of the policy,

(B) the right of the insured individual (or policyholder) to renewal (or to replacement with a substantial equivalent),

(C) the date by which, and the manner in which, the option to renew must be exercised, and

(D) any applicable restrictions or limitations (which may not be inconsistent with the requirements of this part).

(3) REPLACEMENT OF POLICIES.—

(A) IN GENERAL.—Except as provided in subparagraph (B), an insurer shall not be permitted to sell any long-term care insurance policy as a replacement for another such policy unless coverage under such replacement policy is available to an individual insured for benefits covered under the previous policy to the same extent as under such previous policy (including every individual insured under a group policy) on the date of termination of such previous policy, without exclusions or limitations that did not apply under such previous policy.

(B) INSURED'S OPTION TO REDUCE COVERAGE.—In any case where an insured individual covered under a long-term care insurance policy knowingly and voluntarily elects to substitute for such policy a policy that provides less coverage, substitute policy shall be considered a replacement policy for purposes of this part.

(3) CONTINUATION AND CONVERSION RIGHTS WITH RESPECT TO GROUP POLICIES.—

(A) IN GENERAL.—Insurers shall be required to include in each group long-term care insurance policy, a provision affording to each insured individual, when such policy would otherwise terminate, the opportunity (at the insurer's option, subject to approval of the State insurance commissioner) either to continue or to convert coverage under such policy in accordance with this paragraph.

(B) RIGHTS OF RELATED INDIVIDUALS.—In the case of any insured individual whose eligibility for coverage under a group policy is based on relationship to another individual, the insurer shall be required to continue such coverage upon termination of the relationship due to divorce or death.

(C) CONTINUATION OF COVERAGE.—A group policy shall be considered to meet the requirements of this paragraph with respect to rights of an insured individual to continuation of coverage if coverage of the same (or substantially equivalent) benefits for such individual under such policy is maintained, subject only to timely payment of premiums.

(D) CONVERSION OF COVERAGE.—A group policy shall be considered to meet the requirements of this paragraph with respect to conversion if it entitles each individual who has been continuously covered under the policy for at least 6 months before the date of the termination to issuance of a replacement policy providing benefits identical to, substantially equivalent to, or in excess of, the benefits under such terminated group policy—

 (i) without requiring evidence of insurability with respect to benefits covered under such previous policy, and

 (ii) at premium rates no higher than would apply if the insured individual had initially obtained coverage under such replacement policy on the date such insured individual initially obtained coverage under such group policy.

(4) TREATMENT OF SUBSTANTIAL EQUIVALENCE.—

 (A) UNDER SECRETARY'S GUIDELINES.—The Secretary, after considering recommendations by the Advisory Council, shall develop guidelines for comparing long-term care insurance policies for the purpose of determining whether benefits under such policies are substantially equivalent.

 (B) BEFORE EFFECTIVE DATE OF SECRETARY'S GUIDELINES.—During the period prior to the effective date of guidelines published by the Secretary under this paragraph, insurers shall comply with standards for determinations of substantial equivalence established by State insurance commissioners.

(5) ADDITIONAL REQUIREMENTS.—Insurers shall comply with such other requirements relating to continuation, renewal, replacement, and conversion of long-term care insurance policies as the Secretary may establish.

### SEC. 2326. REQUIREMENTS RELATING TO PAYMENT OF BENEFITS.

(a) IN GENERAL.—The Secretary, after considering (where appropriate) recommendations of the Advisory Council, shall promulgate regulations establishing requirements with respect to claims for and payment of benefits under long-term care insurance policies, which shall include at a minimum the requirements specified in this section.

(b) STANDARDS RELATING TO THRESHOLD CONDITIONS FOR RECEIPT OF COVERED BENEFITS.—Each long-term care insurance policy shall meet the following requirements with respect to identification of, and determination of whether an insured individual meets, the threshold conditions for receipt of benefits covered under such policy:

(1) DECLARATION OF THRESHOLD CONDITIONS.—

(A) IN GENERAL.—The policy shall specify the level (or levels) of functional or cognitive mental impairment (or combination of impairments) required as a threshold condition of entitlement to receive benefits under the policy (which threshold condition or conditions shall be consistent with any regulations promulgated by the Secretary pursuant to subsection (B)).

(B) SECRETARIAL RESPONSIBILITY.—The Secretary (after considering the views of the Advisory Council on current practices of insurers concerning, and the appropriateness of standardizing, threshold conditions) may promulgate such regulations as the Secretary finds appropriate establishing standardized thresholds to be used under such policies as preconditions for varying levels of benefits.

(2) INDEPENDENT PROFESSIONAL ASSESSMENT.—The policy shall provide for a procedure for determining whether the threshold conditions specified under paragraph (1) have been met with respect to an insured individual which—

(A) applies such uniform assessment standards, procedures, and formats as the Secretary may specify, after consideration of recommendations by the Advisory Council;

(B) permits an initial evaluation (or, if the initial evaluation was performed by a qualified independent assessor selected by the insurer, a reevaluation) to be made by a qualified independent assessor selected by the insured individual (or designated representative) as to whether the threshold conditions for receipt of benefits have been met;

(C) permits the insurer the option to obtain a reevaluation by a qualified independent assessor selected and reimbursed by the insurer;

(D) provides that the insurer will consider that the threshold conditions have been met in any case where—

(i) the assessment under subparagraph (B) concluded that such conditions had been met, and the insurer declined the option under subparagraph (C), or

(ii) assessments under both subparagraphs (B) and (C) concluded that such conditions had been met; and

(E) provides for final resolution of the question by a State agency or other impartial third party in any case where assessments under subparagraphs (B) and (C) reach inconsistent conclusions.

(3) QUALIFIED INDEPENDENT ASSESSOR.—For purposes of paragraph (2), the term "qualified independent assessor" means a licensed or certified professional, as appropriate, who—

(A) meets such standards with respect to professional qualifications as may be established by the Secretary, after consulting with the Secretary of the Treasury, and

(B) has no significant or controlling financial interest in, is not an employee of, and does not derive more than 5 percent of gross income from, the insurer (or any provider of services for which benefits are available under the policy and in which the insurer has a significant or controlling financial interest).

(c) REQUIREMENTS RELATING TO CLAIMS FOR BENEFITS.—Insurers shall be required—

(1) to promptly pay or deny claims for benefits submitted by (or on behalf of) insured individuals who have been determined pursuant to subsection (b) to meet the threshold conditions for payment of benefits;

(2) to provide an explanation in writing of the reasons for payment, partial payment, or denial of each such claim; and

(3) to provide an administrative procedure under which an insured individual may appeal the denial of any claim.

### Subpart C—Enforcement

**SEC. 2342. STATE PROGRAMS FOR ENFORCEMENT OF STANDARDS.**

(a) REQUIREMENT FOR STATE PROGRAMS IMPLEMENTING FEDERAL STANDARDS.—In order for a State to be eligible for grants under this subpart, the State must have in effect a program (including such laws and procedures as may be necessary) for the regulation of long-term care insurance which the Secretary has determined—

(1) includes the elements required under this subpart, and

(2) is designed to ensure the compliance of long-term care insurance policies sold in the State, and insurers offering such policies and their agents, with the requirements established pursuant to subpart B.

(b) ACTIVITIES UNDER STATE PROGRAM.—A State program approved under this subpart shall provide for the following procedures and activities:

(1) MONITORING OF INSURERS AND POLICIES.—Procedures for ongoing monitoring of the compliance of insurers doing business in the State, and of long-term care insurance policies sold in the State, with requirements under this part, including at least the following:

(A) POLICY REVIEW AND CERTIFICATION.—A program for review and certification (and annual recertification) of each such policy sold in the State.

(B) REPORTING BY INSURERS.—Requirements of annual reporting by insurers selling or servicing long-term care insurance policies in the State, in such form and containing such information as the State may require to determine whether the insurer (and policies) are in compliance with requirements under this part.

(C) DATA COLLECTION.—Procedures for collection, from insurers, service providers, insured individuals, and others, of information required by the State for purposes of carrying out its responsibilities under this part (including authority to compel compliance of insurers with requests for such information).

(D) MARKETING OVERSIGHT.—Procedures for monitoring (through sampling or other appropriate procedures) the sales practices of insurers and agents, including review of marketing literature.

(E) OVERSIGHT OF ADMINISTRATION OF BENEFITS.—Procedures for monitoring (through sampling or other appropriate procedures) insurers' administration of benefits, including monitoring of—

(i) determinations of insured individuals' eligibility to receive benefits, and

(ii) disposition of claims for payment.

(2) INFORMATION TO INSURERS.—Procedures for furnishing, to insurers selling or servicing any long-term care insurance policies in the State, information on conditions of eligibility for, and benefits under, each public long-term care program administered by the State, in order to enable them to comply with the requirement under section 2321(e)(3).

(3) CONSUMER COMPLAINTS AND DISPUTE RESOLUTION.—Administrative procedures for the investigation and resolution of complaints by consumers, and disputes between consumers and insurers, with respect to long-term care insurance, including—

(A) procedures for the filing, investigation, and adjudication of consumer complaints with respect to the compliance of insurers and policies with requirements under this part, or other requirements under State law; and

(B) procedures for resolution of disputes between insured individuals and insurers concerning eligibility for, or the amount of, benefits payable under such policies, and other issues with respect to the rights and responsibilities of insurers and insured individuals under such policies.

(4) TECHNICAL ASSISTANCE TO INSURERS.—Provision of technical assistance to insurers to help them to understand and comply with the requirements of this part, and other State laws, concerning long-term care insurance policies and business practices.

(c) STATE ENFORCEMENT AUTHORITIES.—A State program meeting the requirements of this subpart shall ensure that the State insurance commissioner (or other appropriate official or agency) has the following authority with respect to long-term care insurers and policies:

(1) PROHIBITION OF SALE.—Authority to prohibit the sale, or offering for sale, of any long-term

care insurance policy that fails to comply with all applicable requirements under this part.

(2) PLANS OF CORRECTION.—Authority, in cases where the business practices of an insurer are determined not to comply with requirements under this part, to require the insurer to develop, submit for State approval, and implement a plan of correction which must be fulfilled within the shortest period possible (not to exceed a year) as a condition of continuing to do business in the State.

(3) CORRECTIVE ACTION ORDERS.—Authority, in cases where an insurer is determined to have failed to comply with requirements of this part, or with the terms of a policy, with respect to a consumer or insured individual, to direct the insurer (subject to appropriate due process) to eliminate such noncompliance within 30 days.

(4) CIVIL MONEY PENALTIES.—Authority to assess civil money penalties, in amounts for each violative act up to the greater of $10,000 or three times the amount of any commission involved—

(A) for violations of subsections (d) (concerning compensation or sale of policies), (e) (concerning prohibited sales practices), and (f) (prohibition on sale of duplicate benefits) of section 2324,

　　　　(B) for such other violative acts as the Secretary may specify in regulations, and

　　　　(C) in such other cases as the State finds appropriate.

　　(5) OTHER AUTHORITIES.—Such other authorities as the State finds necessary or appropriate to enforce requirements under this part.

(d) RECORDS, REPORTS, AND AUDITS.—As a condition of approval of its program under this part, a State must agree to maintain such records, make such reports (including expenditure reports), and cooperate with such audits, as the Secretary finds necessary to determine the compliance of such State program (and insurers and policies regulated under such program) with the requirements of this part.

(e) SECRETARIAL RESPONSIBILITIES.—

　　(1) APPROVAL OF STATE PROGRAMS.—The Secretary shall approve a State program meeting the requirements of this part.

　　(2) INFORMATION ON MEDICARE BENEFITS.—The Secretary shall furnish, to the official in each State with chief responsibility for the regulation of long-term care insurance, a description of the Medi-

care programs under title XVIII of the Social Security Act which makes clear the unavailability of long-term benefits under such programs, for distribution by such State official to insurers selling long-term care insurance in the State, in accordance with subsection (b)(2).

**SEC. 2342. AUTHORIZATION OF APPROPRIATIONS FOR STATE PROGRAMS.**

There are authorized to be appropriated $10,000,000 for fiscal year 1996, $10,000,000 for fiscal year 1997, $7,500,000 for fiscal year 1998, and $5,000,000 for fiscal year 1999 and each succeeding fiscal year, for grants to States with programs meeting the requirements of this part, to remain available until expended.

**SEC. 2343. ALLOTMENTS TO STATES.**

The allotment for any fiscal year to a State with a program approved under this part shall be an amount determined by the Secretary, taking into account the numbers of long-term care insurance policies sold, and of elderly individuals residing, in the State, and such other factors as the Secretary finds appropriate.

**SEC. 2344. PAYMENTS TO STATES.**

(a) IN GENERAL.—Each State with a program approved under this part shall be entitled to payment under this title for each fiscal year in an amount equal to its allotment for such fiscal year, for expenditure by such State for up to 50 percent of the cost of activities under such program.

(b) STATE SHARE OF PROGRAM EXPENDITURES.—No Federal funds from any source may be used as any part of the non-Federal share of expenditures under the State program under this subpart.

(c) TRANSFER AND DEPOSIT REQUIREMENTS.—The Secretary shall make payments under this section in accordance with section 6503 of title 31, United States Code.

### SEC. 2345. FEDERAL OVERSIGHT OF STATE ENFORCEMENT.

(a) IN GENERAL.—The Secretary shall periodically review State regulatory programs approved under section 2341 to determine whether they continue to comply with the requirements of this part.

(b) NOTICE OF DETERMINATION OF NONCOMPLIANCE.—The Secretary shall promptly notify the State of a determination that a State program fails to comply with this part, specifying the requirement or requirements not met and the elements of the State program requiring correction.

(c) OPPORTUNITY FOR CORRECTION.—

(1) IN GENERAL.—The Secretary shall afford a State notified of noncompliance pursuant to sub-

section (b) a reasonable opportunity to eliminate such noncompliance.

(2) CORRECTION PLANS.—In a case where substantial corrections are needed to eliminate noncompliance of a State program, the Secretary may—

(A) permit the State a reasonable time after the date of the notice pursuant to subsection (b) to develop and obtain the Secretary's approval of a correction plan, and

(B) permit the State a reasonable time after the date of approval of such plan to eliminate the noncompliance.

(d) WITHDRAWAL OF PROGRAM APPROVAL.—In the case of a State that fails to eliminate noncompliance with requirements under this part by the date specified by the Secretary pursuant to subsection (c), the Secretary shall withdraw the approval of the State program pursuant to section 2341(e).

## SEC. 2346. EFFECT OF FAILURE TO HAVE APPROVED STATE PROGRAM.

(a) RESTRICTION ON SALE OF LONG-TERM CARE INSURANCE.—

(1) IN GENERAL.—No insurer may sell or offer for sale any long-term care insurance policy, on or after the date specified in subsection (c), in a State

that does not have in effect a regulatory program approved under section 2341(e).

(2) APPLICATION OF PROHIBITION.—For purposes of paragraph (1), an insurance policy shall not be considered to be sold or offered for sale in a State solely because it is sold or offered to a resident of such State.

(b) CIVIL MONEY PENALTY.—

(1) IN GENERAL.—An insurer shall be subject to a civil money penalty, in an amount up to the greater of $10,000 or three times any commission involved, for each incident in which the insurer sells, or offers to sell, an insurance policy to an individual in violation of subsection (a).

(2) ENFORCEMENT PROCEDURE.—The Secretary shall enforce the provisions of this subsection in accordance with the procedures provided under section 5412 of this Act.

(c) EFFECTIVE DATE.—

(1) IN GENERAL.—The date specified in this subsection, for purposes of subsection (a), with respect to any requirement under this part, is the date one year after the date the Secretary first promulgates regulations with respect to such requirement.

(2) EXCEPTION.—To the extent that a State demonstrates to the Secretary that State legislation is required to meet any such requirement, the State shall not be regarded as failing to have in effect a program in compliance with this part solely on the basis of its failure to comply with such requirement before the first day of the first calendar quarter beginning after the close of the first regular session of the State legislature that begins after the promulgation of the regulation imposing such requirement. For purposes of the preceding sentence, in the case of a State that has a 2-year legislative session, each year of such session shall be deemed to be a separate regular session of the State legislature.

### Subpart D—Consumer Education Grants

**SEC. 2361. GRANTS FOR CONSUMER EDUCATION.**

(a) GRANT PROGRAM AUTHORIZED.—The Secretary is authorized to make grants—

    (1) to States,

    (2) to regional alliances (at the option of States within which such Alliances are located), and

    (3) to national organizations representing insurance consumers, long-term care providers, and insurers,

for the development and implementation of long-term care information, counseling, and other programs.

(b) APPLICATIONS.—

(1) IN GENERAL.—Each State or organization seeking a grant under this section shall submit to the Secretary an application, in such format and containing such information as the Secretary may require.

(2) GOALS.—Programs under this section shall be directed at the goals of increasing consumers' understanding and awareness of options available to them with respect to long-term care insurance (and alternatives, such as public long-term care programs), including—

(A) the risk of needing long-term care;

(B) the costs associated with long-term care services;

(C) the lack of long-term care coverage under the Medicare program, Medicare supplemental (Medigap) policies, and standard private health insurance;

(D) the limitations on (and conditions of eligibility for) long-term care coverage under State programs;

(E) the availability, and variations in coverage and cost, of private long-term care insurance;

(F) features common to many private long-term care insurance policies; and

(G) pitfalls to avoid when purchasing a long-term care insurance policy.

(3) ACTIVITIES.—An application for a grant under this section shall indicate the activities the State or organization would carry out under such grant, which activities may include—

(A) coordination of the activities of State agencies and private entities as necessary to carry out the State's program under this section;

(B) collection, analysis, publication, and dissemination of information,

(C) conducting or sponsoring of consumer education, outreach, and information programs,

(D) providing (directly or through referral) counseling and consultation services to consumers to assist them in choosing long-term care insurance coverage appropriate to their circumstances, and

(E) other appropriate activities.

(4) PRIORITY FOR INNOVATION.—In awarding grants under this section, the Secretary shall give priority to applications proposing to use innovative approaches to providing information, counseling, and other assistance to individuals who might benefit from, or are considering the purchase of, long-term care insurance.

(c) PERIOD OF GRANTS.—Grants under this section shall be for not longer than 3 years.

(d) EVALUATIONS AND REPORTS.—

(1) BY GRANTEES TO THE SECRETARY.—Each recipient of a grant under this section shall annually evaluate the effectiveness of its program under such grant, and report its conclusions to the Secretary.

(2) BY THE SECRETARY TO THE CONGRESS.—The Secretary shall annually evaluate, and report to the Congress on, the effectiveness of programs under this section, on the basis of reports received under paragraph (1) and such independent evaluation as the Secretary finds necessary.

(e) AUTHORIZATION OF APPROPRIATIONS.—There are authorized to be appropriated, for grants under this section—

(1) $10,000,000 for each of fiscal years 1995 through 1997 for grants to States, and

(2) $1,000,000 for each of fiscal years 1995 through 1997,

for grants to eligible organizations.

## PART 4—TAX TREATMENT OF LONG-TERM CARE INSURANCE AND SERVICES

### SEC. 2401. REFERENCE TO TAX PROVISIONS.

For amendments to the Internal Revenue Code of 1986 relating to the treatment of long-term care insurance and services, see subtitle G of title VII.

## PART 5—TAX INCENTIVES FOR INDIVIDUALS WITH DISABILITIES WHO WORK

### SEC. 2501. REFERENCE TO TAX PROVISION.

For amendment to the Internal Revenue Code of 1986 providing for a tax credit for cost of personal assistance services required by employed individuals, see section 7901.

## PART 6—DEMONSTRATION AND EVALUATION

### SEC. 2601. DEMONSTRATION ON ACUTE AND LONG-TERM CARE INTEGRATION.

(a) PROGRAM AUTHORIZED.—The Secretary of Health and Human Services shall conduct a demonstration program to test the effectiveness of various approaches to financing and providing integrated acute and long-term care services described in subsection (b) for the chronically ill and disabled who meet eligibility criteria under subsection (c).

(b) SERVICES AND BENEFITS.—

    (1) IN GENERAL.—Except as provided in paragraph (2), the following services and benefits shall be provided under each demonstration approved under this section:

        (A) COMPREHENSIVE BENEFIT PACKAGE.—All benefits included in the comprehensive benefit package under title I of this Act.

        (B) TRANSITIONAL BENEFITS.—Specialized benefits relating to the transition from acute to long-term care, including—

            (i) assessment and consultation,

            (ii) inpatient transitional care,

            (iii) medical rehabilitation,

            (iv) home health care and home care,

            (v) caregiver support, and

            (vi) self-help technology.

        (C) LONG-TERM CARE BENEFITS.—Long-term care benefits, including—

            (i) adult day care,

            (ii) personal assistance services,

(iii) homemaker services and chore services;

(iv) home-delivered meals;

(v) respite services;

(vi) nursing facility services in specialized care units;

(vii) services in other residential settings including community supported living arrangements and assisted living facilities; and

(viii) assistive devices and environmental modifications.

(D) HABILITATION SERVICES.—Specialized habilitation services for participants with developmental disabilities.

(2) VARIATIONS IN MINIMUM BENEFITS.—

(A) IN GENERAL.—Subject to the requirement of subparagraph (B), demonstrations may omit specified services listed under subparagraphs (C) and (D) of paragraph (1), or provide additional services, as found appropriate by the Secretary in the case of a particular demonstration, taking into consideration factors such as—

(i) the needs of a specialized group of eligible beneficiaries;

(ii) the availability of the omitted benefits under other programs in the service area; and

(iii) the geographic availability of service providers.

(B) BREADTH REQUIREMENT.—In approving variant demonstrations pursuant to subparagraph (A), the Secretary shall ensure that demonstrations under this section, taken as a group, adequately test financing and delivery models covering the entire array of services and benefits described in paragraph (1).

(c) ELIGIBILITY CRITERIA.—The Secretary shall establish eligibility criteria for individuals who may receive services under demonstrations under this section. Under such criteria, any of the following may be found to be eligible populations for such demonstrations:

(1) Individuals with disabilities who are entitled to services and benefits under a State program under part 1 of this subtitle.

(2) Individuals who are entitled to benefits under parts A and B of title XVIII of the Social Security Act.

(3) Individuals who are entitled to medical assistance under a State plan under title XIX of the Social Security Act, and are also—

 (A) individuals described in paragraph (2), or

 (B) individuals eligible for supplemental security income under title XVI of that Act.

(d) APPLICATION.—

(1) IN GENERAL.—Each entity seeking to participate in a demonstration under this section shall submit an application, in such format and containing such information as the Secretary may require, including the information specified in this subsection.

(2) SERVICE DELIVERY.—The application shall state the services to be provided under the demonstration (either directly by the applicant or under other arrangements approved by the Secretary), which shall include services specified pursuant to subsection (b) and—

 (A) enrollment services;

 (B) client assessment and care planning;

 (C) simplified access to needed services;

(D) integrated management of acute and chronic care, including measures to ensure continuity of care across settings and services;

(E) quality assurance, grievance, and appeals mechanisms; and

(F) such other services as the Secretary may require.

(3) CONSUMER PROTECTION AND PARTICIPATION.—The applicant shall provide evidence of consumer participation—

(A) in the planning of the demonstration (including a showing of support from community agencies or consumer interest groups); and

(B) in the conduct of the demonstration, including descriptions of methods and procedures to be used—

(i) to make available to individuals enrolled in the demonstration information on self-help, health promotion and disability prevention practices, and enrollees' contributions to the costs of care;

(ii) to ensure participation by such enrollees (or their designated representatives, where appropriate) in care planning and in decisions concerning treatment;

(iii) to handle and resolve client grievances and appeals;

(iv) to take enrollee views into account in quality assurance and provider contracting procedures; and

(v) to evaluate enrollee satisfaction with the program.

(4) APPLICANT QUALIFICATIONS.—Applicants for grants under this section shall meet eligibility criteria established by the Secretary, including requirements relating to—

(A) adequate financial controls to monitor administrative and service costs,

(B) demonstrated commitment of the Board of Directors or comparable governing body to the goals of demonstration,

(C) information systems adequate to pay service providers, to collect required utilization and cost data, and to provide data adequate to permit evaluation of program performance, and

(D) compliance with applicable State laws.

(e) PAYMENTS TO PARTICIPANTS.—An entity conducting a demonstration under this section shall be entitled to receive, with respect to each enrollee, for the period during which it is providing to such enrollee services under a demonstration under this section, such amounts as the Secretary shall provide, which amounts—

    (1) may include risk-based payments and non-risk based payments by governmental programs, by third parties, or by project enrollees, or any combination of such payments, and

    (2) may vary by project and by enrollee. .

(f) NUMBER AND DURATION OF DEMONSTRATION PROJECTS.—

    (1) REQUEST FOR APPLICATIONS.—The Secretary shall publish a request for applications under this section not later than one year after enactment of this Act.

    (2) NUMBER AND DURATION.—The Secretary shall authorize not more than 25 demonstrations under this section, each of which shall run for 7 years from the date of the award.

(g) EVALUATION AND REPORTS.—The Secretary shall evaluate the demonstration projects under this section, and shall submit to the Congress—

    (1) an interim report, by three years after enactment, describing the status of the demonstration and characteristics of the approved projects; and

    (2) a final report, by one year after completion of such demonstration projects, evaluating their ef-

fectiveness (including cost-effectiveness), and discussing the advisability of including some or all of the integrated models tested in the demonstration as a benefit under the comprehensive benefit package under title I of this Act, or under the programs under title XVIII of the Social Security Act.

(h) AUTHORIZATION OF APPROPRIATIONS.—

(1) FOR SECRETARIAL RESPONSIBILITIES.—

(A) IN GENERAL.—There are authorized to be appropriated $7,000,000 for fiscal year 1996, and $4,500,000 for each of the 6 succeeding fiscal years, for payment of costs of the Secretary in carrying out this section (including costs for technical assistance to potential service providers, and research and evaluation), which amounts shall remain available until expended.

(B) SET-ASIDE FOR FEASIBILITY STUDIES.—Of the total amount authorized to be appropriated under subparagraph (A), not less than $1,000,000 shall be available for studies of the feasibility of systems to provide integrated care for nonaged populations (including physically disabled children and adults, the chronically mentally ill, and individuals with disabilities, and combinations of these groups).

(2) FOR COVERED BENEFITS.—There are authorized to be appropriated $50,000,000 for the first fiscal year for which grants are awarded under this section, and for each of the four succeeding fiscal years, for payment of costs of benefits for which no public or private program or entity is legally obligated to pay.

## SEC. 2602. PERFORMANCE REVIEW OF THE LONG-TERM CARE PROGRAMS.

(a) IN GENERAL.—The Secretary of Health and Human Services shall prepare and submit to the Congress—

(1) an interim report, not later than the end of the seventh full calendar year beginning after the date of the enactment of this Act, and

(2) a final report, not later than two years after the date of the interim report,

evaluating the effectiveness of the programs established and amendments made by this subtitle (and including at a minimum the elements specified in subsection (b)).

(b) ELEMENTS OF ASSESSMENT.—The evaluations to be made, and included in the reports required pursuant to subsection (a), include at least the following:

(1) STATE SERVICE DELIVERY PROGRAMS.—An evaluation of States' effectiveness in meeting the needs for home and community-based services (including personal assistance services) of individuals with disabilities (including individuals who do, and who do not, meet the eligibility criteria for the service program under part 1, individuals of different ages, type and degree of disability, and income levels, members of minority groups, and individuals residing in rural areas).

(2) SERVICE ACCESS.—An evaluation of the degree of (and obstacles to) access of individuals with disabilities to needed home and community-based services and to inpatient services.

(3) QUALITY.—An evaluation of the quality of long-term care services available.

(4) PRIVATE INSURANCE.—An evaluation of the performance of the private sector in offering affordable long-term care insurance that provides adequate protection against the costs of long-term care, and of the effectiveness of Federal standards and State enforcement, pursuant to part 3, in adequately protecting long-term care insurance consumers.

(5) COST ISSUES.—An evaluation of the effectiveness of amendments made by this subtitle in con-

taining the costs of long-term care, and in limiting the share of such costs borne by individuals with lower incomes.

(6) SERVICE COORDINATION AND INTEGRATION.—An evaluation of the effectiveness of the programs established or amended under this subtitle in achieving coordination and integration of long-term care services, and of such services with acute care services and social services, and in ensuring provision of services in the least restrictive setting possible.

# TITLE III—PUBLIC HEALTH INITIATIVES

### TABLE OF CONTENTS OF TITLE

## Subtitle A—Workforce Priorities Under Federal Payments

PART 1—INSTITUTIONAL COSTS OF GRADUATE MEDICAL EDUCATION; WORKFORCE PRIORITIES

SUBPART A—NATIONAL COUNCIL REGARDING WORKFORCE PRIORITIES

Sec. 3001. National Council on Graduate Medical Education.

SUBPART B—AUTHORIZED POSITIONS IN SPECIALTY TRAINING

Sec. 3011. Cooperation of approved physician training programs.
Sec. 3012. Annual authorization of number of specialty positions; requirements regarding primary health care.
Sec. 3013. Allocations among specialities and programs.

SUBPART C—INSTITUTIONAL COSTS OF GRADUATE MEDICAL EDUCATION

Sec. 3031. Federal formula payments to approved physician training programs.
Sec. 3032. Application for payments.
Sec. 3033. Availability of funds for payments; annual amount of payments.
Sec. 3034. Additional funding provisions.

SUBPART D—GENERAL PROVISIONS

Sec. 3041. Definitions.

SUBPART E—TRANSITIONAL PROVISIONS

Sec. 3051. Transitional payments to institutions.

PART 2—RELATED PROGRAMS

Sec. 3061. Additional funding for certain workforce programs.
Sec. 3062. Programs of the Secretary of Health and Human Services.
Sec. 3063. Programs of the Secretary of Labor.
Sec. 3064. National Institute for Health Care Workforce Development.

## Subtitle B—Academic Health Centers

PART 1—FORMULA PAYMENTS

Sec. 3101. Federal formula payments to academic health centers.
Sec. 3102. Request for payments.
Sec. 3103. Availability of funds for payments; annual amount of payments.
Sec. 3104. Additional funding provisions.

PART 2—ACCESS OF PATIENTS TO ACADEMIC HEALTH CENTERS

Sec. 3131. Contracts for ensuring access to centers.
Sec. 3132. Discretionary grants regarding access to centers.

## Subtitle C—Health Research Initiatives

### PART 1—PROGRAMS FOR CERTAIN AGENCIES

Sec. 3201. Biomedical and behavioral research on health promotion and disease prevention.
Sec. 3202. Health services research.

### PART 2—FUNDING FOR PROGRAMS

Sec. 3211. Authorizations regarding Public Health Service Initiatives Fund.

## Subtitle D—Core Functions of Public Health Programs; National Initiatives Regarding Preventive Health

### PART 1—FUNDING

Sec. 3301. Authorizations regarding Public Health Service Initiatives Fund.

### PART 2—CORE FUNCTIONS OF PUBLIC HEALTH PROGRAMS

Sec. 3311. Purposes.
Sec. 3312. Grants to States for core health functions.
Sec. 3313. Submission of information.
Sec. 3314. Reports.
Sec. 3315. Application for grant.
Sec. 3316. General provisions.
Sec. 3317. Allocations for certain activities.
Sec. 3318. Definitions.

### PART 3—NATIONAL INITIATIVES REGARDING HEALTH PROMOTION AND DISEASE PREVENTION

Sec. 3331. Grants for national prevention initiatives.
Sec. 3332. Priorities.
Sec. 3333. Submission of information.
Sec. 3334. Application for grant.

## Subtitle E—Health Services for Medically Underserved Populations

### PART 1—COMMUNITY AND MIGRANT HEALTH CENTERS

Sec. 3401. Authorizations regarding Public Health Service Initiatives Fund.
Sec. 3402. Use of funds.

### PART 2—INITIATIVES FOR ACCESS TO HEALTH CARE

#### SUBPART A—PURPOSES; FUNDING

Sec. 3411. Purposes.
Sec. 3412. Authorizations regarding Public Health Service Initiatives Fund.

#### SUBPART B—DEVELOPMENT OF QUALIFIED COMMUNITY HEALTH PLANS AND PRACTICE NETWORKS

Sec. 3421. Grants and contracts for development of plans and networks.
Sec. 3422. Preferences in making awards of assistance.
Sec. 3423. Certain uses of awards.
Sec. 3424. Accessibility of services.

Sec. 3425. Additional agreements.
Sec. 3426. Submission of certain information.
Sec. 3427. Reports; audits.
Sec. 3428. Application for assistance.
Sec. 3429. General provisions.

SUBPART C—CAPITAL COST OF DEVELOPMENT OF QUALIFIED COMMUNITY HEALTH PLANS AND PRACTICE NETWORKS

Sec. 3441. Loans and loan guarantees regarding plans and networks.
Sec. 3442. Certain requirements.
Sec. 3443. Defaults; right of recovery.
Sec. 3444. Provisions regarding construction or expansion of facilities.
Sec. 3445. Application for assistance.
Sec. 3446. Administration of programs.

SUBPART D—ENABLING SERVICES

Sec. 3461. Grants and contracts for enabling services.
Sec. 3462. Authorizations regarding Public Health Service Initiatives Fund.

PART 3—NATIONAL HEALTH SERVICE CORPS

Sec. 3471. Authorizations regarding Public Health Service Initiatives Fund.
Sec. 3472. Allocation for participation of nurses in scholarship and loan repayment programs.

PART 4—PAYMENTS TO HOSPITALS SERVING VULNERABLE POPULATIONS

Sec. 3481. Payments to hospitals.
Sec. 3482. Identification of eligible hospitals.
Sec. 3483. Amount of payments.
Sec. 3484. Base year.

## Subtitle F—Mental Health; Substance Abuse

PART 1—FINANCIAL ASSISTANCE

Sec. 3501. Authorizations regarding Public Health Service Initiatives Fund.
Sec. 3502. Supplemental formula grants for States regarding activities under part B of title XIX of Public Health Service Act.
Sec. 3503. Capital costs of development of certain centers and clinics.

PART 2—AUTHORITIES REGARDING PARTICIPATING STATES

SUBPART A—REPORTS

Sec. 3511. Report on integration of mental health systems.

SUBPART B—PILOT PROGRAM

Sec. 3521. Pilot program.

## Subtitle G—Comprehensive School Health Education; School-Related Health Services

PART 1—GENERAL PROVISIONS

Sec. 3601. Purposes.
Sec. 3602. Definitions.

## Part 2—School Health Education; General Provisions

Sec. 3611. Authorizations regarding Public Health Service Initiatives Fund.
Sec. 3612. Waivers of statutory and regulatory requirements.

## Part 3—School Health Education; Grants to States

### Subpart A—Planning Grants for States

Sec. 3621. Application for grant.
Sec. 3622. Approval of Secretary.
Sec. 3623. Amount of grant.
Sec. 3624. Authorized activities.

### Subpart B—Implementation Grants for States

Sec. 3631. Application for grant.
Sec. 3632. Selection of grantees.
Sec. 3633. Amount of grant.
Sec. 3634. Authorized activities; limitation on administrative costs.
Sec. 3635. Subgrants to local educational agencies.

### Subpart C—State and Local Reports

Sec. 3641. State and local reports.

## Part 4—School Health Education; Grants to Certain Local Educational Agencies

### Subpart A—Eligibility

Sec. 3651. Substantial need of area served by agency.

### Subpart B—Planning Grants for Local Education Agencies

Sec. 3661. Application for grant.
Sec. 3662. Selection of grantees.
Sec. 3663. Amount of grant.
Sec. 3664. Authorized activities.

### Subpart C—Implementation Grants for Local Educational Agencies

Sec. 3671. Application for grant.
Sec. 3672. Selection of grantees.
Sec. 3673. Amount of grant.
Sec. 3674. Authorized activities.
Sec. 3675. Reports.

## Part 5—School-Related Health Services

### Subpart A—Development and Operation of Projects

Sec. 3681. Authorizations regarding Public Health Service Initiatives Fund.
Sec. 3682. Eligibility for development and operation grants.
Sec. 3683. Preferences.
Sec. 3684. Grants for development of projects.
Sec. 3685. Grants for operation of projects.
Sec. 3686. Federal administrative costs.

SUBPART B—CAPITAL COSTS OF DEVELOPING PROJECTS

Sec. 3691. Loans and loan guarantees regarding projects.
Sec. 3692. Funding.

### Subtitle H—Public Health Service Initiative

Sec. 3701. Public Health Service Initiative.

### Subtitle I—Coordination With Cobra Continuation Coverage

Sec. 3801. Public Health Service Act; coordination with COBRA continuation coverage.

# Subtitle A—Workforce Priorities Under Federal Payments

## PART 1—INSTITUTIONAL COSTS OF GRADUATE MEDICAL EDUCATION; WORKFORCE PRIORITIES

### Subpart A—National Council Regarding Workforce Priorities

#### SEC. 3001. NATIONAL COUNCIL ON GRADUATE MEDICAL EDUCATION.

(a) IN GENERAL.—There is established within the Department of Health and Human Services a council to be known as the National Council on Graduate Medical Education.

(b) DUTIES.—The Secretary shall carry out subpart B acting through the National Council.

(c) COMPOSITION.—

(1) IN GENERAL.—The membership of the National Council shall include individuals who are appointed to the Council from among individuals who are not officers or employees of the United States. Such individuals shall be appointed by the Secretary,

and shall include individuals from each of the following categories:

(A) Consumers of health care services.

(B) Physicians who are faculty members of medical schools.

(C) Physicians in private practice who are not physicians described in subparagraph (B).

(D) Officers or employees of regional and corporate health alliances.

(E) Officers or employees of health care plans that participate in such alliances.

(F) Such other individuals as the Secretary determines to be appropriate.

(2) EX OFFICIO MEMBERS; OTHER FEDERAL OFFICERS OR EMPLOYEES.—The membership of the National Council shall include individuals designated by the Secretary to serve as members of the Council from among Federal officers or employees who are appointed by the President, or by the Secretary or other Federal officers who are appointed by the President with the advice and consent of the Senate.

(d) CHAIR.—The Secretary shall, from among members of the National Council appointed under subsection (a)(1), designate an individual to serve as the Chair of the Council.

(e) DEFINITIONS.—For purposes of this subtitle:

(1) The term "medical school" means a school of medicine (as defined in section 799 of the Public Health Service Act) or a school of osteopathic medicine (as defined in such section).

(2) The term "National Council" means the council established in subsection (a).

## Subpart B—Authorized Positions in Specialty Training

### SEC. 3011. COOPERATION OF APPROVED PHYSICIAN TRAINING PROGRAMS.

(a) IN GENERAL.—With respect to an approved physician training program in a medical specialty, a funding agreement for payments under section 3031 for a calendar year is that the program will ensure that the number of individuals enrolled in the program in the subsequent academic year is in accordance with this subpart.

(b) DEFINITIONS.—

(1) APPROVED PROGRAM.—

(A) For purposes of this subtitle, the term "approved physician training program", with respect to the medical speciality involved, means a residency or other postgraduate program that trains physicians and meets the following conditions:

(i) Participation in the program may be counted toward certification in the medical specialty.

(ii) The program is accredited by the Accreditation Council on Graduate Medical Education, or approved by the Council on Postgraduate Training of the American Osteopathic Association.

(B) For purposes of this subtitle, the term "approved physician training program" includes any postgraduate program described in subparagraph (A) that provides health services in an ambulatory setting, without regard to whether the program provides inpatient hospital services.

(2) ELIGIBLE PROGRAM; SUBPART DEFINITION.—For purposes of this subpart, the term "eligible program", with respect to an academic year, means an approved physician training program that receives payments under subpart C for the calendar year in which the academic year begins.

(3) OTHER DEFINITIONS.—For purposes of this subtitle:

(A)(i) The term "academic year" means the 1-year period beginning on July 1. The academic year beginning July 1, 1993, is academic year 1993–94.

  (ii) With respect to the funding agreement described in subsection (a), the term "subsequent academic year" means the academic year beginning July 1 of the calendar year for which payments are to be made under the agreement.

 (B) The term "funding agreement", with respect to payments under section 3031 to an approved physician training program, means that the Secretary may make the payments only if the program makes the agreement involved.

 (C) The term "medical specialty" includes subspecialties.

## SEC. 3012. ANNUAL AUTHORIZATION OF NUMBER OF SPECIALTY POSITIONS; REQUIREMENTS REGARDING PRIMARY HEALTH CARE.

(a) ANNUAL AUTHORIZATION OF NUMBER OF POSITIONS.—In the case of each medical specialty, the National Council shall designate for each academic year the number of individuals nationwide who under section 3011 are authorized to be enrolled in eligible programs. The preceding sentence is subject to subsection (c)(2).

(b) PRIMARY HEALTH CARE.—

(1) IN GENERAL.—Subject to paragraph (2), in carrying out subsection (a) for an academic year, the National Council shall ensure that, of the class of training participants entering eligible programs for academic year 2002-03 or any subsequent academic year, the percentage of such class that completes eligible programs in primary health care is not less than 55 percent (without regard to the academic year in which the members of the class complete the programs).

(2) RULE OF CONSTRUCTION.—The requirement of paragraph (1) regarding a percentage applies in the aggregate to training participants entering eligible programs for the academic year involved, and not individually to any eligible program.

(c) DESIGNATIONS REGARDING 3-YEAR PERIODS.—

(1) DESIGNATION PERIODS.—For each medical specialty, the National Council shall make the annual designations under subsection (a) for periods of 3 academic years.

(2) INITIAL PERIOD.—The first designation period established by the National Council after the date of the enactment of this Act shall be the academic years 1998-99 through 2000-01.

(d) CERTAIN CONSIDERATIONS IN DESIGNATING ANNUAL NUMBERS.—

(1) IN GENERAL.—Factors considered by the National Council in designating the annual number of specialty positions for an academic year for a medical specialty shall include the extent to which there is a need for additional practitioners in the speciality, as indicated by the following:

    (A) The incidence and prevalence (in the general population and in various other populations) of the diseases, disorders, or other health conditions with which the specialty is concerned.

    (B) The number of physicians who will be practicing in the specialty in the academic year.

    (C) The number of physicians who will be practicing in the specialty at the end of the 5-year period beginning on the first day of the academic year.

(2) RECOMMENDATIONS OF PRIVATE ORGANIZATIONS.—In designating the annual number of specialty positions for an academic year for a medical specialty, the National Council shall consider the recommendations of organizations representing physicians in the specialty and the recommendations of

organizations representing consumers of the services of such physicians.

(3) MINIMUM TOTAL OF RESPECTIVE ANNUAL NUMBERS.—

(A) Subject to subparagraph (B), for academic year 2003-04 and subsequent academic years, the National Council shall ensure that the total of the respective annual numbers designated under subsection (a) for an academic year is a total that—

(i) bears a relationship to the number of individuals who graduated from medical schools in the United States in the preceding academic year; and

(ii) is consistent with the purposes of this subpart.

(B) For each of the academic years 2003-04 through 2007-08, the total determined under subparagraph (A) shall be reduced by a percentage determined by the National Council.

(e) DEFINITIONS.—For purposes of this subtitle:

(1) The term "annual number of specialty positions", with respect to a medical specialty, means the number designated by the National Council

under subsection (a) for eligible programs for the academic year involved.

(2) The term "designation period" means a 3-year period under subsection (c)(1) for which designations under subsection (a) are made by the National Council.

(3) The term "primary health care" means the following medical specialties: Family medicine, general internal medicine, general pediatrics, and obstetrics and gynecology.

(4) The term "specialty position", with respect to a medical specialty, means a position (designated under subsection (a)) as one of the individuals who may be a training participant in an eligible program.

(5) The term "training participant" means an individual who is enrolled in an approved physician training program.

## SEC. 3013. ALLOCATIONS AMONG SPECIALITIES AND PROGRAMS.

(a) IN GENERAL.—For each academic year, the National Council shall for each medical specialty make allocations among eligible programs of the annual number of specialty positions that the Council has designated for such year. The preceding sentence is subject to subsection (b)(3).

(b) ALLOCATIONS REGARDING 3-YEAR PERIOD.—

(1) IN GENERAL.—For each medical specialty, the National Council shall make the annual allocations under subsection (a) for periods of 3 academic years.

(2) ADVANCE NOTICE TO PROGRAMS.—With respect to the first academic year of an allocation period established by the National Council, the National Council shall, not later than July 1 of the preceding academic year, notify each eligible program of the allocations made for the program for each of the academic years of the period.

(3) INITIAL PERIOD.—The first allocation period established by the National Council after the date of the enactment of this Act shall be the academic years 1998-99 through 2000-01.

(c) CERTAIN CONSIDERATIONS.—

(1) GEOGRAPHIC AREAS; QUALITY OF RESIDENCY PROGRAMS.—In making allocations under subsection (a) for eligible programs of the various geographic areas, the National Council shall include among the factors considered the historical distribution among the areas of approved physician training programs, and the quality of each of the programs.

(2) UNDERREPRESENTATION OF MINORITY GROUPS.—In making an allocation under subsection (a) for an eligible program, the National Council shall include among the factors considered the following:

(A) The extent to which the population of training participants in the program includes training participants who are members of racial or ethnic minority groups.

(B) With respect to a racial or ethnic group represented among the training participants, the extent to which the group is underrepresented in the field of medicine generally and in the various medical specialities.

(3) RECOMMENDATIONS OF PRIVATE ORGANIZATIONS.—In making allocations under subsection (a) for eligible programs, the National Council shall consider the recommendations of organizations representing physicians in the medical specialties and the recommendations of organizations representing consumers of the services of such physicians.

(d) DEFINITIONS.—For purposes of this subtitle, the term "allocation period" means a 3-year period under subsection (b)(1) for which allocations under subsection (a) are made by the National Council.

## Subpart C—Institutional Costs of Graduate Medical Education

### SEC. 3031. FEDERAL FORMULA PAYMENTS TO APPROVED PHYSICIAN TRAINING PROGRAMS.

(a) IN GENERAL.—

(1) FORMULA PAYMENTS.—Subject to paragraph (2), in the case of any approved physician training program that submits to the Secretary an application for a calendar year in accordance with section 3032, the Secretary shall make payments for such year to the program for the purpose specified in subsection (b). The Secretary shall make the payments in an amount determined in accordance with section 3033, and may administer the payments as a contract, grant, or cooperative agreement.

(2) APPLICABLE YEARS.—Payments under paragraph (1) may not be made before calendar year 1998, except that the Secretary may make such payments before such year to eligible programs in any State that has become a participating State under title I.

(b) PAYMENTS FOR OPERATION OF APPROVED PHYSICIAN TRAINING PROGRAMS.—The purpose of payments under subsection (a) is to assist an eligible program with the costs of operation. A funding agreement for such payments is that the program will expend the payments only for such purpose.

(c) ELIGIBLE PROGRAM; SUBPART DEFINITION.—For purposes of this subpart, the term "eligible program", with respect to the calendar year involved, means an approved physician training program that submits to the Secretary an application for such year in accordance with section 3032.

## SEC. 3032. APPLICATION FOR PAYMENTS.

(a) IN GENERAL.—For purposes of section 3031, an application for payments under such section is in accordance with this section if—

> (1) the approved physician training program involved submits the application not later than the date specified by the Secretary;
>
> (2) the condition described in subsection (b) is met with respect to the program;
>
> (3) the application contains each funding agreement described in this part and the application provides assurances of compliance with such agreements that are satisfactory to the Secretary; and
>
> (4) the application is in such form, is made in such manner, and contains such agreements, assurances, and information as the Secretary determines to be necessary to carry out this part.

(b) CERTAIN CONDITIONS.—An approved physician training program meets the condition described in this subsection for receiving payments under section 3031 for a calendar year if the institution within which the program operates agrees that such payments will be made by the Secretary directly to the program (and such agreement is included in the application under subsection (a)), and the Secretary shall ensure that such institution is permitted to participate as a provider in a regional or corporate alliance health plan during such year only if each of the approved physician training programs of the institution meets the requirements for receiving payments under such section for such year.

## SEC. 3033. AVAILABILITY OF FUNDS FOR PAYMENTS; ANNUAL AMOUNT OF PAYMENTS.

(a) DETERMINATION BY SECRETARY OF FUNDS AVAILABLE FOR PAYMENTS.—

(1) ANNUAL HEALTH PROFESSIONS WORKFORCE ACCOUNT.—Subject to paragraph (2) and section 3034, the Secretary shall determine for each calendar year the amount to be made available for the purpose of making payments under section 3031 (and under section 3051, as applicable) for the year. In determining such amount, the Secretary shall consider the amount necessary for making pay-

ments in the amounts determined under subsection (b) (and the amounts necessary for making payments in the amounts determined under section 3051(e) for institutions, in the case of calendar years 1998 through 2001).

(2) LIMITATION.—The amount determined by the Secretary for a calendar year under paragraph (1) may not exceed the following amount, as applicable to the calendar year:

    (A) In the case of calendar year 1996, $3,200,000,000.

    (B) In the case of calendar year 1997, $3,500,000,000.

    (C) In the case of calendar year 1998, $4,800,000,000.

    (D) In the case of each of the calendar years 1999 and 2000, $5,800,000,000.

    (E) In the case of each subsequent calendar year, the amount specified in subparagraph (D) increased by the product of such amount and the general health care inflation factor for such year (as defined in subsection (c)).

(b) AMOUNT OF PAYMENTS FOR INDIVIDUAL ELIGIBLE PROGRAMS.—

(1) IN GENERAL.—Subject to the annual health professions workforce account determined by the Secretary under subsection (a) for the calendar year involved, the amount of payments required in section 3031 to be made to an eligible program for the calendar year is an amount equal to the product of—

    (A) the number of full-time equivalent training participants in the program; and

    (B) the national average of the costs of such programs in training an individual, as determined by consideration of the following factors (and as adjusted under paragraph (2)(B)):

        (i) The national average salary of training participants.

        (ii) The national average costs of such programs in providing for faculty supervision of training participants and for related activities.

(2) ADDITIONAL PROVISIONS REGARDING NATIONAL AVERAGE COST.—

    (A) The Secretary shall in accordance with paragraph (1)(B) determine, for academic year 1992-93, an amount equal to the national average described in such paragraph with respect to training an individual. The national average applicable under such paragraph for a calendar year is, subject to subparagraph (B), the amount determined under the preceding sentence increased by an amount necessary to offset the effects of health care inflation occurring since academic year 1992–93, as determined through use of the general health care inflation factors for such years (or if there is no such factor for a calendar year, the consumer price index for the year).

(B) The national average determined under subparagraph (A) and applicable to a calendar year shall, in the case of the eligible program involved, be adjusted by a factor to reflect regional differences in the applicable wage and wage-related costs.

(c) DEFINITIONS.—For purposes of this subtitle:

(1) The term "annual health professions workforce account", with respect to a calendar year, means the amount determined under subsection (a) for such year.

(2) The term "consumer price index" has the meaning given such term in section 1902.

(3) The term "general health care inflation factor", with respect to a year, has the meaning given such term in section 6001(a)(3) for such year.

**SEC. 3034. ADDITIONAL FUNDING PROVISIONS.**

(a) SOURCES OF FUNDS FOR ANNUAL HEALTH PROFESSIONS WORKFORCE ACCOUNT.—The annual health professions workforce account under section 3033(a) for a calendar year shall be derived from the sources specified in subsection (b).

(b) CONTRIBUTIONS FROM MEDICARE TRUST FUNDS, REGIONAL ALLIANCES, AND CORPORATE ALLIANCES.—For purposes of subsection (a), the sources specified in this subsection for a calendar year are the following:

(1) Transfers made by the Secretary under section 4051.

(2) Payments made by regional alliances under section 1353 and transferred in an amount equal to the aggregate regional alliance portion determined under subsection (c)(2)(A).

(3) The transfer made under section (d)(1).

(c) CONTRIBUTIONS FROM REGIONAL AND CORPORATE ALLIANCES.—

(1) DETERMINATION OF AGGREGATE REGIONAL AND CORPORATE ALLIANCE AMOUNT.—For purposes

regarding the provision of funds for the annual health professions workforce account for a calendar year, the Secretary shall determine an aggregate regional and corporate alliance amount, which amount is to be paid by such alliances pursuant to paragraphs (2) and (3) of subsection (b), respectively, and which amount shall be equal to the difference between—

 (A) the annual health professions workforce account for such year; and

 (B) the amount transferred under section 4051 for the year.

(2) ALLOCATION OF AMOUNT AMONG REGIONAL AND CORPORATE ALLIANCES.—With respect to the aggregate regional and corporate alliance amount determined under paragraph (1) for a calendar year—

 (A) the aggregate regional alliance portion of such amount is the product of such amount and the percentage constituted by the ratio of the total plan payments of regional alliances to the combined total plan payments of regional alliances and corporate alliances; and

 (B) the aggregate corporate alliance portion of such amount is the product of such amount and the percentage constituted by the ratio of the total plan payments of corporate alliances to such combined total plan payments.

(d) COMPLIANCE REGARDING CORPORATE ALLIANCES.—

(1) IN GENERAL.—Effective January 15 of each calendar year, there is hereby transferred to the Secretary, out of any money in the Treasury not otherwise appropriated, an amount equal to the aggregate corporate alliance portion determined under subsection (c)(2)(B) for such year.

(2) MANNER OF COMPLIANCE.—The payment by corporate alliances of the tax imposed under section 3461 of the Internal Revenue Code of 1986 (as added by section 7121 of this Act), together with the transfer made in paragraph (1) for the calendar year involved, is deemed to be the payment required pursuant to subsection (c)(1) for corporate alliances for such year.

(e) DEFINITIONS.—For purposes of this subtitle, the term "plan payments" with respect to a regional or corporate alliance, means the amount paid to health plans by the alliance.

## Subpart D—General Provisions

**SEC. 3041. DEFINITIONS.**

For purposes of this subtitle:

(1) The term "academic year" has the meaning given such term in section 3011(b).

(2) The term "allocation period" has the meaning given such term in section 3013(d).

(3) The term "annual health professions workforce account" has the meaning given such term in section 3033(c).

(4) The term "annual number of specialty positions" has the meaning given such term in section 3012(e).

(5) The term "approved physician training program" has the meaning given such term in section 3011(b).

(6) The term "consumer price index" has the meaning given such term in section 3033(c).

(7) The term "designation period" has the meaning given such term in section 3012(e).

(8) The term "eligible program" has the meaning given such term in section 3011(b), in the case of subpart B; and has the meaning given such term in section 3031(c), in the case of subpart C.

(9) The term "funding agreement" has the meaning given such term in section 3011(b).

(10) The term "general health care inflation factor" has the meaning given such term in section 3033(c).

(11) The term "medical school" has the meaning given such term in section 3001(e).

(12) The term "medical specialty" has the meaning given such term in section 3011(b).

(13) The term "National Council" has the meaning given such term in section 3001(e).

(14) The term "plan payments" has the meaning given such term in section 3034(e).

(15) The term "primary health care" has the meaning given such term in section 3012(e).

(16) The term "specialty position" has the meaning given such term in section 3012(e).

(17) The term "training participant" has the meaning given such term in section 3012(e).

**Subpart E—Transitional Provisions**

**SEC. 3051. TRANSITIONAL PAYMENTS TO INSTITUTIONS.**

(a) PAYMENTS REGARDING EFFECTS OF SUBPART B ALLOCATIONS.—

(1) IN GENERAL.—For each of the calendar years 1998 through 2001, in the case of any eligible institution that submits to the Secretary an application for the year involved in accordance with sub-

section (d), the Secretary shall make payments for such year to the institution for the purpose specified in subsection (c). The Secretary shall make the payments in an amount determined in accordance with subsection (e), and may administer the payments as a contract, grant, or cooperative agreement.

(2) APPLICABLE YEARS.—Payments under paragraph (1) may not be made before calendar year 1998, except that the Secretary may make such payments before such year to eligible institutions in any State that has become a participating State under title I.

(b) ELIGIBLE INSTITUTION.—For purposes of this section, the term "eligible institution", with respect to a calendar year, means an institution—

(1) in which there are one or more programs that—

(A) are approved physician training programs; and

(B) are receiving payments under section 3031 for such year; and

(2) whose number of speciality positions (in the medical specialities with respect to which such payments are made) is below the number of such posi-

tions at the institution for academic year 1993–94 as a result of allocations under subpart B.

(c) PURPOSE OF PAYMENTS.—The purpose of payments under subsection (a) is to assist an eligible institution with the costs of operation. A funding agreement for such payments is that the institution will expend the payments only for such purpose.

(d) APPLICATION FOR PAYMENTS.—For purposes of subsection (a), an application for payments under such subsection is in accordance with this subsection if the institution involved submits the application not later than the date specified by the Secretary; the institution has cooperated with the approved physician training programs of the institution in meeting the condition described in section 3032(b); the application contains each funding agreement described in this section and provides assurances of compliance with such agreements satisfactory to the Secretary; and the application is in such form, is made in such manner, and contains such agreements, assurances, and information as the Secretary determines to be necessary to carry out this section.

(e) AMOUNT OF PAYMENTS.—

(1) IN GENERAL.—Subject to the annual health professions workforce account determined by the Secretary under section 3033(a) for the calendar

year involved, the amount of payments required in subsection (a) to be made to an eligible institution for the calendar year is the product of the amount determined under paragraph (2) and the applicable percentage specified in paragraph (3).

(2) NUMBER OF SPECIALTY POSITIONS LOST; NATIONAL AVERAGE SALARY.—For purposes of paragraph (1), the amount determined under this paragraph for an eligible institution for the calendar year involved is the product of—

(A) an amount equal to the number of full-time equivalent specialty positions lost; and

(B) the national average salary of training participants.

(3) APPLICABLE PERCENTAGE.—For purposes of paragraph (1), the applicable percentage for a calendar year is the following, as applicable to such year:

(A) For calendar year 1998, 100 percent.

(B) For calendar year 1999, 75 percent.

(C) For calendar year 2000, 50 percent.

(D) For calendar year 2001, 25 percent.

(4) DETERMINATION OF SPECIALTY POSITIONS LOST.—

(A) For purposes of this section, the number of specialty positions lost, with respect to a calendar year, is the difference between—

(i) the number of specialty positions described in subparagraph (B) that are estimated for the institution involved for the academic year beginning in such calendar year; and

(ii) the number of such specialty positions at the institution for academic year 1993-94.

(B) For purposes of subparagraph (A), the specialty positions described in this subparagraph are specialty positions in the medical specialities with respect to which payments under section 3031 are made to programs of the institution involved.

(5) ADDITIONAL PROVISION REGARDING NATIONAL AVERAGE SALARY.—

(A) The Secretary shall determine, for academic year 1992-93, an amount equal to the national average described in paragraph (2)(B). The national average applicable under such paragraph for a calendar year is, subject to subparagraph (B), the amount determined under the preceding sentence increased by an amount necessary to offset the effects of health care inflation occurring since academic year 1992–93, as determined through use of the general health care inflation factors for such years (or if there is no such factor for a year, the consumer price index for the year).

(B) The national average determined under subparagraph (A) and applicable to a calendar year shall, in the case of the eligible institution involved, be adjusted by a factor to reflect regional differences in the applicable wage and wage-related costs.

## PART 2—RELATED PROGRAMS

### SEC. 3061. ADDITIONAL FUNDING FOR CERTAIN WORKFORCE PROGRAMS.

(a) IN GENERAL.—For purpose of carrying out the programs described in sections 3062 and 3063, there is authorized to be appropriated $200,000,000 for fiscal year 1994 and each subsequent fiscal year (in addition to amounts that may otherwise be authorized to be appropriated for carrying out the programs).

(b) ALLOCATIONS.—With respect to the amount appropriated under subsection (a) for a fiscal year, the Secretary of Health and Human Services and the Secretary of Labor shall enter into an agreement specifying the aggregate portion of such amount to be made available for the programs described in section 3062 and the aggregate portion to be made available for the programs described in section 3063.

## SEC. 3062. PROGRAMS OF THE SECRETARY OF HEALTH AND HUMAN SERVICES.

(a) IN GENERAL.—The programs described in this section and carried out with amounts made available under section 3061 shall be carried out by the Secretary of Health and Human Services.

(b) PRIMARY CARE PHYSICIAN AND PHYSICIAN ASSISTANT TRAINING.—For purposes of section 3061, the programs described in this section include programs to support projects to train additional numbers of primary care physicians and physician assistants, including projects to enhance community-based generalist training for medical students, residents, and practicing physicians; to retrain mid-career physicians previously certified in a nonprimary care medical specialty; to expand the supply of physicians with special training to serve in rural and inner-city medically underserved areas; to support expansion of service-linked educational networks that train a range of primary care providers in community settings; to provide for training in managed care, cost-effective practice management, and continuous quality improvement; and to develop additional information on primary care workforce issues as required to meet future needs in health care.

(b) TRAINING OF UNDERREPRESENTED MINORITIES AND DISADVANTAGED PERSONS.—For purposes of section 3061, the programs described in this section include a program to support projects to increase the number of underrepresented minority and disadvantaged persons in medicine, osteopathy, dentistry, nursing, public health, and other health professions, including projects to provide continuing financial assistance for such persons entering health professions training programs; to increase support for recruitment and retention of such persons in the health professions; to maintain efforts to foster interest in health careers among such persons at the preprofessional level; and to increase the number of minority health professions faculty.

(c) NURSE TRAINING.—For purposes of section 3061, the programs described in this section include the following:

(1) A program to support projects to support midlevel provider training and address priority nursing workforce needs, including projects to train additional nurse practitioners and nurse midwives; to

support baccalaureate-level nurse training programs providing preparation for careers in teaching, community health service, and specialized clinical care; to train additional nurse clinicians and nurse anesthetists; to support interdisciplinary school-based community nursing programs; and to promote research on nursing workforce issues.

(2) A program to develop and encourage the adoption of model professional practice statutes for advanced practice nurses and physician assistants, and to otherwise support efforts to remove inappropriate barriers to practice by such nurses and such physician assistants.

(d) OTHER PROGRAMS.—For purposes of section 3061, the programs described in this section include a program to train health professionals and administrators in managed care, cost-effective practice management, continuous quality improvement practices, and provision of culturally sensitive care.

(e) RELATIONSHIP TO EXISTING PROGRAMS.—This section may be carried out through programs established in title VII or VIII of the Public Health Service Act, as appropriate and as consistent with the purposes of such programs.

**SEC. 3063. PROGRAMS OF THE SECRETARY OF LABOR.**

(a) IN GENERAL.—The programs described in this section and carried out with amounts made available under section 3061 shall be carried out by the Secretary of Labor (in this section referred to as the "Secretary").

(b) RETRAINING PROGRAMS; ADVANCED CAREER POSITIONS; JOB BANKS.—

(1) IN GENERAL.—For purposes of section 3061, the programs described in this section are the following:

(A) A program to retrain administrative and clerical workers for positions as technicians, nurses, and physician assistants.

(B) A demonstration program to assist workers in health care institutions in obtaining advanced career positions.

(C) A program to support development of health-worker job banks in local employment services agencies.

(D) A program for skills upgrading, occupational retraining, and quality improvement.

(E) A program to facilitate the comprehensive workforce adjustment initiative.

(2) USE OF FUNDS.—Amounts made available under section 3061 for carrying out this section may be expended for program support, faculty develop-

ment, trainee support, workforce analysis, and dissemination of information, as necessary to produce required performance outcomes, and for establishing and operating the Institute authorized in section 3064.

(c) CERTAIN REQUIREMENTS FOR PROGRAMS.—In carrying out the programs described in subsection (b), the Secretary shall, with respect to the organizations and employment positions involved, provide for the following:

(1) Explicit, clearly defined skill requirements developed for all the positions and projections of the number of openings for each position.

(2) Opportunities for internal career movement.

(3) Opportunities to work while training or completing and educational program.

(4) Evaluation and dissemination.

(5) Training opportunities in several forms, as appropriate.

(d) ADMINISTRATIVE REQUIREMENTS.—In carrying out the programs described in subsection (b), the Secretary shall, with respect to the organizations and employment positions involved, provide for the following:

(1) Implementation and administration jointly by management and employees and their representatives.

(2) Discussion with employees as to training needs for career advancement.

(3) Commitment to a policy of internal hirings and promotion.

(4) Provision of support services.

(5) Consultations with employers and with organized labor.

SEC. 3064. NATIONAL INSTITUTE FOR HEALTH CARE WORKFORCE DEVELOPMENT.

(a) ESTABLISHMENT OF INSTITUTE.—The Secretary of Health and Human Services and the Secretary of Labor may jointly establish an office to be known as the National Institute for Health Care Workforce Development. The subsequent provisions of this section apply to any such Institute.

(b) DIRECTOR.—The Institute shall be headed by a director, who shall be appointed jointly by the Secretaries.

(c) DUTIES.—

(1) IN GENERAL.—The Director of the Institute shall make recommendations to the Secretaries regarding—

(A) the supply of health care workers needed for the system of regional and corporate alliance health plans established under title I; and

(B) the impact of such system on health care workers and the needs of such workers with respect to the system, including needs regarding education, training, and other matters relating to career development.

(2) ADMINISTRATION OF PROGRAMS REGARDING RETRAINING, ADVANCED CAREER POSITIONS, AND JOB BANKS.—The Secretary of Labor may carry out section 3063 acting through the Director of the Institute.

(d) ADVISORY BOARD.—

(1) IN GENERAL.—The Secretaries shall establish an advisory board to assist in the develop of recommendations under subsection (c).

(2) COMPOSITION.—The Advisory Board shall be composed of—

(A) the Secretary of Labor;

(B) the Secretary of Health and Human Services;

(C) representatives of health care workers in organized labor;

(D) representatives of health care institutions;

(E) representatives of health care education organizations;

(F) representatives of consumer organizations; and

(G) such other individuals as the Secretaries determine to be appropriate.

(e) STAFF, QUARTERS, AND OTHER ASSISTANCE.—The Secretaries shall provide the Institute and the Advisory Board with such staff, quarters, and other administrative assistance as may be necessary for the Institute and the Advisory Board to carry out this section.

(f) DEFINITIONS.—For purposes of this section:

(1) The term "Advisory Board" means the advisory board established under subsection (c).

(2) The term "Institute" means an Institute established under subsection (a).

(3) The term "Secretaries" means the Secretary of Health and Human Services and the Secretary of Labor.

(g) SUNSET.—Effective upon the end of calendar year 2000, this section is repealed.

# Subtitle B—Academic Health Centers

## PART 1—FORMULA PAYMENTS

### SEC. 3101. FEDERAL FORMULA PAYMENTS TO ACADEMIC HEALTH CENTERS.

(a) IN GENERAL.—

(1) FORMULA PAYMENTS.—In the case of any academic health center that submits to the Secretary a written request for a calendar year in accordance with section 3102, the Secretary shall make payments for such year to the center for the purpose specified in subsection (b). The Secretary shall make the payments in an amount determined in accordance with section 3103, and shall administer the payments as a contract, grant, or cooperative agreement.

(2) APPLICABLE YEARS.—Payments under paragraph (1) may not be made before calendar year 1998, except that the Secretary may make such payments before such year to eligible programs in any State that has become a participating State under title I.

(b) PAYMENTS FOR COSTS ATTRIBUTABLE TO ACADEMIC NATURE OF CENTERS.—The purpose of payments under subsection (a) is to assist academic health centers with costs that are not routinely incurred by other entities in providing health services, but are incurred by such centers in providing health services by virtue of the academic nature of such centers.

(c) ACADEMIC HEALTH CENTERS.—For purposes of this subtitle, the term "academic health center" means an entity that operates a teaching hospital that carries out an approved physician training program (as defined in section 3011(b)).

**SEC. 3102. REQUEST FOR PAYMENTS.**

(a) IN GENERAL.—For purposes of section 3101, a written request for payments under such section is in accordance with this section if the academic health center involved submits the request not later than the date specified by the Secretary; the request is accompanied by each funding agreement described in this part; and the request is in such form, is made in such manner, and contains such agreements, assurances, and information as the Secretary determines to be necessary to carry out this part.

(b) CONTINUED STATUS AS ACADEMIC HEALTH CENTER.—A funding agreement for payments under section 3101 is that the entity involved will maintain status as an academic health center. For purposes of this subtitle, the term "funding agreement", with respect to payments under section 3101 to an entity, means that the Secretary may make the payments only if the entity makes the agreement involved.

**SEC. 3103. AVAILABILITY OF FUNDS FOR PAYMENTS; ANNUAL AMOUNT OF PAYMENTS.**

(a) DETERMINATION BY SECRETARY OF FUNDS AVAILABLE FOR PAYMENTS.—

(1) ANNUAL ACADEMIC HEALTH CENTER ACCOUNT.—Subject to paragraph (2) and section 3104, the Secretary shall determine for each calendar year the amount to be made available for the purpose of making payments under section 3101 for the year to eligible centers. In determining such amount, the Secretary shall consider the need of eligible centers for assistance with the costs described in section 3101(b).

(2) LIMITATION.—The amount determined by the Secretary for a calendar year under paragraph (1) may not exceed the following amount, as applicable to the calendar year:

(A) In the case of calendar year 1996, $3,100,000,000.

(B) In the case of each of the calendar years 1997 and 1998, $3,200,000,000.

(C) In the case of calendar year 1999, $3,700,000,000.

(D) In the case of calendar year 2000, $3,800,000,000.

(E) In the case of each subsequent calendar year, the amount specified in subparagraph (C) increased by the product of such amount and the general health care inflation factor (as defined in subsection (c)).

(b) AMOUNT OF PAYMENTS FOR INDIVIDUAL ELIGIBLE CENTERS.—The amount of payments required in section 3101 to be made to an eligible center for a calendar year is an amount equal to the product of—

(1) the annual academic health center account determined by the Secretary under subsection (a) for the calendar year; and

(2) the percentage constituted by the ratio of—

(A) an amount equal to product of—

(i) the portion of the gross receipts of the center for the preceding calendar year that was derived from providing services to patients (both inpatients and outpatients); and

(ii) the indirect teaching adjustment factor determined under section 1886(d)(5)(B)(ii) of the Social Security Act (as in effect before January 1, 1998) and applicable to patients discharged from the center in such preceding year (or, in the case of patients discharged from the center on or after January 1, 1998, applicable to patients discharged in calendar year 1997); to

(B) the sum of the respective amounts determined under subparagraph (A) for eligible centers.

(c) REPORT REGARDING MODIFICATIONS IN FORMULA.—Not later than July 1, 1996, the Secretary shall submit to the Congress a report containing any recommendations of the Secretary regarding policies for allocating amounts under subsection (a) among eligible centers.

(d) DEFINITION.—For purposes of this subtitle:

(1) The term "eligible center", with respect to the calendar year involved, means an academic health center that submits to the Secretary a written request for such year in accordance with section 3102.

(2) The term "annual academic health center account", with respect to a calendar year, means the amount determined under subsection (a) for such year.

(2) The term "general health care inflation factor", with respect to a year, has the meaning given such term in section 6001(a)(3) for such year.

## SEC. 3104. ADDITIONAL FUNDING PROVISIONS.

(a) SOURCES OF FUNDS FOR ANNUAL ACADEMIC HEALTH CENTER.—The annual academic health center account under section 3103(a) for a calendar year shall be derived from the sources specified in subsection (b).

(b) CONTRIBUTIONS FROM MEDICARE TRUST FUNDS, REGIONAL ALLIANCES, AND CORPORATE ALLIANCES.—For purposes of subsection (a), the sources specified in this subsection for a calendar year are the following:

(1) Transfers made by the Secretary under section 4052.

(2) Payments made by regional alliances under section 1353 and transferred in an amount equal to the aggregate regional alliance portion determined under subsection (c)(2)(A).

(3) The transfer made under section (d)(1).

(c) CONTRIBUTIONS FROM REGIONAL AND CORPORATE ALLIANCES.—

(1) DETERMINATION OF AGGREGATE REGIONAL AND CORPORATE ALLIANCE AMOUNT.—For purposes regarding the provision of funds for the annual academic health center account for a calendar year, the Secretary shall determine an aggregate regional and corporate alliance amount, which amount is to be paid by such alliances pursuant to paragraphs (2)

and (3) of subsection (b), respectively, and which amount shall be equal to the difference between—

 (A) the annual academic health center account for such year; and

 (B) the amount transferred under section 4052 for the year.

 (2) ALLOCATION OF AMOUNT AMONG REGIONAL AND CORPORATE ALLIANCES.—With respect to the aggregate regional and corporate alliance amount determined under paragraph (1) for a calendar year—

 (A) the aggregate regional alliance portion of such amount is the product of such amount and the percentage constituted by the ratio of the total plan payments of regional alliances to the combined total plan payments of regional alliances and corporate alliances; and

 (B) the aggregate corporate alliance portion of such amount is the product of such amount and the percentage constituted by the ratio of the total plan payments of corporate alliances to such combined total plan payments.

(d) COMPLIANCE REGARDING CORPORATE ALLIANCES.—

(1) IN GENERAL.—Effective January 15 of each calendar year, there is hereby transferred to the Secretary, out of any money in the Treasury not otherwise appropriated, an amount equal to the aggregate corporate alliance portion determined under subsection (c)(2)(B) for such year.

(2) MANNER OF COMPLIANCE.—The payment by corporate alliances of the tax imposed under section 3461 of the Internal Revenue Code of 1986 (as added by section 7121 of this Act), together with the transfer made in paragraph (1) for the calendar year involved, is deemed to be the payment required pursuant to subsection (c)(1) for corporate alliances for such year..

(e) DEFINITIONS.—For purposes of this subtitle, the term "plan payments" with respect to a regional or corporate alliance, means the amount paid to health plans by the alliance.

## PART 2—ACCESS OF PATIENTS TO ACADEMIC HEALTH CENTERS

SEC. 3131. CONTRACTS FOR ENSURING ACCESS TO CENTERS.

(a) CONTRACTS WITH HEALTH PLANS.—Regional and corporate health alliances under this Act shall ensure that, in accordance with subsection (b), the health plans of the alliances enter into sufficient contracts with eligible centers to ensure that enrollees in regional or corporate alliance health plans, as appropriate, receive the specialized treatment expertise of such centers, subject to such exceptions as the Secretary may provide.

(b) UTILIZATION OF SPECIALIZED TREATMENT EXPERTISE OF CENTERS.—Contracts under subsection (a) between eligible centers and health plans are in accordance with this subsection if the contracts provide that, with respect to health conditions within the specialized treatment expertise of the centers, health plans will refer medical cases involving such conditions to the centers.

(c) SPECIALIZED TREATMENT EXPERTISE.—For purposes of this subtitle, the term "specialized treatment expertise", with respect to treatment of a health condition by an academic health center, means expertise in treating rare diseases, treating unusually severe conditions, and providing other specialized health care.

## SEC. 3132. DISCRETIONARY GRANTS REGARDING ACCESS TO CENTERS.

(a) RURAL INFORMATION AND REFERRAL SYSTEMS.—The Secretary may make grants to eligible centers for the establishment and operation of information and referral systems to provide the services of such centers to rural regional and corporate health alliance health plans.

(b) OTHER PURPOSES REGARDING URBAN AND RURAL AREAS.—The Secretary may make grants to eligible centers to carry out activities (other than activities carried out under subsection (a)) for the purpose of providing the services of eligible centers to residents of rural or urban communities who otherwise would not have adequate access to such services.

# Subtitle C—Health Research Initiatives

## PART 1—PROGRAMS FOR CERTAIN AGENCIES

### SEC. 3201. BIOMEDICAL AND BEHAVIORAL RESEARCH ON HEALTH PROMOTION AND DISEASE PREVENTION.

Section 402(f) of the Public Health Service Act (42 U.S.C. 282(f)), as amended by section 201 of Public Law 103-43 (107 Stat. 144), is amended—

(1) in paragraph (3), by redesignating subparagraphs (A) and (B) as clauses (i) and (ii), respectively;

(2) by redesignating paragraphs (1) through (3) as subparagraphs (A) through (C);

(3) by inserting "(1)" after "(f)"; and

(4) by adding at the end the following paragraph:

"(2)(A) The Director of NIH, in collaboration with the Associate Director for Prevention and with the heads of the agencies of the National Institutes of Health, shall ensure that such Institutes conduct and support biomedical and behavioral research on promoting health and preventing diseases, disorders, and other health conditions (including Alzheimer's disease, breast cancer, heart disease, and stroke).

"(B) In carrying out subparagraph (A), the Director of NIH shall give priority to conducting and supporting research on child and adolescent health (including birth defects), chronic and recurrent health conditions, reproductive health, mental health, elderly health, substance abuse, infectious diseases, health and wellness promotion, and environmental health, and to resource development related to such research.".

## SEC. 3202. HEALTH SERVICES RESEARCH.

Section 902 of the Public Health Service Act (42 U.S.C. 299a), as amended by section 2(b) of Public Law 102-410 (106 Stat. 2094), is amended by adding at the end the following subsection:

"(f) RESEARCH ON HEALTH CARE REFORM.—

"(1) IN GENERAL.—In carrying out section 901(b), the Administrator shall conduct and support research on the reform of the health care system of the United States, as directed by the National Board.

"(2) PRIORITIES.—In carrying out paragraph (1), the Administrator shall give priority to the following:

"(A) Conducting and supporting research on the appropriateness and effectiveness of alternative clinical strategies; the quality and outcomes of care; and administrative simplification.

"(B) Conducting and supporting research on consumer choice and information resources; the effects of health care reform on health delivery systems; workplace injury and illness prevention; methods for risk adjustment; factors influencing access to health care for underserved populations; and primary care.

"(C) The development of clinical practice guidelines consistent with section 913, the dissemination of such guidelines consistent with section 903, and the assessment of the effectiveness of such guidelines.".

## PART 2—FUNDING FOR PROGRAMS

### SEC. 3211. AUTHORIZATIONS REGARDING PUBLIC HEALTH SERVICE INITIATIVES FUND.

(a) BIOMEDICAL AND BEHAVIORAL RESEARCH ON HEALTH PROMOTION AND DISEASE PREVENTION.—For the purpose of carrying out activities pursuant to the amendments made by section 3201, there are authorized to be appropriated from the Public Health Service Initiatives Fund (established in section 3701) $400,000,000 for fiscal year 1995, and $500,000,000 for each of the fiscal years 1996 through 2000.

(b) HEALTH SERVICES RESEARCH.—For the purpose of carrying out activities pursuant to the amendments made by section 3202, there are authorized to be appropriated from the Public Health Service Initiatives Fund $150,000,000 for fiscal year 1995, $400,000,000 for fiscal year 1996, $500,000,000 for fiscal year 1997, and $600,000,000 for each of the fiscal years 1998 through 2000.

(c) RELATION TO OTHER FUNDS.—The authorizations of appropriations established in subsections (a) and (b) are in addition to any other authorizations of appropriations that are available for the purposes described in such subsections.

# Subtitle D—Core Functions of Public Health Programs; National Initiatives Regarding Preventive Health

## PART 1—FUNDING

### SEC. 3301. AUTHORIZATIONS REGARDING PUBLIC HEALTH SERVICE INITIATIVES FUND.

(a) CORE FUNCTIONS OF PUBLIC HEALTH PROGRAMS.—For the purpose of carrying out part 2, there are authorized to be appropriated from the Public Health Service Initiatives Fund (established in section 3701) $12,000,000 for fiscal year 1995, $325,000,000 for fiscal year 1996, $450,000,000 for fiscal year 1997, $550,000,000 for fiscal year 1998, $650,000,000 for fiscal year 1999, and $750,000,000 for fiscal year 2000.

(b) NATIONAL INITIATIVES REGARDING HEALTH PROMOTION AND DISEASE PREVENTION.—For the purpose of carrying out part 3, there are authorized to be appropriated from the Public Health Service Initiatives Fund (established in section 3701) $175,000,000 for fiscal year 1996, and $200,000,000 for each of the fiscal years 1997 through 2000.

(c) RELATION TO OTHER FUNDS.—The authorizations of appropriations established in subsections (a) and (b) are in addition to any other authorizations of appropriations that are available for the purposes described in such subsections.

## PART 2—CORE FUNCTIONS OF PUBLIC HEALTH PROGRAMS

**SEC. 3311. PURPOSES.**

Subject to the subsequent provisions of this subtitle, the purposes of this part are to strengthen the capacity of State and local public health agencies to carry out the following functions:

(1) To monitor and protect the health of communities against communicable diseases and exposure to toxic environmental pollutants, occupational hazards, harmful products, and poor quality health care.

(2) To identify and control outbreaks of infectious disease and patterns of chronic disease and injury.

(3) To inform and educate health care consumers and providers about their roles in preventing and controlling disease and the appropriate use of medical services.

(4) To develop and test new prevention and public health control interventions.

SEC. 3312. GRANTS TO STATES FOR CORE HEALTH FUNCTIONS.

(a) IN GENERAL.—The Secretary may make grants to States for the purpose of carrying out one or more of the functions described in subsection (b).

(b) CORE FUNCTIONS OF PUBLIC HEALTH PROGRAMS.—For purposes of subsection (a), the functions described in this subsection are, subject to subsection to subsection (c), as follows:

(1) Data collection, activities related to population health measurement and outcomes monitoring, including the regular collection and analysis of public health data, vital statistics, and personal health services data and analysis for planning and needs assessment purposes of data collected from health plans through the information system under title V of this Act.

(2) Activities to protect the environment and to assure the safety of housing, workplaces, food and water, including the following activities:

(A) Monitoring the overall public health quality and safety of communities.

(B) Assessing exposure to high lead levels and water contamination.

(C) Monitoring sewage and solid waste disposal, radiation exposure, radon exposure, and noise levels.

(D) Abatement of lead-related hazards.

(E) Assuring recreation and worker safety.

(F) Enforcing public health safety and sanitary codes.

(G) Other activities relating to promoting the public health of communities.

(3) Investigation and control of adverse health conditions, including improvements in emergency treatment preparedness, cooperative activities to reduce violence levels in communities, activities to control the outbreak of disease, exposure related conditions and other threats to the health status of individuals.

(4) Public information and education programs to reduce risks to health such as use of tobacco, alcohol and other drugs, sexual activities that increase the risk to HIV transmission and sexually transmitted diseases, poor diet, physical inactivity, and low childhood immunization levels.

(5) Accountability and quality assurance activities, including monitoring the quality of personal health services furnished by health plans and provid-

ers of medical and health services in a manner consistent with the overall quality of care monitoring activities undertaken under title V, and monitoring communities' overall access to health services.

(6) Provision of public health laboratory services to complement private clinical laboratory services and that screen for diseases and conditions such as metabolic diseases in newborns, provide toxicology assessments of blood lead levels and other environmental toxins, diagnose sexually transmitted diseases, tuberculosis and other diseases requiring partner notification, test for infectious and food-borne diseases, and monitor the safety of water and food supplies.

(7) Training and education to assure provision of care by all health professionals, with special emphasis placed on the training of public health professions including epidemiologists, biostatisticians, health educators, public health administrators, sanitarians and laboratory technicians.

(8) Leadership, policy development and administration activities, including needs assessment, the setting of public health standards, the development of community public health policies, and the development of community public health coalitions.

(c) RESTRICTIONS ON USE OF GRANT.—

(1) IN GENERAL.—A funding agreement for a grant under subsection (a) for a State is that the grant will not be expended—

(A) to provide inpatient services;

(B) to make cash payments to intended recipients of health services;

(C) to purchase or improve land, purchase, construct, or permanently improve (other than minor remodeling) any building or other facility, or purchase major medical equipment;

(D) to satisfy any requirement for the expenditure of non-Federal funds as a condition for the receipt of Federal funds; or

(E) to provide financial assistance to any entity other than a public or nonprofit private entity.

(2) LIMITATION ON ADMINISTRATIVE EXPENSES.—A funding agreement for a grant under subsection (a) is that the State involved will not expend more than 10 percent of the grant for administrative expenses with respect to the grant.

(d) MAINTENANCE OF EFFORT.—A funding agreement for a grant under subsection (a) is that the State involved will maintain expenditures of non-Federal amounts for core health functions at a level that is not less than the level of such expenditures maintained by the State for the fiscal year preceding the first fiscal year for which the State receives such a grant.

**SEC. 3313. SUBMISSION OF INFORMATION.**

The Secretary may make a grant under section 3312 only if the State involved submits to the Secretary the following information:

(1) A description of existing deficiencies in the State's public health system (at the State level and the local level), using standards of sufficiency developed by the Secretary.

(2) A description of health status measures to be improved within the State (at the State level and the local level) through expanded public health functions.

(3) Measurable outcomes and process objectives for improving health status and core health functions for which the grant is to be expended.

(4) Information regarding each such function, which—

(A) identifies the amount of State and local funding expended on each such function for the fiscal year preceding the fiscal year for which the grant is sought; and

(B) provides a detailed description of how additional Federal funding will improve each such function by both the State and local public health agencies.

(5) A description of the core health functions to be carried out at the local level, and a specification for each such function of—

(A) the communities in which the function will be carried out; and

(B) the amount of the grant to be expended for the function in each community so specified.

### SEC. 3314. REPORTS.

A funding agreement for a grant under section 3312 is that the States involved will, not later than the date specified by the Secretary, submit to the Secretary a report describing—

(1) the purposes for which the grant was expended; and

(2) describing the extent of progress made by the State in achieving measurable outcomes and process objectives described in section 3313(3).

### SEC. 3315. APPLICATION FOR GRANT.

The Secretary may make a grant under section 3312 only if an application for the grant is submitted to the

Secretary, the application contains each agreement described in this part, the application contains the information required in section 3314, and the application is in such form, is made in such manner, and contains such agreements, assurances, and information as the Secretary determines to be necessary to carry out this part.

SEC. 3316. GENERAL PROVISIONS.

(a) UNIFORM DATA SETS.—The Secretary, in consultation with the States, shall develop uniform sets of data for the purpose of monitoring the core health functions carried out with grants under section 3312.

(b) DURATION OF GRANT.—The period during which payments are made to a State from a grant under section 3312 may not exceed 5 years. The provision of such payments shall be subject to annual approval by the Secretary of the payments. This subsection may not be construed as establishing a limitation on the number of grants under such section that may be made to the State.

SEC. 3317. ALLOCATIONS FOR CERTAIN ACTIVITIES.

Of the amounts made available under section 3301 for a fiscal year for carrying out this part, the Secretary may reserve not more than 5 percent for carrying out the following activities:

(1) Technical assistance with respect to planning, development, and operation of core health

functions carried out under section 3312, including provision of biostatistical and epidemiological expertise and provision of laboratory expertise.

(2) Development and operation of a national information network among State and local health agencies.

(3) Program monitoring and evaluation of core health functions carried out under section 3312.

(4) Development of a unified electronic reporting mechanism to improve the efficiency of administrative management requirements regarding the provision of Federal grants to State public health agencies.

### SEC. 3318. DEFINITIONS.

For purposes of this part:

(1) The term "funding agreement", with respect to a grant under section 3312 to a State, means that the Secretary may make the grant only if the State makes the agreement involved.

(2) The term "core health functions", with respect to a State, means the functions described in section 3312(b).

## PART 3—NATIONAL INITIATIVES REGARDING HEALTH PROMOTION AND DISEASE PREVENTION

### SEC. 3331. GRANTS FOR NATIONAL PREVENTION INITIATIVES.

(a) IN GENERAL.—The Secretary may make grants to entities described in subsection (b) for the purpose of carrying out projects to develop and implement innovative community-based strategies to provide for health promotion and disease prevention activities for which there is a significant need, as identified under section 1701 of the Public Health Service Act.

(b) ELIGIBLE ENTITIES.—The entities referred to in subsection (a) are agencies of State or local government, private nonprofit organizations (including research institutions), and coalitions that link two or more of these groups.

(c) CERTAIN ACTIVITIES.—The Secretary shall ensure that projects carried out under subsection (a)—

(1) reflect approaches that take into account the special needs and concerns of the affected populations;

(2) are targeted to the most needy and vulnerable population groups and geographic areas of the Nation;

(3) examine links between various high priority preventable health problems and the potential community-based remedial actions; and

(4) establish or strengthen the links between the activities of agencies engaged in public health activities with those of health alliances, health care providers, and other entities involved in the personal health care delivery system described in title I.

SEC. 3332. PRIORITIES.

(a) ESTABLISHMENT.—

(1) ANNUAL STATEMENT.—After consultation with the advisory board established in section 3335, the Secretary shall for each fiscal year develop a statement of proposed priorities for grants under section 3331 for the fiscal year.

(2) ALLOCATIONS AMONG PRIORITIES.—With respect to the amounts available under section 3301 for the fiscal year for carrying out this part, each statement under paragraph (1) for a fiscal year shall include a specification of the percentage of the amount to be devoted to projects addressing each of the proposed priorities established in the statement.

(3) PROCESS FOR ESTABLISHING PRIORITIES.— Not later than January 1 of each fiscal year, the Secretary shall publish a statement under paragraph

(1) in the Federal Register. A period of 60 days shall be allowed for the submission of public comments and suggestions concerning the proposed priorities. After analyzing and considering comments on the proposed priorities, the Secretary shall publish in the Federal Register final priorities (and associated reservations of funds) for approval of projects for the following fiscal year.

(b) APPLICABILITY TO MAKING OF GRANTS.—

(1) IN GENERAL.—Subject to paragraph (3), the Secretary may make grants under section 3331 for projects that the Secretary determines—

    (A) are consistent with the applicable final statement of priorities and otherwise meets the objectives described in subsection (a); and

    (B) will assist in meeting a health need or concern of a population served by a health plan or health alliance established under title I.

(2) SPECIAL CONSIDERATION FOR CERTAIN PROJECTS.—In making grants under section 3331, the Secretary shall, subject to paragraph (3), give special consideration to applicants that will carry out projects that, in addition to being consistent with the applicable published priorities under subsection (a) and otherwise meeting the requirements of this

part, have the potential for replication in other communities.

### SEC. 3333. SUBMISSION OF INFORMATION.

The Secretary may make a grant under section 3331 only if the applicant involved submits to the Secretary the following information:

(1) A description of the activities to be conducted, and the manner in which the activities are expected to contribute to meeting one or more of the priority health needs specified under section 3332 for the fiscal year for which the grant is initially sought.

(2) A description of the total amount of Federal funding requested, the geographic area and populations to be served, and the evaluation procedures to be followed.

(3) Such other information as the Secretary determines to be appropriate.

### SEC. 3334. APPLICATION FOR GRANT.

The Secretary may make a grant under section 3331 only if an application for the grant is submitted to the Secretary, the application contains each agreement described in this part, the application contains the information required in section 3333, and the application is in such form, is made in such manner, and contains such agreements, assurances, and information as the Secretary determines to be necessary to carry out this part.

# Subtitle E—Health Services for Medically Underserved Populations

## PART 1—COMMUNITY AND MIGRANT HEALTH CENTERS

### SEC. 3401. AUTHORIZATIONS REGARDING PUBLIC HEALTH SERVICE INITIATIVES FUND.

(a) GRANTS TO COMMUNITY AND MIGRANT HEALTH CENTERS.—The Secretary shall make grants in accordance with this part to migrant health centers and community health centers.

(b) AUTHORIZATION OF APPROPRIATIONS.—For the purpose of carrying out subsection (a), there are authorized to be appropriated from the Public Health Service Initiatives Fund (established in section 3701) $100,000,000 for each of the fiscal years 1995 through 2000.

(c) RELATION TO OTHER FUNDS.—The authorizations of appropriations established in subsection (b) for the purpose described in such subsection are in addition to any other authorizations of appropriations that are available for such purpose.

(d) DEFINITIONS.—For purposes of this subtitle, the terms "migrant health center" and "community health center" have the meanings given such terms in sections 329(a)(1) and 330(a) of the Public Health Service Act, respectively.

**SEC. 3402. USE OF FUNDS.**

(a) DEVELOPMENT, OPERATION, AND OTHER PURPOSES REGARDING CENTERS.—Subject to subsection (b), grants under section 3401 to migrant health centers and community health centers may be made only in accordance with the conditions upon which grants are made under sections 329 and 330 of the Public Health Service Act, respectively.

(b) REQUIRED FINANCIAL RESERVES.—The Secretary may authorize migrant health centers and community health centers to expend a grant under section 3401 to establish and maintain the financial reserves required under title I for providers of health services.

## PART 2—INITIATIVES FOR ACCESS TO HEALTH CARE

### Subpart A—Purposes; Funding

**SEC. 3411. PURPOSES.**

Subject to the provisions of subparts B through D, the purposes of this part are as follows:

(1) To improve access to health services for urban and rural medically-underserved populations through a program of flexible grants, contracts, and loans.

(2) To facilitate transition to a system in which medically-underserved populations have an adequate choice of community-oriented providers and health plans.

(3) To promote the development of community practice networks and community health plans that integrate health professionals and health care organizations supported through public funding with other providers in medically underserved areas.

(4) To support linkages between providers of health care for medically-underserved populations and regional and corporate alliance health plans.

(5) To expand the capacity of community practice networks and community health plans in underserved areas by increasing the number of practice sites and by renovating and converting substandard inpatient and outpatient facilities.

(6) To link providers in underserved areas with each other and with regional health care institutions and academic health centers through information systems and telecommunications.

(7) To support activities that enable medically underserved populations to gain access to the health care system and use it effectively.

**SEC. 3412. AUTHORIZATIONS REGARDING PUBLIC HEALTH SERVICE INITIATIVES FUND.**

(a) DEVELOPMENT OF QUALIFIED COMMUNITY HEALTH PLANS AND PRACTICE GROUPS.—For the purpose of carrying out subparts B and C, there are authorized to be appropriated from the Public Health Service Initiatives Fund (established in section 3701) $200,000,000 for fiscal year 1995, $500,000,000 for fiscal year 1996, $600,000,000 for fiscal year 1997, $700,000,000 for fiscal year 1998, $500,000,000 for fiscal year 1999, and $200,000,000 for fiscal year 2000.

(b) RELATION TO OTHER FUNDS.—The authorizations of appropriations established in subsection (a) are in addition to any other authorizations of appropriations that are available for the purpose described in such subsection.

(c) RELATIONSHIP TO PROGRAM REGARDING SCHOOL-RELATED HEALTH SERVICES.—This section is subject to section 3692.

## Subpart B—Development of Qualified Community Health Plans and Practice Networks

### SEC. 3421. GRANTS AND CONTRACTS FOR DEVELOPMENT OF PLANS AND NETWORKS.

(a) IN GENERAL.—The Secretary may make grants to and enter into contracts with consortia of public or private health care providers for the development of qualified community health plans and qualified community practice networks. For purposes of this subtitle, the term "qualified community health group" means such a health plan or such a practice network.

(b) QUALIFIED COMMUNITY HEALTH PLANS.—For purposes of this subtitle, the term "qualified community health plan" means a health plan that meets the following conditions:

(1) The health plan is a public or nonprofit private entity whose principal purpose is, with respect to the items and services included in the comprehensive benefit package under title I, to provide each of such items and services in one or more health professional shortage areas or to provide such items and services to a significant number of individuals who are members of a medically underserved population.

(2) The health plan is a participant in one or more health alliances.

(3) Two or more of the categories specified in subsection (d) are represented among the entities providing health services through the health plan.

(c) QUALIFIED COMMUNITY PRACTICE NETWORKS.—For purposes of this subtitle, the term "qualified community practice network" means a consortium of health care providers meeting the following conditions:

(1) The consortium is a public or nonprofit private entity whose principal purpose is the purpose described in subsection (b)(1).

(2) The consortium has an agreement with one or more health plans that are participating in one or more health alliances.

(3) The participation of health care providers in the consortium is governed by a written agreement to which each of the participating providers is a party.

(4) Two or more of the categories described in subsection (d) are represented among the entities participating in the consortium.

(d) RELEVANT CATEGORIES OF ENTITIES.—For purposes of subsections (b)(3) and (c)(4), the categories described in this subsection are the following categories of entities:

(1) Physicians, other health professionals, or health care institutions that provide health services in one or more health professional shortage areas or provide such services to a significant number of individuals who are members of a medically underserved population, and that do not provide health services under any of the programs specified in paragraphs (2) through (7) or as employees of public entities.

(2) Entities providing health services under grants under sections 329 and 330 of the Public Health Service Act.

(3) Entities providing health services under grants under sections 340 and 340A of such Act.

(4) Entities providing health services under grants under section 1001 or title XXIII of such Act.

(5) Entities providing health services under title V of the Social Security Act.

(6) Entities providing health services through rural health clinics and other federally qualified health centers.

(7) Entities providing health services in urban areas through programs under title V of the Indian Health Care Improvement Act, and entities provid-

ing outpatient health services through programs under the Indian Self-Determination Act.

(8) Programs providing personal health services and operating through State or local public health agencies.

(e) RULE OF CONSTRUCTION.—The consortia to which the Secretary may make an award of financial assistance under subsection (a) for the development of qualified community practice networks include any health plan that participates in one or more health alliances, without regard to whether the health plan is a qualified community health plan.

(f) SERVICE AREA.—In making an award of financial assistance under subsection (a), the Secretary shall designate the geographic area with respect to which the qualified community health group involved is to provide health services. A funding agreement for such an award is that the qualified community health group involved will provide such services in the area so designated.

(g) DEFINITIONS.—For purposes of this subtitle:

(1) The term "health professional shortage areas" means health professional shortage areas designated under section 332 of the Public Health Service Act.

(2) The term "medically underserved population" means a medically underserved population designated under section 330 of the Public Health Service Act.

(3) The term "rural health clinic" has the meaning given such term in section 1861(aa)(2) of the Social Security Act.

(4) The term "federally qualified health centers" has the meaning given such term in section 1861(aa)(4) of the Social Security Act.

(5) The term "service area", with respect to a qualified community health group, means the geographic area designated under subsection (g).

(6) The term "funding agreement", with respect to an award of financial assistance under this section, means that the Secretary may make the award only if the applicant for the award makes the agreement involved.

(7) The term "financial assistance", with respect to awards under subsection (a), means a grant or contract.

## SEC. 3422. PREFERENCES IN MAKING AWARDS OF ASSISTANCE.

In making awards of financial assistance under section 3421, the Secretary shall give preference to applicants in accordance with the following:

(1) The Secretary shall give preference if 3 or more of the categories described in subsection (d) of such section will be represented in the qualified community health group involved (pursuant to subsection (b)(3) or (c)(4), as the case may be).

(2) Of applicants receiving preference under paragraph (1), the Secretary shall give a greater degree of preference according to the extent to which a greater number of categories are represented.

(3) Of applicants receiving preference under paragraph (1), the Secretary shall give a greater degree of preference if one of the categories represented is the category described in subsection (d)(1) of such section.

## SEC. 3423. CERTAIN USES OF AWARDS.

(a) IN GENERAL.—Subject to subsection (b), the purposes for which an award of financial assistance under section 3421 may be expended in developing a qualified community health group include the following:

(1) Planning such group, including entering into contracts between the recipient of the award

and health care providers who are to participate in the group.

(2) Recruitment, compensation, and training of health professionals and administrative staff.

(3) Acquisition, expansion, modernization, and conversion of facilities, including for purposes of providing for sites at which health services are to be provided through such group.

(4) Acquisition and development of information systems (exclusive of systems that the Secretary determines are information highways).

(5) Such other expenditures as the Secretary determines to be appropriate.

(b) TWENTY-YEAR OBLIGATION REGARDING SIGNIFICANT CAPITAL EXPENDITURES; RIGHT OF RECOVERY.—

(1) IN GENERAL.—With respect to a facility for which substantial capital costs are to paid from an award of financial assistance under section 3421, the Secretary may make the award only if the applicant involved agrees that the applicant will be liable to the United States for the amount of the award expended for such costs, together with an amount representing interest, if at any time during the 20-period beginning on the date of completion of the activities involved, the facility—

(A) ceases to be a facility utilized by a qualified community health group, or by another public or nonprofit private entity that provides health services in one or more health professional shortage areas or that provides such services to a significant number of individuals who are members of a medically underserved population; or

(B) is sold or transferred to any entity other than an entity that is—

(i) a qualified community health group or other entity described in subparagraph (A); and

(ii) approved by the Secretary as a purchaser or transferee regarding the facility.

(2) SUBORDINATION; WAIVERS.—The Secretary may subordinate or waive the right of recovery under paragraph (1), and any other Federal interest that may be derived by virtue of an award of financial assistance under section 3421 from which substantial capital costs are to paid from an award, if the Secretary determines that subordination or waiver will further the objectives of this part.

# SEC. 3424. ACCESSIBILITY OF SERVICES.

(a) SERVICES FOR CERTAIN INDIVIDUALS.—A funding agreement for an award of financial assistance under section 3421 is that the qualified community health group involved will ensure that the services of the group will be accessible directly or through formal contractual arrangements with its participating providers regardless of whether individuals who seek care from the applicant are eligible persons under title I.

(b) USE OF THIRD-PARTY PAYORS.—A funding agreement for an award of financial assistance under section 3421 is that the qualified community health group involved will ensure that the health care providers of the group are all approved by the Secretary as providers under title XVIII of the Social Security Act and by the appropriate State agency as providers under title XIX of the Social Security Act, and the applicant has made or will make every reasonable effort to collect appropriate reimbursement for its costs in providing health services to individuals who are entitled to health benefits under title I of this Act, insurance benefits under title XVIII of the Social Security Act, medical assistance under a State plan approved under title XIX of the Social Security Act, or to assistance for medical expenses under any other public assistance program or private health insurance program.

(c) SCHEDULE OF FEES.—A funding agreement for an award of financial assistance under section 3421 is that the qualified community health group involved will—

 (1) prepare a schedule of fees or payments for the provision of health services not covered by title I that is consistent with locally prevailing rates or charges and designed to cover its reasonable costs of operation and has prepared a corresponding schedule of discounts to be applied to the payment of such fees or payments (or payments of cost sharing amounts owed in the case of covered benefits) which discounts are applied on the basis of the patient's ability to pay; and

 (2) make every reasonable effort to secure from patients payment in accordance with such schedules, and to collect reimbursement for services to persons entitled to public or private insurance benefits or other medical assistance on the basis of full fees without application of discounts, except that the applicant will ensure that no person is denied service based on the person's inability to pay therefor.

(d) BARRIERS WITHIN SERVICE AREA.—A funding agreement for an award of financial assistance under section 3421 is that the qualified community health group involved will ensure that the following conditions are met:

(1) In the service area of the group, the group will ensure that—

 (A) the services of the group are accessible to all residents; and

 (B) to the maximum extent possible, barriers to access to the services of the group are eliminated, including barriers resulting from the area's physical characteristics, its residential patterns, its economic, social and cultural groupings, and available transportation.

(2) The group will periodically conduct reviews within the service area of the group to determine whether the conditions described in paragraph (1) are being met.

(e) LIMITED ABILITY TO SPEAK ENGLISH LANGUAGE.—A funding agreement for an award of financial assistance under section 3421 is that, if the service area of the qualified community health group involved serves a substantial number of individuals who have a limited ability to speak the English language, the applicant will—

 (1) maintain arrangements responsive to the needs of such individuals for providing services to the extent practicable in the language and cultural context most appropriate to such individuals; and

(2) maintain a sufficient number of staff members who are fluent in both English and the languages spoken by such individuals, and will ensure that the responsibilities of the employees include providing guidance and assistance to such individuals and to other staff members of the group.

## SEC. 3425. ADDITIONAL AGREEMENTS.

(a) REQUIRED SERVICES.—A funding agreement for an award of financial assistance under section 3421 is that the qualified community health group involved will provide enabling services (as defined in section 3461(g)) and all of the items and services identified by the Secretary in rules regarding qualified community health plans and practice networks.

(b) QUALITY CONTROL SYSTEM.—A funding agreement for an award of financial assistance under section 3421 is that the qualified community health group involved will maintain a community-oriented, patient responsive, quality control system under which the group, in accordance with regulations prescribed by the Secretary—

(1) conducts an ongoing quality assurance program for the health services delivered by participating provider entities;

(2) maintains a continuous community health status improvement process; and

(3) maintains a system for development, compilation, evaluation and reporting of information to the public regarding the costs of operation, service utilization patterns, availability, accessibility and acceptability of services, developments in the health status of the populations served, uniform health and clinical performance measures and financial performance of the network or plan.

(c) USE OF EXISTING RESOURCES.—A funding agreement for an award of financial assistance under section 3421 is that the applicant will, in developing the qualified community health group involved, utilize existing resources to the maximum extent practicable.

SEC. 3426. SUBMISSION OF CERTAIN INFORMATION.

(a) ASSESSMENT OF NEED.—The Secretary may make an award of financial assistance under section 3421 only if the applicant involved submits to the Secretary an assessment of the need that the medically underserved population or populations proposed to be served by the applicant have for health services and for enabling services (as defined in section 3461(g)).

(b) DESCRIPTION OF INTENDED EXPENDITURES; RELATED INFORMATION.—The Secretary may make an award of financial assistance under section 3421 only if the applicant involved submits to the Secretary the following information:

(1) A description of how the applicant will design the proposed quality community health plan or practice network (including the service sites involved) for such populations based on the assessment of need.

(2) A description of efforts to secure, within the proposed service area of such health plan or practice network (including the service sites involved), financial and professional assistance and support for the project.

(3) Evidence of significant community involvement in the initiation, development and ongoing operation of the project.

SEC. 3427. REPORTS; AUDITS.

A funding agreement for an award of financial assistance under section 3421 is that the applicant involved will—

(1) provide such reports and information on activities carried out under this section in a manner and form required by the Secretary; and

(2) provide an annual organization-wide audit that meets applicable standards of the Secretary.

**Health Security Act** *Title III, Subtitle E*

**SEC. 3428. APPLICATION FOR ASSISTANCE.**

The Secretary may make an award of financial assistance under section 3421 only if an application for the award is submitted to the Secretary, the application contains each funding agreement described in this subpart, the application contains the information required in section 3426, and the application is in such form, is made in such manner, and contains such agreements, assurances, and information as the Secretary determines to be necessary to carry out this subpart.

**SEC. 3429. GENERAL PROVISIONS.**

(a) LIMITATION ON NUMBER OF AWARDS.—The Secretary may not make more than two awards of financial assistance under section 3421 for the same project.

(b) AMOUNT.—The amount of any award of financial assistance under section 3421 for any project shall be determined by the Secretary.

**Subpart C—Capital Cost of Development of Qualified Community Health Plans and Practice Networks**

**SEC. 3441. LOANS AND LOAN GUARANTEES REGARDING PLANS AND NETWORKS.**

(a) IN GENERAL.—The Secretary may make loans to, and guarantee the payment of principal and interest to Federal and non-Federal lenders on behalf of, public and private entities for the capital costs of developing qualified community health groups (as defined in section 3421(a)).

(b) PREFERENCES; ACCESSIBILITY OF SERVICES; CERTAIN OTHER PROVISIONS.—The provisions of subpart B apply to loans and loan guarantees under subsection (a) to the same extent and in the same manner as such provisions apply to awards of grants and contracts under section 3421.

(c) USE OF ASSISTANCE.—

(1) IN GENERAL.—With respect to the development of qualified community health groups, the capital costs for which loans made pursuant to subsection (a) may be expended are, subject to paragraphs (2) and (3), the following:

(A) The acquisition, modernization, expansion or construction of facilities, or the conversion of unneeded hospital facilities to facilities that will assure or enhance the provision and accessibility of health care and enabling services to medically underserved populations.

(B) The purchase of major equipment, including equipment necessary for the support of external and internal information systems.

(C) The establishment of reserves required for furnishing services on a prepaid basis.

(D) Such other capital costs as the Secretary may determine are necessary to achieve the objectives of this section.

(2) PRIORITIES REGARDING USE OF FUNDS.—In providing loans or loan guarantees under subsection (a) for an entity, the Secretary shall give priority to authorizing the use of amounts for projects for the renovation and modernization of medical facilities necessary to prevent or eliminate safety hazards, avoid noncompliance with licensure or accreditation standards, or projects to replace obsolete facilities.

(3) LIMITATION.—The Secretary may authorize the use of amounts under subsection (a) for the construction of new buildings only if the Secretary determines that appropriate facilities are not available through acquiring, modernizing, expanding or converting existing buildings, or that construction new buildings will cost less.

(d) AMOUNT OF ASSISTANCE.—The principal amount of loans or loan guarantees under subsection (a) may, when added to any other assistance under this section, cover up to 100 percent of the costs involved.

### SEC. 3442. CERTAIN REQUIREMENTS.

(a) LOANS.—

(1) IN GENERAL.—The Secretary may approve a loan under section 3441 only if—

    (A) the Secretary is reasonably satisfied that the applicant for the project for which the loan would be made will be able to make payments of principal and interest thereon when due; and

    (B) the applicant provides the Secretary with reasonable assurances that there will be available to it such additional funds as may be necessary to complete the project or undertaking with respect to which such loan is requested.

(2) TERMS AND CONDITIONS.—Any loan made under section 3441 shall meet such terms and conditions (including provisions for recovery in case of default) as the Secretary determines to be necessary to carry out the purposes of such section while adequately protecting the financial interests of the United States. Terms and conditions for such loans shall include provisions regarding the following:

    (A) Security.

    (B) Maturity date.

    (C) Amount and frequency of installments.

(D) Rate of interest, which shall be at a rate comparable to the rate of interest prevailing on the date the loan is made.

(b) LOAN GUARANTEES.—The Secretary may not approve a loan guarantee under section 3441 unless the Secretary determines that the terms, conditions, security (if any), schedule and amount of repayments with respect to the loan are sufficient to protect the financial interests of the United States and are otherwise reasonable. Such loan guarantees shall be subject to such further terms and conditions as the Secretary determines to be necessary to ensure that the purposes of this section will be achieved.

(c) USE OF EXISTING RESOURCES.—The Secretary may provide a loan or loan guarantee under section 3441 only if the applicant involved agrees that, in developing the qualified community health group involved, the applicant will utilize existing resources to the maximum extent practicable.

### SEC. 3443. DEFAULTS; RIGHT OF RECOVERY.

(a) DEFAULTS.—

(1) IN GENERAL.—The Secretary may take such action as may be necessary to prevent a default on loans or loan guarantees under section 3441, including the waiver of regulatory conditions, deferral of loan payments, renegotiation of loans, and the ex-

penditure of funds for technical and consultative assistance, for the temporary payment of the interest and principal on such a loan, and for other purposes.

(2) FORECLOSURE.—The Secretary may take such action, consistent with State law respecting foreclosure procedures, as the Secretary deems appropriate to protect the interest of the United States in the event of a default on a loan made pursuant to section 3441, including selling real property pledged as security for such a loan or loan guarantee and for a reasonable period of time taking possession of, holding, and using real property pledged as security for such a loan or loan guarantee.

(3) WAIVERS.—The Secretary may, for good cause, but with due regard to the financial interests of the United States, waive any right of recovery which the Secretary has by reasons of the failure of a borrower to make payments of principal of and interest on a loan made pursuant to section 3441, except that if such loan is sold and guaranteed, any such waiver shall have no effect upon the Secretary's guarantee of timely payment of principal and interest.

(b) TWENTY-YEAR OBLIGATION; RIGHT OF RECOVERY.—

(1) IN GENERAL.—With respect to a facility for which a loan is to be made pursuant to section 3441, the Secretary may provide the loan or loan guarantee only if the applicant involved agrees that the applicant will be liable to the United States for the amount of the loan or loan guarantee, together with an amount representing interest, if at any time during the 20-period beginning on the date of completion of the activities involved, the facility—

    (A) ceases to be a facility utilized by a qualified community health group, or by another public or nonprofit private entity that provides health services in one or more health professional shortage areas or that provides such services to a significant number of individuals who are members of a medically underserved population; or

    (B) is sold or transferred to any entity other than an entity that is—

        (i) a qualified community health group or other entity described in subparagraph (A); and

(ii) approved by the Secretary as a purchaser or transferee regarding the facility.

(2) SUBORDINATION; WAIVERS.—The Secretary may subordinate or waive the right of recovery under paragraph (1), and any other Federal interest that may be derived by virtue of a loan or loan guarantee under subsection (a), if the Secretary determines that subordination or waiver will further the objectives of this part.

## SEC. 3444. PROVISIONS REGARDING CONSTRUCTION OR EXPANSION OF FACILITIES.

(a) SUBMISSION OF INFORMATION.—In the case of a project for construction, conversion, expansion or modernization of a facility, the Secretary may provide loans or loan guarantees under section 3441 only if the applicant submits to the Secretary the following:

(1) A description of the site.

(2) Plans and specifications which meet requirements prescribed by the Secretary.

(3) Information reasonably demonstrating that title to such site is vested in one or more of the entities filing the application (unless the agreement described in subsection (b)(1) is made).

(4) A specification of the type of assistance being requested under section 3441.

(b) AGREEMENTS.—In the case of a project for construction, conversion, expansion or modernization of a facility, the Secretary may provide loans or loan guarantees under section 3441 only if the applicant makes the following agreements:

(1) Title to such site will be vested in one or more of the entities filing the application (unless the assurance described in subsection (a)(3) has been submitted under such subsection).

(2) Adequate financial support will be available for completion of the project and for its maintenance and operation when completed.

(3) All laborers and mechanics employed by contractors or subcontractors in the performance of work on a project will be paid wages at rates not less than those prevailing on similar construction in the locality as determined by the Secretary of Labor in accordance with the Act of March 3, 1931 (40 U.S.C. 276a et seq; commonly known as the Davis-Bacon Act), and the Secretary of Labor shall have with respect to such labor standards the authority and functions set forth in Reorganization Plan

Numbered 14 of 1950 (15 FR 3176; 5 U.S.C. Appendix) and section 276c of title 40.

(4) The facility will be made available to all persons seeking service regardless of their ability to pay.

**SEC. 3445. APPLICATION FOR ASSISTANCE.**

The Secretary may provide loans or loan guarantees under section 3441 only if an application for such assistance is submitted to the Secretary, the application contains each agreement described in this subpart, the application contains the information required in section 3444(a), and the application is in such form, is made in such manner, and contains such agreements, assurances, and information as the Secretary determines to be necessary to carry out this subpart.

**SEC. 3446. ADMINISTRATION OF PROGRAMS.**

This subpart, and any other program of the Secretary that provides loans or loan guarantees, shall be carried out by a centralized loan unit established within the Department of Health and Human Services.

### Subpart D—Enabling Services

**SEC. 3461. GRANTS AND CONTRACTS FOR ENABLING SERVICES.**

(a) IN GENERAL.—

(1) GRANTS AND CONTRACTS.—The Secretary may make grants to and enter into contracts with entities described in paragraph (2) to assist such entities in providing the services described in subsection (b) for the purpose of increasing the capacity of individuals to utilize the items and services included in the comprehensive benefits package under title I.

(2) RELEVANT ENTITIES.—For purposes of paragraph (1), the entities described in this paragraph are qualified community health groups (as defined in section 3421(a)), and other public or nonprofit private entities, that—

 (A) provide health services in one or more health professional shortage areas or that provide such services to a significant number of individuals who are members of a medically underserved population; and

 (B) are experienced in providing services to increase the capacity of individuals to utilize health services.

(b) ENABLING SERVICES.—The services referred to in subsection (a)(1) are transportation, community and patient outreach, patient education, translation services, and such other services as the Secretary determines to be appropriate in carrying out the purpose described in such subsection.

(c) CERTAIN REQUIREMENTS REGARDING PROJECT AREA.—The Secretary may make an award of a grant or contract under subsection (a) only if the applicant involved—

(1) submits to the Secretary—

(A) information demonstrating that the medically underserved populations in the community to be served under the award have a need for enabling services; and

(B) a proposed budget for providing such services; and

(2) the applicant for the award agrees that the residents of the community will be significantly involved in the project carried out with the award.

(d) IMPOSITION OF FEES.—The Secretary may make an award of a grant or contract under subsection (a) only if the applicant involved agrees that, in the project carried out under such subsection, enabling services will be provided without charge to the recipients of the services.

(e) USE OF EXISTING RESOURCES.—The Secretary may make an award of a grant or contract under subsection (a) only if the applicant involved agrees that, in carrying out the project under such subsection, the applicant will utilize existing resources to the maximum extent practicable.

(f) APPLICATION FOR AWARDS OF ASSISTANCE.—The Secretary may make an award of a grant or contract under subsection (a) only if an application for the award is submitted to the Secretary, the application contains each agreement described in this subpart, the application contains the information required in subsection (d)(1), and the application is in such form, is made in such manner, and contains such agreements, assurances, and information as the Secretary determines to be necessary to carry out this subpart.

(g) DEFINITION.—For purposes of this section, the term "enabling services" means services described in subsection (b) that are provided for the purpose described in subsection (a)(1).

## SEC. 3462. AUTHORIZATIONS REGARDING PUBLIC HEALTH SERVICE INITIATIVES FUND.

(a) ENABLING SERVICES.—For the purpose of carrying out section 3461, there are authorized to be appropriated from the Public Health Service Initiatives Fund (established in section 3701) $200,000,000 for fiscal year 1996, $300,000,000 for each of the fiscal years 1997 through 1999, and $100,000,000 for fiscal year 2000.

(b) RELATION TO OTHER FUNDS.—The authorizations of appropriations established in subsection (a) are in addition to any other authorizations of appropriations that are available for the purpose described in such subsection.

## PART 3—NATIONAL HEALTH SERVICE CORPS

SEC. 3471. AUTHORIZATIONS REGARDING PUBLIC HEALTH SERVICE INITIATIVES FUND.

(a) ADDITIONAL FUNDING; GENERAL CORPS PROGRAM; ALLOCATIONS REGARDING NURSES.—For the purpose of carrying out subpart II of part D of title III of the Public Health Service Act, and for the purpose of carrying out section 3472, there are authorized to be appropriated from the Public Health Service Initiatives Fund (established in section 3701) $50,000,000 for fiscal year 1995, $100,000,000 for fiscal year 1996, and $200,000,000 for each of the fiscal years 1997 through 2000.

(b) RELATION TO OTHER FUNDS.—The authorizations of appropriations established in subsection (a) are in addition to any other authorizations of appropriations that are available for the purpose described in such subsection.

(c) AVAILABILITY OF FUNDS.—An appropriation under this section for any fiscal year may be made at any time before that fiscal year and may be included in an Act making an appropriation under an authorization under subsection (a) for another fiscal year; but no funds may be made available from any appropriation under this section for obligation under sections 331 through 335, section 336A, and section 337 before the fiscal year involved.

**SEC. 3472. ALLOCATION FOR PARTICIPATION OF NURSES IN SCHOLARSHIP AND LOAN REPAYMENT PROGRAMS.**

Of the amounts appropriated under section 3471, the Secretary shall reserve such amounts as may be necessary to ensure that, of the aggregate number of individuals who are participants in the Scholarship Program under section 338A of the Public Health Service Act, or in the Loan Repayment Program under section 338B of such Act, the total number who are being educated as nurses or are serving as nurses, respectively, is increased to 20 percent.

**PART 4—PAYMENTS TO HOSPITALS SERVING VULNERABLE POPULATIONS**

**SEC. 3481. PAYMENTS TO HOSPITALS.**

(a) ENTITLEMENT STATUS.—The Secretary shall make payments in accordance with this part to eligible hospitals described in section 3482. The preceding sentence—

(1) is an entitlement in the Secretary on behalf of such eligible hospitals (but is not an entitlement in the State in which any such hospital is located or in any individual receiving services from any such hospital); and

(2) constitutes budget authority in advance of appropriations Acts and represents the obligation of the Federal Government to provide funding for such payments in the amounts, and for the fiscal years, specified in subsection (b).

(b) AMOUNT OF ENTITLEMENT.—

(1) IN GENERAL.—For purposes of subsection (a)(2), the amounts and fiscal years specified in this subsection are (in the aggregate for all eligible hospitals) $800,000,000 for the fiscal year in which the general effective date occurs and for each subsequent fiscal year.

(2) SPECIAL RULE FOR YEARS BEFORE GENERAL EFFECTIVE DATE.—

(A) IN GENERAL.—For any fiscal year that begins prior to the general effective date, the amount specified in this subsection for purposes of subsection (a)(2) shall be equal to the aggregate DSH percentage of the amount otherwise determined under paragraph (1).

(B) AGGREGATE DSH PERCENTAGE DEFINED.—In subparagraph (A), the "aggregate DSH percentage" for a year is the amount (expressed as a percentage) equal to—

(i) the total amount of payment made by the Secretary under section 1903(a) of the Social Security Act during the base year with respect to payment adjustments made under section 1923(c) of such Act for hospitals in the States in which eligible hospitals for the year are located; divided by

(ii) the total amount of payment made by the Secretary under section 1903(a) of such Act during the base year with respect to payment adjustments made under section 1923(c) of such Act for hospitals in all States.

(c) PERIOD OF PAYMENT.—An eligible hospital shall receive a payment under this section for a period of 5 years, without regard to the year for which the hospital first receives a payment.

(d) PAYMENTS MADE ON QUARTERLY BASIS.—Payments to an eligible hospital under this section for a year shall be made on a quarterly basis during the year.

## SEC. 3482. IDENTIFICATION OF ELIGIBLE HOSPITALS.

(a) HOSPITALS IN PARTICIPATING STATES.—In order to be an eligible hospital under this part, a hospital must be located in a State that is a participating State under this Act, except that an eligible hospital remains eligible to receive a payment under this part notwithstanding that, during the 5-year period for which the payment is to be made, the State in which it is located no longer meets the requirements for participating States under this Act.

(b) STATE IDENTIFICATION.—In accordance with the criteria described in subsection (c) and such procedures as the Secretary may require, each State shall identify the hospitals in the State that meet such criteria and provide the Secretary with a list of such hospitals.

(c) CRITERIA FOR ELIGIBILITY.—A hospital meets the criteria described in this subsection if the hospital's low-income utilization rate for the base year under section 1923(b)(3) of the Social Security Act (as such section is in effect on the day before the date of the enactment of this Act) is not less than 25 percent.

## SEC. 3483. AMOUNT OF PAYMENTS.

(a) DISTRIBUTION OF ALLOCATION FOR LOW-INCOME ASSISTANCE.—

(1) ALLOCATION FROM TOTAL AMOUNT.—Of the total amount available for payments under this

section in a year, 75 percent shall be allocated to hospitals for low-income assistance in accordance with this subsection.

(2) DETERMINATION OF HOSPITAL PAYMENT AMOUNT.—The amount of payment to an eligible hospital from the allocation made under paragraph (1) during a year shall be the equal to the hospital's low-income percentage of the allocation for the year.

(b) DISTRIBUTION OF ALLOCATION FOR ASSISTANCE FOR UNCOVERED SERVICES.—

(1) ALLOCATION FROM TOTAL AMOUNT; DETERMINATION OF STATE-SPECIFIC PORTION OF ALLOCATION.—Of the total amount available for payments under this section in a year, 25 percent shall be allocated to hospitals for assistance in furnishing inpatient hospital services that are not covered services under title I (in accordance with regulations of the Secretary) in accordance with this subsection. The amount available for payments to eligible hospitals in a State shall be equal to an amount determined in accordance with a methodology specified by the Secretary.

(2) DETERMINATION OF HOSPITAL PAYMENT AMOUNT.—The amount of payment to an eligible hospital in a State from the amount available for

payments to eligible hospitals in the State under paragraph (1) during a year shall be the equal to the hospital's low-income percentage of such amount for the year.

(c) LOW-INCOME PERCENTAGE DEFINED.—

(1) IN GENERAL.—In this subsection, an eligible hospital's "low-income percentage" for a year is equal to the amount (expressed as a percentage) of the total low-income days for all eligible hospitals for the year that are attributable to the hospital.

(2) LOW-INCOME DAYS DESCRIBED.—For purposes of paragraph (1), an eligible hospital's low-income days for a year shall be equal to the product of—

(A) the total number of inpatient days for the hospital for the year (as reported to the Secretary by the State in which the hospital is located, in accordance with a reporting schedule and procedures established by the Secretary); and

(B) the hospital's low-income utilization rate for the base year under section 1923(b)(3) of the Social Security Act (as such section is in effect on the day before the date of the enactment of this Act).

## SEC. 3484. BASE YEAR.

In this part, the "base year" is, with respect to a State and hospitals in a State, the year immediately prior to the year in which the general effective date occurs.

# Subtitle F—Mental Health; Substance Abuse

## PART 1—FINANCIAL ASSISTANCE

### SEC. 3501. AUTHORIZATIONS REGARDING PUBLIC HEALTH SERVICE INITIATIVES FUND.

(a) IN GENERAL.—For the purpose of carrying out this part, there are authorized to be appropriated from the Public Health Service Initiatives Fund (established in section 3701) $100,000,000 for fiscal year 1995, $150,000,000 for fiscal year 1996, and $250,000,000 for each of the fiscal years 1997 through 2000.

(b) ALLOCATION AMONG PROGRAMS.—Of the amounts made available under subsection (a) for a fiscal year—

    (1) the Secretary may reserve for carrying out section 3503 such amounts as the Secretary determines to be appropriate; and

    (2) the Secretary shall, of the remaining amounts, reserve 50 percent for carrying out subsection (a) of section 3502 and 50 percent for carrying out subsection (b) of such section.

(c) RELATION TO OTHER FUNDS.—The authorizations of appropriations established in subsection (a) are in addition to any other authorizations of appropriations that are available for the purpose described in such subsection.

## SEC. 3502. SUPPLEMENTAL FORMULA GRANTS FOR STATES REGARDING ACTIVITIES UNDER PART B OF TITLE XIX OF PUBLIC HEALTH SERVICE ACT.

(a) MENTAL HEALTH.—

(1) IN GENERAL.—In the case of any State that submits to the Secretary an application in accordance with subsection (e) for a fiscal year with respect to mental health, the Secretary shall make a grant to the State for the purposes authorized in subsection (c) with respect to mental health. The grant shall consist of the allotment determined under paragraph (2) for the State for such year.

(2) DETERMINATION OF ALLOTMENT.—For purposes of paragraph (1), the allotment under this paragraph for a State for a fiscal year shall be determined as follows: With respect to the amount reserved under section 3501(c)(2) for carrying out this subsection, section 1918 of the Public Health Service Act shall be applied to such amount to the same extent and in the same manner as such section 1918

is applied to the amount determined under section 1918(a)(2) of such Act.

(b) SUBSTANCE ABUSE.—

(1) IN GENERAL.—In the case of any State that submits to the Secretary an application in accordance with subsection (e) for a fiscal year with respect to substance abuse, the Secretary shall make a grant to the State for the purposes authorized in subsection (c) with respect to substance abuse. The grant shall consist of the allotment determined under paragraph (2) for the State for such year.

(2) DETERMINATION OF ALLOTMENT.—For purposes of paragraph (1), the allotment under this paragraph for a State for a fiscal year shall be determined as follows: With respect to the amount reserved under section 3501(c)(2) for carrying out this subsection, section 1933 of the Public Health Service Act shall be applied to such amount to the same extent and in the same manner as such section 1933 is applied to the amount determined pursuant to sections 1933(a)(1)(B)(i) and 1918(a)(2)(A) of such Act.

(c) USE OF GRANTS.—

(1) IN GENERAL.—With respect to the expenditure of a grant to a State under subsection (a) or (b), the Secretary—

  (A) shall designate as authorized expenditures such of the activities described in paragraph (2) with respect to mental health and substance abuse, respectively, as the Secretary determines to be appropriate; and

  (B) may make the grant only if the State agrees to expend the grant in accordance with the activities so designated.

(2) DESCRIPTION OF ACTIVITIES.—The activities referred to in paragraph (1) are (as applicable to the grant involved) the following:

  (A) For the purpose of increasing the access of individuals to services relating to mental health and substance abuse, the following services: Transportation, community and patient outreach, patient education, translation services, and such other services as the Secretary determines to be appropriate regarding such purpose.

  (B) Improving the capacity of State and local service systems to coordinate and monitor mental health and substance abuse services, including improvement of management information systems, and establishment of linkages between providers of mental health and substance abuse services and primary care providers and health plans.

(C) Providing incentives to integrate public and private systems for the treatment of mental health and substance abuse disorders.

(D) Any activity for which a grant under section 1911 or section 1921 of the Public Health Service Act is authorized to be expended.

(d) MAINTENANCE OF EFFORT.—

(1) IN GENERAL.—With respect to the activities for which a grant under subsection (a) or (b) is to be made, the Secretary may make the grant only if the State involved agrees to maintain expenditures of non-Federal amounts for such activities at a level that is not less than the level of such expenditures maintained by the State for the fiscal year preceding the first fiscal year for which the State receives such a grant.

(2) WAIVER.—The Secretary may waive all or part of the requirement established for a State under paragraph (1) if—

(A) the State agrees that the amounts that otherwise would have been subject to such requirement will be expended for the purpose of developing community-based systems of care to promote the eventual integration of the public and private systems for treatment of mental health, or substance abuse, as applicable to the grant;

(B) the State submits to the Secretary a request for the waiver and a description of the manner in which the State will carry out such purpose; and

(C) the Secretary approves the waiver.

(e) APPLICATION FOR GRANT.—For purposes of subsection (a)(1) and (b)(1), an application for a grant under this section regarding mental health or substance abuse, respectively, is in accordance with this subsection if the State involved submits the application not later than the date specified by the Secretary, the application contains each applicable agreement described in this section, and the application otherwise is in such form, is made in such manner, and contains such agreements, assurances, and information as the Secretary determines to be necessary to carry out the purpose involved.

## SEC. 3503. CAPITAL COSTS OF DEVELOPMENT OF CERTAIN CENTERS AND CLINICS.

(a) IN GENERAL.—The Secretary may make loans to, and guarantee the payment of principal and interest to Federal and non-Federal lenders on behalf of, public and private entities for the capital costs to be incurred by the entities in the development of non-acute, residential treatment centers and community-based ambulatory clinics.

(b) PRIORITIES REGARDING USE OF FUNDS.—In providing loans or loan guarantees under subsection (a), the Secretary shall give priority to authorizing the use of amounts for projects in health professional shortage areas or in geographic area in which there resides a significant number of individuals who are members of a medically underserved population.

(c) APPLICABILITY OF CERTAIN PROVISIONS.—The Secretary may provide loans or loan guarantees under subsection (a) only if the applicant involved agrees that, except to the extent inconsistent with the purpose described in subsection (a), subpart C of part 2 of subtitle E applies to such assistance to the same extent and in the same manner as such subpart applies to loans and loan guarantees under section 3441.

## PART 2—AUTHORITIES REGARDING PARTICIPATING STATES

### Subpart A—Report

**SEC. 3511. REPORT ON INTEGRATION OF MENTAL HEALTH SYSTEMS.**

(a) IN GENERAL.—As a condition of being a participating State under title I, each State shall, not later than October 1, 1998, submit to the Secretary a plan to achieve the integration of the mental health and substance abuse services of the State and its political subdivisions with the mental health and substance abuse services that are included in the comprehensive benefit package under title I.

(b) REQUIRED CONTENTS.—With respect to the provision of items and services relating to mental health and substance abuse, the report of a State under subsection (a) shall, at a minimum, contain the following information:

(1) Information on the number of individuals served by or through mental health and substance abuse programs administered by State and local agencies and the proportion who are eligible persons under title I.

(2) The following information on services furnished to eligible persons:

(A) Each type of benefit furnished.

(B) The mental health diagnoses for which each type of benefit is covered, the amount, duration and scope of coverage for each covered benefit, and any applicable limits on benefits.

(C) Cost sharing rules that apply.

(3) Information on the extent to which each health provider furnishing mental health and substance abuse services under a State program participates in one or more regional or corporate alliance health plans, and, in the case of providers that do not so participate, the reasons for the lack of participation.

(4) The amount of revenues from health plans received by mental health and substance abuse providers that are participating in such health plans and are funded under one or more State programs.

(5) With respect to the two years preceding the year in which the State becomes a participating State under title I—

(A) the amount of funds expended by the State and its political subdivisions for each of such years for items and services that are included in the comprehensive benefit package under such title;

(B) the amount of funds expended for medically necessary and appropriate items and services not included in such benefit package, including medical care, other health care, and supportive services related to the provision of health care.

    (6) An estimate of the amount that the State will expend to furnish items and services not included in such package once the expansion of coverage for mental health and substance abuse services is implemented in the year 2001.

    (7) A description of how the State will assure that all individuals served by mental health and substance abuse programs funded by the State will be enrolled in a health plan and how mental health and substance abuse services not covered under the benefit package will continue to be furnished to such enrollees.

    (8) A description of the conditions under which the integration of mental health and substance abuse providers into regional and corporate alliances can be achieved, and an identification of changes in participation and certification requirements that are needed to achieve the integration of such programs and providers into health plans.

(9) If the integration of mental health and substance abuse programs operated by the State into one or more health plans is not medically appropriate or feasible for one or more groups of individuals treated under State programs, a description of the reasons that integration is not feasible or appropriate and a plan for assuring the coordination for such individuals of the care and services covered under the comprehensive benefit package with the additional items and services furnished by such programs.

(c) GENERAL PROVISIONS.—Reports under subsection (a) shall be provided at the a time and in the manner prescribed by the Secretary.

### Subpart B—Pilot Program

**SEC. 3521. PILOT PROGRAM.**

(a) IN GENERAL.—The Secretary shall establish a pilot program to demonstrate model methods of achieving the integration of the mental health and substance abuse services of the States with the mental health and substance abuse services that are included in the comprehensive benefit package under title I.

(b) CERTAIN CONSIDERATIONS,—With respect to the provision of items and services relating to mental health and substance abuse, the Secretary, in carrying out subsection (a), shall consider the following:

(1) The types of items and services needed in addition to the items and services included in the comprehensive benefits package under title I.

(2) The optimal methods of treatment for individuals with long-term conditions.

(3) The capacity of alliance health plans to furnish such treatment.

(4) The modifications that should be made in the items and services furnished by such health plans.

(5) The role of publicly-funded health providers in the integration of acute and long-term treatment.

## Subtitle G—Comprehensive School Health Education; School-Related Health Services

### PART 1—GENERAL PROVISIONS

**SEC. 3601. PURPOSES.**

Subject to the subsequent provisions of this subtitle, the purposes of this subtitle are as follows:

(1) To support the provision in kindergarten through grade 12 of sequential, age-appropriate, comprehensive health education programs that address locally relevant priorities.

(2) To establish a national framework within which States can create comprehensive school health education programs that—

  (A) target the health risk behaviors accounting for the majority of the morbidity and mortality among youth and adults, including the following: Tobacco use; alcohol and other drug abuse; sexual behaviors resulting in infection with the human immunodeficiency virus, in other sexually transmitted diseases or in unintended pregnancy; behaviors resulting in intentional and unintentional injuries; dietary patterns resulting in disease; and sedentary lifestyles; and

  (B) are integrated with plans and programs in the State, if any, under title III of the Goals 2000: Educate America Act and those targeting health promotion and disease prevention goals related to the national health objectives set forth in Healthy People 2000.

(3) To pay the initial costs of planning and establishing Statewide comprehensive school health education programs that will be implemented and maintained with local, State, and other Federal resources.

(4) To support Federal activities such as research and demonstrations, evaluations, and training and technical assistance regarding comprehensive school health education.

(5) To motivate youth, especially low-achieving youth, to stay in school, avoid teen pregnancy, and strive for success by providing intensive, high-quality health education programs that include peer-teaching, family, and community involvement.

(6) To improve the knowledge and skills of children and youth by integrating academic and experiential learning in health education with other elements of a comprehensive school health program.

(7) To further the National Education Goals set forth in title I of the Goals 2000: Educate America Act and the national health objectives set forth in Healthy People 2000.

(8) With respect to health services, to make awards of financial assistance to eligible State health agencies and local community partnerships to provide for the development and operation of projects to coordinate and deliver comprehensive health services to children or youth in school-based, school-linked, or community-based locations.

SEC. 3602. DEFINITIONS.

(a) COMPREHENSIVE SCHOOL HEALTH EDUCATION PROGRAM.—For purposes of this subtitle, the term "comprehensive school health education program" means a program that addresses locally relevant priorities and meets the following conditions:

(1) The program is sequential, and age and developmentally appropriate.

(2) The program is provided, in the area served by the program, every year for all students from kindergarten through grade 12.

(3) The program provides comprehensive health education, including the following components:

(A) Community health.

(B) Environmental health.

(C) Personal health.

(D) Family life.

(E) Growth and development.

(F) Nutritional health.

(G) Prevention and control of disease and disorders.

(I) Safety and prevention of injuries.

(J) Substance abuse, including tobacco and alcohol use.

(K) Consumer health, including education to ensure that students understand the benefits and appropriate use of medical services, including immunizations and other clinical preventive services.

(4) The program promotes personal responsibility for a healthy lifestyle and provides the knowledge and skills necessary to adopt a healthy lifestyle, including teaching the legal, social, and health consequences of behaviors that pose health risks.

(5) The program is sensitive to cultural and ethnic issues in the content of instructional materials and approaches.

(6) The program includes activities that support instruction.

(7) The program includes activities to promote involvement by parents, families, community organizations, and other appropriate entities.

(8) The program is coordinated with other Federal, State, and local health education and prevention programs and with other Federal, State and local education programs, including those carried out under title I of the Elementary and Secondary Education Act of 1965.

(9) The program focuses on the particular health concerns of the students in the State, school district, or school, as the case may be.

(b) OTHER DEFINITIONS.—For purposes of this subtitle:

(1) The term "local educational agency" has the meaning given such term in section 1471(12) of the Elementary and Secondary Education Act of 1965.

(2) The term "State educational agency" has the meaning given such term in section 1471(23) of the Elementary and Secondary Education Act of 1965.

## PART 2—SCHOOL HEALTH EDUCATION; GENERAL PROVISIONS

### SEC. 3611. AUTHORIZATIONS REGARDING PUBLIC HEALTH SERVICE INITIATIVES FUND..

(a) FUNDING FOR SCHOOL HEALTH EDUCATION.—For the purpose of carrying out parts 3 and 4, there are authorized to be appropriated from the Public Health Service Initiatives Fund (established in section 3701) $50,000,000 for each of the fiscal year 1995 through 2000.

(b) ALLOCATIONS.—Of the amounts appropriated under subsection (a) for a fiscal year—

(1) the Secretary may reserve not more than $13,000,000 for carrying out part 4;

　　　　(2) the Secretary may reserve not more than $5,000,000 to support national leadership activities, such as research and demonstration, evaluation, and training and technical assistance in comprehensive school health education; and

　　　　(3) the Secretary may reserve not more than 5 percent for administrative expenses regarding parts 3 and 4.

　　(c) RELATION TO OTHER FUNDS.—The authorizations of appropriations established in subsection (a) are in addition to any other authorizations of appropriations that are available for the purpose described in such subsection.

## SEC. 3612. WAIVERS OF STATUTORY AND REGULATORY REQUIREMENTS.

　　(a) IN GENERAL.—

　　　　(1) WAIVERS.—Except as provided in subsection (c), upon the request of an entity receiving funds under part 3 or part 4 and under a program specified in paragraph (2), the Secretary of Health and Human Services or the Secretary of Education (as the case may be, according to which Secretary administers the program so specified) may grant to the entity a waiver of any requirement of such program regarding the use of funds, or of the regula-

tions issued for the program by the Secretary involved, if the following conditions are met with respect to such program:

 (A) The Secretary involved determines that the requirement of such program impedes the ability of the State educational agency or other recipient to achieve more effectively the purposes of part 3 or 4.

 (B) The Secretary involved determines that, with respect to the use of funds under such program, the requested use of the funds by the entity would be consistent with the purposes of part 3 or 4.

 (C) In the case of a request for a waiver submitted by a State educational agency, the State educational agency—

  (i) provides all interested local educational agencies in the State with notice and an opportunity to comment on the proposal; and

  (ii) submits the comments to the Secretary involved.

 (D) In the case of a request for a waiver submitted by a local educational agency or other agency, institution, or organization that receives funds under part 3 from the State educational agency, such request has been reviewed by the State educational agency and is accompanied by the comments, if any, of such agency.

(2) RELEVANT PROGRAMS.—For purposes of paragraph (1), the programs specified in this paragraph are as follows:

(A) In the case of programs administered by the Secretary of Health and Human Services, the following:

(i) The program known as the Prevention, Treatment, and Rehabilitation Model Projects for High Risk Youth, carried out under section 517 of the Public Health Service Act.

(ii) The program known as the State and Local Comprehensive School Health Programs to Prevent Important Health Problems and Improve Educational Outcomes, carried out under such Act.

(B) In the case of programs administered by the Secretary of Education, any program carried out under part B of the Drug-Free Schools and Communities Act of 1986.

(b) WAIVER PERIOD.—

(1) IN GENERAL.—A waiver under this section shall be for a period not to exceed three years.

(2) EXTENSIONS.—The Secretary involved under subsection (a) may extend such period if the Secretary determines that—

    (A) the waiver has been effective in enabling the State or affected recipients to carry out the activities for which it was requested and has contributed to improved performance; and

    (B) such extension is in the public interest.

(c) WAIVERS NOT AUTHORIZED.—The Secretary involved under subsection (a) may not waive, under this section, any statutory or regulatory requirement relating to—

    (1) comparability of services;

    (2) maintenance of effort;

    (3) the equitable participation of students attending private schools;

    (4) parental participation and involvement;

    (5) the distribution of funds to States or to local educational agencies or other recipients of funds under the programs specified in subsection (a)(2);

    (6) maintenance of records;

    (7) applicable civil rights requirements; or

(8) the requirements of sections 438 and 439 of the General Education Provisions Act.

(d) TERMINATION OF WAIVER.—The Secretary involved under subsection (a) shall terminate a waiver under this section if the Secretary determines that the performance of the State or other recipient affected by the waiver has been inadequate to justify a continuation of the waiver or if it is no longer necessary to achieve its original purposes.

## PART 3—SCHOOL HEALTH EDUCATION; GRANTS TO STATES

### Subpart A—Planning Grants for States

**SEC. 3621. APPLICATION FOR GRANT.**

(a) IN GENERAL.—Any State educational agency that wishes to receive a planning grant under this subpart shall submit an application to the Secretary of Health and Human Services, at such time and in such manner as the Secretary may require.

(b) APPLICATION; JOINT DEVELOPMENT; CONTENTS.—An application under subsection (a) shall be jointly developed by the State educational agency and the State health agencies of the State involved, and shall contain the following:

(1) An assessment of the State's need for comprehensive school health education, using goals es-

tablished by the Department of Health and Human Services and the Department of Education and goals established under Goals 2000: Educate America Act.

(2) A description of how the State educational agency will collaborate with the State health agency in the planning and development of a comprehensive school health education program in the State, including coordination of existing health education programs and resources.

(3) A plan to build capacity at the State and local levels to provide staff development and technical assistance to local educational agency and local health agency personnel involved with comprehensive school health education.

(4) A preliminary plan for evaluating comprehensive school health education activities.

(5) Information demonstrating that the State has established a State-level advisory council whose membership includes representatives of the State agencies with principal responsibilities for programs regarding health, education, and mental health.

(6) A timetable and proposed budget for the planning process.

(7) Such other information and assurances as the Secretary may require.

(c) NUMBER OF GRANTS.—States may receive one planning grant annually and no more than two planning grants may be awarded to any one State.

**SEC. 3622. APPROVAL OF SECRETARY.**

The Secretary may approve the application of a State under section 3621 if the Secretary determines that—

  (1) the application meets the requirements of this subpart; and

  (2) there is a substantial likelihood that the State will be able to develop and implement a comprehensive school health education plan that complies with the requirements of subpart B.

**SEC. 3623. AMOUNT OF GRANT.**

For any fiscal year, the minimum grant to any State under this subpart is an amount determined by the Secretary to be necessary to enable the State to conduct the planning process, and the maximum such grant is $500,000.

**SEC. 3624. AUTHORIZED ACTIVITIES.**

A State may use funds received under this subpart only for the following:

  (1) To establish and carry out the State planning process.

  (2) To conduct Statewide or sub-State regional coordination and collaboration activities for local

educational agencies, local health agencies, and other agencies and organizations, as appropriate.

(3) To conduct activities to build capacity to provide staff development and technical assistance services to local educational agency and local health agency personnel involved with comprehensive school health education.

(4) To develop student learning objectives and assessment instruments.

(5) To work with State and local health agencies and State and local educational agencies to reduce barriers to the implementation of comprehensive school health education programs in schools.

(6) To prepare the plan required to receive an implementation grant under subpart B.

(7) To adopt, validate, and disseminate curriculum models and program strategies, if the Secretary determines that such activities are necessary to achieving the objectives of the State's program.

**Subpart B—Implementation Grants for States**

SEC. 3631. APPLICATION FOR GRANT.

(a) IN GENERAL.—Any State that wishes to receive an implementation grant under this subpart shall submit an application to the Secretary of Health and Human

Services, at such time, in such manner, and containing such information and assurances as the Secretary may require.

(b) APPLICATION AND STATE PLAN; JOINT DEVELOPMENT; CONTENTS.—An application under subsection (a) shall be jointly developed by the State educational agency and the State health agencies of the State involved, and shall include a State plan for comprehensive school health education programs (as defined in section 3602) that describes the following:

> (1) The State's goals and objectives for those programs.
>
> (2) How the State will allocate funds, if any, to local educational agencies in accordance with section 3634.
>
> (3) How the State will coordinate programs under this subpart with other local, State and Federal health education programs.
>
> (4) How comprehensive school health education programs will be coordinated with other local, State and Federal education programs, such as programs under title I of the Elementary and Secondary Education Act of 1965, with the State's school improvement plan, if any, under title III of the Goals 2000:

Educate America Act, and with any similar programs.

(5) How the State has worked with State and local education agencies and with State and local health agencies to reduce barriers to implementing comprehensive school health education programs.

(6) How the State will monitor the implementation of such programs by local educational agencies.

(7) How the State will build capacity for professional development of health educators.

(8) How the State will provide staff development and technical assistance to local educational agencies.

(9) The respective roles of the State educational agency, local educational agencies, the State health agency, and the local health agencies in developing and implementing such school health education programs.

(10) How such school health education programs will be tailored to the extent practicable to be culturally and linguistically sensitive and responsive to the various needs of the students served, including individuals with disabilities, and individuals from disadvantaged backgrounds (including racial and ethnic minorities).

(11) How the State will evaluate and report on the State's progress toward attaining the goals and objectives described in paragraph (1).

**SEC. 3632. SELECTION OF GRANTEES.**

(a) SELECTION OF GRANTEES.—The Secretary shall establish criteria for the competitive selection of grantees under this subpart.

(b) OPPORTUNITY FOR PLANNING GRANT.—If the Secretary does not approve a State's application under this subpart and determines that the State could benefit from a planning grant under subpart A, the Secretary shall inform the State of any planning grant funds that may be available to it under subpart A, subject to section 3621(c).

**SEC. 3633. AMOUNT OF GRANT.**

(a) IN GENERAL.—For any fiscal year, the minimum grant to any State under this subpart is an amount determined by the Secretary to be necessary to enable the State to conduct the implementation process.

(b) CRITERIA.—In determining the amount of any such grant, the Secretary may consider such factors as the number of children enrolled in schools in the State, the number of school-aged children living in poverty in the State, and the scope and quality of the State's plan.

## SEC. 3634. AUTHORIZED ACTIVITIES; LIMITATION ON ADMINISTRATIVE COSTS.

(a) SUBGRANTS TO LOCAL EDUCATIONAL AGENCIES.—Each State that receives funds under this subpart for any fiscal year shall retain not more than 75 percent of those funds in the first year, 50 percent of those funds in the second and third years, and 25 percent of those funds in each succeeding year. Those funds not retained by the State shall be used to make grants to local educational agencies in accordance with section 3635.

b) STATE-LEVEL ACTIVITIES.—Each State shall use retained funds for any fiscal year for the following purposes:

(1) To conduct Statewide or sub-State regional coordination and collaboration activities.

(2) To adapt, validate, or disseminate program models or strategies for comprehensive school health education.

(3) To build capacity to deliver staff development and technical assistance services to local educational agencies, and State and local health agencies.

(4) To promote program activities involving families and coordinating program activities with community groups and agencies.

(5) To evaluate and report to the Secretary on the progress made toward attaining the goals and objectives described in section 3621(b)(1).

(6) To conduct such other activities to achieve the objectives of this subpart as the Secretary may by regulation authorize.

(c) STATE ADMINISTRATION.—Of the amounts received by a State for a fiscal year under this subpart and remaining after any grants to local educational agencies made from such amounts, the State may use up to 10 percent for the costs of administering such amounts, including the activities of the State advisory council and monitoring the performance of local educational agencies.

## SEC. 3635. SUBGRANTS TO LOCAL EDUCATIONAL AGENCIES.

(a) APPLICATION FOR GRANT.—Any local educational agency that wishes to receive a grant under this subpart shall submit an application to the State, containing such information and assurances as the State may require, including a description of the following:

(1) The local educational agency's goals and objectives for comprehensive school health education programs.

(2) How the local educational agency will concentrate funds in high-need schools and provide suf-

ficient funds to targeted schools to ensure the implementation of comprehensive programs.

(3) How the local educational agency will monitor the implementation of these programs.

(4) How the local educational agency will ensure that school health education programs are tailored to the extent practicable to be culturally and linguistically sensitive and responsive to the various needs of the students served, including individuals with disabilities, and individuals from disadvantaged backgrounds (including racial and ethnic minorities).

(5) How the local educational agency, in consultation with the local health agency, will evaluate and report on its progress toward attaining the goals and objectives described in paragraph (1).

(b) SELECTION OF SUBGRANTEES.—Each State shall give priority to applications from local educational agencies serving areas with high needs, as indicated by criteria developed by the State, which shall include, but need not be limited to, high rates of any of the following:

(1) Poverty among school-aged youth.

(2) Births to adolescents.

(3) Sexually transmitted diseases among school-aged youth.

(4) Drug and alcohol use among school-aged youth.

(5) Violence among school-aged youth.

(c) AUTHORIZED ACTIVITIES.—Each local educational agency that receives a grant under this subpart shall use the grant funds to implement comprehensive school health education programs, as defined in section 3602.

### Subpart C—State and Local Reports

**SEC. 3641. STATE AND LOCAL REPORTS.**

(a) STATE REPORTS.—Each State that receives a grant under this part shall collect and submit to the Secretary such data and other information on State and local programs as the Secretary may require.

(b) IN GENERAL.— Each local educational agency that receives a grant under subpart B shall collect and report to the State such data and other information as the Secretary may require.

## PART 4—SCHOOL HEALTH EDUCATION; GRANTS TO CERTAIN LOCAL EDUCATIONAL AGENCIES

### Subpart A—Eligibility

**SEC. 3651. SUBSTANTIAL NEED OF AREA SERVED BY AGENCY.**

Any local educational agency is eligible for a grant under this part for any fiscal year if—

(1) the agency enrolls at least 25,000 students; and

(2) the geographic area served by the agency has a substantial need for such a grant, relative to other geographic areas in the United States.

## Subpart B—Planning Grants for Local Education Agencies

**SEC. 3661. APPLICATION FOR GRANT.**

(a) IN GENERAL.—Any local educational agency that wishes to receive a planning grant under this subpart shall submit an application to the Secretary of Health and Human Services at such time and in such manner as the Secretary may require.

(b) STATE EDUCATIONAL AGENCY REVIEW.—Each such local educational agency, before submitting its application to the Secretary, shall submit the application to the State educational agency for comment by such agency and by the State health agencies of the State.

(c) CONTENTS OF APPLICATIONS.—Each such application shall contain the following:

(1) An assessment of the local educational agency's need for comprehensive school health education, using goals established by the Department of Health and Human Services and the Department of Education, as well as local health and education

strategies, such as State school improvement plans, if any, under title III of the Goals 2000: Educate America Act.

(2) Information demonstrating that the local educational agency has established or selected a community-level advisory council, which shall include representatives of relevant community agencies such as those that administer education, child nutrition, health, and mental health programs.

(3) A description of how the local educational agency will collaborate with the State educational agency, the State health agency, and the local health agency in the planning and development of a comprehensive school health education program in the local educational agency, including coordination of existing health education programs and resources.

(4) A plan to build capacity at the local educational agency to provide staff development and technical assistance to local educational agency and local health agency personnel involved with comprehensive school health education.

(5) A preliminary plan for evaluating comprehensive school health education activities.

(6) A timetable and proposed budget for the planning process.

(7) Such other information and assurances as the Secretary may require.

(d) NUMBER OF GRANTS.—Local educational agencies may receive at a maximum two annual planning grants.

SEC. 3662. SELECTION OF GRANTEES.

(a) SELECTION CRITERIA.—The Secretary shall establish criteria for the competitive selection of grantees under this part.

(b) LIMITATION.—The Secretary shall not approve an application from a local educational agency in a State that has an approved plan under subpart A or B of part 3 of this subtitle unless the Secretary determines, after consultation with the State that the local application is consistent with the State plan, if one exists.

SEC. 3663. AMOUNT OF GRANT.

For any fiscal year, the minimum grant to any local educational agency under this subpart is an amount determined by the Secretary to be necessary to enable the local educational agency to conduct the planning process, and the maximum such grant is $500,000.

SEC. 3664. AUTHORIZED ACTIVITIES.

A local educational agency may use funds received under this subpart only for the following:

(1) To establish and carry out the local educational agency planning process.

(2) To undertake joint training, staffing, administration, and other coordination and collaboration activities for local educational agencies, local health agencies, and other agencies and organizations, as appropriate.

(3) To conduct activities to build capacity to provide staff development and technical assistance services to local educational agency and local health agency personnel involved with comprehensive school health education.

(4) To develop student learning objectives and assessment instruments.

(5) To work with State and local health agencies and State educational agencies to reduce barriers to the implementation of comprehensive school health education programs in schools, by, for example, ensuring that adequate time is a available during the school day for such programs.

(6) To prepare the plan required to receive an implementation grant under subpart C.

## Subpart C—Implementation Grants for Local Educational Agencies

**SEC. 3671. APPLICATION FOR GRANT.**

(a) IN GENERAL.—Any local educational agency that wishes to receive an implementation grant under this subpart shall submit an application to the Secretary of Health and Human Services, at such time, in such manner, and containing such information and assurances as the Secretary may require.

(b) STATE EDUCATIONAL AGENCY REVIEW.—Each such local educational agency shall submit its application to the State educational agency for comment before submitting it to the Secretary.

(c) LOCAL EDUCATIONAL AGENCY PLAN.—Each such application shall include a local educational agency plan for comprehensive school health education programs (as defined in section 3602) that describes the following:

    (1) The local educational agency's goals and objectives for those programs.

    (2) How the local educational agency will coordinate programs under this subpart with other local, State and Federal health education programs.

    (3) How comprehensive school health education programs will be coordinated with other local, State and Federal education programs, such as programs under title I of the Elementary and Secondary Edu-

cation Act of 1965, and with State's school improvement plan, if any, under title III of the Goals 2000: Educate America Act.

(4) How the local educational agency has worked with State educational agencies and with State and local health agencies to reduce barriers to implementing comprehensive school health education programs.

(5) How local educational agencies will monitor the implementation of such programs.

(6) How the local educational agency, in consultation with the State educational agency and State and local health agencies and in conjunction with other local professional development activities, will build capacity for professional development of health educators.

(7) How the local educational agency, in consultation with the State educational agency and State and local health agencies, will provide staff development and technical assistance.

(8) The respective roles of the State educational agency, local educational agencies, the State health agency, and the local health agencies in developing and implementing such school health education programs.

(9) How such school health education programs will be tailored to the extent practicable to be culturally and linguistically sensitive and responsive to the various needs of the students served, including individuals with disabilities, and individuals from disadvantaged backgrounds (including racial and ethnic minorities).

(10) How the local educational agency, in consultation with the local health agency, will evaluate and report on the local educational agency's progress toward attaining the goals and objectives described in paragraph (1).

**SEC. 3672. SELECTION OF GRANTEES.**

(a) SELECTION OF GRANTEES.—The Secretary shall establish criteria for the competitive selection of grantees under this subpart.

(b) LIMITATION.—The Secretary shall not approve an application from a local educational agency in a State that has an approved plan under subpart A or B of part 3 unless the Secretary determines, after consultation with the State that the local application is consistent with such State plan.

(c) OPPORTUNITY FOR PLANNING GRANT.—If the Secretary does not approve a local educational agency's application under this subpart and determines that the local educational agency could benefit from a planning grant under subpart B, the Secretary shall inform the local educational agency of any planning grant funds that may be available to it under subpart B, subject to section 3661(d).

## SEC. 3673. AMOUNT OF GRANT.

(a) IN GENERAL.—For any fiscal year, the minimum grant to any local educational agency under this subpart is an amount determined by the Secretary to be necessary to enable the local educational agency to conduct the implementation process.

(b) CRITERIA.—In determining the amount of any such grant, the Secretary may consider such factors as the number of children enrolled in schools in the local educational agency, the number of school-aged children living in poverty in the local educational agency, and the scope and quality of the local educational agency's plan.

## SEC. 3674. AUTHORIZED ACTIVITIES.

Each local educational agency that receives a grant under this subpart shall use the grant funds as follows:

(1) To implement comprehensive school health education programs, as defined in section 3602.

(2) To conduct local or regional coordination and collaboration activities.

(3) To provide staff development and technical assistance to schools, local health agencies, and other community agencies involved in providing comprehensive school health education programs.

(4) To administer the program and monitor program implementation at the local level.

(5) To evaluate and report to the Secretary on the local educational agency's progress toward attaining the goals and objectives described in section 3671(c)(1).

(6) To conduct such other activities as the Secretary may by regulation authorize.

### SEC. 3675. REPORTS.

Each local educational agency that receives a grant under this subpart shall collect and report to the Secretary and the State such data and other information as the Secretary may require.

## PART 5—SCHOOL-RELATED HEALTH SERVICES

### Subpart A—Development and Operation of Projects

### SEC. 3681. AUTHORIZATIONS REGARDING PUBLIC HEALTH SERVICE INITIATIVES FUND.

(a) FUNDING FOR SCHOOL-RELATED HEALTH SERVICES.—For the purpose of carrying out this subpart, there are authorized to be appropriated from the Public Health Service Initiatives Fund (established in section 3701)

$100,000,000 for fiscal year 1996, $275,000,000 for fiscal year 1997, $350,000,000 for fiscal year 1998, and $400,000,000 for each of the fiscal years 1999 and 2000.

(b) RELATION TO OTHER FUNDS.—The authorizations of appropriations established in subsection (a) are in addition to any other authorizations of appropriations that are available for the purpose described in such subsection.

## SEC. 3682. ELIGIBILITY FOR DEVELOPMENT AND OPERATION GRANTS.

(a) IN GENERAL.—Entities eligible to apply for and receive grants under section 3484 or 3485 are:

 (1) State health agencies that apply on behalf of local community partnerships and other communities in need of adolescent health services within the State.

 (2) Local community partnerships in States in which health agencies have not applied.

(b) LOCAL COMMUNITY PARTNERSHIPS.—

 (1) IN GENERAL.—A local community partnership under subsection (a)(2) is an entity that, at a minimum, includes—

  (A) a local health care provider with experience in delivering services to adolescents;

  (B) one or more local public schools; and

(C) at least one community based organization located in the community to be served that has a history of providing services to at-risk youth in the community.

(2) PARTICIPATION.—A partnership described in paragraph (1) shall, to the maximum extent feasible, involve broad based community participation from parents and youth to be served, health and social service providers (including regional alliance health plans and corporate alliance health plans in which families in the community are enrolled), teachers and other public school and school board personnel, the regional health alliance in which the schools participating in the partnership are located, youth development and service organizations, and interested business leaders. Such participation may be evidenced through an expanded partnership, or an advisory board to such partnership.

## SEC. 3683. PREFERENCES

(a) IN GENERAL.—In making grants under sections 3484 and 3485, the Secretary shall give preference to applicants whose communities to be served show the most substantial level of need for such services among individuals who are between the ages of 10 and 19 (inclusive), as measured by indicators of community health including the following:

(1) High levels of poverty.

(2) The presence of a medically underserved area or population (as defined under section 330(a) of the Public Health Service Act).

(3) A health professional shortage area, as designated under section 332 of the Public Health Service Act.

(4) High rates of indicators of health risk among children and youth, including a high proportion of children receiving services through the Individuals with Disabilities Education Act, adolescent pregnancy, sexually transmitted disease (including infection with the human immunodeficiency virus), preventable disease, communicable disease, intentional and unintentional injuries among children and youth, community and gang violence, youth unemployment, juvenile justice involvement, and high rates of drug and alcohol exposure.

(b) LINKAGE TO QUALIFIED COMMUNITY HEALTH GROUPS.—In making grants under sections 3484 and 3485, the Secretary shall give preference to applicants that demonstrate a linkage to qualified community health groups (as defined in section 3421(a)).

## SEC. 3684. GRANTS FOR DEVELOPMENT OF PROJECTS.

(a) IN GENERAL.—The Secretary may make grants to State health agencies or to local community partnerships to develop school health service sites.

(b) USE OF FUNDS.—A project for which a grant may be made under subsection (a) may include but not be limited to the cost of the following:

   (1) Planning for the provision of school health services.

   (2) Recruitment, compensation, and training of health and administrative staff.

   (3) The development of agreements with regional and corporate alliance health plans and the acquisition and development of equipment and information services necessary to support information exchange between school health service sites and health plans, health providers, and other entities authorized to collect information under this Act.

   (4) In the case of communities described in subsection (d)(2)(B), funds to aid in the establishment of local community partnerships.

   (5) Other activities necessary to assume operational status.

(c) AUTHORITY REGARDING QUALIFIED COMMUNITY HEALTH GROUPS.—A project under subsection (a) may require that, in order to receive services from the project, an individual be enrolled in a health plan of a qualified community health group (as defined in section 3421(a)).

(d) APPLICATION FOR GRANT.—

(1) IN GENERAL.—Applicants shall submit applications in a form and manner prescribed by the Secretary.

(2) APPLICATIONS BY STATE HEALTH AGENCIES.—

(A) In the case of applicants that are State health agencies, the application shall contain assurances that the State health agency is applying for funds—

(i) on behalf of at least one local community partnership; and

(ii) on behalf of at least one other community identified by the State as in need of the services funded under this part but without a local community partnership.

(B) In the case of communities identified in applications submitted by State health agencies that do not yet have local community partnerships, the State shall describe the steps that will be taken to aid the community in developing a local community partnership.

(C) A State applying on behalf of local community partnerships and other communities may retain not more than 10 percent of grants awarded under this part for administrative costs.

(e) CONTENTS OF APPLICATION.—In order to receive a grant under this section, an applicant must include in the application the following information:

(1) An assessment of the need for school health services in the communities to be served, using the latest available health data and health goals and objectives established by the Secretary.

(2) A description of how the applicant will design the proposed school health services to reach the maximum number of school-aged children and youth at risk for poor health outcome.

(3) An explanation of how the applicant will integrate its services with those of other health and social service programs within the community.

(4) An explanation of how the applicant will link its activities to the regional and corporate alliance health plans serving the communities in which the applicant's program is to be located.

(5) Evidence of linkages with regional and corporate health alliances in whose areas the applicant's program is to be located.

(6) A description of a quality assurance program which complies with standards that the Secretary may prescribe.

(f) NUMBER OF GRANTS.—Not more than two planning grants may be made to a single applicant.

## SEC. 3685. GRANTS FOR OPERATION OF PROJECTS.

(a) IN GENERAL.—The Secretary may make grants to State health agencies or to local community partnerships for the cost of operating school health service sites

(b) USE OF GRANT.—The costs for which a grant may be made under this section include but are not limited to the following:

(1) The cost of furnishing health services that are not covered under title I of this Act or by any other public or private insurer.

(2) The cost of furnishing enabling services, as defined in section 3461(h).

(3) Training, recruitment and compensation of health professionals and other staff.

(4) Outreach services to at-risk youth and to parents.

(5) Linkage of individuals to health plans, community health services and social services.

(6) Other activities deemed necessary by the Secretary.

(c) APPLICATION FOR GRANT.—Applicants shall submit applications in a form and manner prescribed by the Secretary. In order to receive a grant under this section, an applicant must include in the application the following information:

(1) A description of the services to be furnished by the applicant.

(2) The amounts and sources of funding that the applicant will expend, including estimates of the amount of payments the applicant will received from alliance health plans and from other sources.

(3) Such other information as the Secretary determines to be appropriate.

(d) ADDITIONAL CONTENTS OF APPLICATION.—In order to receive a grant under this section, an applicant must meet the following conditions:

(1) The applicant furnishes the following services:

(A) Diagnosis and treatment of simple illnesses and minor injuries.

(B) Preventive health services, including health screenings.

(C) Enabling services, as defined in section 3461(h).

(D) Referrals and followups in situations involving illness or injury.

(E) Health and social services, counseling services, and necessary referrals, including referrals regarding mental health and substance abuse.

(F) Such other services as the Secretary determines to be appropriate.

(2) The applicant maintains agreements with all regional and corporate alliance health plans offering services in the applicant's service area.

(3) The applicant is a participating provider in the State's program for medical assistance under title XIX of the Social Security Act.

(4) The applicant does not impose charges on students or their families for services (including collection of any cost-sharing for services under the comprehensive benefit package that otherwise would be required).

(5) The applicant has reviewed and will periodically review the needs of the population served by

the applicant in order to ensure that its services are accessible to the maximum number of school age children and youth in the area, and that, to the maximum extent possible, barriers to access to services of the applicant are removed (including barriers resulting from the area's physical characteristics, its economic, social and cultural grouping, the health care utilization patterns of children and youth, and available transportation).

(6) In the case of an applicant which serves a population that includes a substantial proportion of individuals of limited English speaking ability, the applicant has developed a plan to meet the needs of such population to the extent practicable in the language and cultural context most appropriate to such individuals.

(7) The applicant will provide non-Federal contributions toward the cost of the project in an amount determined by the Secretary.

(8) The applicant will operate a quality assurance program consistent with section 3684(e)(6).

(e) DURATION OF GRANT.—A grant under this section shall be for a period determined by the Secretary.

(f) REPORTS.—A recipient of funding under this section shall provide such reports and information as are required in regulations of the Secretary.

SEC. 3686. FEDERAL ADMINISTRATIVE COSTS.

Of the amounts made available under section 3681, the Secretary may reserve not more than 5 percent for administrative expenses regarding this subpart.

## Subpart B—Capital Costs of Developing Projects

SEC. 3691. LOANS AND LOAN GUARANTEES REGARDING PROJECTS.

(a) IN GENERAL.—The Secretary may make loans to, and guarantee the payment of principal and interest to Federal and non-Federal lenders on behalf of, State health agencies and local community partnerships for the capital costs of developing projects in accordance with subpart A.

(b) APPLICABILITY OF CERTAIN PROVISIONS.—The provisions of subpart A apply to loans and loan guarantees under subsection (a) to the same extent and in the same manner as such provisions apply to grants under subpart A. Except for any provision inconsistent with the purpose described in subsection (a), the provisions of subpart C of part 2 of subtitle E apply to loans and loan guarantees under subsection (a) to the same extent and in the same manner as such provisions apply to loans and loan guarantees under section 3441.

SEC. 3692. FUNDING.

Amounts available to the Secretary under section 3412 for the purpose of carrying out subparts B and C of part 2 of subtitle E are, in addition to such purpose, available to the Secretary for the purpose of carrying out this subpart.

# Subtitle H—Public Health Service Initiative

SEC. 3701. PUBLIC HEALTH SERVICE INITIATIVE.

(a) IN GENERAL.—There is established pursuant to this title a Public Health Service Initiative consisting of the total amounts authorized and described in subsection (b). The Initiative includes all the programs authorized under the previous provisions of this title.

(b) TOTAL OF THE AMOUNTS AUTHORIZED TO BE APPROPRIATED.—The following is the total of the amounts authorized to be appropriated for the Initiative under the previous subtitles of this title:

(1) For fiscal year 1995, $1,125,000,000.

(2) For fiscal year 1996, $2,984,000,000.

(3) For fiscal year 1997, $3,830,000,000.

(4) For fiscal year 1998, $4,205,000,000.

(5) For fiscal year 1999, $4,055,000,000.

(6) For fiscal year 2000, $3,655,000,000.

(c) USE OF AMOUNTS; AVAILABILITY.—

(1) USE; ANNUAL APPROPRIATIONS.—Amounts appropriated to carry out the Initiative, including subtitles A through F of this title, are available to carry out the specific programs for which the amounts are appropriated.

(2) AVAILABILITY OF APPROPRIATED AMOUNTS.—Amounts appropriated for programs in the Initiative are available until expended.

# Subtitle I—Coordination With Cobra Continuation Coverage

SEC. 3801. PUBLIC HEALTH SERVICE ACT; COORDINATION WITH COBRA CONTINUATION COVERAGE.

(a) PERIOD OF COVERAGE.—Subparagraph (D) of section 2202(2) of the Public Health Service Act (42 U.S.C. 300bb–2(2)) is amended—

(1) by striking "or" at the end of clause (i), by striking the period at the end of clause (ii) and inserting ", or", and by adding at the end the following new clause:

"(iii) eligible for comprehensive health coverage described in section 1101 of the Health Security Act.", and

(2) by striking "OR MEDICARE ENTITLEMENT" in the heading and inserting ", MEDICARE ENTITLEMENT, OR HEALTH SECURITY ACT ELIGIBILITY".

(b) QUALIFIED BENEFICIARY.—Section 2208(3) of such Act (42 U.S.C. 300bb–8(3)) is amended by adding at the end the following new subparagraph:

"(C) SPECIAL RULE FOR INDIVIDUALS COVERED BY HEALTH SECURITY ACT.—The term 'qualified beneficiary' shall not include any individual who, upon termination of coverage under a group health plan, is eligible for comprehensive health coverage described in section 1101 of the Health Security Act.".

(c) REPEAL UPON IMPLEMENTATION OF HEALTH SECURITY ACT.—

(1) IN GENERAL.—Title XXII of such Act (42 U.S.C. 300bb–1 et seq.) is hereby repealed.

(2) CONFORMING AMENDMENT.—The table of contents of such Act is amended by striking the item relating to title XXII.

(3) EFFECTIVE DATE.—The amendments made by this subsection shall take effect on the earlier of—

(A) January 1, 1998, or

(B) the first day of the first calendar year following the calendar year in which all States have in effect plans under which individuals are eligible for comprehensive health coverage described in section 1101 of this Act.

# TITLE IV—MEDICARE AND MEDICAID

TABLE OF CONTENTS OF TITLE

Sec. 4000. References in title.

## Subtitle A—Medicare and the Alliance System

### PART 1—ENROLLMENT OF MEDICARE BENEFICIARIES IN REGIONAL ALLIANCE PLANS

Sec. 4001. Optional State integration of medicare beneficiaries into regional alliance plans.
Sec. 4002. Individual election to remain in certain health plans.
Sec. 4003. Treatment of certain medicare beneficiaries.
Sec. 4004. Prohibiting employers from taking into account status as medicare beneficiary on any grounds.

### PART 2—ENCOURAGING MANAGED CARE UNDER MEDICARE PROGRAM; COORDINATION WITH MEDIGAP PLANS

Sec. 4011. Enrollment and termination of enrollment.
Sec. 4012. Uniform informational materials.
Sec. 4013. Outlier payments.
Sec. 4014. Point of service option.

### PART 3—MEDICARE COVERAGE EXPANSIONS

Sec. 4021. Reference to coverage of outpatient prescription drugs.
Sec. 4022. Coverage of services of advanced practice nurses.

### PART 4—COORDINATION WITH ADMINISTRATIVE SIMPLIFICATION AND QUALITY MANAGEMENT INITIATIVES

Sec. 4031. Repeal of separate medicare peer review program.
Sec. 4032. Mandatory assignment for all part B services.
Sec. 4033. Elimination of complexities caused by dual funding sources and rules for payment of claims.
Sec. 4034. Repeal of PRO precertification requirement for certain surgical procedures.
Sec. 4035. Requirements for changes in billing procedures.

### PART 5—AMENDMENTS TO ANTI-FRAUD AND ABUSE PROVISIONS

Sec. 4041. Anti-kickback provisions.
Sec. 4042. Revisions to limitations on physician self-referral.
Sec. 4043. Civil monetary penalties.
Sec. 4044. Exclusions from program participation.
Sec. 4045. Sanctions against practitioners and persons for failure to comply with statutory obligations relating to quality of care.
Sec. 4046. Effective date.

# Health Security Act

## Title IV

### PART 6—FUNDING OF GRADUATE MEDICAL EDUCATION AND ACADEMIC HEALTH CENTERS

Sec. 4051. Transfers from medicare trust funds for graduate medical education.
Sec. 4052. Transfers from hospital insurance trust fund for academic health centers.

### PART 7—COVERAGE OF SERVICES PROVIDED BY FACILITIES AND PLANS OF DEPARTMENTS OF DEFENSE AND VETERANS AFFAIRS

Sec. 4061. Treatment of uniformed services health plan as eligible organization under medicare.
Sec. 4062. Coverage of services provided to medicare beneficiaries by plans and facilities of Department of Veterans Affairs.
Sec. 4063. Conforming amendments.

## Subtitle B—Savings in Medicare Program

### PART 1—SAVINGS RELATING TO PART A

Sec. 4101. Reduction in update for inpatient hospital services.
Sec. 4102. Reduction in adjustment for indirect medical education.
Sec. 4103. Reduction in payments for capital-related costs for inpatient hospital services.
Sec. 4104. Revisions to payment adjustments for disproportionate share hospitals in participating States.
Sec. 4105. Moratorium on designation of additional long-term care hospitals.
Sec. 4106. Extension of freeze on updates to routine service costs of skilled nursing facilities.

### PART 2—SAVINGS RELATING TO PART B

Sec. 4111. Establishment of cumulative expenditure goals for physician services.
Sec. 4112. Use of real GDP to adjust for volume and intensity; repeal of restriction on maximum reduction permitted in default update.
Sec. 4113. Reduction in conversion factor for physician fee schedule for 1995.
Sec. 4114. Limitations on payment for physicians' services furnished by high-cost hospital medical staffs.
Sec. 4115. Medicare incentives for physicians to provide primary care.
Sec. 4116. Elimination of formula-driven overpayments for certain outpatient hospital services.
Sec. 4117. Imposition of coinsurance on laboratory services.
Sec. 4118. Application of competitive bidding process for Part B items and services.
Sec. 4119. Application of competitive acquisition procedures for laboratory services.

### PART 3—SAVINGS RELATING TO PARTS A AND B

Sec. 4131. Medicare secondary payer changes.
Sec. 4132. Payment limits for HMOs and CMPs with risk-sharing contracts.
Sec. 4133. Reduction in routine cost limits for home health services.
Sec. 4134. Imposition of copayment for certain home health visits.
Sec. 4135. Expansion of centers of excellence.

### PART 4—PART B PREMIUM

Sec. 4141. General Part B premium.

### Subtitle C—Medicaid

PART 1—COMPREHENSIVE BENEFIT PACKAGE

Sec. 4201. Limiting coverage under medicaid of items and services covered under comprehensive benefit package.

PART 2—EXPANDING ELIGIBILITY FOR NURSING FACILITY SERVICES; LONG-TERM CARE INTEGRATION OPTION

Sec. 4211. Spenddown eligibility for nursing facility residents.
Sec. 4212. Increased income and resource disregards for nursing facility residents.
Sec. 4213. New State long-term care integration option.
Sec. 4214. Informing nursing home residents about availability of assistance for home and community-based services.

PART 3—OTHER BENEFITS

Sec. 4221. Treatment of items and services not covered under the comprehensive benefit package.
Sec. 4222. Establishment of program for poverty-level children with special needs.

PART 4—DISCONTINUATION OF CERTAIN PAYMENT POLICIES

Sec. 4231. Discontinuation of medicaid DSH payments.
Sec. 4232. Discontinuation of reimbursement standards for inpatient hospital services.

PART 5—COORDINATION WITH ADMINISTRATIVE SIMPLIFICATION AND QUALITY MANAGEMENT INITIATIVES

Sec. 4241. Requirements for changes in billing procedures.

PART 6—MEDICAID COMMISSION

Sec. 4251. Medicaid commission.

### Subtitle D—Increase in SSI Personal Needs Allowance

Sec. 4301. Increase in ssi personal needs allowance.

# TITLE IV—MEDICARE AND MEDICAID

**SEC. 4000. REFERENCES IN TITLE.**

(a) AMENDMENTS TO SOCIAL SECURITY ACT.—Except as otherwise specifically provided, whenever in this title an amendment is expressed in terms of an amendment to or repeal of a section or other provision, the reference shall be considered to be made to that section or other provision of the Social Security Act.

(b) REFERENCES TO OBRA.—In this title, the terms "OBRA–1986", "OBRA–1987", "OBRA–1989", "OBRA–1990", and "OBRA–1993" refer to the Omnibus Budget Reconciliation Act of 1986 (Public Law 99–509), the Omnibus Budget Reconciliation Act of 1987 (Public Law 100–203), the Omnibus Budget Reconciliation Act of 1989 (Public Law 101–239), the Omnibus Budget Reconciliation Act of 1990 (Public Law 101–508), and the Omnibus Budget Reconciliation Act of 1993 (Public Law 103–66), respectively.

# Subtitle A—Medicare and the Alliance System

## PART 1—ENROLLMENT OF MEDICARE BENEFICIARIES IN REGIONAL ALLIANCE PLANS

### SEC. 4001. OPTIONAL STATE INTEGRATION OF MEDICARE BENEFICIARIES INTO REGIONAL ALLIANCE PLANS.

Title XVIII is amended by adding at the end the following:

### "INTEGRATION OF MEDICARE INTO STATE HEALTH SECURITY PROGRAMS

"SEC. 1893. (a) PAYMENT TO STATES.—The Secretary shall pay a participating State that has submitted an application, as specified by subsection (b) which the Secretary has approved under subsection (c), the amount specified by subsection (d) for the period specified by subsection (e) for covered medicare beneficiaries. This section shall apply without regard to whether or not a State is a single-payer State.

"(b) APPLICATION BY STATE.—An application submitted by a participating State shall contain the following assurances:

"(1) DESIGNATION OF CLASSES COVERED.—

"(A) DESIGNATION OF CLASSES OF MEDICARE BENEFICIARIES COVERED.—In the application the State shall designate which of the following classes of medicare beneficiaries are to be covered:

"(i) Individuals who are 65 years of age or older.

"(ii) Individuals who are eligible for benefits under part A by reason of section 226(b) or section 1818A (relating to disabled individuals).

"(iii) Individuals who are eligible for benefits under part A only by reason of section 226A (relating to individuals with end stage renal disease).

A State may not restrict the individuals within such a class who are to be covered under this section.

"(B) LIMITATION.—An individual may not be covered under the application unless the individual is entitled to benefits under part A and is enrolled under part B.

"(2) ENROLLMENT IN AND SELECTION OF HEALTH PLANS.—

"(A) ENROLLMENT.—Each medicare-eligible individual (within a class of medicare beneficiaries covered under the application) who is a resident of the State will be enrolled in a regional alliance health plan serving the area in which the individual resides (or, in the case of an individual who is a resident of a single-payer State, in the Statewide single-payer system operated under part 2 of subtitle C of title I of the Health Security Act).

"(B) SELECTION.—Each such individual will have the same choice among applicable health plans as other individuals in the State who are eligible individuals under the Health Security Act.

"(C) OFFER OF FEE-FOR-SERVICE PLAN.—
Each such individual shall be offered enrollment in at least one health plan that is a fee-for-service plan (or, in the case of an indivdiual who is a resident of a single-payer State, the Statewide single-payer system under part 2 of subtitle B of title I of the Health Security Act) that meets the following requirements:

"(i) The plan's premium rate, and the actuarial value of the plan's deductibles, coinsurance, and copayments, charged to the individual do not exceed the actuarial value of the premium rate, coinsurance, and deductibles that would be applicable on the average to such individuals if this section did not apply to those individuals.

"(ii) The plan's payment rates for hospital services, post-hospital extended care services, home health services, home intravenous drug therapy services, comprehensive outpatient rehabilitation facility services, hospice care, dialysis services for individuals with end stage renal disease, and facility services furnished in connection with ambulatory surgical procedures are accepted as payment in full.

"(iii) The plan's payment rates for physicians' services are no less a percentage of the amounts accepted as payment in full than are the payment rates for physicians' services under part B.

"(3) COVERAGE OF FULL MEDICARE BENEFITS.—For each health plan providing coverage under this section—

"(A) the plan shall cover at least the items and services for which payment would otherwise be made under this title, and

"(B) coverage determinations under the plan are made under rules that are no more restrictive than otherwise applicable under this title.

"(4) PREMIUM.—During the period for which payments are made to a State under this section, the requirements of the Health Security Act relating to premiums that are otherwise applicable with respect to individuals enrolled in health plans in a State shall not apply with respect to medicare-eligible individuals in the State who are covered under the State's application under this section. Nothing in the previous sentence shall operate to permit a State or health plans in a State to charge different premiums among medicare-eligible individuals within the same premium class under the Health Security Act.

"(5) QUALITY ASSURANCE.—For each health plan providing coverage under this section there are quality assurance mechanisms for covered medicare individuals that equal, or exceed, such mechanisms otherwise applicable under this title.

"(6) REVIEW RIGHTS.—Covered medicare individuals have review, reconsideration, and appeal rights (including appeals to courts of the State) that equal or exceed such rights otherwise applicable under this title.

"(7) DATA REPORTING AND ACCESS TO DOCUMENTS.—The State will—

"(A) provide such utilization and statistical data as the Secretary determines are needed for purposes of the programs established under this title, and

"(B) the State will ensure access by the Secretary or the Comptroller General to relevant documents.

"(8) USE OF PAYMENTS.—Payments made to the State under subsection (a) will be used only to carry out the purposes of this section.

"(c) APPROVAL BY SECRETARY.—The Secretary shall approve an application under subsection (b) if the Secretary finds—

"(1) that the individuals covered under the State's application shall receive at least the benefits provided under this title (including cost sharing);

"(2) that the amount of expenditures that will be made under this title will not exceed the amount of expenditures that will be made if the State's application is not accepted; and

"(3) that the State is able and willing to carry out the assurances provided in its application.

"(d) AMOUNT AND SOURCE OF PAYMENT.—

"(1) AMOUNT OF PAYMENT.—For purposes of subsection (a), the amount of payments to a State—

"(A) for the first year for which payments are made to the State under this section shall be determined by the applicable rate specified in section 1876(a)(1)(C) (but at 100 percent, rather than 95 percent, of the applicable amount) for each medicare-eligible individual who is a resident of the State (but without regard to any reduction based on payments to be made under section 1876(a)(1)(G)), and

"(B) for each succeeding year, shall be determined by the applicable rate determined under subparagraph (A) or this subparagraph for the preceding year for each such individual, adjusted by the regional alliance inflation factor applicable to regional alliances in the State (as determined in accordance with subtitle A of title VI of the Health Security Act) for the year.

"(2) SOURCE OF PAYMENT.—Payment shall be made from the Federal Hospital Insurance Trust Fund and the Federal Supplementary Medical Insurance Trust Fund as provided under paragraph (5) of section 1876(a) (other than as provided under subparagraph (B) of that paragraph).

"(e) PERIOD FOR WHICH PAYMENT MADE.—The period for which payment may be made under subsection (a) to a State—

"(1) begins with January 1 of the first calendar year for which the Secretary approves under subsection (c) the application of the State; and

"(2) ends—

"(A) on December 31 of the year in which the State notifies the Secretary (before April of that year) that the State no longer intends to receive payments under this section, or

"(B) if the Secretary finds that the State is no longer in substantial compliance with the requirements under paragraphs (2) or (3) of subsection (c), at the time specified by the Secretary.

No termination is effective under paragraph (2) unless notice has been provided to medicare covered individuals, health providers, and health plans affected by the termination.

"(f) PAYMENTS UNDER THIS SECTION AS SOLE MEDICARE BENEFITS.—Payments to a State under subsection (a) shall be instead of the amounts that would otherwise be payable, pursuant to sections 1814(b) and 1833(a), for services furnished to medicare-eligible residents of the State covered under the application.

"(g) EVALUATION.—The Secretary shall evaluate on an ongoing basis the compliance of a State with the requirements of this section.

"(h) DEFINITIONS.—In this section the terms 'applicable health plan', 'fee-for-service plan', 'health care budget', 'health plan', 'medicare-eligible individual', 'participating State', 'single-payer State', and 'Statewide single-payer system' have the meanings of those terms in the Health Security Act.".

**SEC. 4002. INDIVIDUAL ELECTION TO REMAIN IN CERTAIN HEALTH PLANS.**

(a) IN GENERAL.—Section 1876 (42 U.S.C. 1395mm) is amended by adding at the end the following new subsection:

"(k)(1) Notwithstanding any other provision of this section, each eligible organization with a risk-sharing contract that is the sponsor of a health plan under subtitle E of title I of the Health Security Act shall provide each individual who meets the requirements of paragraph (2) with the opportunity to elect (by submitting an application at such time and in such manner as specified by the Secretary) to continue enrollment in such plan and to have payments made by the Secretary to the plan on the individual's behalf in accordance with paragraph (3).

"(2) An individual meets the requirements of this paragraph if the individual is—

"(A) enrolled in the health plan of an eligible organization in a month in which the individual is either not entitled to benefits under part A, or is an eligible employee (as defined in the Health Security Act) or the spouse of an eligible employee,

"(B) entitled to benefits under part A and enrolled under part B in the succeeding month,

"(C) an eligible individual under the Health Security Act in that succeeding month, and

"(D) not an eligible employee (as defined in the Health Security Act) or the spouse of an eligible employee in that succeeding month.

"(3) The Secretary shall make a payment to an eligible organization on behalf of each individual enrolled with the organization for whom an election is in effect under this subsection in an amount determined by the rate specified by subsection (a)(1)(C). Such payment shall be made from the Federal Hospital Insurance Trust Fund and the Federal Supplementary Medical Insurance Trust Fund as provided under subsection (a)(5) (other than as provided under subparagraph (B) of that paragraph).

"(4) The period for which payment may be made under paragraph (3)—

"(A) begins with the first month for which the individual meets the requirements of paragraph (2) (or a later month, in the case of a late application, as may be specified by the Secretary); and

"(B) ends with the earliest of—

"(i) the month following the month—

"(I) in which the individual notifies the Secretary that the individual no longer wishes to be enrolled in the health plan of the eligible organization and to have payment made on the individual's behalf under this subsection; and

"(II) which is a month specified by the Secretary as a uniform open enrollment period under subsection (c)(3)(A)(i), or

"(ii) the month in which the individual ceases to meet the requirements of paragraph (2).

"(5) Notwithstanding any other provision of this title, payments to a health plan under this subsection on behalf of an individual shall be the sole payments made with respect to items and services furnished to the individual during the period for which the indivdual's election under this subsection is in effect.".

(b) CONFORMING AMENDMENT.—Section 1838(b) (42 U.S.C. 1395q(b)) is amended by inserting after "section 1843(e)" the following: ", 1876(c)(3)(B), 1876(k)(4)(B), or 1890(j)(1)(B)(iv)".

## SEC. 4003. TREATMENT OF CERTAIN MEDICARE BENEFICIARIES.

Title XVIII, as amended by section 4001, is further amended by adding at the end the following new section:

"TREATMENT OF CERTAIN MEDICARE-ELIGIBLE INDIVIDUALS UNDER HEALTH SECURITY ACT

"SEC. 1894. (a) NO MEDICARE COVERAGE FOR CERTAIN MEDICARE-ELIGIBLE INDIVIDUALS.—Notwithstanding any other provision of this title or title II, an individual is not entitled to receive payment or have payment made on the individual's behalf under this title for items and services furnished during a year if the individual is not treated as a medicare-eligible individual under the Health Security Act during the year through the application of section 1012(a) of such Act.

"(b) TRANSFERS TO REGIONAL ALLIANCES.—The Secretary shall provide for a transfer from the Federal Hospital Insurance Trust Fund and the Federal Supplementary Medical Insurance Trust Fund, in appropriate proportions, to each regional alliance in each year of the amount of the reductions in liability owed to the alliance in the year resulting from the application of section 6115 of the Health Security Act.".

## SEC. 4004. PROHIBITING EMPLOYERS FROM TAKING INTO ACCOUNT STATUS AS MEDICARE BENEFICIARY ON ANY GROUNDS.

(a) EXTENSION OF PROTECTIONS FOR WORKING AGED TO GROUP HEALTH PLANS OF ALL EMPLOYERS.—Section 1862(b)(1)(A) (42 U.S.C. 1395y(b)(1)(A)) is amended by striking clauses (ii) and (iii).

(b) EXTENSION OF PROTECTIONS FOR DISABLED ACTIVE INDIVIDUALS TO ALL GROUP HEALTH PLANS.—

(1) IN GENERAL.—Section 1862(b)(1)(B) (42 U.S.C. 1395y(b)(1)(B)), as amended by section 13561(e) of OBRA–1993, is amended—

    (A) in clause (i)—

        (i) by striking "large group health plan (as defined in clause (iv)(II))" and inserting "group health plan (as defined in subparagraph (A)(v))", and

        (ii) by striking "clause (iv)(I)" and inserting "clause (iv)"; and

    (B) by striking clause (iv).

(2) CONFORMING AMENDMENT.—Section 1862(b)(1)(A)(v) (42 U.S.C. 1395y(b)(1)(A)(v)) is amended by striking "this subparagraph, and subparagraph (C)" and inserting "this paragraph".

(c) REPEAL OF LIMITATION ON PERIOD OF PROTECTION FOR INDIVIDUALS WITH END STAGE RENAL DISEASE.—

(1) IN GENERAL.—Section 1862(b)(1)(C) (42 U.S.C. 1395y(b)(1)(C)), as amended by section 13561(c) of OBRA–1993, is amended—

    (A) in clause (i), by striking "during the 12-month period" and all that follows through "such benefits";

    (B) in clause (ii), by striking the semicolon at the end and inserting a period; and

    (C) by striking the matter following clause (ii).

(2) CONFORMING AMENDMENT.—Section 1862(b)(1) is amended—

    (A) in subparagraph (A), by striking clause (iv); and

    (B) in subparagraph (B), by striking clause (ii).

(d) EFFECTIVE DATE.—The amendments made by this section shall apply with respect to medicare-eligible individuals residing in a participating State as of January 1 of the first year for which the State is a participating State.

# PART 2—ENCOURAGING MANAGED CARE UNDER MEDICARE PROGRAM; COORDINATION WITH MEDIGAP PLANS

### SEC. 4011. ENROLLMENT AND TERMINATION OF ENROLLMENT.

(a) UNIFORM OPEN ENROLLMENT PERIODS.—

(1) FOR CAPITATED PLANS.—The first sentence of section 1876(c)(3)(A)(i) (42 U.S.C. 1395mm(c)(3)(A)(i)) is amended by inserting "(which may be specified by the Secretary)" after "open enrollment period".

(2) FOR MEDIGAP PLANS.—Section 1882(s) (42 U.S.C. 1395ss(s)) is amended—

(A) in paragraph (3), by striking "paragraphs (1) and (2)" and inserting "paragraph (1), (2), or (3)",

(B) by redesignating paragraph (3) as paragraph (4), and

(C) by inserting after paragraph (2) the following new paragraph:

"(3) Each issuer of a medicare supplemental policy shall have an open enrollment period (which may be specified by the Secretary), of at least 30 days duration every year, during which the issuer may not deny or condition the issuance or effectiveness of a medicare supplemental policy, or discriminate in the pricing of the policy, because of age, health status, claims experience, receipt of health care, or medical condition. The policy may not provide any time period applicable to pre-existing conditions, waiting periods, elimination periods, and probationary periods (except as provided by paragraph (2)(B)). The Secretary may require enrollment through a third party.".

(b) ENROLLMENTS FOR NEW MEDICARE BENEFICIARIES AND THOSE WHO MOVE.—Section 1876(c)(3)(A) (42 U.S.C. 1395mm(c)(3)(A)) is amended—

(1) in clause (i), by striking "clause (ii)" and inserting "clauses (ii) through (iv)", and

(2) by adding at the end the following:

"(iii) Each eligible organization shall have an open enrollment period for each individual eligible to enroll under subsection (d) during any enrollment period specified by section 1837 that applies to that individual. Enrollment under this clause shall be effective as specified by section 1838.

"(iv) Each eligible organization shall have an open enrollment period for each individual eligible to enroll under subsection (d) who has previously resided outside the geographic area which the organization serves. The enrollment period shall begin with the beginning of the month that precedes the month in which the individual becomes a resident of that geographic area and shall end at the end of the following month. Enrollment under this clause shall be effective as of the first of the month following the month in which the individual enrolls.''.

(c) ENROLLMENT THROUGH THIRD PARTY; UNIFORM TERMINATION OF ENROLLMENT.—The first sentence of section 1876(c)(3)(B) (42 U.S.C. 1395mm(c)(3)(B)) is amended—

    (1) by inserting ''(including enrollment through a third party)'' after ''regulations'', and

    (2) by striking everything after ''with the eligible organization'' and inserting ''during an annual period as prescribed by the Secretary, and as specified by the Secretary in the case of financial insolvency of the organization, if the individual moves from the geographic area served by the organization, or in other special circumstances that the Secretary may prescribe.''.

(d) EFFECTIVE DATE.—The amendments made by the previous subsections apply to enrollments and terminations of enrollments occurring after 1995 (but only after the Secretary of Health and Human Services has prescribed the relevant annual period), except that the amendments made by subsection (a)(2) apply to enrollments for a medicare supplemental policy made after 1995.

SEC. 4012. UNIFORM INFORMATIONAL MATERIALS.

(a) FOR CAPITATION PLANS.—Section 1876(c)(3)(C) (42 U.S.C. 1395mm(c)(3)(C)) is amended by adding at the end the following: "In addition, the Secretary shall develop and distribute comparative materials about all eligible organizations. Each eligible organization shall reimburse the Secretary for its pro rata share (as determined by the Secretary) of the costs incurred by the Secretary in carrying out the requirements of the preceding sentence and other enrollment activities.".

(b) FOR MEDIGAP PLANS.—Paragraph (1) of section 1882(f) (42 U.S.C. 1395ss(f)) is amended to read as follows:

"(f)(1) The Secretary shall develop and distribute comparative materials about all medicare supplemental policies issued in a State. Each issuer of such a policy shall reimburse the Secretary for its pro rata share (as determined by the Secretary) of the costs incurred by the Secretary in carrying out the requirements of the preceding sentence and other enrollment activities, or the issuer shall no longer be considered as meeting the requirements of this section.".

(c) EFFECTIVE DATE.—The amendments made by this section shall apply with respect to materials for enrollment in years after 1995.

**SEC. 4013. OUTLIER PAYMENTS.**

(a) GENERAL RULE.—Section 1876(a)(1) (42 U.S.C. 1395mm(a)(1)) is amended by adding at the end the following:

"(G)(i) In the case of an eligible organization with a risk-sharing contract, the Secretary may make additional payments to the organization equal to not more than 50 percent of the imputed reasonable cost (or, if so requested by the organization, the reasonable cost) above the threshold amount of services covered under parts A and B and provided (or paid for) in a year by the organization to any individual enrolled with the organization under this section.

"(ii) For purposes of clause (i), the 'imputed reasonable cost' is an amount determined by the Secretary on a national, regional, or other basis that is related to the reasonable cost of services.

"(iii) For purposes of clause (i), the 'threshold amount' is an amount determined by the Secretary from time to time, adjusted by the geographic factor utilized in determining payments to the organization under subparagraph (C) and rounded to the nearest multiple of

$100, such that the total amount to be paid under this subparagraph for a year is estimated to be 5 percent or less of the total amount to be paid under risk-sharing contracts for services furnished for that year.

"(iv) An eligible organization shall submit a claim for additional payments under subsection (i) within such time as the Secretary may specify.".

(b) CONFORMING AMENDMENT.—Section 1876(a)(1)(C) (42 U.S.C. 1395mm(a)(1)(C)), as amended by section 4122(a), is further amended by inserting ", and reduced (by a uniform percentage) determined by the Secretary so that the total reduction is estimated to equal the amount to be paid under subparagraph (G) for a particular year" before the period.

(c) EFFECTIVE DATE.—The amendments made by the preceding subsections apply to services furnished after 1994.

SEC. 4014. POINT OF SERVICE OPTION.

(a) POINT OF SERVICE CONTRACTS.—Part C of title XVIII is amended by inserting after section 1889 the following:

"POINT OF SERVICE OPTION

"SEC. 1890. (a) ESTABLISHMENT OF PROGRAM.—Not later than July 1, 1995, the Secretary shall promulgate regulations establishing a point-of-service program under which individuals entitled to benefits under this title may enroll in a point-of-service network that meets such criteria as the Secretary may establish and may obtain such benefits through providers and suppliers who are members of the network.

"(b) CRITERIA FOR NETWORKS.—In establishing criteria for point-of-service networks under the program under this section, the Secretary shall—

"(1) designate appropriate geographic service areas for such networks to ensure that each network has a sufficient number of participating members to provide items and services under this title to beneficiaries;

"(2) establish qualifications relating to the business structure and ownership of networks;

"(3) establish requirements for participating members;

"(4) establish a schedule of payments for services furnished by networks, including a schedule of bundled payment arrangements for selected medical and surgical procedures;

"(5) delineate permissible incentive arrangements to encourage physicians and other suppliers to join the network;

"(6) specify the rules under which carriers under section 1842 may administer the program;

"(7) identify certain illnesses and conditions for which the use of case management by the network will result in savings;

"(8) standards for the processing and payment of claims for payment for services furnished by the network, including standards for the apportionment of payments among the Trust Funds established under this title; and

"(9) such other criteria as the Secretary considers appropriate.".

(b) CONFORMING AMENDMENTS.—

(1) Section 1812(a) (42 U.S.C. 1395d(a)) is amended—

    (A) by striking "and" at the end of paragraph (3),

    (B) by substituting "; and" for the period at the end of paragraph (4), and

    (C) by adding at the end the following:

"(5) such additional items and services furnished by a provider of services to an individual subject to case management as may be specified under a point-of-service network arrangement under section 1890.".

(2)(A) Section 1814(b) (42 U.S.C. 1395f(b)) is amended—

(i) in paragraph (1), by inserting "or (4)" after "paragraph (3)",

(ii) by striking "or" at the end of paragraph (2),

(iii) by substituting "; and" for the period at the end of paragraph (3), and

(iv) by inserting after paragraph (3) the following:

"(4) in the case of items and services furnished through a point of service network (as described in section 1890), the payment basis specified under the arrangement established for such network, plus any bonus payments as determined under subsection (i) of that section.".

(B) The matter in section 1886(d)(1)(A) (42 U.S.C. 1395ww(d)(1)(A)) preceding clause (i) is amended by inserting "(other than paragraph (4))" after "1814(b)".

(3) Section 1832(a)(2) (42 U.S.C. 1395k(a)(2)) is amended—

(A) by striking "and" at the end of subparagraph (I),

(B) by substituting "; and" for the period at the end of subparagraph (J), and

(C) by adding at the end the following:

"(K) such additional items and services (other than inpatient services furnished by providers of services) as may be specified in an arrangement for a point-of-service network under section 1890.".

(4) Section 1833 (42 U.S.C. 1395l), as amended by section 4032, is amended by adding at the end the following new subsection:

"(u) In the case of items and services furnished through a point of service network (as described in section 1890), there shall be paid (subject to subsection (b)) amounts equal to 80 percent of the payment basis specified in an agreement entered into pursuant to that section, plus any bonus payments as determined under subsection (i) of that section.".

(5) Section 1862(a)(1)(B) (42 U.S.C. 1395y(a)(1)(B)) is amended by inserting "or section 1890(h)" after "section 1861(s)(10)".

(6) Section 1862(a) (42 U.S.C. 1395y(a)), as amended by sections 4034(b)(4), 4118(b), and 2001(c), is further amended—

(A) in paragraph (7), by striking "or under paragraph (1)(F)" and inserting ", under paragraph (1)(F), or under a contract under section 1890",

(B) by striking "or" at the end of paragraph (16),

(C) by striking the period at the end of paragraph (17) and inserting "; or", and

(D) by inserting after paragraph (17) the following new paragraph:

"(18) which are furnished to an individual and related to a health condition with respect to which he is subject to case management through a point-of-service network under section 1890 but which are not included in the plan of care developed for such individual and agreed to by him and the case manager.".

(c) EFFECTIVE DATE.—The amendments made by this subsection shall take effect January 1, 1996.

## PART 3—MEDICARE COVERAGE OF OUTPATIENT PRESCRIPTION DRUGS

### SEC. 4021. REFERENCE TO COVERAGE OF OUTPATIENT PRESCRIPTION DRUGS.

For provisions adding a new outpatient prescription drug benefit to the medicare program, see subtitle A of title II.

## SEC. 4022. COVERAGE OF SERVICES OF ADVANCED PRACTICE NURSES.

(a) COVERAGE.—Section 1861(s)(2)(K) (42 U.S.C. 1395x(s)(2)(K)) is amended—

(1) by striking "and" at the end of clause (iii);

(2) in clause (iv), by striking "(i) or (ii)" and inserting "(i), (ii), or (iv)";

(3) by redesignating clause (iv) as clause (v); and

(4) by inserting after clause (iii) the following new clause:

"(iv) services which would be physicians' services if furnished by a physician (as defined in subsection (r)(1)) and which are performed by an advanced practice nurse (as defined in subsection (aa)(5)) working in collaboration (as defined in subsection (aa)(6)) with such a physician which the advanced practice nurse is legally authorized to perform by the State in which the services are performed, and".

(b) APPLICATION OF PAYMENT RULES AND METHODOLOGY USED FOR SERVICES OF NURSE PRACTITIONERS AND CLINICAL NURSE SPECIALISTS IN RURAL AREAS.—

(1) DIRECT PAYMENT.—Section 1832(a)(2)(B)(iii) (42 U.S.C. 1395k(a)(2)(B)(iii)) is amended by striking

"1861(s)(2)(K)(i)," and inserting "1861(s)(2)(K)(i) or section 1861(s)(2)(K)(iv),".

(2) AMOUNT OF PAYMENT.—Section 1833(a)(1)(O) (42 U.S.C. 1395l(a)(1)(M)), as amended by section 13544(b)(2)(B) of OBRA–1993, is amended by striking "rural area)," and inserting "rural area) or section 1861(s)(2)(K)(iv) (relating to services of advanced practice nurses),".

(3) MANDATORY ASSIGNMENT.—The section 1833(r) added by section 4155(b)(3) of OBRA–1990 is amended—

    (1) in paragraph (1)—

        (A) by striking "rural area)," and inserting "rural area) or section 1861(s)(2)(K)(iv) (relating to services of advanced practice nurses),", and

        (B) by striking "nurse practitioner or clinical nurse specialist" each place it appears and inserting "nurse practitioner, clinical nurse specialist, or advanced practice nurse"; and

    (2) by inserting "or section 1861(s)(2)(K)(iv)" after "section 1861(s)(2)(K)(iii)" each place it appears.

(c) SERVICES DEFINED.—Section 1861(aa)(5) (42 U.S.C. 1395x(aa)(5)) is amended—

(1) by striking "and the term 'clinical nurse specialist'" and inserting ", the term 'clinical nurse specialist', and the term 'advanced practice nurse'"; and

(2) by striking "or clinical nurse specialist" and inserting "clinical nurse specialist, or advanced practice nurse".

(d) EFFECTIVE DATE.—The amendments made by this section shall apply to services furnished on or after January 1, 1995.

## PART 4—COORDINATION WITH ADMINISTRATIVE SIMPLIFICATION AND QUALITY MANAGEMENT INITIATIVES

### SEC. 4031. REPEAL OF SEPARATE MEDICARE PEER REVIEW PROGRAM.

Part B of title XI of the Social Security Act (42 U.S.C. 1301 et seq.) is amended by adding at the end the following new section:

"TERMINATION

"SEC. 1165. The provisions of this part shall terminate effective upon the adoption of the National Quality Management Program under subtitle A of title V of the Health Security Act. Any reference to this part or any section in this part shall not be effective after such date.".

## SEC. 4032. MANDATORY ASSIGNMENT FOR ALL PART B SERVICES.

Section 1833 (42 U.S.C. 1395l) is amended—

(1) by redesignating the subsection (r) added by section 4206(b)(2) of OBRA–1990 as subsection (s); and

(2) by adding at the end the following new subsection:

"(t)(1) Notwithstanding any other provision of this part, payment under this part for any item or service furnished on or after January 1, 1996, may only be made on an assignment-related basis.

"(2) Except for deductible, coinsurance, or copayment amounts applicable under this part, no physician, supplier, or other person may bill or collect any amount from an individual enrolled under this part a bill for an item or service for which payment may be made under this part. No such individual is liable for payment of any amounts billed in violation of the previous sentence.

"(3) If a physician, supplier, or other person knowingly and willfully bills or collects an amount in violation of paragraph (2), the Secretary may apply sanctions against such physician, supplier, or other person in accordance with section 1842(j)(2). Paragraph (4) of section 1842(j) shall apply in this paragraph in the same manner as such paragraph applies to such section.".

## SEC. 4033. ELIMINATION OF COMPLEXITIES CAUSED BY DUAL FUNDING SOURCES AND RULES FOR PAYMENT OF CLAIMS.

(a) IN GENERAL.—The Secretary of Health and Human Services shall take such steps as may be necessary to consolidate the administration (including processing systems) of parts A and B of the medicare program (under title XVIII of the Social Security Act).

(b) COMBINATION OF INTERMEDIARY AND CARRIER FUNCTIONS.—In taking such steps, the Secretary shall contract with a single entity that combines the fiscal intermediary and carrier functions in each area except where the Secretary finds that special regional or national contracts are appropriate.

(c) SUPERSEDING CONFLICTING REQUIREMENTS.—The provisions of sections 1816 and 1842 of the Social Security Act (including provider nominating provisions in such section 1816) are superseded to the extent required to carry out this section.

## SEC. 4034. REPEAL OF PRO PRECERTIFICATION REQUIREMENT FOR CERTAIN SURGICAL PROCEDURES.

(a) IN GENERAL.—Section 1164 (42 U.S.C. 1320c–13) is repealed.

(b) CONFORMING AMENDMENTS.—

(1) Section 1154 (42 U.S.C. 1320c–3) is amended—

 (A) in subsection (a), by striking paragraph (12), and

 (B) in subsection (d), by striking "(and except as provided in section 1164)".

(2) Section 1833 (42 U.S.C. 1395l) is amended—

 (A) in subsection (a)(1)(D)(i), by striking ", or for tests furnished in connection with obtaining a second opinion required under section 1164(c)(2) (or a third opinion, if the second opinion was in disagreement with the first opinion)";

 (B) in subsection (a)(1), by striking clause (G);

 (C) in subsection (a)(2)(A), by striking ", to items and services (other than clinical diagnostic laboratory tests) furnished in connection with obtaining a second opinion required under section 1164(c)(2) (or a third opinion, if the second opinion was in disagreement with the first opinion),";

 (D) in subsection (a)(2)(D)(i)—

                    (i) by striking "basis," and inserting
                "basis or", and
                    (ii) by striking ", or for tests fur-
                nished in connection with obtaining a sec-
                ond opinion required under section
                1164(c)(2) (or a third opinion, if the sec-
                ond opinion was in disagreement with the
                first opinion)";
            (E) in subsection (a)(3), by striking "and
        for items and services furnished in connection
        with obtaining a second opinion required under
        section 1164(c)(2), or a third opinion, if the
        second opinion was in disagreement with the
        first opinion)"; and
            (F) in the first sentence of subsection (b),
        by striking "(4)" and all that follows through
        "and (5)" and inserting and "(4)".
    (3) Section 1834(g)(1)(B) (42 U.S.C. 1395m(g)(1)(B)) is amended by striking "and for items and services furnished in connection with obtaining a second opinion required under section 1164(c)(2), or a third opinion, if the second opinion was in disagreement with the first opinion)".
    (4) Section 1862(a) (42 U.S.C. 1395y(a)) is amended—

(A) by adding "or" at the end of paragraph (14),

(B) by striking "; or" at the end of paragraph (15) and inserting a period, and

(C) by striking paragraph (16).

(5) The third sentence of section 1866(a)(2)(A) (42 U.S.C. 1395w(a)(2)(A)) is amended by striking ", with respect to items and services furnished in connection with obtaining a second opinion required under section 1164(c)(2) (or a third opinion, if the second opinion was in disagreement with the first opinion),".

(c) EFFECTIVE DATE.—The amendments made by this section shall apply to services provided on or after the date of the enactment of this Act.

## SEC. 4035. REQUIREMENTS FOR CHANGES IN BILLING PROCEDURES.

(a) LIMITATION ON FREQUENCY OF SYSTEM CHANGES.—The Secretary of Health and Human Services may not implement any change in the system used for the billing and processing of claims for payment for items and services furnished under title XVIII of the Social Security Act within 6 months of implementing any previous change in such system.

(b) ADVANCE NOTIFICATION TO PROVIDERS AS REQUIREMENT FOR CARRIERS AND FISCAL INTERMEDIARIES.—

(1) FISCAL INTERMEDIARIES.—Section 1816(c) (42 U.S.C. 1395h(c)) is amended by adding at the end the following new paragraph:

"(4) Each agreement with an agency or organization under this section shall provide that the agency or organization shall notify providers of services of any major change in the procedures for billing for services furnished under this part at least 120 days before such change is to take effect.".

(2) CARRIERS.—Section 1842(b)(3) (42 U.S.C. 1395u(b)(3)) is amended—

 (A) by striking "and" at the end of subparagraph (G) and the end of subparagraph (H); and

 (B) by inserting after subparagraph (H) the following new subparagraph:

"(I) will notify individuals and entities furnishing items and services for which payment may be made under this part of any major change in the procedures for billing for such items and services at least 120 days before such change is to take effect; and".

(3) EFFECTIVE DATE.—The amendments made by paragraphs (1) and (2) shall apply to agreements with fiscal intermediaries under section 1816 of the Social Security Act and to contracts with carriers under section 1842 of such Act for years beginning after the expiration of the 9-month period beginning on the date of the enactment of this Act.

## PART 5—AMENDMENTS TO ANTI-FRAUD AND ABUSE PROVISIONS

SEC. 4041. ANTI-KICKBACK PROVISIONS.

(a) REVISION TO PENALTIES.—

(1) PERMITTING SECRETARY TO IMPOSE CIVIL MONETARY PENALTY.—Section 1128A(a) (42 U.S.C. 1320a–7a(a)) is amended—

(A) by striking "or" at the end of paragraphs (1) and (2);

(B) by striking the semicolon at the end of paragraph (3) and inserting "; or"; and

(C) by inserting after paragraph (3) the following new paragraph:

"(4) carries out any activity in violation of paragraph (1) or (2) of section 1128B(b);".

(2) DESCRIPTION OF CIVIL MONETARY PENALTY APPLICABLE.—Section 1128A(a) (42 U.S.C. 1320a–7a(a)) is amended—

(A) by striking "given)." at the end of the first sentence and inserting the following: "given or, in cases under paragraph (4), $50,000 for each such violation).": and

(B) by striking "claim." at the end of the second sentence and inserting the following: "claim (or, in cases under paragraph (4), an assessment of not more than three times the total amount of remuneration offered, paid, solicited, or received, without regard to whether a portion of such remuneration was offered, paid solicited, or received for a lawful purpose).".

(3) INCREASE IN CRIMINAL PENALTY.—Paragraphs (1) and (2) of section 1128B(b) (42 U.S.C. 1320a–7b(b)) are each amended—

(A) by striking "$25,000" and inserting "$50,000"; and

(B) by striking the period at the end and inserting the following: ", and shall be subject to an assessment of not more than three times the total remuneration offered, paid, solicited, or received, without regard to whether a portion of such remuneration was offered, paid solicited, or received for a lawful purpose.".

(4) CIVIL REMEDY.—Section 1128B(b) (42 U.S.C. 1320a–7b(b)) is amended by adding at the end the following new paragraph:

"(4) Any person who carries out any activity in violation of paragraph (1) or (2) shall be subject to a penalty of not more than $50,000 fo reach such violation, and shall be subject to an assessment of not more than three times the total remuneration offered, paid, solicited, or received, without regard to whether a portion of such remuneration was offered, paid solicited, or received for a lawful purpose.".

(b) REVISIONS TO EXCEPTIONS.—

(1) EXCEPTION FOR DISCOUNTS.—Section 1128B(b)(3)(A) (42 U.S.C. 1320a-7b(b)(3)(A)) is amended by striking "program;" and inserting "program and is not—

"(i) for the furnishing of one item or service without charge or at a reduced charge in exchange for any agreement to buy a different item or service;

"(ii) applicable to one payor but not to providers of services or other entities under title XVIII or a State health care program; or

"(iii) in the form of a cash payment;".

(2) EXCEPTION FOR PAYMENTS TO EMPLOY-EES.—Section 1128B(b)(3)(B) (42 U.S.C. 1320a-7b(b)(3)(B)) is amended by inserting at the end "if the amount of remuneration under the arrangement is consistent with the fair market value of the services and is not determined in a manner that takes into account (directly or indirectly) the volume or value of any referrals, except that such employees can be paid remuneration in the form of a productivity bonus based on services personally performed by the employee.

(3) EXCEPTION FOR WAIVER OF COINSURANCE BY CERTAIN PROVIDERS.—Section 1128B(b)(3)(D) (42 U.S.C. 1320a-7b(b)(3)(D)) is amended to read as follows:

"(D) a waiver or reduction of any coinsurance or other copayment—

"(i) if the waiver or reduction is made pursuant to a public schedule of discounts which the person is obligated as a matter of law to apply to certain individuals, or

"(ii) under part B of title XVIII by any person if the person does not routinely waive coinsurance or deductible amounts and the person—

"(I) waives the coinsurance and deductible amounts after determining in good faith that the individual is indigent;

"(II) fails to collect coinsurance or deductible amounts after making reasonable collection efforts; or

"(III) provides for any permissible waiver as specified in section 1128B(b)(3) or in regulations issued by the Secretary.".

(4) NEW EXCEPTION FOR CERTAIN PROVIDERS.—Section 1128B(b)(3) (42 U.S.C. 1320a–7b(b)(3)) is amended—

(A) by striking "and" at the end of subparagraph (D);

(B) by striking the period at the end of subparagraph (E) and inserting "; and"; and

(C) by adding at the end the following new subparagraph:

"(F) any remuneration obtained by or given to an individual or entity who is obligated as a matter of law to waive or reduce coinsurance or other copayment for certain individuals pursuant to a public schedule of discounts, if the remuneration is pursuant to a written arrangement for the use or procurement of space, equipment, goods or services or for the referral of patients if—

"(i) the arrangement does not result in private inurement to any current employee, officer, member of the Board of Directors, or agent of the recipient or any other person involved in recommending or negotiating the arrangement; and

"(ii) the arrangement does not preclude the referral of patients to other providers of service of the patient's own choosing and does not interfere with the ability of health professionals to refer patients to providers of services they believe are the most appropriate, except to the extent such choices or referrals are limited by the terms of a health plan in which the patient has enrolled or the terms of the Federal grant or cooperative agreement.".

(5) NEW EXCEPTION FOR CAPITATED PAYMENTS.—Section 1128B(b)(3) (42 U.S.C. 1320a-7b(b)(3)), as amended by paragraph (4), is further amended—

(A) by striking "and" at the end of subparagraph (E);

(B) by striking the period at the end of subparagraph (F) and inserting "; and"; and

(C) by adding at the end the following new subparagraph—

"(G) any reduction in cost sharing or increased benefits given to an individual, any amounts paid to a provider of services for items or services furnished to an individual, or any discount or reduction in price given by the provider for such items or services, if the individual is enrolled with and such items and services are covered under any of the following:

"(i) A health plan which is furnishing items or services under title XVIII or a State health care program to individuals on an at-risk, prepaid, capitated basis pursuant to a written agreement with the Secretary or a State health care program.

"(ii) An organization receiving payments on a prepaid basis, under a demonstration project under section 402(a) of the Social Security Amendments of 1967 or under section 222(a) of the Social Security Amendments of 1972.

"(iii) Any other plan or insurer under which a participating provider is paid wholly on an at-risk, prepaid, capitated basis for such items or services pursuant to a written arrangement between the plan and the provider.''.

(c) CLARIFICATION OF COVERAGE OF EMPLOYERS AND EMPLOYEES.—Section 1128B(b) (42 U.S.C. 1320a–7b(b)), as amended by subsection (a)(4), is further amended by adding at the end the following new paragraph:

"(5) In this subsection, the term 'referral' includes the referral by an employee to his or her employer of any item or service for which payment may be made in whole or in part under title XVIII or a State health care program."

(d) AUTHORIZATION FOR THE SECRETARY TO ISSUE REGULATIONS.—Section 1128B(b) (42 U.S.C. 1320a–7b(b)), as amended by subsections (a)(4) and (c), is further amended by adding at the end the following new paragraph—

"(6) The Secretary is authorized to impose by regulation such other requirements as needed to protect against program or patient abuse with respect to any of the exceptions described in paragraph (3).''.

(e) CLARIFICATION OF OTHER ELEMENTS OF OFFENSE.—Section 1128B(b) (42 U.S.C. 1320a–7b(b)) is amended—

(1) in paragraph (1) in the matter preceding subparagraph (A), by striking "kind—" and inserting "kind with intent to be influenced—";

(2) in paragraph (1)(A), by striking "in return for referring" and inserting "to refer";

(3) in paragraph (1)(B), by striking "in return for purchasing, leasing, ordering, or arranging for or recommending" and inserting "to purchase, lease, order, or arrange for or recommend"; and

(4) in paragraph (2) in the matter preceding subparagraph (A), by striking "to induce such person" and inserting "with intent to influence such person".

**SEC. 4042. REVISIONS TO LIMITATIONS ON PHYSICIAN SELF-REFERRAL.**

(a) CLARIFICATION OF PAYMENT BAN.—Section 1877(a)(1)(B) (42 U.S.C. 1395nn(a)(1)(B)) is amended to read as follows:

"(B) no physician or entity may present or cause to be presented a claim under this title or bill to any third party payor or other entity for designated health services furnished pursuant to a referral prohibited under subparagraph (A).".

(b) CLARIFICATION OF COVERAGE OF HOLDING COMPANY TYPE ARRANGEMENTS AND LOANS.—The last sentence of section 1877(a)(2) (42 U.S.C. 1395nn(a)(2)) is amended by striking "an interest in an entity that holds an ownership or investment interest in any entity providing the designated health service" and inserting the following: "a loan from the entity, and an interest held indirectly through means such as (but not limited to) having a family member hold such investment interest or holding a legal or beneficial interest in another entity (such as a trust or holding company) that holds such investment interest".

(c) REVISIONS TO GENERAL EXCEPTIONS TO BOTH OWNERSHIP AND COMPENSATION ARRANGEMENT PROHIBITIONS.—

    (1) REPEAL OF EXCEPTION FOR PHYSICIANS' SERVICES.—Section 1877(b) (42 U.S.C. 1395nn(b)) is amended—

        (A) by striking paragraph (1); and

        (B) by redesignating paragraphs (2) and (3) as paragraphs paragraphs (1) and (2).

    (2) REVISION TO IN-OFFICE ANCILLARY SERVICES EXCEPTION.—Section 1877(b)(1) (42 U.S.C. 1395nn(b)(1)), as redesignated by paragraph (1), is amended—

        (A) in the matter preceding subparagraph (A), by striking "services (other than durable medical equipment (excluding infusion pumps) and parenteral and enteral nutrients, equipment, and supplies)" and inserting "clinical laboratory services, x-ray and ultrasound services that are provided at low-cost (as determined in accordance with regulations of the Secretary)"; and

 (B) in subparagraph (A)—

  (i) in clause (ii)(I), by striking "(or another physician who is a member of the same group practice)",

  (ii) in clause (ii)(II) by inserting "the same or" before "another building", and

  (iii) in clause (ii)(II)(bb), by inserting "all of" after "centralized provision of".

(3) REVISION TO PREPAID PLAN EXCEPTION.—Section 1877(b)(2), (42 U.S.C. 1395nn(b)(2)), as redesignated by paragraph (1), is amended to read as follows:

 "(2) PREPAID PLANS.—In the case of services furnished by an organization—

  "(A) with a risk sharing contract under section 1876(g) to an individual enrolled with the organization,

"(B) receiving payments on a prepaid basis, under a demonstration project under section 402(a) of the Social Security Amendments of 1967 or under section 222(a) of the Social Security Amendments of 1972, to an individual enrolled with the organization, or

"(C) that is a qualified health maintenance organization (within the meaning of section 1310(d) of the Public Health Service Act) to an individual enrolled with the organization.".

(4) NEW EXCEPTION FOR CAPITATED PAYMENTS.—Section 1877(b) (42 U.S.C. 1395nn(b)), as amended by paragraph (1), is amended by inserting after paragraph (2) the following new paragraph:

"(3) CAPITATED PAYMENTS.—In the case of a designated health service, if the designated health service is included in the services for which a physician or physician group is paid wholly on an at-risk, prepaid, capitated basis by a health plan or insurer pursuant to a written arrangement between the plan or insurer and the physician or physician group.".

(d) REVISION TO PUBLICLY TRADED SECURITIES EXCEPTION.—Section 1877(c)(1) (42 U.S.C. 1395nn(c)(1)) is amended by inserting "at the time acquired by the physician" after "which may be purchased on terms generally available to the public".

(e) REVISION TO RURAL PROVIDER EXCEPTION.—Section 1877(d)(2) (42 U.S.C. 1395nn(d)(2)) is amended by striking "substantially all" and inserting "not less than 85 percent (as determined in accordance with regulations of the Secretary)".

(f) REVISIONS TO EXCEPTIONS RELATING TO OTHER COMPENSATION ARRANGEMENTS.—

(1) EXCEPTION FOR PERSONAL SERVICES ARRANGEMENTS.—(A) Section 1877(e)(3)(B)(i)(II) (42 U.S.C. 1395nn(e)(3)(B)(i)(II)) is amended to read as follows:

"(II) If the plan places a physician or physician group at substantial financial risk (as determined by the Secretary pursuant to section 1876(i)(8)(A)(ii)), for services not provided by the physician, the entity complies with the provisions of subclauses (I) and (II) of section 1876(i)(8)(A)(ii).";

(B) Section 1877(e)(3)(B)(ii), 42 U.S.C. 1395nn(e)(3)(B)(ii) is amended by striking "may directly or indirectly have the effect of" and inserting "has the purpose of".

(2) REPEAL OF EXCEPTION FOR REMUNERATION UNRELATED TO THE PROVISION OF DESIGNATED HEALTH SERVICES.—Section 1877(e) (42 U.S.C. 1395nn(e)) is amended—

(A) by striking paragraph (4); and

(B) by redesignating paragraphs (5), (6), (7), and (8) as paragraphs (4), (5), (6), and (7).

(3) EXCEPTION FOR CERTAIN PHYSICIAN RECRUITMENT.—Section 1877(e)(4) (42 U.S.C. 1395nn(e)(4)), as redesignated by paragraph (2), is amended to read as follows:

"(4) PHYSICIAN RECRUITMENT.—In the case of remuneration which is provided by an entity located in a rural area (as defined in section 1886(d)(2)(D)) or a health professional shortage areas (designated under section 332 of the Public Health Service Act), or an entity that serves a significant number of individuals who are members of a medically underserved population (designated under section 330 of the Public Health Service Act), in order to induce a physician who has been practicing within the physician's current specialty for less than one year to establish staff privileges at the entity, or to induce any other physician to relocate his or her primary place of practice to the geographic area served by the entity, if the following standards are met:

"(A) The arrangement is set forth in a written agreement that specifies the benefits provided by the entity to the physician, the terms under which the benefits are to be provided, and the obligations of each party.

"(B) If a physician is leaving an established practice, the physical location of the new primary place of practice must be not less than 100 miles from the location of the established primary place of practice and at least 85 percent of the revenues of the physician's new practice must be generated from new patients for whom the physician did not previously provide services at the former practice.

"(C) The benefits are provided by the entity for a period not in excess of 3 years, and the terms of the agreement are not renegotiated during this 3-year period in any substantial aspect, unless the physician's new primary place of practice is designated as a health professional shortage area (pursuant to section 332 of the Public Health Service Act) for the physician's specialty category during the entire duration of the relationship between the physician and the entity.

"(D) There is no requirement that the physician make referrals to, be in a position to make or influence referrals to, or otherwise generate business for the entity as a condition for receiving the benefits.

"(E) The physician is not restricted from establishing staff privileges at, referring any service to, or otherwise generating any business for any other entity of the physician's choosing.

"(F) The amount or value of the benefits provided by the entity may not vary (or be adjusted or renegotiated) in any manner based on the volume or value of any expected referrals to or business otherwise generated for the entity by the physician for which payment may be made in whole or in part under this title or a State health care program (as defined in section 1128(h)).

"(G) The physician agrees to treat patients entitled to benefits under this title or enrolled in a State plan for medical assistance under title XIX.".

(4) EXCEPTION FOR ISOLATED TRANSACTIONS.—Section 1877(e)(5) (42 U.S.C. 1395nn(e)(6)), as redesignated by paragraph (2), is amended—

    (A) by redesignating subparagraph (B) as subparagraph (C);

    (B) by striking "and" at the end of subparagraph (A); and

    (C) by inserting after subparagraph (A) the following new subparagraph:

    "(B) there is no financing of the sale between the parties, and".

(5) EXCEPTION FOR PAYMENTS BY A PHYSICIAN.—Section 1877(e)(7) (42 U.S.C. 1395nn(e)(7)), as redesignated by paragraph (2), is amended to read as follows:

"(7) PAYMENTS BY A PHYSICIAN FOR ITEMS AND SERVICES.—Payments made by a physician to a laboratory in exchange for the provision of clinical laboratory services furnished at a price that is consistent with fair market value.".

(6) ADDITIONAL EXCEPTION FOR DISCOUNTS OR OTHER REDUCTIONS IN PRICE.—Section 1877(e)

(42 U.S.C. 1395nn(e)), as amended by paragraph (2), is amended by adding at the end the following new paragraph:

"(8) DISCOUNTS OR OTHER REDUCTIONS IN PRICE.—Discounts or other reductions in price between a physician and an entity for items or services for which payment may be made under this title so long as the discount or other reduction in price is properly disclosed and appropriately reflected in the costs claimed or charges made by the physician or entity under this title and is not—

"(A) for the furnishing of one item or service without charge or at a reduced charge in exchange for any agreement to buy a different item or service,

"(B) applicable to one or more payers but not to all individuals and entities providing services for which payment may be made under this title, or

"(C) in the form of a cash payment.".

(g) CLARIFICATION OF SANCTION AUTHORITY.—Section 1877(g)(4) (42 U.S.C. 1395nn(g)(4)) is amended by striking "Any physician" and all that follows through "to such entity," and inserting the following: "Any physician or other entity that enters into an arrangement or scheme (such as a cross-referral arrangement or an arrangement with multiple leases overlapping in time for the same or similar rental space or equipment) which the physician or entity knows or should know has a principal purpose of inducing referrals to another entity, which referrals, if made directly by the physician or entity to such other entity,".

(h) CLARIFICATION OF DEFINITION OF REMUNERATION.—Section 1877(h)(1)(B) (42 U.S.C. 1395nn(h)(1)(B)) is amended to read as follows:

"(B) The term 'remuneration' includes any payment, discount or other reduction in price, forgiveness of debt or other benefit made directly or indirectly, overtly or covertly, in cash or in kind.".

(i) REVISION TO DEFINITION OF GROUP PRACTICE.—Section 1877(h)(4) (42 U.S.C. 1395nn(h)(4)) is amended—

(1) in subparagraph (A)(vi), by striking the period at the end and inserting the following: ", including a requirement for the physical grouping of physician practices as may be reasonably required to prevent the abuse of any exceptions provided to group practices under this section."; and

(2) in subparagraph (B)(i), by striking "or services incident to such personally performed services".

(j) REVISION OF DEFINITION OF REFERRAL; REFERRING PHYSICIAN.—

(1) IN GENERAL.—Section 1877(h)(5) (42 U.S.C. 1395nn(h)(5)) is amended by striking subparagraph (C).

(2) CONFORMING AMENDMENTS.—Section 1877(h)(5) (42 U.S.C. 1395nn(h)(5)) is amended—

(A) in subparagraph (A), by striking "Except as provided in subparagraph (C), in" and inserting "In"; and

(B) in subparagraph (B), by striking "Except as provided in subparagraph (C), the" and inserting "The".

(k) EXPANSION TO COVER ADDITIONAL ITEMS AND SERVICES.—Section 1877(h)(6) (42 U.S.C. 1395nn(h)(6)), as amended by section 2006(c)(3), is amended—

(1) in subparagraph (D), by striking "or other"; and

(2) by adding at the end the following new subparagraphs:

"(M) Diagnostic services.

"(N) Any other item or service not rendered by the physician personally or by a person under the physician's direct supervision.".

(l) AUTHORIZATION FOR THE SECRETARY TO ISSUE REGULATIONS.—Section 1877 (42 U.S.C. 1395nn) is amended by adding the following new subsection:

"(i) ADDITIONAL REQUIREMENTS.—The Secretary is authorized to impose by regulation such other requirements as needed to protect against program or patient abuse with respect to any of the exceptions under this section.".

(m) INCORPORATION OF AMENDMENTS MADE UNDER OBRA–1993.—In this section, any reference to section 1877 of the Social Security Act shall be considered a reference to such section as amended by section 13562(a) of OBRA–1993.

## SEC. 4043. CIVIL MONETARY PENALTIES.

(a) PROHIBITION AGAINST OFFERING INDUCEMENTS TO INDIVIDUALS ENROLLED UNDER PLANS.—

(1) OFFER OF REMUNERATION.—Section 1128A(a) (42 U.S.C. 1320a–7a(a)) (as amended by section 4041(a)(1)) is amended—

(A) by striking "; or" at the end of paragraph (3) and inserting a semicolon;

(B) by striking the semicolon at the end of paragraph (4) and inserting "; or"; and

(C) by inserting after paragraph (4) the following new paragraph:

"(5) offers, pays, or transfers remuneration to any individual eligible for benefits under title XVIII of this Act, or under a State health care program (as defined in section 1128(h)) that such person knows or should know is likely to influence such individual to order or receive from a particular provider, practitioner, or supplier any item or service for which payment may be made, in whole or in part, under title XVIII, or a State health care program;".

(2) REMUNERATION DEFINED.—Section 1128A(i) (42 U.S.C. 1320a–7a(i)) is amended by adding at the end the following new paragraph:

"(6) The term 'remuneration' includes the waiver of coinsurance and deductible amounts (or any part thereof), and transfers of items or services for free or for other than fair market value, except that such term does not include the waiver of coinsurance or deductible amounts by a person or entity, if—

"(A) the waiver is not offered as part of any advertisement or solicitation;

"(B) the person does not routinely waive coinsurance or deductible amounts; and

"(C) the person—

"(i) waives the coinsurance and deductible amounts after determining in good faith that the individual is indigent;

"(ii) fails to collect coinsurance or deductible amounts after making reasonable collection efforts; or

"(iii) provides for any permissible waiver as specified in section 1128B(b)(3) or in regulations issued by the Secretary.".

(b) CLAIM FOR ITEM OR SERVICE BASED ON INCORRECT CODING OR MEDICALLY UNNECESSARY SERVICES.—Section 1128A(a)(1) (42 U.S.C. 1320a-7a(a)(1)) is amended—

(1) in subparagraph (A), by striking "claimed," and inserting the following: "claimed, including any person who presents or causes to be presented a claim for an item or service which includes a procedure or diagnosis code that the person knows or should know will result in a greater payment to the person than the code applicable to the item or service actually provided or actual patient medical condition,";

(2) in subparagraph (C), by striking "or" at the end;

(3) in subparagraph (D), by striking "; or" and inserting ", or"; and

(4) by inserting after subparagraph (D) the following new subparagraph:

"(E) is for a medical or other item or service that a person knows or should know is not medically necessary; or".

(c) EXCLUDED INDIVIDUAL RETAINING OWNERSHIP OR CONTROL INTEREST IN PARTICIPATING ENTITY.—Section 1128A(a) of such Act, as amended by section 4041(a)(1) and subsection (a)(1), is further amended—

(1) by striking "or" at the end of paragraph (4);

(2) by striking the semicolon at the end of paragraph (5) and inserting "; or"; and

(3) by inserting after paragraph (5) the following new paragraph:

"(6) in the case of a person who is not an organization, agency, or other entity, who is excluded from participating in a program under title XVIII or a State health care program in accordance with this section, section 1128, or section 1156 and who, during the period of exclusion, retains either a direct or indirect ownership or control interest of 5 percent or more in, or an ownership or control interest (as defined in section 1124(a)(3)) in, or who is an officer, director, agent, or managing employee (as defined in section 1126(b)) of, an entity that is participating in a program under title XVIII or a State health care program;".

(d) ADDITIONAL OFFENSES RELATING TO ALLIANCE SYSTEM.—Section 1128A(a) of such Act, as amended by section 4041(a)(1) and subsections (a)(1) and (c), is further amended—

(1) by striking "or" at the end of paragraph (5);

(2) by striking the semicolon at the end of paragraph (6) and inserting "; or"; and

(3) by inserting after paragraph (6) the following new paragraphs:

"(7) engages in a practice that circumvents a payment methodology intended to reimburse for two or more discreet medical items or services at a single or fixed amount, including but not limited to, multiple admissions or readmission to hospitals and other institutions reimbursed on a diagnosis reimbursement grouping basis;

"(8) engages in a practice which has the effect of limiting or discouraging (as compared to other plan enrollees) the utilization of health care services covered by law or under the service contract by title XIX or other publicly subsidized patients, including but not limited to differential standards for the location and hours of service offered by providers participating in the plan;

"(9) substantially fails to cooperate with a quality assurance program or a utilization review activity;

"(10) fails substantially to provide or authorize medically necessary items and services that are required to be provided to an individual covered under a health plan or public program for the delivery of or payment for health care items or services, if the failure has adversely affected (or had a substantial likelihood of adversely affecting) the individual;

"(11) employs or contracts with any individual or entity who is excluded from participating in a program under title XVIII or a State health care program in accordance with this section, section 1128, or section 1156, for the provision of any services (including but not limited to health care, utilization review, medical social work, or administrative), or employs or contracts with any entity for the direct or indirect provision of such services, through such an excluded individual or entity; or

"(12) submits false or fraudulent statements, data or information or claims to the National Health Board established under part 1 of subtitle F of title I of the Health Security Act, any other federal agency, a state health care agency, a health alliance, or any other Federal, state or local agency charged with implementation or oversight of the plan that the person knows or should know is fraudulent;".

(e) MODIFICATIONS OF AMOUNTS OF PENALTIES AND ASSESSMENTS.—Section 1128A(a) (42 U.S.C. 1320a-7a(a)), as amended by section 4041(a), subsection (a)(1), subsection (c), and subsection (d), is amended in the matter following paragraph (6)—

(1) by striking "$2,000" and inserting "$10,000";

(2) by inserting after "under paragraph (4), $50,000 for each such violation" the following: "; in cases under paragraph (5), $10,000 for each such offer of transfer; in cases under paragraph (6), $10,000 for each day the prohibited relationship occurs; in cases under paragraphs (7) through (12),

an amount not to exceed $50,000 for each such determination by the Secretary''; and

(3) by striking "twice the amount" and inserting "three times the amount".

(f) INTEREST ON PENALTIES.—Section 1128A(f) (42 U.S.C. 1320a-7a(f)) is amended by adding after the first sentence the following: "Interest shall accrue on the penalties and assessments (as defined in subsection (g)) imposed by a final determination of the Secretary in accordance with an annual rate established by the Secretary under the Federal Claims Collection Act. The rate of interest charged shall be the rate in effect on the date the determination becomes final and shall remain fixed at that rate until the entire amount due is paid. In addition, the Secretary is authorized to recover the costs of collection in any case where the penalties and assessments are not paid within 30 days after the determination becomes final, or in the case of a compromised amount, where payments are more than 90 days past due. In lieu of actual costs, the Secretary is authorized to impose a charge of up to 10 percent of the amount of penalties and assessments owed to cover the costs of collection.".

(g) AUTHORIZATION TO ACT.—

(1) IN GENERAL.—The first sentence of section 1128A(c)(1) (42 U.S.C. 1320a-7a(c)(1)) is amended

by striking all that follows "(b)" and inserting the following: "unless, within one year after the date the Secretary presents a case to the Attorney General for consideration, the Attorney General brings an action in a district court of the United States.".

(2) EFFECTIVE DATE.—The amendment made by this paragraph (1) shall apply to cases presented by the Secretary of Health and Human Services for consideration on or after the date of the enactment of this Act.

(h) DEPOSIT OF PENALTIES COLLECTED INTO ALL-PAYER TRUST FUND.—Section 1128A(f)(3) (42 U.S.C. 1320a–7a(f)(3)) is amended by striking "as miscellaneous receipts of the Treasury of the United States" and inserting "in the All-Payer Health Care Fraud and Abuse Control Trust Fund established under section 5402 of the Health Security Act".

(i) CLARIFICATION OF PENALTY IMPOSED ON EXCLUDED PROVIDER FURNISHING SERVICES.—Section 1128A(a)(1)(D) (42 U.S.C. 1320a–7a(a)(1)(D)) is amended by inserting "who furnished the service" after "in which the person was".

SEC. 4044. EXCLUSIONS FROM PROGRAM PARTICIPATION.

(a) MANDATORY EXCLUSION FOR INDIVIDUAL CONVICTED OF CRIMINAL OFFENSE RELATED TO HEALTH

CARE FRAUD.—Section 1128 (42 U.S.C. 1320a-7) is amended—

(1) by amending paragraph (1) of subsection (a) to read as follows:

"(1) CONVICTIONS OF PROGRAM-RELATED CRIMES AND HEALTH CARE FRAUD.—

"(A) Any individual or entity that has been convicted of a criminal offense related to the delivery of an item or service under title XVIII or under any State health care program; or

"(B) Any individual or entity that has been convicted, under Federal or State law, in connection with the delivery of a health care item or service of a criminal offense relating to fraud, theft, embezzlement, breach of fiduciary responsibility, or other financial misconduct.";

and

(2) in subsection (b)(1), by striking "in connection with the delivery of a health care item or service or".

(b) ESTABLISHMENT OF MINIMUM PERIOD OF EXCLUSION FOR CERTAIN INDIVIDUALS AND ENTITIES SUBJECT TO PERMISSIVE EXCLUSION FROM MEDICARE AND STATE HEALTH CARE PROGRAMS.—Section 1128(c)(3)

(42 U.S.C. 1320a–7(c)(3)) is amended by adding at the end the following new subparagraphs:

"(D) In the case of an exclusion of an individual or entity under paragraphs (1), (2), or (3) of subsection (b), the period of exclusion shall be a minimum of 3 years, unless the Secretary determines that a longer period is appropriate because of aggravating circumstances.

"(E) In the case of an exclusion of an individual or entity under paragraph (4) or (5) of subsection (b), the period of the exclusion shall not be less than the period during which the individual's or entity's license to provide health care is revoked, suspended, or surrendered, or the individual or the entity is excluded or suspended from a Federal or State health care program.

"(F) In the case of an exclusion of an individual or entity under subsection (b)(6)(B), the period of the exclusion shall be not less than 1 year.".

(c) REVISION TO EXCLUSION FOR DEFAULT ON HEALTH EDUCATION LOAN OR SCHOLARSHIP OBLIGATIONS.—Section 1128(b)(14) (42 U.S.C. 1320a–7(b)(14)) is amended by striking "all reasonable steps" and inserting "reasonable steps".

(d) PERMISSIVE EXCLUSION OF INDIVIDUALS WITH OWNERSHIP OR CONTROL INTEREST IN SANCTIONED ENTITIES.—Section 1128(b) (42 U.S.C. 1320a-7(b)), is amended by adding at the end the following new paragraph:

"(15) INDIVIDUALS CONTROLLING A SANCTIONED ENTITY.—Any individual who has a direct or indirect ownership or control interest of 5 percent or more, or an ownership or control interest (as defined in section 1124(a)(3)) in, or who is an officer, director, agent, or managing employee (as defined in section 1126(b)) of, an entity—

"(A) that has been convicted of any offense described in subsection (a) or in paragraph (1), (2), or (3) of this subsection;

"(B) against which a civil monetary penalty has been assessed under section 1128A; or

"(C) that has been excluded from participation under a program under title XVIII or under a State health care program.".

(e) EXCLUSIONS BASED ON ACTIONS UNDER ALLIANCE SYSTEM.—Section 1128(b) (42 U.S.C. 1320a–7(b)), as amended by subsections (a) and (d), is amended—

(1) in paragraph (1), by striking "XVIII or under a State health care program" and inserting "XVIII, a State health care program, or under an applicable health plan (as defined in section 1902(6) of the Health Security Act)";

(2) in paragraph (7), by striking the period at the end and inserting ", or in section 5412 of the Health Security Act.";

(3) in paragraph (8)(B)—

(A) in clause (ii), by striking "1128A" and inserting "1128A or under section 5412 of the Health Security Act", and

(B) in clause (iii), by striking "XVIII or under a State health care program" and inserting "XVIII, a State health care program, or under an applicable health plan (as defined in section 1902(6) of the Health Security Act)";

(4) in paragraph (9), by striking the period at the end and inserting ", or any information requested by the Inspector General of the Department of Health and Human Services to carry out the All-Payer Health Care Fraud and Abuse Control Program established under section 5401 of the Health Security Act.";

(5) in paragraph (11)—

(A) by striking "title XVIII or a State health care program" and inserting "title XVIII, a State health care program, or an applicable health plan (as defined in section 1902(6) of the Health Security Act)",

(B) by striking "Secretary or the appropriate State agency" and inserting "Secretary, the appropriate State agency, or plan sponsor", and

(C) by striking "Secretary or that agency" and inserting "Secretary, that agency, or that sponsor";

(6) in paragraph (12), by adding at the end the following new subparagraph:

"(E) Any entity authorized by law to (i) conduct on-site health, safety or patient care reviews and surveys or (ii) to investigate whether any actions have occurred that would subject an individual or entity to the imposition of any sanctions under this section, section 1128A, section 1128B, or part 2 of subtitle E of title V of the Health Security Act."; and

(7) in paragraph (15)—

(A) in subparagraph (B), by striking "1128A" and inserting "1128A or section 54.. of the Health Security Act", and

(B) in subparagraph (C), by striking "title XVIII or under a State health care program" and inserting "title XVIII, a State health care program, or an applicable health plan (as defined in section 1902(6) of the Health Security Act''.

(f) APPEAL OF EXCLUSIONS TO COURT OF APPEALS.—Section 1128(f)(1) (42 U.S.C. 1320a–7(f)(1)) is amended by striking the period at the end and inserting the following: ", except that any action brought to appeal such decision shall be brought in the United States Court of Appeals for the judicial circuit in which the individual or entity resides or has a principal place of business (or, if the individual or entity does not reside or have a principal place of business within any such judicial circuit, in the United States Court of Appeals for the District of Columbia Circuit).''.

### SEC. 4045. SANCTIONS AGAINST PRACTITIONERS AND PERSONS FOR FAILURE TO COMPLY WITH STATUTORY OBLIGATIONS RELATING TO QUALITY OF CARE.

(a) MINIMUM PERIOD OF EXCLUSION FOR PRACTITIONERS AND PERSONS FAILING TO MEET STATUTORY OBLIGATIONS.—

(1) IN GENERAL.—The second sentence of section 1156(b)(1) (42 U.S.C. 1320c-5(b)(1)) is amended by striking "may prescribe)" and inserting "may prescribe, except that such period may not be less than one year)".

(2) CONFORMING AMENDMENT.—Section 1156(b)(2) (42 U.S.C. 1320c-5(b)(2)) is amended by striking "shall remain" and inserting "shall (subject to the minimum period specified in the second sentence of paragraph (1)) remain".

(b) REPEAL OF "UNWILLING OR UNABLE" CONDITION FOR IMPOSITION OF SANCTION.—Section 1156(b)(1) (42 U.S.C. 1320c-5(b)(1)) is amended—

(1) in the second sentence, by striking "and determines" and all that follows through "such obligations," and

(2) by striking the third sentence.

(c) AMOUNT OF CIVIL MONEY PENALTY.—Section 1156(b)(3) (42 U.S.C. 1320c-5(b)(3)) is amended by striking "the actual or estimated cost" and inserting the following: "$50,000 for each instance".

**SEC. 4046. EFFECTIVE DATE.**

The amendments made by this part shall take effect January 1, 1995.

## PART 6—FUNDING OF GRADUATE MEDICAL EDUCATION AND ACADEMIC HEALTH CENTERS

**SEC. 4051. TRANSFERS FROM MEDICARE TRUST FUNDS FOR GRADUATE MEDICAL EDUCATION.**

(a) IN GENERAL.—For purposes of complying with section 3034(a), there shall be transferred to the Secretary from the Federal Hospital Insurance Trust Fund (established under section 1817 of the Social Security Act) and the Federal Supplementary Medical Insurance Trust Fund (established under section 1841 of such Act) the following amount (in the aggregate), as applicable to a calendar year:

(1) In the case of a calendar year prior to 1998, the proportion of the amounts expended from such Trust Funds during the most recent fiscal year ending before the first day of such calendar year for payments for the direct costs of graduate medical education under section 1886(h) of such Act that is attributable to payments to hospitals located in the States that are participating States for the calendar year.

(2) In the case of calendar year 1998, the amount expended from such Trust Funds during fiscal year 1997 for payments for such direct costs of graduate medical education.

(3) In the case of each subsequent calendar year, the amount specified in paragraph (2) increased by the product of such amount and the general health care inflation factor (as defined in section 6001(a)(3), except that for purposes of this subparagraph the increases provided for in sub-

paragraphs (A) through (C) of such section shall not be made).

(b) ALLOCATION OF AMOUNT AMONG FUNDS.—With respect to the amount required under subsection (a) to be transferred for an academic year from the Federal Hospital Insurance Trust Fund and the Federal Supplementary Medical Insurance Trust Fund, the Secretary shall determine an equitable allocation of such amount among the funds.

(c) TERMINATION OF GRADUATE MEDICAL EDUCATION PAYMENTS UNDER MEDICARE.—

(1) IN GENERAL.— Section 1886(h) (42 U.S.C. 1395ww(h)) is amended by adding at the end the following new paragraph:

"(6) TERMINATION OF PAYMENTS ATTRIBUTABLE TO COSTS OF TRAINING PHYSICIANS.—Notwithstanding any other provision of this section or section 1861(v), no payment may be made under this title for direct graduate medical education costs attributable to an approved medical residency training program for any cost reporting period (or portion thereof) beginning on or after January 1, 1998 (or, in the case of costs of a program operating in a State that is a participating State under the Health Security Act for a year prior to 1998, on or after January 1 of the first year for which the State is such a participating State).".

(2) PROHIBITION AGAINST RECOGNITION OF COSTS.—Section 1861(v)(1) (42 U.S.C. 1395x(v)(1)) is amended by adding at the end the following new subparagraph:

"(T) Such regulations shall not include any provision for specific recognition of the costs of graduate medical education for hospitals for any cost reporting period (or portion thereof) beginning on or after January 1, 1998 (or, in the case of a hospital located in a State that is a participating State under the Health Security Act for a year prior to 1998, ending on or before December 31 of the year prior to the first year for which the State is such a participating State). Nothing in the previous sentence shall be construed to affect in any way payments to hospitals for the costs of any approved educational activities that are not described in such sentence.".

**SEC. 4052. TRANSFERS FROM HOSPITAL INSURANCE TRUST FUND FOR ACADEMIC HEALTH CENTERS.**

(a) IN GENERAL.—For purposes of complying with section 3104(a), there shall be transferred to the Secretary from the Federal Hospital Insurance Trust Fund (established under section 1817 of the Social Security Act) the following amount (in the aggregate), as applicable to a calendar year:

(1) In the case of a calendar year prior to 1998, the proportion of the amounts expended from such Trust Fund during the most recent fiscal year ending before the first day of such calendar year for payments for the indirect costs of medical education under section 1886(d)(5)(B) of such Act that is attributable to discharges of hospitals located in the States that are participating States for the calendar year.

(2) In the case of calendar year 1998, the amount expended from such Trust Fund during fiscal year 1997 for payments for such indirect costs of medical education.

(3) In the case of each subsequent calendar year, the amount specified in paragraph (2) increased by the product of such amount and the general health care inflation factor (as defined in section 6001(a)(3), except that for purposes of this subparagraph the increases provided for in subparagraphs (A) through (C) of such section shall not be made).

(b) TERMINATION OF PAYMENTS UNDER MEDICARE.—

(1) IN GENERAL.—Section 1886(d)(5)(B) (42 U.S.C. 1395ww(d)(5)(B)) is amended in the matter preceding clause (i) by striking "The Secretary" and inserting "For discharges occurring before January 1, 1998 (or, in the case of discharges of a hospital located in a State that is a participating State under the Health Security Act for a year prior to 1998, before January 1 of the first year for which the State is such a participating State), the Secretary".

(2) ADJUSTMENT TO STANDARDIZED AMOUNTS.—Section 1886(d)(2)(C)(i) (42 U.S.C. 1395ww(d)(2)(C)(i)) is amended by striking "excluding" and inserting "for discharges occurring before January 1, 1998, (or, in the case of discharges of a hospital located in a State that is a participating State under the Health Security Act for a year prior to 1998, before January 1 of the first year for which the State is such a participating State) excluding".

# PART 7—COVERAGE OF SERVICES PROVIDED BY FACILITIES AND PLANS OF DEPARTMENTS OF DEFENSE AND VETERANS AFFAIRS

### SEC. 4061. TREATMENT OF UNIFORMED SERVICES HEALTH PLAN AS ELIGIBLE ORGANIZATION UNDER MEDICARE.

(a) IN GENERAL.—Section 1876 (42 U.S.C. 1395mm), as amended by section 4002(a), is further amended by adding at the end the following new subsection:

"(l) Notwithstanding any other provision of this section, a Uniformed Services Health Plan of the Department of Defense under chapter 55 of title 10, United States Code, shall be considered an eligible organization under this section, and the Secretary shall make payments to such Plan during a year on behalf of any individuals entitled to benefits under this title who are enrolled with such a Plan during the year in such amounts and under such terms and conditions as may be imposed under an agreement between the Secretary and the Secretary of Defense.".

(b) EFFECTIVE DATE.—The amendment made by subsection (a) shall apply to items and services furnished under title XVIII of the Social Security Act on or after January 1, 1998.

## SEC. 4062. COVERAGE OF SERVICES PROVIDED TO MEDICARE BENEFICIARIES BY PLANS AND FACILITIES OF DEPARTMENT OF VETERANS AFFAIRS.

(a) IN GENERAL.—Title XVIII, as amended by sections 4001 and 4003, is further amended by adding at the end the following new section:

"TREATMENT OF PLANS AND FACILITIES OF DEPARTMENT OF VETERANS AFFAIRS AS PROVIDERS

"SEC. 1895. (a) IN GENERAL.—Notwithstanding any other provision of this title—

"(1) a VA health plan (as defined in section 1801(2) of title 38, United States Code) shall be considered an eligible organization for purposes of section 1876; and

"(2) a health care facility of the Department of Veterans Affairs shall be considered a provider of services under section 1861(u).

"(b) ELIGIBILITY FOR PAYMENTS.—

"(1) VA HEALTH PLANS.—The Secretary shall make payments to a VA health plan during a year on behalf of any individuals entitled to benefits under this title who are enrolled with such a plan during the year in the same amounts and under the same terms and conditions under which the Secretary makes payments to eligible organizations with a risk-sharing contract under section 1876.

"(2) HEALTH CARE FACILITIES.—The Secretary shall make payments to a health care facility of the Department of Veterans Affairs for services provided to an individual entitled to benefits under this title in the same amounts and under the same terms and conditions under which the Secretary makes payments to provider of services under this title.".

(b) EFFECTIVE DATE.—The amendment made by subsection (a) shall apply to items and services furnished under title XVIII of the Social Security Act on or after January 1, 1998.

**SEC. 4063. CONFORMING AMENDMENTS.**

(a) PART A.—Section 1814 (42 U.S.C. 1395f) is amended by striking subsection (c).

(b) PART B.—Section 1835 (42 U.S.C. 1395n) is amended by striking subsection (d).

(c) ADDITIONAL CONFORMING AMENDMENT.—Section 1880(a) (42 U.S.C. 1395qq(a)) is amended by striking ", notwithstanding sections 1814(c) and 1835(d),".

(d) EFFECTIVE DATE.—The amendments made by this section shall take effect January 1, 1998.

# Subtitle B—Savings in Medicare Program

## PART 1—SAVINGS RELATING TO PART A

### SEC. 4101. REDUCTION IN UPDATE FOR INPATIENT HOSPITAL SERVICES.

Section 1886(b)(3)(B)(i) (42 U.S.C. 1395ww(b)(3)(B)(i)), as amended by section 13501(a)(1) of OBRA–1993, is amended—

    (1) in subclause (XII)—

        (A) by striking "fiscal year 1997" and inserting "for each of the fiscal years 1997 through 2000", and

        (B) by striking "0.5 percentage point" and inserting "2.0 percentage points"; and

    (2) in subclause (XIII), by striking "fiscal year 1998" and inserting "fiscal year 2001".

### SEC. 4102. REDUCTION IN ADJUSTMENT FOR INDIRECT MEDICAL EDUCATION.

Section 1886(d)(5)(B)(ii) (42 U.S.C. 1395ww(d)(5)(B)(ii)) is amended to read as follows:

    "(ii) For purposes of clause (i)(II), the indirect teaching adjustment factor is equal to c * (((1+r) to the nth power) - 1), where 'r' is the ratio of the hospital's full-time equivalent interns and residents to beds and 'n' equals .405. For discharges occurring on or after—

"(I) May 1, 1986, and before October 1, 1994, 'c' is equal to 1.89,

"(II) October 1, 1994, and before October 1, 1995, 'c' is equal to 1.395, and

"(III) October 1, 1995, 'c' is equal to 0.74.".

## SEC. 4103. REDUCTION IN PAYMENTS FOR CAPITAL-RELATED COSTS FOR INPATIENT HOSPITAL SERVICES.

(a) PPS HOSPITALS.—

(1) REDUCTION IN BASE PAYMENT RATES.—Section 1886(g)(1)(A) (42 U.S.C. 1395ww(g)(1)(A)), as amended by section 13501(a)(3) of OBRA–1993, is amended by adding at the end the following new sentence: "In addition to the reduction described in the preceding sentence, the Secretary shall reduce by 7.31 percent the unadjusted standard Federal capital payment rate (as described in 42 CFR 412.308(c), as in effect on the date of the enactment of the Health Security Act) and shall reduce by 10.41 percent the unadjusted hospital-specific rate (as described in 42

CFR 412.328(e)(1), as in effect on the date of the enactment of the Health Security Act).".

(2) REDUCTION IN UPDATE.—Section 1886(g)(1) (42 U.S.C. 1395ww(g)(1)) is amended—

    (A) in subparagraph (B)(i)—

        (i) by striking "and (II)" and inserting "(II)", and

        (ii) by striking the semicolon at the end and inserting the following: ", and (III) an annual update factor established for the prospective payment rates applicable to discharges in a fiscal year which (subject to reduction under subparagraph (C)) will be based upon such factor as the Secretary determines appropriate to take into account amounts necessary for the efficient and effective delivery of medically appropriate and necessary care of high quality;";

    (B) by redesignating subparagraph (C) as subparagraph (D); and

    (C) by inserting after subparagraph (B) the following new subparagraph:

"(C)(i) With respect to payments attributable to portions of cost reporting periods or discharges occurring during each of the fiscal years 1996 through 2000, the Secretary shall include a reduction in the annual update factor established under subparagraph (B)(i)(III) for discharges in the year equal to the applicable update reduction described in clause (ii) to adjust for excessive increases in capital costs per discharge for fiscal years prior to fiscal year 1992 (but in no event may such reduction result in an annual update factor less than zero).

"(ii) In clause (i), the term 'applicable update reduction' means, with respect to the update factor for a fiscal year—

"(I) 4.9 percentage points; or

"(II) if the annual update factor for the previous fiscal year was less than the applicable update reduction for the previous year, the sum of 4.9 percentage points and the difference between the annual update factor for the previous year and the applicable update reduction for the previous year.".

(b) PPS-EXEMPT HOSPITALS.—Section 1861(v)(1) (42 U.S.C. 1395x(v)(1)), as amended by section 4051(c)(2), is further amended by adding at the end the following new subparagraph:

"(U) Such regulations shall provide that, in determining the amount of the payments that may be made under this title with respect to the capital-related costs of inpatient hospital services furnished by a hospital that is not a subsection (d) hospital (as defined in section 1886(d)(1)(B)) or a subsection (d) Puerto Rico hospital (as defined in section 1886(d)(9)(A)), the Secretary shall reduce the amounts of such payments otherwise established under this title by 15 percent for payments attributable to portions of cost reporting periods occurring during each of the fiscal years 1996 through 2000.".

## SEC. 4104. REVISIONS TO PAYMENT ADJUSTMENTS FOR DISPROPORTIONATE SHARE HOSPITALS IN PARTICIPATING STATES.

(a) APPLICATION OF ALTERNATIVE ADJUSTMENTS.—Section 1886(d)(5) (42 U.S.C. 1395ww(d)(5)) is amended—

(1) by redesignating subparagraphs (H) and (I) as subparagraphs (I) and (J); and

(2) by inserting after subparagraph (G) the following new subparagraph:

"(H)(i) In accordance with this subparagraph, the Secretary shall provide for an additional payment for each subsection (d) hospital that is located in a participating State under subtitle C of title I of the Health Security

Act during a cost reporting period and that meets the eligibility requirements described in clause (iii).

"(ii) The amount of the additional payment made under clause (i) for each discharge shall be determined by multiplying—

"(I) the sum of the amount determined under paragraph (1)(A)(ii)(II) (or, if applicable, the amount determined under paragraph (1)(A)(iii)) and the amount paid to the hospital under subparagraph (A) for the discharge, by

"(II) the SSI adjustment percentage for the cost reporting period in which the discharge occurs (as defined in clause (iv)).

"(iii) A hospital meets the eligibility requirements described in this clause with respect to a cost reporting period if—

"(I) in the case of a hospital that is located in an urban area and that has more than 100 beds, the hospital's SSI patient percentage (as defined in clause (v)) for the cost reporting period is not less than 5 percent;

"(II) in the case of a hospital that is located in an urban area and that has less than 100 beds, the hospital's SSI patient percentage is not less than 17 percent;

"(III) in the case of a hospital that is classified as a rural referral center under subparagraph (C) or a sole community hospital under subparagraph (D), the hospital's SSI patient percentage for the cost reporting period is not less than 23 percent; and

"(IV) in the case of any other hospital, the hospital's SSI patient percentage is not less than 23 percent.

"(iv) For purposes of clause (ii), the 'SSI adjustment percentage' applicable to a hospital for a cost reporting period is equal to—

"(I) in the case of a hospital described in clause (iii)(I), the percentage determined in accordance with the following formula: e to the nth power, where 'e' is the natural antilog of 1 and where 'n' is equal to (.5642 * (the hospital's SSI patient percentage for the cost reporting period - .055)) - 1;

"(II) in the case of a hospital described in clause (iii)(II) or clause (iii)(IV), 2 percent; and

"(III) in the case of a hospital described in clause (iii)(III), the sum of 2 percent and .30 percent of the difference between the hospital's SSI patient percentage for the cost reporting period and 23 percent.

"(v) In this subparagraph, a hospital's 'SSI patient percentage' with respect to a cost reporting period is equal to the fraction (expressed as a percentage)—

"(I) the numerator of which is the number of the hospital's patient days for such period which were made up of patients who (for such days) were entitled to benefits under part A and were entitled to supplementary security income benefits (excluding State supplementation) under title XVI; and

"(II) the denominator of which is the number of the hospital's patient days for such period which were made up of patients who (for such days) were entitled to benefits under part A.".

(b) NO STANDARDIZATION RESULTING FROM REDUCTION.—Section 1886(d)(2)(C)(iv) (42 U.S.C. 1395ww(d)(2)(C)(iv)) is amended—

(1) by striking "exclude additional payments" and inserting "adjust such estimate for changes in payments";

(2) by striking "1989 or" and inserting "1989,"; and

(3) by striking the period at the end and inserting the following: ", or the enactment of section 4104 of the Health Security Act.".

(c) CONFORMING AMENDMENT.—Section 1886(d)(5)(F)(i) (42 U.S.C. 1395ww(d)(5)(F)(i)) is amended in the matter preceding subclause (I) by inserting after "hospital" the following: "that is not located in a State that is a participating State under subtitle C of title I of the Health Security Act".

### SEC. 4105. MORATORIUM ON DESIGNATION OF ADDITIONAL LONG-TERM CARE HOSPITALS.

Notwithstanding clause (iv) of section 1886(d)(1)(B) of the Social Security Act, a hospital which has an average inpatient length of stay (as determined by the Secretary of Health and Human Services) of greater than 25 days shall not be treated as a hospital described in such clause for purposes of title XVIII of such Act unless the hospital was treated as a hospital described in such clause for purposes of such title as of the date of the enactment of this Act.

### SEC. 4106. EXTENSION OF FREEZE ON UPDATES TO ROUTINE SERVICE COSTS OF SKILLED NURSING FACILITIES.

(a) PAYMENTS BASED ON COST LIMITS.—Section 1888(a) (42 U.S.C. 1395yy(a)) is amended by striking "112 percent" each place it appears and inserting "100 percent (adjusted by such amount as the Secretary determines to be necessary to preserve the savings resulting from the enactment of section 13503(a)(1) of the Omnibus Budget Reconciliation Act of 1993)".

(b) PAYMENTS DETERMINED ON PROSPECTIVE BASIS.—Section 1888(d)(2)(B) (42 U.S.C. 1395yy(d)(2)(B)) is amended by striking "105 percent" and inserting "100 percent (adjusted by such amount as the Secretary determines to be necessary to preserve the savings resulting from the enactment of section 13503(b) of the Omnibus Budget Reconciliation Act of 1993)".

(c) EFFECTIVE DATE.—The amendments made by subsections (a) and(b) shall apply to cost reporting periods beginning on or after October 1, 1995.

## PART 2—SAVINGS RELATING TO PART B

### SEC. 4111. ESTABLISHMENT OF CUMULATIVE EXPENDITURE GOALS FOR PHYSICIAN SERVICES.

(a) USE OF CUMULATIVE PERFORMANCE STANDARD.—Section 1848(f)(2) (42 U.S.C. 1395w–4(f)(2)) is amended—

　　(1) in subparagraph (A)—

　　　　(A) in the heading, by striking "IN GENERAL" and inserting "FISCAL YEARS 1991 THROUGH 1993.—",

　　　　(B) in the matter preceding clause (i), by striking "a fiscal year (beginning with fiscal year 1991)" and inserting "fiscal years 1991, 1992, and 1993", and

    (C) in the matter following clause (iv), by striking "subparagraph (B)" and inserting "subparagraph (C)";

  (2) in subparagraph (B), by striking "subparagraph (A)" and inserting "subparagraphs (A) and (B)";

  (3) by redesignating subparagraphs (B) and (C) as subparagraphs (C) and (D); and

  (4) by inserting after subparagraph (A) the following new subparagraph:

    "(B) FISCAL YEARS BEGINNING WITH FISCAL YEAR 1994.—Unless Congress otherwise provides, the performance standard rate of increase, for all physicians' services and for each category of physicians's services, for a fiscal year beginning with fiscal year 1994 shall be equal to the performance standard rate of increase determined under this paragraph for the previous fiscal year, increased by the product of—

      "(i) 1 plus the Secretary's estimate of the weighted average percentage increase (divided by 100) in the fees for all physicians' services or for the category of physicians' services, respectively, under this part for portions of calendar years included in the fiscal year involved,

"(ii) 1 plus the Secretary's estimate of the percentage increase or decrease (divided by 100) in the average number of individuals enrolled under this part (other than HMO enrollees) from the previous fiscal year to the fiscal year involved,

"(iii) 1 plus the Secretary's estimate of the average annual percentage growth (divided by 100) in volume and intensity of all physicians' services or of the category of physicians' services, respectively, under this part for the 5-fiscal-year period ending with the preceding fiscal year (based upon information contained in the most recent annual report made pursuant to section 1841(b)(2)), and

"(iv) 1 plus the Secretary's estimate of the percentage increase or decrease (divided by 100) in expenditures for all physicians' services or of the category of physicians' services, respectively, in the fiscal year (compared with the previous fiscal year) which are estimated to result from changes in law or regulations affecting the percentage increase described in clause (i) and which is not taken into account in the percentage increase described in clause (i), minus 1, multiplied by 100, and reduced by the performance standard factor (specified in subparagraph (C)).".

(b) TREATMENT OF DEFAULT UPDATE.—

(1) IN GENERAL.—Section 1848(d)(3)(B) (42 U.S.C. 1395w–4(d)(3)(B)) is amended—

(A) in clause (i)—

(i) in the heading, by striking "IN GENERAL" and inserting "1992 THROUGH 1995", and

(ii) by striking "for a year" and inserting "for 1992, 1993, 1994, and 1995"; and

(B) by adding after clause (ii) the following new clause:

"(iii) YEARS BEGINNING WITH 1996.—

"(I) IN GENERAL.—The update for a category of physicians' services for a year beginning with 1996 provided under subparagraph (A) shall be increased or decreased by the same percentage by which the cumulative percentage increase in actual expenditures for such category of physicians' services for such year was less or greater, respectively, than the performance standard rate of increase (established under subsection (f)) for such category of services for such year.

"(II) CUMULATIVE PERCENTAGE INCREASE DEFINED.—In subclause (I), the 'cumulative percentage increase in actual expenditures' for a year shall be equal to the product of the adjusted increases for each year beginning with 1994 up to and including the year involved, minus 1 and multiplied by 100. In the previous sentence, the 'adjusted increase' for a year is equal to 1 plus the percentage increase in actual expenditures for the year.".

(2) CONFORMING AMENDMENT.—Section 1848(d)(3)(A)(i) (42 U.S.C. 1395w–4(d)(3)(A)(i)) is amended by striking "subparagraph (B)" and inserting "subparagraphs (B) and (C)".

**SEC. 4112. USE OF REAL GDP TO ADJUST FOR VOLUME AND INTENSITY; REPEAL OF RESTRICTION ON MAXIMUM REDUCTION PERMITTED IN DEFAULT UPDATE.**

(a) USE OF REAL GDP TO ADJUST FOR VOLUME AND INTENSITY.—Section 1848(f)(2)(B)(iii) (42 U.S.C. 1395w–4(f)(2)(B)(iii)), as added by section 4111(a), is amended to read as follows:

"(iii) 1 plus the average per capita growth in the real gross domestic product (divided by 100) for the 5-fiscal-year period ending with the previous fiscal year (increased by 1.5 percentage points for the category of services consisting of primary care services), and".

(b) REPEAL OF RESTRICTION ON MAXIMUM REDUCTION.—Section 1848(d)(3)(B)(ii) (42 U.S.C. 1395w–4(d)(3)(B)(ii)), as amended by section 13512(b) of OBRA–1993, is amended—

(1) in the heading, by inserting "IN CERTAIN YEARS" after "ADJUSTMENT";

(2) in the matter preceding subclause (I), by striking "for a year";

(3) in subclause (I), by adding "and" at the end;

(4) in subclause (II), by striking ", and" and inserting a period; and

(5) by striking subclause (III).

## SEC. 4113. REDUCTION IN CONVERSION FACTOR FOR PHYSICIAN FEE SCHEDULE FOR 1995.

Section 1848(d)(1) (42 U.S.C. 1395w–4(d)(1)) is amended—

(1) in subparagraph (A), by inserting after "subparagraph (B)" the following: ", and, in the case of 1995, specified in subparagraph (C)";

(2) by redesignating subparagraph (C) as subparagraph (D); and

(3) by inserting after subparagraph (B) the following new subparagraph:

"(C) SPECIAL PROVISION FOR 1995.—For purposes of subparagraph (A), the conversion factor specified in this subparagraph for 1995 is—

"(i) in the case of physicians' services included in the category of primary care services (as defined in subsection (j)(1)), the conversion factor established under this subsection for 1994 adjusted by the update established under paragraph (3) for 1995; and

"(ii) in the case of any other physicians' services, the conversion factor established under this subsection for 1994 reduced by 3 percentage points.".

## SEC. 4114. LIMITATIONS ON PAYMENT FOR PHYSICIANS' SERVICES FURNISHED BY HIGH-COST HOSPITAL MEDICAL STAFFS.

(a) IN GENERAL.—

(1) LIMITATIONS DESCRIBED.—Part B of title XVIII, as amended by section 2003(a), is amended by inserting after section 1848 the following new section:

"LIMITATIONS ON PAYMENT FOR PHYSICIANS' SERVICES FURNISHED BY HIGH-COST HOSPITAL MEDICAL STAFFS

"SEC. 1849. (a) SERVICES SUBJECT TO REDUCTION.—

"(1) DETERMINATION OF HOSPITAL-SPECIFIC PER ADMISSION RELATIVE VALUE.—Not later than October 1 of each year (beginning with 1997), the Secretary shall determine for each hospital—

"(A) the hospital-specific per admission relative value under subsection (b)(2) for the following year; and

"(B)(i) whether such hospital-specific relative value is projected to exceed the allowable average per admission relative value applicable to the hospital for the following year under subsection (b)(1), and, if so, (ii) the hospital's projected excess relative value for the year under subsection (b)(3).

"(2) REDUCTION FOR SERVICES AT HOSPITALS EXCEEDING ALLOWABLE AVERAGE PER ADMISSION RELATIVE VALUE.—If the Secretary determines (under paragraph (1)) that a medical staff's hospital-specific per admission relative value for a year (beginning with 1998) is projected to exceed the allowable average per admission relative value applicable to the medical staff for the year, the Secretary shall reduce (in accordance with subsection (c)) the amount of payment otherwise determined under this part for each physicians' service furnished during the year to an inpatient of the hospital by an individual who is a member of the hospital's medical staff.

"(3) TIMING OF DETERMINATION; NOTICE TO HOSPITALS AND CARRIERS.—Not later than October 1 of each year (beginning with 1997), the Secretary shall notify the medical executive committee of each hospital (as set forth in the Standards of the Joint Commission on the Accreditation of Health Organizations) of the determinations made with respect to the medical staff under paragraph (1).

"(b) DETERMINATION OF ALLOWABLE AVERAGE PER ADMISSION RELATIVE VALUE AND HOSPITAL-SPECIFIC PER ADMISSION RELATIVE VALUES.—

"(1) ALLOWABLE AVERAGE PER ADMISSION RELATIVE VALUE.—

"(A) URBAN HOSPITALS.—In the case of a hospital located in an urban area, the allowable average per admission relative value established under this subsection—

"(i) for 1998 and 1999, is equal to 125 percent of the median of the 1996 hospital-specific per admission relative values determined under paragraph (2) for all hospital medical staffs; and

"(ii) for 2000 and each succeeding year, is equal to 120 percent of the median of such relative values for all hospital medical staffs.

"(B) RURAL HOSPITALS.—In the case of a hospital located in a rural area, the allowable average per admission relative value established under this subsection for 1998 and each succeeding year, is equal to 140 percent of the median of the 1996 hospital-specific per admission relative values determined under paragraph (2) for all hospital medical staffs.

"(2) HOSPITAL-SPECIFIC PER ADMISSION RELATIVE VALUE.—

"(A) IN GENERAL.—The hospital-specific per admission relative value for a hospital (other than a teaching hospital), shall be equal to the average per admission relative value (as determined under section 1848(c)(2)) for each physician's service furnished to inpatients of the hospital by the hospital's medical staff (excluding interns and residents) during 1996, adjusted for variations in case-mix and disproportionate share status among hospitals (as determined by the Secretary under subparagraph (C)).

"(B) SPECIAL RULE FOR TEACHING HOSPITALS.—The hospital-specific relative value for a teaching hospital shall be equal to the sum of—

"(i) the average per admission relative value (as determined under section 1848(c)(2)) for each physician's service furnished to inpatients of the hospital by the hospital's medical staff (excluding interns and residents) during 1996, adjusted for variations in case-mix, disproportionate share status, and teaching status among hospitals (as determined by the Secretary under subparagraph (C)); and

"(ii) the equivalent per admission relative value (as determined under section 1848(c)(2)) for each physician's service furnished to inpatients of the hospital by interns and residents of the hospital during 1996, adjusted for variations in case-mix, disproportionate share status, and teaching status among hospitals (as determined by the Secretary under subparagraph (C)). The Secretary shall determine such equivalent relative value unit per admission for interns and residents based on the best available data for teaching hospitals and may make such adjustment in the aggregate.

"(C) ADJUSTMENT FOR TEACHING AND DISPROPORTIONATE SHARE HOSPITALS.—The Secretary shall adjust the allowable per admission relative values otherwise determined under this paragraph to take into account the needs of teaching hospitals and hospitals receiving additional payments under subparagraphs (F) and (G) of section 1886(d)(5). The adjustment for teaching status or disproportionate share shall not be less than zero.

"(3) PROJECTED EXCESS RELATIVE VALUE DEFINED.—The 'projected excess relative value' with respect to a hospital's medical staff for a year means the number of percentage points by which the Secretary determines (under subsection (a)(1)(B)) that the medical staff's hospital-specific per admission relative value (determined under paragraph (2)) will exceed the allowable average per admission relative value applicable to the hospital medical staff for the year (as determined under paragraph (1)).

"(c) AMOUNT OF REDUCTION.—The amount of payment otherwise made under this part for a physician's service that is subject to a reduction under subsection (a) during a year shall be reduced 15 percent, in the case of a service furnished by a member of the medical staff of a hospital for which the Secretary determines under subsection (a)(1) that the hospital medical staff's projected relative value per admission exceeds the allowable average per admission relative value.

"(d) RECONCILIATION OF REDUCTIONS BASED ON HOSPITAL-SPECIFIC RELATIVE VALUE PER ADMISSION WITH ACTUAL RELATIVE VALUES.—

"(1) DETERMINATION OF ACTUAL AVERAGE PER ADMISSION RELATIVE VALUE.—Not later than October 1 of each year (beginning with 1999), the Secretary shall determine the actual average per admission relative value (as determined pursuant to section 1848(c)(2)) for the physicians' services furnished by members of a hospital's medical staff to inpatients of the hospital during the previous year, on the basis of claims for payment for such services that are submitted to the Secretary not later than 90 days after the last day of such previous year. The actual average per admission shall be adjusted by the appropriate case-mix, disproportionate share factor, and teaching factor for the hospital medical staff (as determined by the Secretary under subsection (b)(2)(C)).

"(2) RECONCILIATION WITH REDUCTIONS TAKEN.—In the case of a hospital for which the payment amounts for physicians' services furnished by members of the hospital's medical staff to inpatients of the hospital were reduced under this section for a year—

"(A) if the actual average per admission relative value for such hospital's medical staff during the year (as determined by the Secretary under paragraph (1)) did not exceed the allowable average per admission relative value applicable to the hospital's medical staff under subsection (b)(1) for the year, the Secretary shall reimburse the fiduciary agent for the medical staff by the amount by which payments for such services were reduced for the year under subsection (c);

"(B) if the actual average per admission relative value for such hospital's medical staff during the year is less than 10 percentage points above the allowable average per admission relative value applicable to the hospital's medical staff under subsection (b)(1) for the year, the Secretary shall reimburse the fiduciary agent for the medical staff, as a percent of the total allowed charges for physicians' services performed in such hospital (prior to the withhold), the difference between 10 percentage points and the actual number of percentage points that the staff exceeds the limit;

"(C) if the actual average per admission relative value for such hospital's medical staff during the year exceeded the allowable average per admission relative value applicable to the hospital's medical staff by 10 percentage points or more, none of the withhold is paid to the fiduciary agent for the medical staff.

"(3) MEDICAL EXECUTIVE COMMITTEE OF A HOSPITAL.—Each medical executive committee of a hospital whose medical staff is projected to exceed the allowable relative value per admission for a year, shall have one year from the date of notification that such medical staff is projected to exceed the allowable relative value per admission to designate a fiduciary agent for the medical staff to receive and disburse any appropriate withhold amount made by the carrier.

"(4) ALTERNATIVE REIMBURSEMENT TO MEMBERS OF STAFF.—At the request of a fiduciary agent for the medical staff, if the fiduciary agent for the medical staff is owed the reimbursement described in paragraph (2)(B) for excess reductions in payments during a year, the Secretary shall make such reimbursement to the members of the hospital's medical staff.

"(e) DEFINITIONS.—In this section, the following definitions apply:

"(1) MEDICAL STAFF.—An individual furnishing a physician's service is considered to be on the medical staff of a hospital—

"(A) if (in accordance with requirements for hospitals established by the Joint Commission on Accreditation of Health Organizations)—

"(i) the individual is subject to bylaws, rules, and regulations established by the hospital to provide a framework for the self-governance of medical staff activities;

"(ii) subject to such bylaws, rules, and regulations, the individual has clinical privileges granted by the hospital's governing body; and "(iii) under such clinical privileges, the individual may provide physicians' services independently within the scope of the individual's clinical privileges, or

"(B) if such physician provides at least one service to a Medicare beneficiary in such hospital.

"(2) RURAL AREA; URBAN AREA.—The terms 'rural area' and 'urban area' have the meaning given such terms under section 1886(d)(2)(D).

"(3) TEACHING HOSPITAL.—The term 'teaching hospital' means a hospital which has a teaching program approved as specified in section 1861(b)(6).".

(2) CONFORMING AMENDMENTS.—(A) Section 1833(a)(1)(N) (42 U.S.C. 1395l(a)(1)(N)) is amended by inserting "(subject to reduction under section 1849)" after "1848(a)(1)".

(B) Section 1848(a)(1)(B) (42 U.S.C. 1395w–4(a)(1)(B)) is amended by striking "this subsection," and inserting "this subsection and section 1849,".

(b) REQUIRING PHYSICIANS TO IDENTIFY HOSPITAL AT WHICH SERVICE FURNISHED.—Section 1848(g)(4)(A)(i) (42 U.S.C. 1395w–4(g)(4)(A)(i)) is amended by striking "beneficiary," and inserting "beneficiary (and, in the case of a service furnished to an inpatient of a hospital, report the hospital identification number on such claim form),".

(c) EFFECTIVE DATE.—The amendments made by this section shall apply to services furnished on or after January 1, 1998.

### SEC. 4115. MEDICARE INCENTIVES FOR PHYSICIANS TO PROVIDE PRIMARY CARE.

(a) RESOURCE-BASED PRACTICE EXPENSE RELATIVE VALUE UNITS.—

(1) INCREASE IN PRACTICE EXPENSE RELATIVE VALUE UNITS FOR CERTAIN SERVICES.—Section 1848(c)(2) (42 U.S.C. 1395w–4(c)(2)), as amended by sections 13513 and 13514 of OBRA–93, is amended by adding at the end the following new subparagraph:

"(G) INCREASE IN PRACTICE EXPENSE RELATIVE VALUE UNITS FOR CERTAIN SERVICES.—The Secretary shall increase the practice expense relative value units applied in primary care services, as defined in section 1842(i)(4), by 10 percent, beginning with 1996.".

(2) ASSURING BUDGET NEUTRALITY.—Section 1842(c)(2)(F) (42 U.S.C. 1395u(c)(2)(F)), as added by section 13513 and amended by section 13514 of

OBRA-93, is amended by adding at the end the following new clause:

"(iii) shall reduce the relative values for all services (other than anesthesia services and primary care services, as defined in section 1842(i)(4)) established under this paragraph (and, in the case of anesthesia services, the conversion factor established by the Secretary for such services) by such percentage as the Secretary determines to be necessary so that, beginning in 1996, the amendment made by section 4115(a)(1) of the Health Security Act would not result in expenditures under this section that exceed the amount of such expenditures that would have been made if such amendment had not been made.".

 (3) STUDY.—The Secretary of Health and Human Services shall—

  (A) develop a methodology for implementing in 1997 a resource-based system for determining practice expense relative values unit for each physician's service, and

  (B) transmit a report by June 30, 1996, on the methodology developed under paragraph

(1) to the Committees on Ways and Means and Energy and Commerce of the House of Representatives and the Committee on Fiance of the Senate. The reported shall include a presentation of the data utilized in developing the methodology and an explanation of the methodology.

(b) OFFICE VISIT PRE- AND POST-TIME.—

(1) INCREASE IN WORK RELATIVE VALUE UNITS FOR OFFICE VISITS.—Section 1848(c)(2) (42 U.S.C. 1395w–4(c)(2)) is amended by adding at the end the following new subparagraph:

"(H) INCREASE IN WORK RELATIVE VALUE UNITS FOR CERTAIN SERVICES.—The Secretary shall increase the work relative value units applied to office visits by 10 percent, beginning with 1996.".

(2) ASSURING BUDGET NEUTRALITY.—Section 1842(c)(2)(F)(iii) is amended by striking "section 4115(a)" and substituting "sections 4115(a)(1) and (b)(1)".

(c) OFFICE CONSULTATIONS.—Section 1848(c)(2) (42 U.S.C. 1395w–4(c)(2)) is amended by adding at the end the following new subparagraph:

"(1) AMENDMENT IN RELATIVE VALUES FOR OFFICE CONSULTATIONS.—The Secretary shall reduce the work, practice expense and malpractice relative value components of office consultations to be equal to the work, practice expense and malpractice relative value components for comparable office visits beginning with 1996. In making such adjustment, the Secretary shall apply the savings from such reduction to increase each of the relative value components for office visits in a manner that would not result in expenditures under this section that exceed the amount of such expenditures that would have been made if such amendment had not been made.".

(d) OUTLIER INTENSITY RELATIVE VALUE ADJUSTMENTS.—

(1) ADJUSTMENT OF OUTLIER INTENSITY OF RELATIVE VALUES.—Section 1848(c)(2) (42 U.S.C. 1395w–4(c)(2)) is amended by adding at the end the following new subparagraph:

"(J) ADJUSTMENT OF OUTLIER INTENSITY OF RELATIVE VALUES.—Beginning with 1996, the Secretary shall reduce the work relative value components of procedures, or classes of procedures, where the intensity exceeds thresholds established by the Secretary. In the previous sentence, intensity shall mean the work relative value units for the procedure divided by the time for the procedure. The Secretary shall apply the savings from such reductions to increase the work relative value components of primary care services, as defined in section 1842(i)(4), such that the changes made by this subsection would not result in expenditures under this section that exceed the amount of such expenditures that would have been made if such amendment had not been made.".

(e) CHANGES IN UNDERSERVED AREA BONUS PAYMENTS.—

(1) Section 1833(m) (42 U.S.C. 1395l(m)) is amended by—

(A) striking "10 percent" and inserting "a percent",

(B) striking "service" the last time it appears and inserting "services", and

(C) adding the following new sentence: "The percent referred to in the previous sentence is 20 percent in the case of primary care services, as defined in section 1842(i)(4), and 10 percent for services other than primary care services furnished in health professional shortage areas located in rural areas as defined in section 1886(d).".

(2) The amendments made by subparagraph (A) are effective for services furnished on or after January 1, 1996.

## SEC. 4116. ELIMINATION OF FORMULA-DRIVEN OVERPAYMENTS FOR CERTAIN OUTPATIENT HOSPITAL SERVICES.

(a) AMBULATORY SURGICAL CENTER PROCEDURES.—Section 1833(i)(3)(B)(i)(II) (42 U.S.C. 1395l(i)(3)(B)(i)(II)) is amended—

(1) by striking "of 80 percent"; and

(2) by striking the period at the end and inserting the following: ", less the amount a provider may charge as described in clause (ii) of section 1866(a)(2)(A).".

(b) RADIOLOGY SERVICES AND DIAGNOSTIC PROCEDURES.—Section 1833(n)(1)(B)(i)(II) (42 U.S.C. 1395l(n)(1)(B)(i)(II)) is amended—

(1) by striking "of 80 percent"; and

(2) by striking the period at the end and inserting the following: ", less the amount a provider may charge as described in clause (ii) of section 1866(a)(2)(A).".

(c) EFFECTIVE DATE.—The amendments made by this section shall apply to services furnished during portions of cost reporting periods occurring on or after July 1, 1994.

## SEC. 4117. IMPOSITION OF COINSURANCE ON LABORATORY SERVICES.

(a) IN GENERAL.—Paragraphs (1)(D) and (2)(D) of section 1833(a) (42 U.S.C. 1395l(a)) are each amended—

 (1) by striking "(or 100 percent" and all that follows through "the first opinion))"; and

 (2) by striking "100 percent of such negotiated rate" and inserting "80 percent of such negotiated rate".

(b) EFFECTIVE DATE.—The amendments made by subsection (a) shall apply to tests furnished on or after January 1, 1995.

## SEC. 4118. APPLICATION OF COMPETITIVE BIDDING PROCESS FOR PART B ITEMS AND SERVICES.

(a) GENERAL RULE.—Part B of title XVIII of the Social Security Act is amended by inserting after section 1846 the following:

"COMPETITION ACQUISITION FOR ITEMS AND SERVICES

"SEC. 1847. (a) ESTABLISHMENT OF BIDDING AREAS.—

 "(1) IN GENERAL.—The Secretary shall establish competitive acquisition areas for the purpose of awarding a contract or contracts for the furnishing under this part of the items and services described in subsection (c) on or after January 1, 1995. The Secretary may establish different competitive acquisition areas under this subsection for different classes of items and services under this part.

"(2) CRITERIA FOR ESTABLISHMENT.—The competitive acquisition areas established under paragraph (1) shall—

    "(A) initially be, or be within, metropolitan statistical areas; and

    "(B) be chosen based on the availability and accessibility of suppliers and the probable savings to be realized by the use of competitive bidding in the furnishing of items and services in the area.

"(b) AWARDING OF CONTRACTS IN AREAS.—

    "(1) IN GENERAL.—The Secretary shall conduct a competition among individuals and entities supplying items and services under this part for each competitive acquisition area established under subsection (a) for each class of items and services.

    "(2) CONDITIONS FOR AWARDING CONTRACT.— The Secretary may not award a contract to any individual or entity under the competition conducted pursuant to paragraph (1) to furnish an item or service under this part unless the Secretary finds that the individual or entity—

"(A) meets quality standards specified by the Secretary for the furnishing of such item or service; and

"(B) offers to furnish a total quantity of such item or service that is sufficient to meet the expected need within the competitive acquisition area.

"(3) CONTENTS OF CONTRACT.—A contract entered into with an individual or entity under the competition conducted pursuant to paragraph (1) shall specify (for all of the items and services within a class)—

"(A) the quantity of items and services the entity shall provide; and

"(B) such other terms and conditions as the Secretary may require.

"(c) SERVICES DESCRIBED.—The items and services to which the provisions of this section shall apply are as follows:

"(1) Magnetic resonance imaging tests and computerized axial tomography scans, including a physician's interpretation of the results of such tests and scans.

"(2) Oxygen and oxygen equipment.

"(3) Enteral and parenteral nutrients, supplies, and equipment.

"(4) Such other items and services for which the Secretary determines that the use of competitive acquisition under this section will be appropriate and cost-effective.".

(b) ITEMS AND SERVICES TO BE FURNISHED ONLY THROUGH COMPETITIVE ACQUISITION.—Section 1862(a) (42 U.S.C. 1395y(a)), as amended by section 4034(b)(4), is amended—

(1) by striking "or" at the end of paragraph (14);

(2) by striking the period at the end of paragraph (15) and inserting "; or"; and

(3) by inserting after paragraph (15) the following new paragraph:

"(16) where such expenses are for an item or service furnished in a competitive acquisition area (as established by the Secretary under section 1847(a)) by an individual or entity other than the supplier with whom the Secretary has entered into a contract under section 1847(b) for the furnishing of such item or service in that area, unless the Secretary finds that such expenses were incurred in a case of urgent need.".

(c) REDUCTION IN PAYMENT AMOUNTS IF COMPETITIVE ACQUISITION FAILS TO ACHIEVE MINIMUM REDUCTION IN PAYMENTS.—Notwithstanding any other provision of title XVIII of the Social Security Act, if the establishment of competitive acquisition areas under section 1847 of such Act (as added by subsection (a)) and the limitation of coverage for items and services under part B of such title to items and services furnished by providers with competitive acquisition contracts under such section does not result in a reduction of at least 10 percent in the payment amount under part B during a year for any such item or service from the payment amount for the previous year, the Secretary shall reduce the payment amount by such percentage as the Secretary determines necessary to result in such a reduction.

(d) EFFECTIVE DATE.—The amendments made by this section shall apply to items and services furnished under part B of title XVIII of the Social Security Act on or after January 1, 1995.

## SEC. 4119. APPLICATION OF COMPETITIVE ACQUISITION PROCEDURES FOR LABORATORY SERVICES.

(a) IN GENERAL.—Section 1847(c), as added by section 4117(a), is amended—

(1) by redesignating paragraph (4) as paragraph (5); and

(2) by inserting after paragraph (3) the following new paragraph:

"(4) Clinical diagnostic laboratory tests.".

(b) REDUCTION IN FEE SCHEDULE AMOUNTS IF COMPETITIVE ACQUISITION FAILS TO ACHIEVE SAVINGS.—Section 1833(h) (42 U.S.C. 1395l(h)) is amended by adding at the end the following new paragraph:

"(7) Notwithstanding any other provision of this subsection, if the Secretary applies the authority provided under section 1847 to establish competitive acquisition areas for the furnishing of clinical diagnostic laboratory tests in a year and the application of such authority does not result in a reduction of at least 10 percent in the fee schedules and negotiated rates established under this subsection for such tests under this part during the year from the fee schedules and rates for the previous year, the Secretary shall reduce each payment amount otherwise determined under the fee schedules and negotiated rates established under this subsection by such percentage as the

Secretary determines necessary to result in such a reduction.''.

## PART 3—SAVINGS RELATING TO PARTS A AND B

### SEC. 4131. MEDICARE SECONDARY PAYER CHANGES.

(a) EXTENSION OF DATA MATCH.—

(1) Section 1862(b)(5)(C) (42 U.S.C. 1395y(b)(5)(C)) is amended by striking clause (iii).

(2) Section 6103(l)(12) of the Internal Revenue Code of 1986 is amended by striking subparagraph (F).

(b) REPEAL OF SUNSET ON APPLICATION TO DISABLED EMPLOYEES OF EMPLOYERS WITH MORE THAN 20 EMPLOYEES.—Section 1862(b)(1)(B)(iii) (42 U.S.C. 1395y(b)(1)(B)(iii)), as amended by section 13561(b) of OBRA–1993, is amended—

(1) in the heading, by striking "SUNSET" and inserting "EFFECTIVE DATE"; and

(2) by striking ", and October 1, 1998".

(c) EXTENSION OF PERIOD FOR END STAGE RENAL DISEASE BENEFICIARIES.—Section 1862(b)(1)(C) (42 U.S.C. 1395y(b)(1)(C)), as amended by section 13561(c) of OBRA–1993, is amended in the second sentence by striking "and on or before October 1, 1998,".

## SEC. 4132. PAYMENT LIMITS FOR HMOS AND CMPS WITH RISK-SHARING CONTRACTS.

(a) IN GENERAL.—Section 1876(a)(1)(C) (42 U.S.C. 1395mm(a)(1)(C)) is amended—

(1) by inserting ", subject to adjustment to take into account the provisions of the succeeding clauses" before the period,

(2) by striking "(C)" and inserting "(C)(i)", and

(3) by adding at the end the following new clauses:

"(ii) The portion of the annual per capita rate of payment for each such class attributable to payments made from the Federal Supplementary Medical Insurance Trust Fund may not exceed 95 percent of the following amount (unless the portion of the annual per capita rate of payment for each such class attributable to payments made from the Federal Hospital Insurance Trust Fund is less than 95 percent of the weighted national average of all adjusted average per capita costs determined under paragraph (4) for that class that are attributable to payments made from the Federal Hospital Insurance Trust Fund):

"(I) For 1995, 150 percent of the weighted national average of all adjusted average per capita costs determined under paragraph (4) for that class that are attributable to payments made from such

Trust Fund, plus 80 percent of the amount by which (if any) the adjusted average per capita cost for that class exceeds 150 percent of that weighted national average.

"(II) For 1996, 150 percent of the weighted national average of all adjusted average per capita costs determined under paragraph (4) for that class that are attributable to payments made from such Trust Fund, plus 60 percent of the amount by which (if any) the adjusted average per capita cost for that class exceeds 150 percent of that weighted national average.

"(III) For 1997, 150 percent of the weighted national average of all adjusted average per capita costs determined under paragraph (4) for that class that are attributable to payments made from such Trust Fund, plus 40 percent of the amount by which (if any) the adjusted average per capita cost for that class exceeds 150 percent of that weighted national average.

"(IV) For 1998, 150 percent of the weighted national average of all adjusted average per capita costs determined under paragraph (4) for that class that are attributable to payments made from such Trust Fund, plus 20 percent of the amount by which (if any) the adjusted average per capita cost for that class exceeds 150 percent of that weighted national average.

"(V) For 1999 and each succeeding year (subject to the establishment by the Secretary of alternative limits under clause (vi)), 150 percent of the weighted national average of all adjusted average per capita costs determined under paragraph (4) for that class that are attributable to payments made from such Trust Fund.

"(iii) The portion of the annual per capita rate of payment for each such class attributable to payments made from the Federal Hospital Insurance Trust Fund may not exceed 95 percent of the following amount (unless the portion of the annual per capita rate of payment for each such class attributable to payments made from the Federal Supplementary Medical Insurance Trust Fund is less than 95 percent of the weighted national average of all adjusted average per capita costs determined under paragraph (4) for that class that are attributable to payments made from the Federal Supplementary Medical Insurance Trust Fund):

"(I) For 1995, 170 percent of the weighted national average of all adjusted average per capita costs determined under paragraph (4) for that class that are attributable to payments made from such Trust Fund, plus 80 percent of the amount by which (if any) the adjusted average per capita cost for that class exceeds 170 percent of that weighted national average.

"(II) For 1996, 170 percent of the weighted national average of all adjusted average per capita costs determined under paragraph (4) for that class that are attributable to payments made from such Trust Fund, plus 60 percent of the amount by which (if any) the adjusted average per capita cost for that class exceeds 170 percent of that weighted national average.

"(III) For 1997, 170 percent of the weighted national average of all adjusted average per capita costs determined under paragraph (4) for that class that are attributable to payments made from such Trust Fund, plus 40 percent of the amount by which (if any) the adjusted average per capita cost for that class exceeds 170 percent of that weighted national average.

"(IV) For 1998, 170 percent of the weighted national average of all adjusted average per capita costs determined under paragraph (4) for that class that are attributable to payments made from such

Trust Fund, plus 20 percent of the amount by which (if any) the adjusted average per capita cost for that class exceeds 170 percent of that weighted national average.

"(V) For 1999 and each succeeding year (subject to the establishment by the Secretary of alternative limits under clause (vi)), 170 percent of the weighted national average of all adjusted average per capita costs determined under paragraph (4) for that class that are attributable to payments made from such Trust Fund.

"(iv) The portion of the annual per capita rate of payment for each such class attributable to payments made from the Federal Supplementary Medical Insurance Trust Fund may not be less than 80 percent of 95 percent of the weighted national average of all adjusted average per capita costs determined under paragraph (4) for that class that are attributable to payments made from such Trust Fund, unless the portion of the annual per capita rate of payment for each such class attributable to payments made from the Federal Hospital Insurance Trust Fund is greater than 95 percent of the weighted national average of all adjusted average per capita costs determined under paragraph (4) for that class that are attributable to payments made from the Federal Hospital Insurance Trust Fund.

"(v) The portion of the annual per capita rate of payment for each such class attributable to payments made from the Federal Hospital Insurance Trust Fund may not be less than 80 percent of 95 percent of the weighted national average of all adjusted average per capita costs determined under paragraph (4) for that class that are attributable to payments made from such Trust Fund, unless the portion of the annual per capita rate of payment for each such class attributable to payments made from the Federal Supplementary Medical Insurance Trust Fund is greater than 95 percent of the weighted national average of all adjusted average per capita costs determined under paragraph (4) for that class that are attributable to payments made from the Federal Supplementary Medical Insurance Trust Fund.

"(vi) For 2000 and succeeding years, the Secretary may revise any of the percentages otherwise applicable during a year under the preceding clauses (other than clause (i)), but only if the aggregate payments made under this title to eligible organizations under risk-sharing contracts during the year is not greater than the aggregate payments that would have been made under this title to such organizations during the year if the Secretary had not revised the percentages.".

(b) CONFORMING AMENDMENT.—Section 1876(a)(5)(A) (42 U.S.C. 1395mm(a)(5)(A)) is amended by inserting ", adjusted to take into account the limitations imposed by clauses (ii) through (vi) of paragraph (1)(C)" before the period.

## SEC. 4133. REDUCTION IN ROUTINE COST LIMITS FOR HOME HEALTH SERVICES.

(a) REDUCTION IN UPDATE TO MAINTAIN FREEZE IN 1996.—Section 1861(v)(1)(L)(i) (42 U.S.C. 1395x(v)(1)(L)(i)) is amended—

(1) in subclause (II), by striking "or" at the end;

(2) in subclause (III), by striking "112 percent," and inserting "and before July 1, 1996, 112 percent, or"; and

(3) by inserting after subclause (III) the following new subclause:

"(IV) July 1, 1996, 100 percent (adjusted by such amount as the Secretary determines to be necessary to preserve the savings resulting from the enactment of section 13564(a)(1) of the Omnibus Budget Reconciliation Act of 1993),".

(b) BASING LIMITS IN SUBSEQUENT YEARS ON MEDIAN OF COSTS.—

(1) IN GENERAL.—Section 1861(v)(1)(L)(i) (U.S.C. 1395x(v)(1)(L)(i)), as amended by subsection (a), is amended in the matter following subclause (IV) by striking "the mean" and inserting "the median".

(2) EFFECTIVE DATE.—The amendment made by paragraph (1) shall apply to cost reporting periods beginning on or after July 1, 1997.

## SEC. 4134. IMPOSITION OF COPAYMENT FOR CERTAIN HOME HEALTH VISITS.

(a) IN GENERAL.—

(1) PART A.—Section 1813(a) (42 U.S.C. 1395e(a)) is amended by adding at the end the following new paragraph:

"(5) The amount payable for home health services furnished to an individual under this part shall be reduced by a copayment amount equal to 10 percent of the average of all per visit costs for home health services furnished under this title determined under section 1861(v)(1)(L) (as determined by the Secretary on a prospective basis for services furnished during a calendar year), unless such services were furnished to the individual during the 30-

day period that begins on the date the individual is discharged as an inpatient from a hospital.".

(2) PART B.—Section 1833(a)(2) (42 U.S.C. 1395l(a)(2)) is amended—

(A) in subparagraph (A), by striking "to home health services," and by striking the comma after "opinion)";

(B) in subparagraph (D), by striking "and" at the end;

(C) in subparagraph (E), by striking the semicolon at the end and inserting "; and"; and

(D) by adding at the end the following new subparagraph:

"(F) with respect to home health services—

"(i) the lesser of —

"(I) the reasonable cost of such services, as determined under section 1861(v), or

"(II) the customary charges with respect to such services,

less the amount a provider may charge as described in clause (ii) of section 1866(a)(2)(A), "(ii) if such services are furnished by a public provider of services, or by another provider which demonstrates to the satisfaction of the Secretary that a significant portion of its patients are low-income (and requests that payment be made under this clause), free of charge or at nominal charges to the public, the amount determined in accordance with section 1814(b)(2), or

"(iii) if (and for so long as) the conditions described in section 1814(b)(3) are met, the amounts determined under the reimbursement system described in such section,

less a copayment amount equal to 10 percent of the average of all per visit costs for home health services furnished under this title determined under section 1861(v)(1)(L) (as determined by the Secretary on a prospective basis for services furnished during a calendar year), unless such services were furnished to the individual during the 30-day period that begins on the date the individual is discharged as an inpatient from a hospital;".

(3) PROVIDER CHARGES.—Section 1866(a)(2)(A)(i) (42 U.S.C. 1395cc(a)(2)(A)(i)) is amended—

(A) by striking "deduction or coinsurance" and inserting "deduction, coinsurance, or copayment"; and

(B) by striking "or (a)(4)" and inserting "(a)(4), or (a)(5)".

(b) EFFECTIVE DATE.—The amendments made by subsection (a) shall apply to home health services furnished on or after July 1, 1995.

## SEC. 4135. EXPANSION OF CENTERS OF EXCELLENCE.

(a) IN GENERAL.—The Secretary of Health and Human Services shall use a competitive process to contract with centers of excellence for cataract surgery and such other services as the Secretary determines to be appropriate. Payment under title XVIII of the Social Security Act will be made for services subject to such contracts on the basis of negotiated or all-inclusive rates as follows:

(1) The center shall cover services provided in an urban area (as defined in section 1886(d)(2)(D) of the Social Security Act) for years beginning with fiscal year 1995.

(2) The amount of payment made by the Secretary to the center under title XVIII of the Social

Security Act for services covered under the project shall be less than the aggregate amount of the payments that the Secretary would have made to the center for such services had the project not been in effect.

(3) The Secretary shall make payments to the center on such a basis for the following services furnished to individuals entitled to benefits under such title:

>(A) Facility, professional, and related services relating to cataract surgery.

>(B) Coronary artery bypass surgery and related services.

>(C) Such other services as the Secretary and the center may agree to cover under the agreement.

(b) REBATE OF PORTION OF SAVINGS.—In the case of any services provided under a demonstration project conducted under subsection (a), the Secretary shall make a payment to each individual to whom such services are furnished (at such time and in such manner as the Secretary may provide) in an amount equal to 10 percent of the amount by which—

>(1) the amount of payment that would have been made by the Secretary under title XVIII of the

Social Security Act to the center for such services if the services had not been provided under the project, exceeds

(2) the amount of payment made by the Secretary under such title to the center for such services.

### PART 4—PART B PREMIUM

### SEC. 4141. GENERAL PART B PREMIUM.

Section 1839(e) (42 U.S.C. 1395r(e)), as amended by section 13571 of OBRA–1993, is amended—

(1) in paragraph (1)(A), by striking "and prior to January 1999"; and

(2) in paragraph (2), by striking "prior to January 1998".

## Subtitle C—Medicaid

### PART 1—COMPREHENSIVE BENEFIT PACKAGE

### SEC. 4201. LIMITING COVERAGE UNDER MEDICAID OF ITEMS AND SERVICES COVERED UNDER COMPREHENSIVE BENEFIT PACKAGE.

(a) REMOVAL OF COMPREHENSIVE BENEFITS PACKAGE FROM STATE PLAN.—Title XIX is amended by redesignating section 1931 as section 1932 and by inserting after section 1930 the following new section:

## "TREATMENT OF COMPREHENSIVE BENEFIT PACKAGE UNDER HEALTH SECURITY ACT

"SEC. 1931. (a) ITEMS AND SERVICES COVERED UNDER COMPREHENSIVE BENEFIT PACKAGE.—If a State plan for medical assistance under this title provides for payment in accordance with section 1902(a)(63) for a year, notwithstanding any other provision of this title, the State plan under this title is not required to provide medical assistance consisting of payment for items and services in the comprehensive benefit package under subtitle B of title I of the Health Security Act for alliance eligible individuals (as defined in section 1902(5) of such Act).

"(b) CONSTRUCTION.—(1) Payment under section 1902(a)(63) shall not constitute medical assistance for purposes of section 1903(a).

"(2) This section shall not be construed as affecting the provision of medical assistance under this title for items and services included in the comprehensive benefit package for—

    "(A) medicare-eligible individuals, or

    "(B) certain emergency services to certain aliens under section 1903(v)(2).".

(b) SUBSTITUTE REQUIREMENT OF STATE PAYMENT.—Section 1902(a) (42 U.S.C. 1396a(a)) is amended—

(1) by striking "and" at the end of paragraph (61),

(2) by striking the period at the end of paragraph (62) and inserting "; and", and

(3) by inserting after paragraph (62) the following new paragraph:

"(63) provide for payment to regional alliances of the amounts required under part 1 of subtitle C of title VI of such Act.".

(c) NO FEDERAL FINANCIAL PARTICIPATION.—Section 1903(i) (42 U.S.C. 1396b(i)) is amended—

(1) by striking "or" at the end of paragraph (14),

(2) by striking the period at the end of paragraph (15) and inserting "; or", and

(3) by inserting after paragraph (15) the following new paragraph:

"(16) with respect to items and services covered under the comprehensive benefit package under subtitle B of title I of the Health Security Act for alliance eligible individuals (as defined in section 1902(5) of such Act).".

(d) EFFECTIVE DATE.—The amendments made by this section shall apply with respect to items or services furnished in a State on or after January 1 of the first year (as defined in section 1902(17)) for the State.

# PART 2—EXPANDING ELIGIBILITY FOR NURSING FACILITY SERVICES; LONG-TERM CARE INTEGRATION OPTION

## SEC. 4211. SPENDDOWN ELIGIBILITY FOR NURSING FACILITY RESIDENTS.

(a) IN GENERAL.—Section 1902(a)(10)(A)(i) (42 U.S.C. 1396a(a)(10)(A)(i)) is amended—

(1) by striking "or" at the end of subclause (VI);

(2) by striking the semicolon at the end of subclause (VII) and inserting ", or"; and

(3) by inserting after subclause (VII) the following new subclause:

"(VIII) who are individuals who would meet the income and resource requirements of the appropriate State plan described in subclause (I) or the supplemental security income program (as the case may be), if incurred expenses for medical care as recognized under State law were deducted from income;".

(b) LIMITATION TO BENEFITS FOR NURSING FACILITY SERVICES.—Section 1902(a)(10)(A) of such Act (42 U.S.C. 1396a(a)(10)(A)), as amended by section

13603(c)(1) of OBRA–1993, is amended in the matter following subparagraph (F)—

>(1) by striking "and (XIII)" and inserting "(XIII)"; and

>(2) by inserting before the semicolon at the end the following: ", and (XIV) the medical assistance made available to an individual described in subparagraph (A)(i)(VIII) shall be limited to medical assistance for nursing facility services, except to the extent that assistance is provided in accordance with the option described in section 1932 in the case of a State exercising such option".

(c) EFFECTIVE DATE.—The amendments made by subsections (a) and (b) shall apply with respect to a State as of January 1, 1996.

## SEC. 4212. INCREASED INCOME AND RESOURCE DISREGARDS FOR NURSING FACILITY RESIDENTS.

(a) INCREASED DISREGARDS FOR PERSONAL NEEDS ALLOWANCE; RESOURCES.—Section 1902(a)(10) (42 U.S.C. 1396a(a)(1)) is amended—

>(1) by striking "and" at the end of paragraph (F); and

>(2) by adding at the end the following new paragraph:

"(G) that, in determining the eligibility of any individual who is an inpatient in a nursing facility or intermediate care facility for the mentally retarded—

"(i) the first $70 of income for each month shall be disregarded; and

"(ii) in the case of an unmarried individual, the first $12,000 of resources may, at the option of the State, be disregarded;".

(b) CONFORMING SSI PERSONAL NEEDS ALLOWANCE.—For provision increasing SSI personal needs allowance, see section 4301.

(c) FEDERAL REIMBURSEMENT FOR REDUCTIONS IN STATE FUNDS ATTRIBUTABLE TO INCREASED DISREGARD.—Section 1903(a) (42 U.S.C. 1396b(a)) is amended—

(1) by striking "plus" at the end of paragraph (6);

(2) by striking the period at the end of paragraph (7) and inserting "; plus"; and

(3) by adding at the end the following new paragraph:

"(8) an amount equal to 100 percent of the difference between the amount of expenditures made by the State for nursing facility services and services in an intermediate care facility for the mentally retarded during the quarter and the amount of expenditures that would have been made by the State for such services during the quarter if the amendment made by subsection (a) had not taken effect (as estimated by the Secretary).''.

(d) EFFECTIVE DATE.—The amendments made by subsection (a) shall apply with respect to months beginning with January 1996.

## SEC. 4213. NEW STATE LONG-TERM CARE INTEGRATION OPTION.

Title XIX, as amended by section 4201(a), is amended by redesignating section 1932 as section 1933 and by inserting after section 1931 the following new section:

"STATE LONG-TERM CARE OPTION

"SEC. 1932. (a) IN GENERAL.—A State under this title may make an election under and subject to the succeeding provisions of this section. Under such an election instead of being entitled to receive payment under section 1903(a) for medical assistance for nursing facility services and intermediate care facilities for the mentally retarded, for one or more defined populations, the State is entitled to receive, subject to subsection (e), payment under section 1903(a) for long-term care services described in subsection (b)(2) for such populations under this section.

"(b) PLAN AMENDMENT REQUIRED.—A State making an election under subsection (a) shall submit a State plan amendment describing—

"(1) the category (or categories) of defined populations (otherwise eligible for medical assistance with respect to nursing facility services or home and community-based services or described in subsection (d)) with respect to whom this section shall apply;

"(2) the long-term care services (within the range of services described in subsection (c)(1)) for which medical assistance is available under the State plan for eligible individuals within each such category of individuals;

"(3) how the provision of such services, and expenditures under this section, will be coordinated with the provision of services and expenditures under part 1 of subtitle B of title II of the Health Security Act (relating to State programs for home and community-based services for individuals with disabilities); and

"(4) such other information as the Secretary determines as necessary to carry out this section.

"(c) CARE AND SERVICES.—

"(1) CONTINUUM OF CARE REQUIRED.—The services described in this paragraph shall represent a continuum of long-term care, and shall include (as appropriate based upon a plan of care described in paragraph (2))—

"(A) nursing facility services and other services described in section 1905(a),

"(B) home and community-based services described in section 1915(c) or 1915(d),

"(C) home and community care for functionally disabled elderly individuals described in section 1929, and

"(D) community supported living arrangements services (as defined in section 1930(a)).

"(2) PLAN OF CARE AND SERVICE EVALUATION.—A plan of care described in this paragraph shall—

"(A) be developed in consultation with the individual or, in the case of an individual incapable of participating in the development of the plan of care, the individual's family members or guardian;

"(C) be based on a comprehensive assessment of the individual's need for the continuum of services described in paragraph (1), and

"(D) be periodically updated based upon the individual's needs (but in no event less frequently than every 6 months).

"(3) INTAKE AND ASSESSMENT PROCESS.—A State shall use an intake and assessment process meeting standards established by the Secretary to develop the plan of care required under paragraph (2).

"(4) DISSEMINATION OF INFORMATION.—The State shall provide information about the availability of services under this section, and how to obtain them, in a manner that ensures that such information is widely disseminated to all eligible providers, agencies, and organizations providing services to the population of individuals receiving assistance under this section.

"(d) ADDITIONAL ELIGIBLE POPULATIONS.—

"(1) IN GENERAL.—A State may provide medical assistance under this section, in addition to individuals otherwise eligible for medical assistance, to individuals who would be so eligible but for—

"(A) failure to meet the disability criteria otherwise applicable, or

"(B) subject to paragraph (2), failure to meet income or resource requirements otherwise applicable.

"(2) LIMITATION ON INCOME.—A State may not provide under this subsection medical assistance to an individual whose income (as determined under section 1612 for purposes of the supplemental security income program) exceeds the greater of—

"(A) the income official poverty line (as defined by the Office of Management and Budget, and revised annually in accordance with section 673(2) of the Omnibus Budget Reconciliation Act of 1981), or

"(B) the maximum level of State supplementary payment under section 1616 (or under section 212 of Public Law 93–66).

"(e) RULES RELATING TO FEDERAL FINANCIAL PARTICIPATION.—

"(1) IN GENERAL.—With respect to medical assistance provided under this section for a category of individuals (specified under subsection (b)(1))—

"(A) the amount of medical assistance that may otherwise be taken into account in making payment under section 1903(a)(1) shall not exceed the amount specified in paragraph (2) for the category;

"(B) the amount of State expenditures (other than for medical assistance) that may otherwise be taken into account in making payment under section 1903(a) (other than paragraph (1)) shall not exceed the amount specified in paragraph (3) for the category; and

"(C) a State may include (as expenditures for medical assistance under the State plan) expenditures for room and board and other community-assisted residential services furnished in settings that meet standards established by the Secretary and that otherwise may not qualify as settings for which Federal financial participation is available under this title.

"(2) LIMIT ON MEDICAL ASSISTANCE.—The amount specified in this paragraph (for a calendar quarter or other period) is as follows:

"(A) BASE MEDICAL ASSISTANCE.—The total medical assistance provided under the State plan for the services described in subsection (c)(1) for the category of individuals in the base period (specified by the Secretary).

"(B) UPDATE.—The amount determined under subparagraph (A) shall be updated (to the calendar quarter or other period involved)—

"(i) for periods through fiscal year 2002, by the rate of growth (estimated by the Secretary) in the medical assistance described in subparagraph (A) under the State plan if the election in subsection (a) had not been made, and

"(ii) beginning in fiscal year 2003, by a factor (for each such fiscal year) equivalent to the product of the factors described in subparagraph (A) and (B) of section 2109(a)(2) of the Health Security Act for the fiscal year.

"(3) LIMIT ON ADMINISTRATION.—The amount specified in this paragraph is such amount as the State establishes, to the satisfaction of the Secretary, does not exceed the amount of expenditures that would have been made for administrative expenditures with respect to services covered under this section if the election in subsection (a) had not been made.

"(4) EFFECT ON ENTITLEMENT.—In the case of a State that has made an election under subsection (a), notwithstanding any other provision of this title, no individual is entitled to medical assistance under the State plan for nursing facility services and intermediate care facilities for the mentally retarded except as the State provides under this section.

"(f) OTHER REQUIREMENTS.—

"(1) SAFEGUARDS.—The State must establish necessary safeguards (including adequate standards for provider participation) have been taken to protect the health and welfare of individuals provided services under this section and to assure financial accountability of funds. Nothing in this section shall be construed as waiving requirements otherwise applicable under this title with respect to providers of covered services.

"(2) FINANCIAL COORDINATION.—The State must provide for the financial coordination of expenditures for medical assistance under this section with expenditures under any State program for home and community-based services for individuals with disabilities under part 1 of subtitle B of title II of the Health Security Act.".

## SEC. 4214. INFORMING NURSING HOME RESIDENTS ABOUT AVAILABILITY OF ASSISTANCE FOR HOME AND COMMUNITY-BASED SERVICES.

(a) IN GENERAL.—Section 1902(a) (42 U.S.C. 1396a(a)) is amended—

(1) by striking "and" at the end of paragraph (61),

(2) by striking the period at the end of paragraph (62) and inserting "; and", and

(3) by inserting after paragraph (62) the following new paragraph:

"(63) provide, in the case of an individual who is a resident (or who is applying to become a resident) of a nursing facility or intermediate care facility for the mentally retarded, at the time of application for medical assistance and periodically thereafter, the individual (or a designated representative) with information on the range of home and community-based services for which assistance is available in the State either under the plan under this title, under the program under part 1 of subtitle B of title II of the Health Security Act, or any other public program.".

(b) EFFECTIVE DATE.—The amendments made by this section shall apply to quarters beginning on or after January 1, 1996.

# PART 3—OTHER BENEFITS

## SEC. 4221. TREATMENT OF ITEMS AND SERVICES NOT COVERED UNDER THE COMPREHENSIVE BENEFIT PACKAGE.

(a) CONTINUATION OF ELIGIBILITY FOR ASSISTANCE FOR AFDC AND SSI RECIPIENTS.—With respect to an individual who is described in section 1933(b) of the Social Security Act (as added by subsection (b)(1)), nothing in this Act shall be construed as—

 (1) changing the eligibility of the individual for medical assistance under title XIX of the Social Security Act for items and services not covered under the comprehensive benefit package, or

 (2) subject to the amendments made by this subtitle, changing the amount, duration, or scope of medical assistance required (or permitted) to be provided to the individual under such title.

(b) LIMITATION ON SCOPE OF ASSISTANCE FOR OTHER MEDICAID BENEFICIARIES.—

 (1) IN GENERAL.—Title XIX, as amended by sections 4201 and 4213, is amended by redesignating section 1933 as section 1934 and by inserting after section 1932 the following new section:

## "LIMITATION ON SCOPE OF ASSISTANCE FOR MOST NON-CASH BENEFICIARIES

"SEC 1933. (a) LIMITATION.—Notwithstanding any other provision of this title, the medical assistance made available under section 1902(a) to an individual not described in subsection (b) shall be limited to medical assistance for—

"(1) long-term care services (as defined in subsection (c)); and

"(2) medicare cost-sharing (as defined in section 1905(p)(3)), in accordance with the requirements of section 1902(a)(10)(E).

"(b) INDIVIDUALS EXEMPT FROM LIMITATION.—The individuals described in this subsection are the following:

"(1) AFDC recipients (as defined in section 1902(3) of the Health Security Act) 18 years of age or older.

"(2) SSI recipients (as defined in section 1902(33) of the Health Security Act) 18 years of age or older.

"(3) Individuals entitled to benefits under title XVIII.

"(c) LONG-TERM CARE SERVICES DEFINED.—In subsection (a), the term 'long-term care services' means the following items and services, but only to the extent they are not included as an item or service under the comprehensive benefit package under the Health Security Act:

"(1) Nursing facility services and intermediate care facility services for the mentally retarded (including items and services that may be included in such services pursuant to regulations in effect as of October 26, 1993).

"(2) Personal care services.

"(3) Home or community-based services provided under a waiver granted under subsection (c), (d), or (e) of section 1915.

"(4) Home and community care provided to functionally disabled elderly individuals under section 1929.

"(5) Community supported living arrangements services provided under section 1930.

"(6) Case-management services (as described in section 1915(g)(2)).

"(7) Home health care services, clinic services, and rehabilitation services that are furnished to an individual who has a condition or disability that qualifies the individual to receive any of the services described in paragraphs (1) through (6).

"(8) Hospice care.".

(2) CONFORMING AMENDMENT.—Section 1902(a)(10) of such Act (42 U.S.C. 1396a(a)(10)), as amended by section 13603(c)(1) of OBRA–1993 and section 4211(b), is amended in the matter following subparagraph (G) (as inserted by section 4212(a))—

>(A) by striking "and (XIV)" and inserting "(XIV)"; and

>(B) by inserting before the semicolon at the end the following: ", and (XV) the medical assistance made available to an individual who is not described in section 1933(b) shall be limited in accordance with section 1933".

(c) CONFORMING AMENDMENTS RELATING TO SECONDARY PAYER.—(1) Section 1902(a)(25)(A) (42 U.S.C. 1396a(a)(25)(A)), as amended by section 13622(a) of OBRA–1993, is amended by inserting "health plans (as defined in section 1400 of the Health Security Act)," after "of 1974),".

(2) Section 1903(o) (42 U.S.C. 1396b(o)), as so amended, is amended by inserting "and a health plan (as defined in section 1400 of the Health Security Act)" after "of 1974)".

(d) EFFECTIVE DATE.—The amendments made by this section shall apply to items and services furnished in a State on or after January 1 of the first year for which the State is a participating State under the Health Security Act.

**SEC. 4222. ESTABLISHMENT OF PROGRAM FOR POVERTY-LEVEL CHILDREN WITH SPECIAL NEEDS.**

(a) ESTABLISHMENT OF PROGRAM.—Title XIX, as amended by sections 4201 and 4213 and by subsection (b), is amended by redesignating section 1934 as section 1935 and by inserting after section 1933 the following new section:

"SERVICES FOR POVERTY-LEVEL CHILDREN WITH SPECIAL NEEDS

"SEC 1934. (a) ESTABLISHMENT OF PROGRAM.—There is hereby established a program under which the Secretary shall make payments on behalf of each qualified child (as defined in subsection (b)) during a year for all medically necessary items and services described in section 1905(a) (including items and services described in section 1905(r) but excluding long-term care services described in section 1933(c)) that are not included in the comprehensive benefit package under subtitle B of title I of the Health Security Act.

"(b) QUALIFIED CHILD DEFINED.—

"(1) IN GENERAL.—In this section, a 'qualified child' is an eligible individual (as defined in section 1001(c)) who—

"(A) for years prior to 1998, is a resident of a participating State under the Health Security Act;

"(B) is under the age of 18; and

"(C) meets the requirements relating to financial eligibility described in paragraph (2).for kids over 6, is 100%: missing date; at 100% (vo. 133%); also excluded children eligible by virtue of medcailly needy;

"(2) REQUIREMENTS RELATING TO FINANCIAL ELIGIBILITY.—An individual meets the requirements of this paragraph if—

"(A) the individual is an AFDC recipient or an SSI recipient (as such terms are defined in section 1902 of the Health Security Act);

"(B) the individual is eligible to receive medical assistance under the State plan under section 1902(a)(10)(C); or

"(C) the individual is—

"(i) under one year of age and has adjusted family income at or below 133 percent of the applicable poverty level (as defined in section 1902(25)(A) of the Health Security Act) (or, in the case of a State that established an income level greater than 133 percent for individuals under 1 year of age for purposes of section 1902(l)(2)(A) as of October 1, 1993, an income level which is a percentage of such level not greater than 185 percent),

"(ii) the individual has attained 1 year of age but is under 6 years of age and has adjusted family income at or below 133 percent of the applicable poverty level (as defined in section 1902(25)(A) of the Health Security Act), or

"(iii) the individual was born after September 30, 1983, has attained 6 years of age, and has adjusted family income at or below 100 percent of the applicable poverty level (as defined in section 1902(25)(A) of the Health Security Act).

"(3) ENROLLMENT PROCEDURES.—

"(A) IN GENERAL.—Not later than July 1, 1995, the Secretary shall establish procedures for the enrollment of qualified children in the program under this section under which—

"(i) essential community providers certified by the Secretary under subpart B of part 2 of subtitle F of title I of the

Health Security Act serve as enrollment sites for the program; and

"(ii) any forms used for enrollment purposes are designed to make the enrollment as simple as practicable.

"(B) INDIVIDUALS UNDER ALLIANCE PLANS AUTOMATICALLY ENROLLED.—The Secretary shall establish a process under which an individual who is a qualified child under paragraph (1) and is enrolled in an alliance health plan (as defined in section 1300 of the Health Security Act) shall automatically be deemed to have met any enrollment requirements established under paragraph (1).

"(c) ADDITIONAL RESPONSIBILITIES OF SECRETARY.—Not later than July 1, 1995, the Secretary shall promulgate such regulations as are necessary to establish and operate the program under this section, including regulations with respect to the following:

"(1) The benefits to be provided and the circumstances under which such benefits shall be considered medically necessary.

"(2) Procedures for the periodic redetermination of an individual's eligibility for benefits.

"(3) Qualification criteria for providers participating in the program.

"(4) Payment amounts for services provided under the program, the methodology used to determine such payment amounts, and the procedures for making payments to providers.

"(5) Standards to ensure the quality of services and the coordination of services under the program with services under the comprehensive benefit package, as well as services under parts B and H of the Individuals With Disabilities Education Act, title V, and any other program providing health care, remedial, educational, and social services to qualified children as the Secretary may identify.

"(6) Hearing and appeals for individuals adversely affected by any determination by the Secretary under the program.

"(7) Such other requirements as the Secretary determines to be necessary for the proper and efficient administration of the program.

"(d) FEDERAL PAYMENT FOR PROGRAM.—

"(1) IN GENERAL.—Subject to paragraph (2), the Secretary shall pay 100 percent of the costs of providing benefits under this program in a year, including all administrative expenses.

"(2) ANNUAL LIMIT ON EXPENDITURES.—The total amount of Federal expenditures that may be made under this section in a year may not exceed—

"(A) for a year prior to 1998, an amount equal to the percentage of total expenditures for medical assistance under State plans under this title during fiscal year 1993 for services described in subsection (a) furnished to qualified children that is attributable to States in which the program is in operation during the year (adjusted to take into account the operation of the program under this section on a calendar year basis)—

"(i) adjusted to take into account any increases or decreases in the number of qualified children under the most recent decennial census, as adjusted by the most recent current population survey for the year in question, and

"(ii) adjusted by the applicable percentage applied to the State non-cash baseline amount for the year under section 9003(a) of the Health Security Act; and

"(B) for 1998, the total expenditures for medical assistance under State plans under this title during 1993 for services described in subsection (a) furnished to qualified children (adjusted to take into account the operation of the program under this section on a calendar year basis)—

"(i) adjusted to take into account any increases or decreases in the number of qualified children under the most recent decennial census, as adjusted by the most recent current population survey for the year in question, and

"(ii) adjusted by the update applied to the State non-cash baseline amount for the year under section 9003(b) of the Health Security Act; and

"(C) for each succeeding year, the limit established under this paragraph for the previous year (adjusted to take into account the operation of the program under this section on a calendar year basis), adjusted by the update applied to the State non-cash baseline amount for the year under section 9003(b) of the Health Security Act.".

(b) REPEAL OF ALTERNATIVE ELIGIBILITY STANDARDS FOR CHILDREN IN PARTICIPATING STATES.—Section 1902(r)(2) (42 U.S.C. 1396a(r)(2)) is amended by adding at the end the following new subparagraph:

"(C) Subparagraph (A) shall not apply with respect to the determination of income and resources for children under age 18 under the State plan of a State (other than under the State plan of a State that utilized an alternative methodology pursuant to such subparagraph as of October 1, 1993)—

"(i) in the case of a State that is a participating State under the Health Security Act for a year prior to 1998, for quarters beginning on or after January 1 of the first year for which the State is such a participating State; and

"(ii) in the case of any State not described in clause (i), for quarters beginning on or after January 1, 1998.".

## PART 4—DISCONTINUATION OF CERTAIN PAYMENT POLICIES

### SEC. 4231. DISCONTINUATION OF MEDICAID DSH PAYMENTS.

(a) ELIMINATION OF SPECIFIC OBLIGATION.—Section 1923(a) (42 U.S.C. 1396r–4(a)) is amended by adding at the end the following new paragraph:

"(5) Notwithstanding any other provision of this title, the requirement of this subsection shall not apply—

"(A) with respect to a State for any portion of a fiscal year during which the State is a participating State within the meaning of section 1200 of the Health Security Act; or

"(B) with respect to any State for any months beginning on or after January 1, 1997.".

(b) ELIMINATION OF STATE PLAN REQUIREMENT.—Section 1902(a)(13)(A) (42 U.S.C. 1396a(a)(13)(A)) is amended by inserting after "special needs" the following: "(but only with respect to a quarters during which the State is not a participating State within the meaning of section 1200 of the Health Security Act or with respect to any quarters ending on or before December 31, 1996)".

(c) ELIMINATION OF STATE DSH ALLOTMENTS AND FEDERAL FINANCIAL PARTICIPATION.—Section 1923(f) (42 U.S.C. 1396r–4(f)) is amended—

(1) in paragraph (2), by inserting "and paragraph (5)" after "subparagraph (B)", and

(2) by adding at the end the following new paragraph:

"(5) ELIMINATION OF ALLOTMENTS FOR PARTICIPATING STATES AND SUNSET FOR ALL STATES.—

"(A) IN GENERAL.—Notwithstanding any other provision of this section, the State DSH allotment shall be zero with respect to—

"(i) any participating State within the meaning of section 1200 of the Health Security Act; and

"(ii) any State for any portion of a fiscal year that occurs on or after January 1, 1997.

"(B) NO REDISTRIBUTION OF REDUCTIONS.—In the computation of State supplemental amounts under paragraph (3), the State DSH allotments shall be determined under subparagraph (A)(ii) of such paragraph as if this paragraph did not apply.".

**SEC. 4232. DISCONTINUATION OF REIMBURSEMENT STANDARDS FOR INPATIENT HOSPITAL SERVICES.**

Section 1902(a)(13)(A) (42 U.S.C. 1396a(a)(13)(A)), as amended by section 4231(b), is amended by inserting "(in the case of services other than hospital services in a State that is a participating State under the Health Security Act)" before "are reasonable and adequate".

## PART 5—COORDINATION WITH ADMINISTRATIVE SIMPLIFICATION AND QUALITY MANAGEMENT INITIATIVES

### SEC. 4241. REQUIREMENTS FOR CHANGES IN BILLING PROCEDURES.

(a) LIMITATION ON FREQUENCY OF SYSTEM CHANGES; ADVANCE NOTIFICATION TO PROVIDERS.—Section 1902(a) (42 U.S.C. 1396a(a)), as amended by section 4213, is amended—

(1) by striking "and" at the end of paragraph (62),

(2) by striking the period at the end of paragraph (63) and inserting "; and", and

(3) by inserting after paragraph (63) the following new paragraph:

"(64) provide that the State—

"(A) will not implement any change in the system used for the billing and processing of claims for payment for items and services furnished under the State plan within 6 months of implementing any previous change in such system; and

"(B) shall notify individuals and entities providing medical assistance under the State plan of any major change in the procedures for billing for services furnished under the plan at least 120 days before such change is to take effect.".

(b) EFFECTIVE DATE.—The amendments made by subsection (a) shall apply to a State as of January 1 of the first year for which the State is a participating State.

## PART 6—MEDICAID COMMISSION

**SEC. 4251. MEDICAID COMMISSION.**

(a) ESTABLISHMENT.—There is established a commission to be known as the "Medicaid Commission" (in this section referred to as the "Commission").

(b) MEMBERSHIP.—(1) The Commission shall be composed of 15 members appointed by the Secretary for the life of the Commission.

(2) Members shall include representatives of the Federal Government and State Governments.

(3) The Administrator of the Health Care Financing Administration shall be an ex officio member of the Commission.

(4) Individuals, while serving as members of the Commission, shall not be entitled to compensation, other than travel expenses, including per diem in lieu of subsist-

ence, in accordance with sections 5702 and 5703 of title 5, United States Code.

(c) STUDY.—The Commission shall study options with respect to each of the following in relation to the medicaid program under title XIX of the Social Security Act:

    (1) USE OF BLOCK GRANT.—Whether, and (if so) how, to convert payments for services not covered in the comprehensive benefit package (for all recipients, including AFDC and SSI recipients defined in section 1902 of the Health Security Act) into new financing mechanisms that give the States greater flexibility in targeting and delivering needed services.

    (2) INTEGRATION OF ACUTE AND LONG-TERM CARE SERVICES FOR HEALTH PLANS.—Whether, and (if so) how, to integrate long-term care services and the home and community-based services program under part 1 of subtitle B of title II with the services covered under the comprehensive benefit package offered by health plans.

    (3) CONSOLIDATING INSTITUTIONAL AND HOME AND COMMUNITY-BASED LONG-TERM CARE.—Whether, and (if so) how, to offer States an option to combine together expenditures under the home and com-

munity-based services program (under part 1 of subtitle B of title II) with continuing home and community-based services and institutional care under the medicaid program into a global budget for long-term care services, and how such a combined program could be implemented.

(d) REPORT AND RECOMMENDATIONS.—The Commission shall submit to the Secretary and the National Health Board, not later than 1 year after the date of the enactment of this Act, a report on its study under subsection (c). The Commission shall include in such report such recommendations for changes in the medicaid program, and the programs under this Act, as it deems appropriate.

(e) OPERATIONS.—(1) The Commission shall appoint a chair from among its members.

(2) Upon request of the Chair of the Commission, the head of any Federal department or agency may detail, on a reimbursable basis, any of the personnel of that department or agency to the Commission to assist it in carrying out its duties under this section.

(3) The Commission may secure directly from any department or agency of the United States information necessary to enable it to carry out this section. Upon request of the Chair of the Commission, the head of that depart-

ment or agency shall furnish that information to the Commission.

(4) Upon the request of the Commission, the Administrator of General Services shall provide to the Commission, on a reimbursable basis, the administrative support services necessary for the Commission to carry out its responsibilities under this section.

(e) TERMINATION.—The Commission shall terminate 90 days after the date of submission of its report under subsection (d).

(f) AUTHORIZATION OF APPROPRIATIONS.—There are authorized to be appropriate such sums as may be necessary to carry out this section.

# Subtitle D—Increase in SSI Personal Needs Allowance

SEC. 4301. INCREASE IN SSI PERSONAL NEEDS ALLOWANCE.

(a) IN GENERAL.—Section 1611(e)(1)(B) (42 U.S.C. 1382(e)(1)(B)) is amended—

(1) in clauses (i) and (ii)(I), by striking "$360" and inserting "$840"; and

(2) in clause (iii), by striking "$720" and inserting "$1,680".

(b) EFFECTIVE DATE.—The amendments made by subsection (a) shall apply with respect to months beginning with January 1996.

# TITLE V—QUALITY AND CONSUMER PROTECTION

TABLE OF CONTENTS OF TITLE

## Subtitle A—Quality Management and Improvement

Sec. 5001. National Quality Management Program.
Sec. 5002. National Quality Management Council.
Sec. 5003. National measures of quality performance.
Sec. 5004. Consumer surveys.
Sec. 5005. Evaluation and reporting of quality performance.
Sec. 5006. Development and dissemination of practice guidelines.
Sec. 5007. Research on health care quality.
Sec. 5008. Regional professional foundations.
Sec. 5009. National Quality Consortium.
Sec. 5010. Eliminating CLIA requirement for certificate of waiver for simple laboratory examinations and procedures.
Sec. 5012. Role of alliances in quality assurance.
Sec. 5013. Role of health plans in quality management.

## Subtitle B—Information Systems, Privacy, and Administrative Simplification

### PART 1—HEALTH INFORMATION SYSTEMS

Sec. 5101. Establishment of health information system.
Sec. 5102. Additional requirements for health information system.
Sec. 5103. Electronic data network.
Sec. 5104. Unique identifier numbers.
Sec. 5105. Health security cards.
Sec. 5106. Technical assistance in the establishment of health information systems.

### PART 2—PRIVACY OF INFORMATION

Sec. 5120. Health information system privacy standards.
Sec. 5121. Other duties with respect to privacy.
Sec. 5122. Comprehensive health information privacy protection act.
Sec. 5123. Definitions.

### PART 3—INTERIM REQUIREMENTS FOR ADMINISTRATIVE SIMPLIFICATION

Sec. 5130. Standard benefit forms.

### PART 4—GENERAL PROVISIONS

Sec. 5140. National Privacy and Health Data Advisory Council.
Sec. 5141. Civil money penalties.
Sec. 5142. Relationship to other laws.

## Subtitle C—Remedies and Enforcement

### PART 1—REVIEW OF BENEFIT DETERMINATIONS FOR ENROLLED INDIVIDUALS

### SUBPART A—GENERAL RULES

Sec. 5201. Health plan claims procedure.
Sec. 5202. Review in regional alliance complaint review offices of grievances based on acts or practices by health plans.
Sec. 5203. Initial proceedings in complaint review offices.
Sec. 5204. Hearings before hearing officers in complaint review offices.
Sec. 5205. Review by Federal Health Plan Review Board.
Sec. 5206. Civil money penalties.

### SUBPART B—EARLY RESOLUTION PROGRAMS

Sec. 5211. Establishment of early resolution programs in complaint review offices.
Sec. 5212. Initiation of participation in mediation proceedings.
Sec. 5213. Mediation proceedings.
Sec. 5214. Legal effect of participation in mediation proceedings.
Sec. 5215. Enforcement of settlement agreements.

### PART 2—ADDITIONAL REMEDIES AND ENFORCEMENT PROVISIONS

Sec. 5231. Judicial review of Federal action on State systems.
Sec. 5232. Administrative and judicial review relating to cost containment.
Sec. 5233. Civil enforcement.
Sec. 5234. Priority of certain bankruptcy claims.
Sec. 5235. Private right to enforce State responsibilities.
Sec. 5236. Private right to enforce Federal responsibilities in operating a system in a State.
Sec. 5237. Private right to enforce responsibilities of alliances.
Sec. 5238. Discrimination claims.
Sec. 5239. Nondiscrimination in federally assisted programs.
Sec. 5240. Civil action by essential community provider.
Sec. 5241. Facial constitutional challenges.
Sec. 5242. Treatment of plans as parties in civil actions.
Sec. 5243. General nonpreemption of existing rights and remedies.

## Subtitle D—Medical Malpractice

### PART 1—LIABILITY REFORM

Sec. 5301. Federal tort reform.
Sec. 5302. Plan-based alternative dispute resolution mechanisms.
Sec. 5303. Requirement for certificate of merit.
Sec. 5304. Limitation on amount of attorney's contingency fees.
Sec. 5305. Reduction of awards for recovery from collateral sources.
Sec. 5306. Periodic payment of awards.

### PART 2—OTHER PROVISIONS RELATING TO MEDICAL MALPRACTICE LIABILITY

Sec. 5311. Enterprise liability demonstration project.
Sec. 5312. Pilot program applying practice guidelines to medical malpractice liability actions.

## Subtitle E—Fraud and Abuse

### PART 1—ESTABLISHMENT OF ALL-PAYER HEALTH CARE FRAUD AND ABUSE CONTROL PROGRAM

Sec. 5401. All-Payer Health Care Fraud and Abuse Control Program.
Sec. 5402. Establishment of All-Payer Health Care Fraud and Abuse Control Account.
Sec. 5403. Use of funds by Inspector General.

PART 2—APPLICATION OF FRAUD AND ABUSE AUTHORITIES UNDER THE SOCIAL SECURITY ACT TO ALL PAYERS

Sec. 5411. Exclusion from participation.
Sec. 5412. Civil monetary penalties.
Sec. 5413. Limitations on physician self-referral.
Sec. 5414. Construction of Social Security Act references.

PART 3—AMENDMENTS TO ANTI-FRAUD AND ABUSE PROVISIONS UNDER THE SOCIAL SECURITY ACT

Sec. 5421. Reference to amendments.

PART 4—AMENDMENTS TO CRIMINAL LAW

Sec. 5431. Health care fraud.
Sec. 5432. Forfeitures for violations of fraud statutes.
Sec. 5433. False statements.
Sec. 5434. Bribery and graft.
Sec. 5435. Injunctive relief relating to health care offenses.
Sec. 5436. Grand jury disclosure.
Sec. 5437. Theft or embezzlement.
Sec. 5438. Misuse of health security card or unique identifier.

PART 5—AMENDMENTS TO CIVIL FALSE CLAIMS ACT

Sec. 5441. Amendments to Civil False Claims Act.

**Subtitle F—McCarran-Ferguson Reform**

Sec. 5501. Repeal of exemption for health insurance.

# Subtitle A—Quality Management and Improvement

### SEC. 5001. NATIONAL QUALITY MANAGEMENT PROGRAM.

Not later than 1 year after the date of the enactment of this Act, the National Health Board shall establish and oversee a performance-based program of quality management and improvement designed to enhance the quality, appropriateness, and effectiveness of health care services and access to such services. The program shall be known as the National Quality Management Program and shall be administered by the National Quality Management Council established under section 5002.

**SEC. 5002. NATIONAL QUALITY MANAGEMENT COUNCIL.**

(a) ESTABLISHMENT.—There is established a council to be known as the National Quality Management Council.

(b) DUTIES.—The Council shall—

    (1) administer the National Quality Management Program;

    (2) perform any other duty specified as a duty of the Council in this subtitle; and

    (3) advise the National Health Board with respect its duties under this subtitle.

(c) NUMBER AND APPOINTMENT.—The Council shall be composed of 15 members appointed by the President. The Council shall consist of members who are broadly representative of the population of the United States and shall include—

    (1) individuals representing the interests of governmental and corporate purchasers of health care;

    (2) individuals representing the interests of health plans;

    (3) individuals representing the interests of States;

(4) individuals representing the interests of health care providers and academic health centers (as defined in section 3101(c)); and

(5) individuals distinguished in the fields of public health, health care quality, and related fields of health services research.

(d) TERMS.—

(1) IN GENERAL.—Except as provided in paragraph (2), members of the Council shall serve for a term of 3 years.

(2) STAGGERED ROTATION.—Of the members first appointed to the Council under subsection (c), the President shall appoint 5 members to serve for a term of 3 years, 5 members to serve for a term of 2 years, and 5 members to serve for a term of 1 year.

(3) SERVICE BEYOND TERM.—A member of the Council may continue to serve after the expiration of the term of the member until a successor is appointed.

(e) VACANCIES.—If a member of the Council does not serve the full term applicable under subsection (d), the individual appointed to fill the resulting vacancy shall be appointed for the remainder of the term of the predecessor of the individual.

(f) CHAIR.—The President shall designate an individual to serve as the chair of the Council.

(g) MEETINGS.—The Council shall meet not less than once during each discrete 4-month period and shall otherwise meet at the call of the President or the chair.

(h) COMPENSATION AND REIMBURSEMENT OF EXPENSES.—Members of the Council shall receive compensation for each day (including travel time) engaged in carrying out the duties of the Council. Such compensation may not be in an amount in excess of the maximum rate of basic pay payable for level IV of the Executive Schedule under section 5315 of title 5, United States Code.

(i) STAFF.—The National Health Board shall provide to the Council such staff, information, and other assistance as may be necessary to carry out the duties of the Council.

(j) HEALTH CARE PROVIDER.—For purposes of this subtitle, the term "health care provider" means an individual who, or entity that, provides an item or service to an individual that is covered under the health plan (as defined in section 1400) in which the individual is enrolled.

SEC. 5003. NATIONAL MEASURES OF QUALITY PERFORMANCE.

(a) IN GENERAL.—The National Quality Management Council shall develop a set of national measures of quality performance, which shall be used to assess the provision of health care services and access to such services.

(b) SUBJECT OF MEASURES.—National measures of quality performance shall be selected in a manner that provides information on the following subjects:

(1) Access to health care services by consumers.

(2) Appropriateness of health care services provided to consumers.

(3) Outcomes of health care services and procedures.

(4) Health promotion.

(5) Prevention of diseases, disorders, and other health conditions.

(6) Consumer satisfaction with care.

(c) SELECTION OF MEASURES.—

(1) CONSULTATION.—In developing and selecting the national measures of quality performance, the National Quality Management Council shall consult with appropriate interested parties, including—

(A) States;

(B) health plans;

(C) employers and individuals purchasing health care through regional and corporate alliances;

(D) health care providers;

(E) the National Quality Consortium established under section 5009;

(F) individuals distinguished in the fields of law, medicine, economics, public health, and health services research;

(G) the Administrator for Health Care Policy and Research;

(H) the Director of the National Institutes of Health; and

(I) the Administrator of the Health Care Financing Administration.

(2) CRITERIA.—The following criteria shall be used in developing and selecting national measures of quality performance:

(A) SIGNIFICANCE.—When a measure relates to a specific disease, disorder, or other health condition, the disease, disorder, or condition shall be of significance in terms of prevalence, morbidity, mortality, or the costs associated with the prevention, diagnosis, treatment, or clinical management of the disease, disorder, or condition.

(B) RANGE OF SERVICES.—The set of measures, taken as a whole, shall be representative of the range of services provided to consumers of health care by the individuals and entities described in subsection (a).

(C) RELIABILITY AND VALIDITY.—The measures shall be reliable and valid.

(D) UNDUE BURDEN.—The data needed to calculate the measures shall be obtained without undue burden on the entity or individual providing the data.

(E) VARIATION.—Performance with respect to measures that are applicable to each category of individual or entity described in subsection (a) shall be expected to vary widely among individuals or entities in the category.

(F) LINKAGE TO HEALTH OUTCOME.—When a measure is a rate of a process of care, the process shall be linked to a health outcome based upon the best available scientific evidence.

(G) PROVIDER CONTROL AND RISK ADJUSTMENT.—When a measure is an outcome of the provision of care, the outcome shall be within the control of the provider and one with respect to which an adequate risk adjustment can be made.

(H) PUBLIC HEALTH.—The measures may incorporate standards identified by the Secretary of Health and Human Services for meeting public health objectives.

(d) UPDATING.—The National Quality Management Council shall review and update the set of national measures of quality performance annually to reflect changing goals for quality improvement. The Board shall establish and maintain a priority list of performance measures that within a 5-year period it intends to consider for inclusion within the set through the updating process.

## SEC. 5004. CONSUMER SURVEYS.

(a) IN GENERAL.—The National Quality Management Council shall conduct periodic surveys of health care consumers to gather information concerning access to care, use of health services, health outcomes, and patient satisfaction. The surveys shall monitor consumer reaction to the implementation of this Act and be designed to assess the impact of this Act on the general population of the United States and potentially vulnerable populations.

(b) SURVEY ADMINISTRATION.—The National Quality Management Council shall develop and approve a standard design for the surveys, which shall be administered by the Administrator for Health Care Policy and Research on a plan-by-plan and State-by-State basis. A State may add survey questions on quality measures of local interest to surveys conducted in the State.

(c) SAMPLING STRATEGIES.—The National Quality Management Council shall develop sampling strategies that ensure that survey samples adequately measure populations that are considered to be at risk of receiving inadequate health care and may be difficult to reach through consumer-sampling methods, including individuals who—

(1) fail to enroll in a health plan;

(2) resign from a plan; or

(3) are members of a vulnerable population.

## SEC. 5005. EVALUATION AND REPORTING OF QUALITY PERFORMANCE.

(a) NATIONAL GOALS.—In subject matter areas with respect to which the National Quality Management Council determines that sufficient information and consensus exist, the Council will recommend to the Board that it establish goals for performance by health plans and health care providers on a subset of the set of national measures of quality performance.

(b) IMPACT OF REFORM.—The National Quality Management Council shall evaluate the impact of the implementation of this Act on the quality of health care services in the United States and the access of consumers to such services.

(c) PERFORMANCE REPORTS.—

(1) ALLIANCE AND HEALTH PLAN REPORTS.—Each health alliance annually shall publish and make available to the public a performance report outlining in a standard format the performance of each health plan offered in the alliance on the set of national measures of quality performance. The report shall include the results of a smaller number of such measures for health care providers who are members of provider networks of such plans (as defined in section 1402(f)), if the available information is statistically meaningful. The report also shall include the results of consumer surveys described in section 5004 that were conducted in the alliance during the year that is the subject of the report.

(2) NATIONAL QUALITY REPORTS.—The National Quality Management Council annually shall provide to the Congress and to each health alliance a report that—

    (A) outlines in a standard format the performance of each regional alliance, corporate alliance, and health plan;

    (B) discusses State-level and national trends relating to health care quality; and

(C) presents data for each health alliance from consumer surveys described in section 5004 that were conducted during the year that is the subject of the report.

## SEC. 5006. DEVELOPMENT AND DISSEMINATION OF PRACTICE GUIDELINES.

(a) DEVELOPMENT OF GUIDELINES.—

(1) IN GENERAL.—The National Quality Management Council shall direct the Administrator for Health Care Policy and Research to develop and periodically review and update clinically relevant guidelines that may be used by health care providers to assist in determining how diseases, disorders, and other health conditions can most effectively and appropriately be prevented, diagnosed, treated, and managed clinically.

(2) CERTAIN REQUIREMENTS.—Guidelines under paragraph (1) shall—

(A) be based on the best available research and professional judgment regarding the effectiveness and appropriateness of health care services and procedures;

(B) be presented in formats appropriate for use by health care providers, medical educators, medical review organizations, and consumers of health care;

(C) include treatment-specific or condition-specific practice guidelines for clinical treatments and conditions in forms appropriate for use in clinical practice, for use in educational programs, and for use in reviewing quality and appropriateness of medical care;

(D) include information on risks and benefits of alternative strategies for prevention, diagnosis, treatment, and management of a given disease, disorder, or other health condition;

(E) include information on the costs of alternative strategies for the prevention, diagnosis, treatment, and management of a given disease, disorder, or other health condition, where cost information is available and reliable; and

(F) be developed in accordance with priorities that shall be established by the National Quality Management Council based on the research priorities that are established under section 5007(b) and the 5-year priority list of performance measures described in section 5003(d).

(3) HEALTH SERVICE UTILIZATION PROTOCOLS.—The National Quality Management Council shall establish standards and procedures for evaluating the clinical appropriateness of protocols used to manage health service utilization.

(4) USE IN MEDICAL MALPRACTICE LIABILITY PILOT PROGRAM.—Guidelines developed under this subsection may be used by the Secretary of Health and Human Services in the pilot program applying practice guidelines to medical malpractice liability under section 5312.

(b) EVALUATION AND CERTIFICATION OF OTHER GUIDELINES.—

(1) METHODOLOGY.—The National Quality Management Council shall direct the Administrator for Health Care Policy and Research to develop and publish standards relating to methodologies for developing the types of guidelines described in subsection (a)(1).

(2) EVALUATION AND CERTIFICATION.—The National Quality Management Council shall direct the Administrator for Health Care Policy and Research to establish a procedure by which individuals and entities may submit guidelines of the type described in subsection (a)(1) to the Council for eval-

uation and certification by the Council using the standards developed under paragraph (1).

(3) USE IN MEDICAL MALPRACTICE LIABILITY PILOT PROGRAM.—Guidelines certified under paragraph (2) may be used by the Secretary of Health and Human Services in the pilot program applying practice guidelines to medical malpractice liability under section 5312.

(c) GUIDELINE CLEARINGHOUSE.—The National Quality Management Council shall direct the Administrator for Health Care Policy and Research to establish and oversee a clearinghouse and dissemination program for practice guidelines that are developed or certified under this section.

(d) DISSEMINATION OF INFORMATION ON INEFFECTIVE TREATMENTS.—The National Quality Management Council shall disseminate information documenting clinically ineffective treatments and procedures.

**SEC. 5007. RESEARCH ON HEALTH CARE QUALITY.**

(a) RESEARCH SUPPORT.—The National Quality Management Council shall direct the Administrator for Health Care Policy and Research to support research directly related to the 5-year priority list of performance measures described in section 5003(d), including research with respect to—

(1) outcomes of health care services and procedures;

(2) effective and efficient dissemination of information, standards, and guidelines;

(3) methods of measuring quality and shared decisionmaking; and

(4) design and organization of quality of care components of automated health information systems.

(b) RESEARCH PRIORITIES.—The National Quality Management Council shall establish priorities for research with respect to the quality, appropriateness, and effectiveness of health care and make recommendations concerning research projects. In establishing the priorities, the National Quality Management Council shall emphasize research involving diseases, disorders, and health conditions as to which—

(1) there is the highest level of uncertainty concerning treatment;

(2) there is the widest variation in practice patterns;

(3) the costs associated with prevention, diagnosis, treatment, or clinical management are significant; and

(4) the rate of incidence or prevalence is high for the population as a whole or for particular subpopulations.

SEC. 5008. REGIONAL PROFESSIONAL FOUNDATIONS.

(a) ESTABLISHMENT.—The National Health Board shall establish and oversee regional professional foundations to perform the duties specified in subsection (c).

(b) STRUCTURE AND MEMBERSHIP.—

(1) IN GENERAL.—The National Quality Consortium established under section 5009 shall oversee the establishment of regional professional foundations, the membership requirements for each foundation, and any other requirement for the internal operation of each foundation.

(2) ENTITIES ELIGIBLE FOR MEMBERSHIP.—Each regional professional foundation shall include at least one academic health center (as defined in section 3101(c)). The following entities also shall be eligible to serve as members of the regional professional foundation for the region in which the entity is located:

(A) Schools of public health (as defined in section 799 of the Public Health Service Act).

(B) Other schools and programs defined in such section.

(C) Health plans.

(D) Regional alliances.

(E) Corporate alliances.

(F) Health care providers.

(c) DUTIES.—A regional professional foundation shall carry out the following duties for the region in which the foundation is located (such region to be demarcated by the National Health Board with the advice of the National Quality Consortium established under section 5009):

(1) Developing programs in lifetime learning for health professionals (as defined in section 1112(c)(1)) to ensure the delivery of quality health care.

(2) Fostering collaboration among health plans and health care providers to improve the quality of primary and specialized health care.

(3) Disseminating information about successful quality improvement programs, practice guidelines, and research findings.

(4) Disseminating information on innovative uses of health professionals.

(5) Developing innovative patient education systems that enhance patient involvement in decisions relating their health care.

(6) Applying for and conducting research described in section 5007.

(d) PROGRAMS IN LIFETIME LEARNING.—The programs described in subsection (c)(1) shall ensure that health professionals remain abreast of new knowledge, acquire new skills, and adopt new roles as technology and societal demands change.

**SEC. 5009. NATIONAL QUALITY CONSORTIUM.**

(a) ESTABLISHMENT.—The National Health Board shall establish a consortium to be known as the National Quality Consortium.

(b) DUTIES.—The Consortium shall—

(1) establish programs for continuing education for health professionals;

(2) advise the National Quality Management Council and the Administrator for Health Care Policy and Research on research priorities;

(3) oversee the development of the regional professional foundations established under section 5008;

(4) advise the National Quality Management Council with respect to the funding of proposals to establish such foundations;

(5) consult with the National Quality Management Council regarding the selection of national

measures of quality performance under section 5003(c); and

(6) advise the National Health Board and the National Quality Management Council with respect to any other duty of the Board or the Council under this subtitle.

(c) MEMBERSHIP.—The Consortium shall be composed of 11 members appointed by the National Health Board. The members of the Consortium shall include—

(1) 5 individuals representing the interests of academic health centers; and

(2) 6 other individuals representing the interests of one of the following persons:

(A) Schools of public health.

(B) Other schools and programs defined in section 799 of the Public Health Service Act (including medical schools, nursing schools, and allied health professional schools).

(d) TERMS.—

(1) IN GENERAL.—Except as provided in paragraph (2), members of the Consortium shall serve for a term of 3 years.

(2) STAGGERED ROTATION.—Of the members first appointed to the Consortium under subsection (c), the National Health Board shall appoint 4 mem-

bers to serve for a term of 3 years, 3 members to serve for a term of 2 years, and 4 members to serve for a term of 1 year.

(e) CHAIR.—The National Health Board shall designate an individual to serve as the chair of the Consortium.

SEC. 5010. ELIMINATING CLIA REQUIREMENT FOR CERTIFICATE OF WAIVER FOR SIMPLE LABORATORY EXAMINATIONS AND PROCEDURES.

(a) IN GENERAL.—Section 353 of the Public Health Service Act (42 U.S.C. 263a) is amended—

(1) in subsection (b), by inserting before the period at the end the following: "or unless the laboratory is exempt from the certificate requirement under subsection (d)(2)";

(2) by amending paragraph (2) of subsection (d) to read as follows:

"(2) EXEMPTION FROM CERTIFICATE REQUIREMENT FOR LABORATORIES PERFORMING ONLY SIMPLE EXAMINATIONS AND PROCEDURES.—A laboratory which performs only laboratory examinations and procedures described in paragraph (3) is not required to have in effect a certificate under this section."; and

(3) by striking paragraph (4) of subsection (d).

(b) EFFECTIVE DATE.—The amendments made by this section shall take effect on the first day of the first month beginning after the date of the enactment of this Act.

## SEC. 5012. ROLE OF ALLIANCES IN QUALITY ASSURANCE.

Each regional alliance and each corporate alliance shall—

    (1) disseminate to consumers information related to quality and access to aid in their selection of plans in accordance with section 1325;

    (2) disseminate information on the quality of health plans and health care providers contained in reports of the National Quality Management Council section 5005(d);

    (3) ensure through negotiations with health plans that performance and quality standards are continually improved; and

    (4) conduct educational programs in cooperation with regional quality foundations to assist consumers in using quality and other information in choosing health plans.

## SEC. 5013. ROLE OF HEALTH PLANS IN QUALITY MANAGEMENT.

Each health plan shall—

(1) measure and disclose performance on quality measures used by—

 (A) participating States in which the plan does business;

 (B) regional alliances and corporate alliances that offer the plan; and

 (C) the National Quality Management Council;

(2) furnish information required under subtitle B of this title and provide such other reports and information on the quality of care delivered by health care providers who are members of a provider network of the plan (as defined in section 1402(f)) as may be required under this Act; and

(3) maintain quality management systems that—

 (A) use the national measures of quality performance developed by the National Quality Management Council under section 5003; and

 (B) measure the quality of health care furnished to enrollees under the plan by all health care providers who are members of a provider network of the plan.

# Subtitle B—Information Systems, Privacy, and Administrative Simplification

## PART 1—HEALTH INFORMATION SYSTEMS

### SEC. 5101. ESTABLISHMENT OF HEALTH INFORMATION SYSTEM.

(a) IN GENERAL.—Not later than 2 years after the date of the enactment of this Act, the National Health Board shall develop and implement a health information system by which the Board shall collect, report, and regulate the collection and dissemination of the health care information described in subsection (e) pursuant to standards promulgated by the Board and (if applicable) consistent with policies established as part of the National Information Infrastructure Act of 1993.

(b) PRIVACY.—The health information system shall be developed and implemented in a manner that is consistent with the privacy and security standards established under section 5120.

(c) REDUCTION IN ADMINISTRATIVE COSTS.—The health information system shall be developed and implemented in a manner that is consistent with the objectives of reducing wherever practicable and appropriate—

    (1) the costs of providing and paying for health care;

(2) the time, effort, and financial resources expended by persons to provide information to States and the Federal Government.

(d) USES OF INFORMATION.—The health care information described in subsection (e) shall be collected and reported in a manner that facilitates its use for the following purposes:

(1) Health care planning, policy development, policy evaluation, and research by Federal, State, and local governments and regional and corporate alliances.

(2) Establishing and monitoring payments for health services by the Federal Government, States, regional alliances, and corporate alliances.

(3) Assessing and improving the quality of health care.

(4) Measuring and optimizing access to health care.

(5) Evaluating the cost of specific clinical or administrative functions.

(6) Supporting public health functions and objectives.

(7) Improving the ability of health plans, health care providers, and consumers to coordinate, improve, and make choices about health care.

(8) Managing and containing costs at the alliance and plan levels.

(e) HEALTH CARE INFORMATION.—The health care information referred to in subsection (a) shall include data on—

(1) enrollment and disenrollment in health plans;

(2) clinical encounters and other items and services provided by health care providers;

(3) administrative and financial transactions and activities of participating States, regional alliances, corporate alliances, health plans, health care providers, employers, and individuals that are necessary to determine compliance with this Act or an Act amended by this Act;

(4) the characteristics of regional alliances, including the number, and demographic characteristics of eligible individuals residing in each alliance area;

(5) the characteristics of corporate alliances, including the number, and demographic characteristics of individuals who are eligible to be enrolled in each corporate alliance health plan and individuals with respect to whom a large employer has exercised an option under section 1311 to make ineligible for such enrollment;

(6) terms of agreement between health plans and the health care providers who are members of provider networks of the plans (as defined in section 1402(f));

(7) payment of benefits in cases in which benefits may be payable under a health plan and any other insurance policy or health program;

(8) utilization management by health plans and health care providers;

(9) the information collected and reported by the Board or disseminated by other individuals or entities as part of the National Quality Management Program under subtitle A;

(10) grievances filed against regional alliances, corporate alliances, and health plans and the resolutions of such grievances; and

(11) any other fact that may be necessary to determine whether a health plan or a health care provider has complied with a Federal statute pertaining to fraud or misrepresentation in the provision or purchasing of health care or in the submission of a claim for benefits or payment under a health plan.

## SEC. 5102. ADDITIONAL REQUIREMENTS FOR HEALTH INFORMATION SYSTEM.

(a) CONSULTATION.—The health information system shall be developed in consultation with—

    (1) Federal agencies that—

        (A) collect health care information;

        (B) oversee the collection of information or records management by other Federal agencies;

        (C) directly provide health care services;

        (D) provide for payments for health care services; or

        (E) enforce a provision of this Act or any Act amended by this Act;

    (2) the National Quality Management Council established under section 5002;

    (3) participating States;

    (4) regional alliances and corporate alliances;

    (5) health plans;

    (6) representatives of health care providers;

    (7) representatives of employers;

    (8) representatives of consumers of health care;

    (9) experts in public health and health care information and technology; and

    (10) representatives of organizations furnishing health care supplies, services, and equipment.

(b) COLLECTION AND TRANSMISSION REQUIREMENTS.—In establishing standards under section 5101, the National Health Board shall specify the form and manner in which individuals and entities are required to collect or transmit health care information for or to the Board. The Board also shall specify the frequency with which individuals and entities are required to transmit such information to the Board. Such specifications shall include, to the extent practicable—

   (1) requirements for use of uniform paper forms containing standard data elements, definitions, and instructions for completion in cases where the collection or transmission of data in electronic form is not specified by the Board;

   (2) requirements for use of uniform health data sets with common definitions to standardize the collection and transmission of data in electronic form;

   (3) uniform presentation requirements for data in electronic form; and

   (4) electronic data interchange requirements for the exchange of data among automated health information systems.

(c) PREEMPTION OF STATE "PEN & QUILL" LAWS.—A standard established by the National Health Board relating to the form in which medical or health plan records are required to be maintained shall supercede any contrary provision of State law, except where the Board determines that the provision is necessary to prevent fraud and abuse, with respect to controlled substances, or for other purposes.

SEC. 5103. ELECTRONIC DATA NETWORK.

(a) IN GENERAL.—As part of the health information system, the National Health Board shall oversee the establishment of an electronic data network consisting of regional centers that collect, compile, and transmit information.

(b) CONSULTATION.—The electronic data network shall be developed in consultation with—

    (1) Federal agencies that—

        (A) collect health care information;

        (B) oversee the collection of information or records management by other Federal agencies;

        (C) directly provide health care services;

        (D) provide for payments for health care services; or

        (E) enforce a provision of this Act or any Act amended by this Act;

    (2) the National Quality Management Council established under section 5002;

    (3) participating States;

(4) regional alliances and corporate alliances; and

(5) health plans.

(c) DEMONSTRATION PROJECTS.—The electronic data network shall be tested prior to full implementation through the establishment of demonstration projects.

(d) DISCLOSURE OF INDIVIDUALLY IDENTIFIABLE INFORMATION.—The electronic data network may be used to disclose individually identifiable health information (as defined in section 5123(3)) to any individual or entity only in accordance with the health information system privacy standards promulgated by the National Health Board under section 5120.

## SEC. 5104. UNIQUE IDENTIFIER NUMBERS.

(a) IN GENERAL.—As part of the health information system, the Board shall establish a system to provide for a unique identifier number for each—

(1) eligible individual;

(2) employer;

(3) health plan; and

(4) health care provider.

(b) IMPERMISSIBLE DATA LINKS.—In establishing the system under subsection (a), the National Health Board shall ensure that a unique identifier number may not be used to connect individually identifiable health information (as defined in section 5123(3)) that is collected as part of the health information system or that otherwise may be accessed through the number with individually identifiable information from any other source, except in cases where the National Health Board determines that such connection is necessary to carry out a duty imposed on any individual or entity under this Act.

(c) PERMISSIBLE USES OF IDENTIFIER.—The National Health Board shall by regulation establish the purposes for which a unique identifier number provided pursuant to this section may be used.

**SEC. 5105. HEALTH SECURITY CARDS.**

(a) PERMISSIBLE USES OF CARD.—A health security card that is issued to an eligible individual under section 1001(b) may be used by an individual or entity, in accordance with regulations promulgated by the Board, only for the purpose of providing or assisting the eligible individual in obtaining an item or service that is covered under—

   (1) the applicable health plan in which the individual is enrolled (as defined in section 1902);

   (2) a policy consisting of a supplemental health benefit policy (described in part 2 of subtitle E of title I), a cost sharing policy (described in such part), or both;

(3) a FEHBP supplemental plan (described in subtitle C of title VIII);

(4) a FEHBP medicare supplemental plan (described in such subtitle); or

(5) such other programs as the Board may specify.

(b) FORM OF CARD AND ENCODED INFORMATION.—The National Health Board shall establish standards respecting the form of health security cards and the information to be encoded in electronic form on the cards. Such information shall include—

(1) the identity of the individual to whom the card is issued;

(2) the applicable health plan in which the individual is enrolled;

(3) any policy described in paragraph (2), (3), or (4) of subsection (a) in which the individual is enrolled; and

(4) any other information that the National Health Board determines to be necessary in order for the card to serve the purpose described in subsection (a).

(c) UNIQUE IDENTIFIER NUMBERS.—The unique identifier number system developed by the National

Health Board under section 5104 shall be used in encoding the information described in subsection (b).

(d) REGISTRATION OF CARD.—The Board shall take appropriate steps to register the card, the name of the card, and other indicia relating to the card as a trademark or service mark (as appropriate) under the Trademark Act of 1946. For purposes of this subsection, the "Trademark Act of 1946" refers to the Act entitled "An Act to provide for the registration and protection of trademarks used in commerce, to carry out the provisions of international conventions, and for other purposes", approved July 5, 1946 (15 U.S.C. et seq.).

(e) REFERENCE TO CRIME.—For a provision relating to criminal penalties for misuse of a health security card or a unique identifier number, see section 5438.

## SEC. 5106. TECHNICAL ASSISTANCE IN THE ESTABLISHMENT OF HEALTH INFORMATION SYSTEMS.

The National Health Board shall provide information and technical assistance to participating States, regional alliances, corporate alliances, health plans, and health care providers with respect to the establishment and operation of automated health information systems. Such assistance shall focus on—

    (1) the promotion of community-based health information systems; and

(2) the promotion of patient care information systems that collect data at the point of care or as a by-product of the delivery of care.

## PART 2—PRIVACY OF INFORMATION

**SEC. 5120. HEALTH INFORMATION SYSTEM PRIVACY STANDARDS.**

(a) HEALTH INFORMATION SYSTEM STANDARDS.—Not later than 2 years after the date of the enactment of this Act, the National Health Board shall promulgate standards respecting the privacy of individually identifiable health information that is in the health information system described in part 1 of this subtitle. Such standards shall include standards concerning safeguards for the security of such information. The Board shall develop and periodically revise the standards in consultation with—

(1) Federal agencies that—

(A) collect health care information;

(B) oversee the collection of information or records management by other Federal agencies;

(C) directly provide health care services;

(D) provide for payments for health care services; or

(E) enforce a provision of this Act or any Act amended by this Act;

(2) the National Quality Management Council established under section 5002;

(3) participating States;

(4) regional alliances and corporate alliances;

(5) health plans; and

(6) representatives of consumers of health care.

(b) INFORMATION COVERED.—The standards established under subsection (a) shall apply to individually identifiable health information collected for or by, reported to or by, or the dissemination of which is regulated by, the National Health Board under section 5101.

(c) PRINCIPLES.—The standards established under subsection (a) shall incorporate the following principles:

(1) UNAUTHORIZED DISCLOSURE.—All disclosures of individually identifiable health information by an individual or entity shall be unauthorized unless—

(A) the disclosure is by the enrollee identified in the information or whose identity can be associated with the information;

(B) the disclosure is authorized by such enrollee in writing in a manner prescribed by the Board;

(C) the disclosure is to Federal, State, or local law enforcement agencies for the purpose of enforcing this Act or an Act amended by this Act; or

(D) the disclosure otherwise is consistent with this Act and specific criteria governing disclosure established by the Board.

(2) MINIMAL DISCLOSURE.—All disclosures of individually identifiable health information shall be restricted to the minimum amount of information necessary to accomplish the purpose for which the information is being disclosed.

(3) RISK ADJUSTMENT.—No individually identifiable health information may be provided by a health plan to a regional alliance or a corporate alliance for the purpose of setting premiums based on risk adjustment factors.

(4) REQUIRED SAFEGUARDS.—Any individual or entity who maintains, uses, or disseminates individually identifiable health information shall implement administrative, technical, and physical safeguards for the security of such information.

(5) RIGHT TO KNOW.—An enrollee (or an enrollee representative of the enrollee) has the right to know—

(A) whether any individual or entity uses or maintains individually identifiable health information concerning the enrollee; and

(B) for what purposes the information may be used or maintained.

(6) RIGHT TO ACCESS.—Subject to appropriate procedures, an enrollee (or an enrollee representative of the enrollee) has the right, with respect to individually identifiable health information concerning the enrollee that is recorded in any form or medium—

(A) to see such information;

(B) to copy such information; and

(C) to have a notation made with or in such information of any amendment or correction of such information requested by the enrollee or enrollee representative.

(7) RIGHT TO NOTICE.—An enrollee and an enrollee representative have the right to receive a written statement concerning—

(A) the purposes for which individually identifiable health information provided to a health care provider, a health plan, a regional alliance, a corporate alliance, or the National Health Board may be used or disclosed by, or disclosed to, any individual or entity; and

(B) the right of access described in paragraph (6).

(8) USE OF UNIQUE IDENTIFIER.—When individually identifiable health information concerning an enrollee is required to accomplish the purpose for which information is being transmitted between or among the National Health Board, regional and corporate alliances, health plans, and health care providers, the transmissions shall use the unique identifier number provided to the enrollee pursuant to section 5104 in lieu of the name of the enrollee.

(9) USE FOR EMPLOYMENT DECISIONS.—Individually identifiable health care information may not be used in making employment decisions.

## SEC. 5121. OTHER DUTIES WITH RESPECT TO PRIVACY.

(a) RESEARCH AND TECHNICAL SUPPORT.—The National Health Board may sponsor—

(1) research relating to the privacy and security of individually identifiable health information;

(2) the development of consent forms governing disclosure of such information; and

(3) the development of technology to implement standards regarding such information.

(c) EDUCATION.—The National Health Board shall establish education and awareness programs—

(1) to foster adequate security practices by States, regional alliances, corporate alliances, health plans, and health care providers;

(2) to train personnel of public and private entities who have access to individually identifiable health information respecting the duties of such personnel with respect to such information; and

(3) to inform individuals and employers who purchase health care respecting their rights with respect to such information.

### SEC. 5122. COMPREHENSIVE HEALTH INFORMATION PRIVACY PROTECTION ACT.

(a) IN GENERAL.—Not later than 3 years after the date of the enactment of this Act, the National Health Board shall submit to the President and the Congress a detailed proposal for legislation to provide a comprehensive scheme of Federal privacy protection for individually identifiable health information.

(b) CODE OF FAIR INFORMATION PRACTICES.—The proposal shall include a Code of Fair Information Practices to be used to advise enrollees to whom individually identifiable health information pertains of their rights with respect to such information in an easily understood and useful form.

(c) ENFORCEMENT.—The proposal shall include provisions to enforce effectively the rights and duties that would be created by the legislation.

**SEC. 5123. DEFINITIONS.**

For purposes of this part:

(1) ENROLLEE.—The term "enrollee" means an individual who enrolls or has enrolled under a health plan. The term includes a deceased individual who was enrolled under a health plan.

(2) ENROLLEE REPRESENTATIVE.—The term "enrollee representative" means any individual legally empowered to make decisions concerning the provision of health care to an enrollee or the administrator or executor of the estate of a deceased enrollee.

(3) INDIVIDUALLY IDENTIFIABLE HEALTH INFORMATION.—The term "individually identifiable health information" means any information, whether oral or recorded in any form or medium, that—

(A) identifies or can readily be associated with the identity of an enrollee; and

(B) relates to—

(i) the past, present, or future physical or mental health of the enrollee;

(ii) the provision of health care to the enrollee; or

(iii) payment for the provision of health care to the enrollee.

## PART 3—INTERIM REQUIREMENTS FOR ADMINISTRATIVE SIMPLIFICATION

**SEC. 5130. STANDARD BENEFIT FORMS.**

(a) DEVELOPMENT.—Not later than 1 year after the date of the enactment of this Act, the National Health Board shall develop, promulgate, and publish in the Federal Register the following standard health care benefit forms:

(1) An enrollment and disenrollment form to be used to record enrollment and disenrollment in a health benefit plan.

(2) A clinical encounter record to be used by health benefit plans and health service providers.

(3) A claim form to be used in the submission of claims for benefits or payment under a health benefit plan.

(b) INSTRUCTIONS, DEFINITIONS, AND CODES.—Each standard form developed under subsection (a) shall include instructions for completing the form that—

(1) specifically define, to the extent practicable, the data elements contained in the form; and

(2) standardize any codes or data sets to be used in completing the form.

(c) REQUIREMENTS FOR ADOPTION OF FORMS.—

(1) HEALTH SERVICE PROVIDERS.—On or after the date that is 270 days after the publication of the standard forms developed under subsection (a), a health service provider that furnishes items or services in the United States for which payment may be made under a health benefit plan may not—

(A) maintain records of clinical encounters involving such items or services that are required to be maintained by the National Health Board in a paper form that is not the clinical encounter record promulgated by the Board; or

(B) submit any claim for benefits or payment for such services to such plan in a paper form that is not the claim form promulgated by the National Health Board.

(2) HEALTH BENEFIT PLANS.—On or after the date that is 270 days after the publication of the standard forms developed under subsection (a), a health benefit plan may not—

(A) record enrollment and disenrollment in a paper form that is not the enrollment and disenrollment form promulgated by the National Health Board;

(B) maintain records of clinical encounters that are required to be maintained by the National Health Board in a paper form that is not the clinical encounter record promulgated by the Board; or

(C) reject a claim for benefits or payment under the plan on the basis of the form or manner in which the claim is submitted if—

(i) the claim is submitted on the claim form promulgated by the National Health Board; and

(ii) the plan accepts claims submitted in paper form.

(d) DEFINITIONS.—For purposes of this subtitle:

(1) HEALTH BENEFIT PLAN.—

(A) IN GENERAL.—The term "health benefit plan" means, except as provided in subparagraphs (B) through (D), any public or private entity or program that provides for payments for health care services, including—

(i) a group health plan (as defined in section 5000(b)(1) of the Internal Revenue Code of 1986); and

(ii) any other health insurance arrangement, including any arrangement consisting of a hospital or medical expense incurred policy or certificate, hospital or medical service plan contract, or health maintenance organization subscriber contract.

(B) PLANS EXCLUDED.—Such term does not include—

(i) accident-only, credit, or disability income insurance;

(ii) coverage issued as a supplement to liability insurance;

(iii) an individual making payment on the individual's own behalf (or on behalf of a relative or other individual) for deductibles, coinsurance, or services not covered under a health benefit plan; and

(iv) such other plans as the National Health Board may determine, because of the limitation of benefits to a single type or kind of health care, such as dental services or hospital indemnity plans, or other reasons should not be subject to the requirements of this section.

(C) PLANS INCLUDED.—Such term includes—

(i) workers compensation or similar insurance insofar as it relates to workers compensation medical benefits (as defined in section 10000(3)) provided by or through health plans; and

(ii) automobile medical insurance insofar as it relates to automobile insurance medical benefits (as defined in section 10100(2)) provided by or through health plans.

(D) TREATMENT OF DIRECT PROVISION OF SERVICES.—Such term does not include a Federal or State program that provides directly for the provision of health services to beneficiaries.

(2) HEALTH SERVICE PROVIDER.—The term "health service provider" includes a provider of services (as defined in section 1861(u) of the Social Security Act), physician, supplier, and other person furnishing health care services. Such term includes a Federal or State program that provides directly for the provision of health services to beneficiaries.

(e) INTERIM NATURE OF REQUIREMENTS.—The National Health Board may modify, update, or supercede any standard form or requirement developed, promulgated, or imposed under this section through the establishment of a standard under section 5101.

## PART 4—GENERAL PROVISIONS

### SEC. 5140. NATIONAL PRIVACY AND HEALTH DATA ADVISORY COUNCIL.

(a) ESTABLISHMENT.—There is established an advisory council to be known as the National Privacy and Health Data Advisory Council.

(b) DUTIES.—The Council shall advise the National Health Board with respect its duties under this subtitle.

(c) NUMBER AND APPOINTMENT.—The Council shall be composed of 15 members appointed by the National Health Board. The members of the Council shall include—

 (1) individuals representing the interests of consumers, employers, and other purchasers of health care;

 (2) individuals representing the interests of health plans, health care providers, corporate alliances, regional alliances, public health agencies, and participating States; and

 (3) individuals distinguished in the fields of data collection, data protection and privacy, law, ethics, medical and health services research, public health, and civil liberties and patient advocacy.

(d) TERMS.—

(1) IN GENERAL.—Except as provided in paragraph (2), members of the Council shall serve for a term of 3 years.

(2) STAGGERED ROTATION.—Of the members first appointed to the Council under subsection (c), the National Health Board shall appoint 5 members to serve for a term of 3 years, 5 members to serve for a term of 2 years, and 5 members to serve for a term of 1 year.

(3) SERVICE BEYOND TERM.—A member of the Council may continue to serve after the expiration of the term of the member until a successor is appointed.

(e) VACANCIES.—If a member of the Council does not serve the full term applicable under subsection (d), the individual appointed to fill the resulting vacancy shall be appointed for the remainder of the term of the predecessor of the individual.

(f) CHAIR.—The National Health Board shall designate an individual to serve as the chair of the Council.

(g) MEETINGS.—The Council shall meet not less than once during each discrete 4-month period and shall otherwise meet at the call of the National Health Board or the chair.

(h) COMPENSATION AND REIMBURSEMENT OF EXPENSES.—Members of the Council shall receive compensation for each day (including travel time) engaged in carrying out the duties of the Council. Such compensation may not be in an amount in excess of the maximum rate of basic pay payable for level IV of the Executive Schedule under section 5315 of title 5, United States Code.

(i) STAFF.—The National Health Board shall provide to the Council such staff, information, and other assistance as may be necessary to carry out the duties of the Council.

(j) DURATION.—Notwithstanding section 14(a) of the Federal Advisory Committee Act, the Council shall continue in existence until otherwise provided by law.

**SEC. 5141. CIVIL MONEY PENALTIES.**

(a) VIOLATION OF HEALTH INFORMATION SYSTEM STANDARDS.—Any person who the Secretary of Health and Human Services determines—

   (1) is required, but has substantially failed, to comply with a standard established by the National Health Board under section 5101 or 5120;

   (2) has required the display of, has required the use of, or has used a health security card for any purpose other than a purpose described in section 5105(a); or

(3) has required the disclosure of, has required the use of, or has used a unique identifier number provided pursuant to section 5104 for any purpose that is not authorized by the National Health Board pursuant to such section

shall be subject, in addition to any other penalties that may be prescribed by law, to a civil money penalty of not more than $10,000 for each such violation.

(b) STANDARD BENEFIT FORMS.—Any health service provider or health benefit plan that the Secretary of Health and Human Services determines is required, but has substantially failed, to comply with section 5130(c) shall be subject, in addition to any other penalties that may be prescribed by law, to a civil money penalty of not more than $10,000 for each such violation.

(c) PROCESS.—The process for the imposition of a civil money penalty under the All-Payer Health Care Fraud and Abuse Control Program under part 1 of subtitle E of this title shall apply to a civil money penalty under this section in the same manner as such process applies to a penalty or proceeding under such program.

**SEC. 5142. RELATIONSHIP TO OTHER LAWS.**

(a) COURT ORDERS.—Nothing in this title shall be construed to invalidate or limit the power or authority of any court of competent jurisdiction with respect to health care information.

(b) PUBLIC HEALTH REPORTING.—Nothing in this title shall be construed to invalidate or limit the authorities, powers, or procedures established under any law that provides for the reporting of disease, child abuse, birth, or death.

# Subtitle C—Remedies and Enforcement

## PART 1—REVIEW OF BENEFIT DETERMINATIONS FOR ENROLLED INDIVIDUALS

### Subpart A—General Rules

SEC. 5201. HEALTH PLAN CLAIMS PROCEDURE.

(a) DEFINITIONS.—For purposes of this section—

(1) CLAIM.—The term "claim" means a claim for payment or provision of benefits under a health plan or a request for preauthorization of items or services which is submitted to a health plan prior to receipt of the items or services.

(2) INDIVIDUAL CLAIMANT.—The term "individual claimant" with respect to a claim means any individual who submits the claim to a health plan in connection with the individual's enrollment under the plan, or on whose behalf the claim is submitted to the plan by a provider.

(3) PROVIDER CLAIMANT.—The term "provider claimant" with respect to a claim means any provider who submits the claim to a health plan with respect to items or services provided to an individual enrolled under the plan.

(b) GENERAL RULES GOVERNING TREATMENT OF CLAIMS.—

(1) ADEQUATE NOTICE OF DISPOSITION OF CLAIM.—In any case in which a claim is submitted in complete form to a health plan, the plan shall provide to the individual claimant and any provider claimant with respect to the claim a written notice of the plan's approval or denial of the claim within 30 days after the date of the submission of the claim. The notice to the individual claimant shall be written in language calculated to be understood by the typical individual enrolled under the plan and in a form which takes into account accessibility to the information by individuals whose primary language is not English. In the case of a denial of the claim, the notice shall be provided within 5 days after the date of the determination to deny the claim, and shall set forth the specific reasons for the denial. The notice of a denial shall include notice of the right to appeal the denial under paragraph (2). Fail-

ure by any plan to comply with the requirements of this paragraph with respect to any claim submitted to the plan shall be treated as approval by the plan of the claim.

(2) PLAN'S DUTY TO REVIEW DENIALS UPON TIMELY REQUEST.—The plan shall review its denial of the claim if an individual claimant or provider claimant with respect to the claim submits to the plan a written request for reconsideration of the claim after receipt of written notice from the plan of the denial. The plan shall allow any such claimant not less than 60 days, after receipt of written notice from the plan of the denial, to submit the claimant's request for reconsideration of the claim.

(3) TIME LIMIT FOR REVIEW.—The plan shall complete any review required under paragraph (2), and shall provide the individual claimant and any provider claimant with respect to the claim written notice of the plan's decision on the claim after reconsideration pursuant to the review, within 30 days after the date of the receipt of the request for reconsideration.

(4) DE NOVO REVIEWS.—Any review required under paragraph (2)—

(A) shall be de novo,

(B) shall be conducted by an individual who did not make the initial decision denying the claim and who is authorized to approve the claim, and

(C) shall include review by a qualified physician if the resolution of any issues involved requires medical expertise.

(c) TREATMENT OF URGENT REQUESTS TO PLANS FOR PREAUTHORIZATION.—

(1) IN GENERAL.—This subsection applies in the case of any claim submitted by an individual claimant or a provider claimant consisting of a request for preauthorization of items or services which is accompanied by an attestation that—

(A) failure to immediately provide the items or services could reasonably be expected to result in—

(i) placing the health of the individual claimant (or, with respect to an individual claimant who is a pregnant woman, the health of the woman or her unborn child) in serious jeopardy,

(ii) serious impairment to bodily functions, or

(iii) serious dysfunction of any bodily organ or part,

or

(B) immediate provision of the items or services is necessary because the individual claimant has made or is at serious risk of making an attempt to harm such individual claimant or another individual.

(2) SHORTENED TIME LIMIT FOR CONSIDERATION OF REQUESTS FOR PREAUTHORIZATION.—Notwithstanding subsection (b)(1), a health plan shall approve or deny any claim described in paragraph (1) within 24 hours after submission of the claim to the plan. Failure by the plan to comply with the requirements of this paragraph with respect to the claim shall be treated as approval by the plan of the claim.

(3) EXPEDITED EXHAUSTION OF PLAN REMEDIES.—Any claim described in paragraph (1) which is denied by the plan shall be treated as a claim with respect to which all remedies under the plan provided pursuant to this section are exhausted, irrespective of any review provided under subsection (b)(2).

(4) DENIAL OF PREVIOUSLY AUTHORIZED CLAIMS NOT PERMITTED.—In any case in which a health plan approves a claim described in paragraph (1)—

    (A) the plan may not subsequently deny payment or provision of benefits pursuant to the claim, unless the plan makes a showing of an intentional misrepresentation of a material fact by the individual claimant, and

    (B) in the case of a violation of subparagraph (A) in connection with the claim, all remedies under the plan provided pursuant to this section with respect to the claim shall be treated as exhausted.

(d) TIME LIMIT FOR DETERMINATION OF INCOMPLETENESS OF CLAIM.—For purposes of this section—

    (1) any claim submitted by an individual claimant and accepted by a provider serving under contract with a health plan and any claim described in subsection (b)(1) shall be treated with respect to the individual claimant as submitted in complete form, and

    (2) any other claim for benefits under the plan shall be treated as filed in complete form as of 10 days after the date of the submission of the claim,

unless the plan provides to the individual claimant and any provider claimant, within such period, a written notice of any required matter remaining to be filed in order to complete the claim.

Any filing by the individual claimant or the provider claimant of additional matter requested by the plan pursuant to paragraph (2) shall be treated for purposes of this section as an initial filing of the claim.

(e) ADDITIONAL NOTICE AND DISCLOSURE REQUIREMENTS FOR HEALTH PLANS.—In the case of a denial of a claim for benefits under a health plan, the plan shall include, together with the specific reasons provided to the individual claimant and any provider claimant under subsection (b)(1)—

   (1) if the denial is based in whole or in part on a determination that the claim is for an item or service which is not covered by the comprehensive benefit package or exceeds payment rates under the applicable alliance or State fee schedule, the factual basis for the determination,

   (2) if the denial is based in whole or in part on exclusion of coverage with respect to services because the services are determined to comprise an experimental treatment or investigatory procedure, the medical basis for the determination and a descrip-

tion of the process used in making the determination, and

 (3) if the denial is based in whole or in part on a determination that the treatment is not medically necessary or appropriate or is inconsistent with the plan's practice guidelines, the medical basis for the determination, the guidelines used in making the determination, and a description of the process used in making the determination.

(f) WAIVER OF RIGHTS PROHIBITED.—A health plan may not require any party to waive any right under the plan or this Act as a condition for approval of any claim under the plan, except to the extent otherwise specified in a formal settlement agreement.

## SEC. 5202. REVIEW IN REGIONAL ALLIANCE COMPLAINT REVIEW OFFICES OF GRIEVANCES BASED ON ACTS OR PRACTICES BY HEALTH PLANS.

(a) COMPLAINT REVIEW OFFICES.—

 (1) IN GENERAL.—In accordance with rules which shall be prescribed by the Secretary of Labor, each State shall establish and maintain a complaint review office for each regional alliance established by such State. According to designations which shall be made by each State under regulations of the Secretary of Labor, the complaint review office for a re-

gional alliance established by such State shall also serve as the complaint review office for corporate alliances operating in the State with respect to individuals who are enrolled under corporate alliance health plans maintained by such corporate alliances and who reside within the area of the regional alliance.

(2) REGIONAL ALLIANCES NOT ESTABLISHED BY STATES.—In the case of any regional alliance established in any State by the Secretary of Health and Human Services, the Secretary of Health and Human Services shall assume all duties and obligations of such State under this part in accordance with the applicable regulations of the Secretary of Labor under this part.

(b) FILINGS OF COMPLAINTS BY AGGRIEVED PERSONS.—In the case of any person who is aggrieved by—

(1) any act or practice engaged in by any health plan which consists of or results in denial of payment or provision of benefits under the plan or delay in the payment or provision of benefits, or

(2) any act or practice engaged in by any other plan maintained by a regional alliance or a corporate alliance which consists of or results in denial of payment or provision of benefits under a cost sharing

policy described in section 1421(b)(2) or delay in the
payment or provision of the benefits,
if the denial or delay consists of a failure to comply with
the terms of the plan (including the provision of benefits
in full when due in accordance with the terms of the plan),
or with the applicable requirements of this Act, such person may file a complaint with the appropriate complaint review office.

(c) EXHAUSTION OF PLAN REMEDIES.—Any complaint including a claim to which section 5201 applies may not be filed until the complainant has exhausted all remedies provided under the plan with respect to the claim in accordance with such section.

(d) EXCLUSIVE MEANS OF REVIEW FOR PLANS MAINTAINED BY CORPORATE ALLIANCES.—Proceedings under sections 5203 and 5204 pursuant to complaints filed under subsection (b), and review under section 5205 of determinations made under section 5204, shall be the exclusive means of review of acts or practices described in subsection (b) which are engaged in by a corporate alliance health plan or by any plan maintained by a corporate alliance with respect to benefits under a cost sharing policy described in section 1421(b)(2).

(e) FORM OF COMPLAINT.—The complaint shall be in writing under oath or affirmation, shall set forth the complaint in a manner calculated to give notice of the nature of the complaint, and shall contain such information as may be prescribed in regulations of the Secretary of Labor.

(f) NOTICE OF FILING.—The complaint review office shall serve by certified mail a notice of the complaint (including the date, place, and circumstances of the alleged violation) on the person or persons alleged in the complaint to have committed the violation within 10 days after the filing of the complaint.

(g) TIME LIMITATION.—Complaints may not be brought under this section with respect to any violation later than one year after the date on which the violation occurs. This subsection shall not prevent the subsequent amending of a complaint.

## SEC. 5203. INITIAL PROCEEDINGS IN COMPLAINT REVIEW OFFICES.

(a) ELECTIONS.—Whenever a complaint is brought to the complaint review office under section 5202(b), the complaint review office shall provide the complainant with an opportunity, in such form and manner as shall be prescribed in regulations of the Secretary of Labor, to elect one of the following:

(1) to forego further proceedings in the complaint review office and rely on remedies available in

a court of competent jurisdiction, except with respect to any matter in the complaint with respect to which proceedings under this section and section 5204, and review under section 5205, are not under section 5202(d) the exclusive means of review,

(2) to submit the complaint as a dispute under the Early Resolution Program established under subpart B and thereby suspend further review proceedings under this section pending termination of proceedings under the Program, or

(3) in any case in which an election under paragraph (2) is not made, or such an election was made but resolution of all matters in the complaint was not obtained upon termination of proceedings pursuant to the election by settlement agreement or otherwise, to proceed with the complaint to a hearing in the complaint review office under section 5204 regarding the unresolved matters.

(b) EFFECT OF PARTICIPATION IN EARLY RESOLUTION PROGRAM.—Any matter in a complaint brought to the complaint review office which is included in a dispute which is timely submitted to the Early Resolution Program established under subpart B shall not be assigned to a hearing under this section unless the proceedings under the Program with respect to the dispute are terminated without settlement or resolution of the dispute with respect to such matter. Upon termination of any proceedings regarding a dispute submitted to the Program, the applicability of this section to any matter in a complaint which was included in the dispute shall not be affected by participation in the proceedings, except to the extent otherwise required under the terms of any settlement agreement or other formal resolution obtained in the proceedings.

## SEC. 5204. HEARINGS BEFORE HEARING OFFICERS IN COMPLAINT REVIEW OFFICES.

(a) HEARING PROCESS.—

(1) ASSIGNMENT OF COMPLAINTS TO HEARING OFFICERS AND NOTICE TO PARTIES.—

(A) IN GENERAL.—In the case of an election under section 5203(a)(3)—

(i) the complaint review office shall assign the complaint, and each motion in connection with the complaint, to a hearing officer employed by the State in the office; and

(ii) the hearing officer shall have the power to issue and cause to be served upon the plan named in the complaint a copy of the complaint and a notice of hearing before the hearing officer at a place fixed in the notice, not less than 5 days after the serving of the complaint.

(B) QUALIFICATIONS FOR HEARING OFFICERS.—No individual may serve in a complaint review office as a hearing officer unless the individual meets standards which shall be prescribed by the Secretary of Labor. Such standards shall include experience, training, affiliations, diligence, actual or potential conflicts of interest, and other qualifications deemed relevant by the Secretary of Labor. At no time shall a hearing officer have any official, financial, or personal conflict of interest with respect to issues in controversy before the hearing officer.

(2) AMENDMENT OF COMPLAINTS.—Any such complaint may be amended by the hearing officer conducting the hearing, upon the motion of the complainant, in the hearing officer's discretion at any time prior to the issuance of an order based thereon.

(3) ANSWERS.—The party against whom the complaint is filed shall have the right to file an answer to the original or amended complaint and to

appear in person or otherwise and give testimony at the place and time fixed in the complaint.

(b) ADDITIONAL PARTIES.—In the discretion of the hearing officer conducting the hearing, any other person may be allowed to intervene in the proceeding and to present testimony.

(c) HEARINGS.—

(1) DE NOVO HEARING.—Each hearing officer shall hear complaints and motions de novo.

(2) TESTIMONY.—The testimony taken by the hearing officer shall be reduced to writing. Thereafter, the hearing officer, in his or her discretion, upon notice may provide for the taking of further testimony or hear argument.

(3) AUTHORITY OF HEARING OFFICERS.—The hearing officer may compel by subpoena the attendance of witnesses and the production of evidence at any designated place or hearing. In case of contumacy or refusal to obey a subpoena lawfully issued under this paragraph and upon application of the hearing officer, an appropriate district court may issue an order requiring compliance with the subpoena and any failure to obey the order may be punished by the court as a contempt thereof. The hear-

ing officer may also seek enforcement of the subpoena in a State court of competent jurisdiction.

(4) EXPEDITED HEARINGS.—Notwithstanding section 5203 and the preceding provisions of this section, upon receipt of a complaint containing a claim described in section 5201(c)(1), the complaint review office shall promptly provide the complainant with the opportunity to make an election under section 5203(a)(3) and assignment to a hearing on the complaint before a hearing officer. The complaint review office shall ensure that such a hearing commences not later than 24 hours after receipt of the complaint by the complaint hearing office.

(d) DECISION OF HEARING OFFICER.—

(1) IN GENERAL.—The hearing officer shall decide upon the preponderance of the evidence whether to decide in favor of the complainant with respect to each alleged act or practice. Each such decision—

(A) shall include the hearing officer's findings of fact, and

(B) shall constitute the hearing officer's final disposition of the proceedings.

(2) DECISIONS FINDING IN FAVOR OF COMPLAINANT.—

(A) IN GENERAL.—If the hearing officer's decision includes a determination that any party named in the complaint has engaged in or is engaged in an act or practice described in section 5202(b), the hearing officer shall issue and cause to be served on such party an order which requires such party—

(i) to cease and desist from such act or practice,

(ii) to provide the benefits due under the terms of the plan and to otherwise comply with the terms of the plan and the applicable requirements of this Act,

(iii) to pay to the complainant prejudgment interest on the actual costs incurred in obtaining the items and services at issue in the complaint, and

(iv) to pay to the prevailing complainant a reasonable attorney's fee, reasonable expert witness fees, and other reasonable costs relating to the hearing on the charges on which the complainant prevails.

(3) DECISIONS NOT IN FAVOR OF COMPLAINANT.—If the hearing officer's decision includes a determination that the party named in the complaint

has not engaged in or is not engaged in an act or practice referred to in section 5202(b), the hearing officer—

>(A) shall include in the decision a dismissal of the charge in the complaint relating to the act or practice, and

>(B) upon a finding that such charge is frivolous, shall issue and cause to be served on the complainant an order which requires the complainant to pay to such party a reasonable attorney's fee, reasonable expert witness fees, and other reasonable costs relating to the proceedings on such charge.

(4) SUBMISSION AND SERVICE OF DECISIONS.—The hearing officer shall submit each decision to the complaint review office at the conclusion of the proceedings and the office shall cause a copy of the decision to be served on the parties to the proceedings.

(e) REVIEW.—

(1) IN GENERAL.—The decision of the hearing officer shall be final and binding upon all parties. Except as provided in paragraph (2), any party to the complaint may, within 30 days after service of the decision by the complaint review office, file an appeal of the decision with the Federal Health Plan

Review Board under section 5205 in such form and manner as may be prescribed by such Board.

(2) EXCEPTION.—The decision in the case of an expedited hearing under subsection (c)(4) shall not be subject to review.

(f) COURT ENFORCEMENT OF ORDERS.—

(1) IN GENERAL.—If a decision of the hearing officer in favor of the complainant is not appealed under section 5205, the complainant may petition any court of competent jurisdiction for enforcement of the order. In any such proceeding, the order of the hearing officer shall not be subject to review.

(2) AWARDING OF COSTS.—In any action for court enforcement under this subsection, a prevailing complainant shall be entitled to a reasonable attorney's fee, reasonable expert witness fees, and other reasonable costs relating to such action.

**SEC. 5205. REVIEW BY FEDERAL HEALTH PLAN REVIEW BOARD.**

(a) ESTABLISHMENT AND MEMBERSHIP.—The Secretary of Labor shall establish by regulation a Federal Health Plan Review Board (hereinafter in this subtitle referred to as the "Review Board"). The Review Board shall be composed of 5 members appointed by the Secretary of Labor from among persons who by reason of training, education, or experience are qualified to carry out the functions of the Review Board under this subtitle. The Secretary of Labor shall prescribe such rules as are necessary for the orderly transaction of proceedings by the Review Board. Every official act of the Review Board shall be entered of record, and its hearings and records shall be open to the public.

(b) REVIEW PROCESS.—The Review Board shall ensure, in accordance with rules prescribed by the Secretary of Labor, that reasonable notice is provided for each appeal before the Review Board of a hearing officer's decision under section 5304, and shall provide for the orderly consideration of arguments by any party to the hearing upon which the hearing officer's decision is based. In the discretion of the Review Board, any other person may be allowed to intervene in the proceeding and to present written argument. The National Health Board may intervene in the proceeding as a matter of right.

(c) SCOPE OF REVIEW.—The Review Board shall review the decision of the hearing officer from which the appeal is made, except that the review shall be only for the purposes of determining—

(1) whether the determination is supported by substantial evidence on the record considered as a whole,

(2) in the case of any interpretation by the hearing officer of contractual terms (irrespective of the extent to which extrinsic evidence was considered), whether the determination is supported by a preponderance of the evidence,

(3) whether the determination is in excess of statutory jurisdiction, authority, or limitations, or in violation of a statutory right, or

(4) whether the determination is without observance of procedure required by law.

(d) DECISION OF REVIEW BOARD.—The decision of the hearing officer as affirmed or modified by the Review Board (or any reversal by the Review Board of the hearing officer's final disposition of the proceedings) shall become the final order of the Review Board and binding on all parties, subject to review under subsection (e). The Review Board shall cause a copy of its decision to be served on the parties to the proceedings not later than 5 days after the date of the proceeding.

(e) REVIEW OF FINAL ORDERS.—

(1) IN GENERAL.—Not later than 60 days after the entry of the final order, any person aggrieved by any such final order under which the amount or value in controversy exceeds $10,000 may seek a review of the order in the United States court of ap-

peals for the circuit in which the violation is alleged to have occurred or in which the complainant resides.

(2) FURTHER REVIEW.—Upon the filing of the record with the court, the jurisdiction of the court shall be exclusive and its judgment shall be final, except that the judgment shall be subject to review by the Supreme Court of the United States upon writ of certiorari or certification as provided in section 1254 of title 28 of the United States Code.

(3) ENFORCEMENT DECREE IN ORIGINAL REVIEW.—If, upon appeal of an order under paragraph (1), the United States court of appeals does not reverse the order, the court shall have the jurisdiction to make and enter a decree enforcing the order of the Review Board.

(f) DETERMINATIONS.—Determinations made under this section shall be in accordance with the provisions of this Act, the comprehensive benefit package as provided by this Act, the rules and regulations of the National Health Board prescribed under this Act, and decisions of the National Health Board published under this Act.

(g) AWARDING OF ATTORNEYS' FEES AND OTHER COSTS AND EXPENSES.—In any proceeding before the Review Board under this section or any judicial proceeding under subsection (e), the Review Board or the court (as the case may be) shall award to a prevailing complainant reasonable costs and expenses (including a reasonable attorney's fee) on the causes on which the complainant prevails.

## SEC. 5206. CIVIL MONEY PENALTIES.

(a) DENIAL OR DELAY IN PAYMENT OR PROVISION OF BENEFITS.—

(1) IN GENERAL.—The Secretary of Labor may assess a civil penalty against any health plan, or against any other plan in connection with benefits provided thereunder under a cost sharing policy described in section 1421(b)(2), for unreasonable denial or delay in the payment or provision of benefits thereunder, in an amount not to exceed—

(A) $25,000 per violation, or $75,000 per violation in the case of a finding of bad faith on the part of the plan, and

(B) in the case of a finding of a pattern or practice of such violations engaged in by the plan, $1,000,000 in addition to the total amount of penalties assessed under subparagraph (A) with respect to such violations.

For purposes of subparagraph (A), each violation with respect to any single individual shall be treated as a separate violation.

(2) CIVIL ACTION TO ENFORCE CIVIL PENALTY.—The Secretary of Labor may commence a civil action in any court of competent jurisdiction to enforce a civil penalty assessed under subsection (a).

(b) CIVIL PENALTIES FOR CERTAIN OTHER ACTIONS.—The Secretary of Labor may assess a civil penalty described in section 5412(b)(1) against any corporate alliance health plan, or against any other plan sponsored by a corporate alliance in connection with benefits provided thereunder under a cost sharing policy described in section 1421(b)(2), for any action described in section 5412(a). The Secretary of Labor may initiate proceedings to impose such penalty in the same manner as the Secretary of Health and Human Services may initiate proceedings under section 5412 with respect to actions described in section 5412(a).

## Subpart B—Early Resolution Programs

### SEC. 5211. ESTABLISHMENT OF EARLY RESOLUTION PROGRAMS IN COMPLAINT REVIEW OFFICES.

(a) ESTABLISHMENT OF PROGRAMS.—Each State shall establish and maintain an Early Resolution Program in each complaint review office in such State. The Program shall include—

    (1) the establishment and maintenance of forums for mediation of disputes in accordance with this subpart, and

    (2) the establishment and maintenance of such forums for other forms of alternative dispute resolution (including binding arbitration) as may be prescribed in regulations of the Secretary of Labor.

Each State shall ensure that the standards applied in Early Resolution Programs administered in such State which apply to any form of alternative dispute resolution described in paragraph (2) and which relate to time requirements, qualifications of facilitators, arbitrators, or other mediators, and confidentiality are at least equivalent to the standards which apply to mediation proceedings under this subpart.

  (b) DUTIES OF COMPLAINT REVIEW OFFICES.—Each complaint review office in a State—

    (1) shall administer its Early Resolution Program in accordance with regulations of the Secretary of Labor,

    (2) shall, pursuant to subsection (a)(1)—

        (A) recruit and train individuals to serve as facilitators for mediation proceedings under the Early Resolution Program from attorneys who have the requisite expertise for such service, which shall be specified in regulations of the Secretary of Labor,

(B) provide meeting sites, maintain records, and provide facilitators with administrative support staff, and

(C) establish and maintain attorney referral panels,

(3) shall ensure that, upon the filing of a complaint with the office, the complainant is adequately apprised of the complainant's options for review under this part, and

(4) shall monitor and evaluate the Program on an ongoing basis.

## SEC. 5212. INITIATION OF PARTICIPATION IN MEDIATION PROCEEDINGS.

(a) ELIGIBILITY OF CASES FOR SUBMISSION TO EARLY RESOLUTION PROGRAM.—A dispute may be submitted to the Early Resolution Program only if the following requirements are met with respect to the dispute:

(1) NATURE OF DISPUTE.—The dispute consists of an assertion by an individual enrolled under a health plan of one or more claims against the health plan for payment or provision of benefits, or

against any other plan maintained by the regional alliance or corporate alliance sponsoring the health plan with respect to benefits provided under a cost sharing policy described in section 1421(b)(2), based on alleged coverage under the plan, and a denial of the claims, or a denial of appropriate reimbursement based on the claims, by the plan.

(2) NATURE OF DISPUTED CLAIM.—Each claim consists of—

(A) a claim for payment or provision of benefits under the plan; or

(B) a request for information or documents the disclosure of which is required under this Act (including claims of entitlement to disclosure based on colorable claims to rights to benefits under the plan).

(b) FILING OF ELECTION.—A complainant with a dispute which is eligible for submission to the Early Resolution Program may make the election under section 5203(a)(2) to submit the dispute to mediation proceedings under the Program not later than 15 days after the date the complaint is filed with the complaint review office under subpart A.

(c) AGREEMENT TO PARTICIPATE.—

(1) ELECTION BY CLAIMANT.—A complainant may elect participation in the mediation proceedings only by entering into a written agreement (including an agreement to comply with the rules of the Program and consent for the complaint review office to contact the health plan regarding the agreement), and by releasing plan records to the Program for the exclusive use of the facilitator assigned to the dispute.

(2) PARTICIPATION BY PLANS OR HEALTH BENEFITS CONTRACTORS.—Each party whose participation in the mediation proceedings has been elected by a claimant pursuant to paragraph (1) shall participate in, and cooperate fully with, the proceedings. The claims review office shall provide such party with a copy of the participation agreement described in paragraph (1), together with a written description of the Program. Such party shall submit the copy of the agreement, together with its authorized signature signifying receipt of notice of the agreement, to the claims review office, and shall include in the submission to the claims review office a copy of the written record of the plan claims procedure completed pursuant to section 5201 with respect to the dispute and all relevant plan documents. The rel-

evant documents shall include all documents under which the health plan is or was administered or operated, including copies of any insurance contracts under which benefits are or were provided and any fee or reimbursement schedules for health care providers.

**SEC. 5213. MEDIATION PROCEEDINGS.**

(a) ROLE OF FACILITATOR.—In the course of mediation proceedings under the Early Resolution Program, the facilitator assigned to the dispute shall prepare the parties for a conference regarding the dispute and serve as a neutral mediator at such conference, with the goal of achieving settlement of the dispute.

(b) PREPARATIONS FOR CONFERENCE.—In advance of convening the conference, after identifying the necessary parties and confirming that the case is eligible for the Program, the facilitator shall analyze the record of the claims procedure conducted pursuant to section 5201 and any position papers submitted by the parties to determine if further case development is needed to clarify the legal and factual issues in dispute, and whether there is any need for additional information and documents.

(c) CONFERENCE.—Upon convening the conference, the facilitator shall assist the parties in identifying undisputed issues and exploring settlement. If settlement is reached, the facilitator shall assist in the preparation of a written settlement agreement. If no settlement is reached, the facilitator shall present the facilitator's evaluation, including an assessment of the parties' positions, the likely outcome of further administrative action or litigation, and suggestions for narrowing the issues in dispute.

(d) TIME LIMIT.—The facilitator shall ensure that mediation proceedings with respect to any dispute under the Early Resolution Program shall be completed within 120 days after the election to participate. The parties may agree to one extension of the proceedings by not more than 30 days if the proceedings are suspended to obtain an agency ruling or to reconvene the conference in a subsequent session.

(e) INAPPLICABILITY OF FORMAL RULES.—Formal rules of evidence shall not apply to mediation proceedings under the Early Resolution Program. All statements made and evidence presented in the proceedings shall be admissible in the proceedings. The facilitator shall be the sole judge of the proper weight to be afforded to each submission. The parties to mediation proceedings under the Program shall not be required to make statements or present evidence under oath.

(f) REPRESENTATION.—Parties may participate pro se or be represented by attorneys throughout the proceedings of the Early Resolution Program.

(g) CONFIDENTIALITY.—

(1) IN GENERAL.—Under regulations of the Secretary of Labor, rules similar to the rules under section 574 of title 5, United States Code (relating to confidentiality in dispute resolution proceedings) shall apply to the mediation proceedings under the Early Resolution Program.

(2) CIVIL REMEDIES.—The Secretary of Labor may assess a civil penalty against any person who discloses information in violation of the regulations prescribed pursuant to subsection (a) in the amount of three times the amount of the claim involved. The Secretary of Labor may bring a civil action to enforce such civil penalty in any court of competent jurisdiction.

### SEC. 5214. LEGAL EFFECT OF PARTICIPATION IN MEDIATION PROCEEDINGS.

(a) PROCESS NONBINDING.—Findings and conclusions made in the mediation proceedings of the Early Resolution Program shall be treated as advisory in nature and nonbinding. Except as provided in subsection (b), the rights of the parties under subpart A shall not be affected by participation in the Program.

(b) RESOLUTION THROUGH SETTLEMENT AGREEMENT.—If a case is settled through participation in mediation proceedings under the Program, the facilitator shall assist the parties in drawing up an agreement which shall constitute, upon signature of the parties, a binding contract between the parties, which shall be enforceable under section 5215.

(c) PRESERVATION OF RIGHTS OF NON-PARTIES.—The settlement agreement shall not have the effect of waiving or otherwise affecting any rights to review under subpart A, or any other right under this Act or the plan, with respect to any person who is not a party to the settlement agreement.

## SEC. 5215. ENFORCEMENT OF SETTLEMENT AGREEMENTS.

(a) ENFORCEMENT.—Any party to a settlement agreement entered pursuant to mediation proceedings under this subpart may petition any court of competent jurisdiction for the enforcement of the agreement, by filing in the court a written petition praying that the agreement be enforced. In such a proceeding, the order of the hearing officer shall not be subject to review.

(b) COURT REVIEW.—It shall be the duty of the court to advance on the docket and to expedite to the greatest possible extent the disposition of any petition filed under this section, with due deference to the role of settlement agreements under this part in achieving prompt resolution of disputes involving health plans.

(d) AWARDING OF ATTORNEY'S FEES AND OTHER COSTS AND EXPENSES.—In any action by an individual enrolled under a health plan for court enforcement under this section, a prevailing plaintiff shall be entitled to reasonable costs and expenses (including a reasonable attorney's fee and reasonable expert witness fees) on the charges on which the plaintiff prevails.

## PART 2—ADDITIONAL REMEDIES AND ENFORCEMENT PROVISIONS

### SEC. 5231. JUDICIAL REVIEW OF FEDERAL ACTION ON STATE SYSTEMS.

(a) IN GENERAL.—Any State or an alliance that is aggrieved by a determination by the National Health Board under subpart B of part 1 of subtitle F of title I shall be entitled to judicial review of such determination in accordance with this section.

(b) JUDICIAL REVIEW.—

(1) JURISDICTION.—The courts of appeals of the United States (other than the United States Court of Appeals for the Federal Circuit) shall have jurisdiction to review a determination described in

subsection (a), to affirm the determination, or to set it aside, in whole or in part. A judgment of a court of appeals in such an action shall be subject to review by the Supreme Court of the United States upon certiorari or certification as provided in section 1254 of title 28, United States Code.

(2) PETITION FOR REVIEW.—A State or an alliance that desires judicial review of a determination described in subsection (a) shall, within 30 days after it has been notified of such determination, file with the United States court of appeals for the circuit in which the State or alliance is located a petition for review of such determination. A copy of the petition shall be transmitted by the clerk of the court to the National Health Board, and the Board shall file in the court the record of the proceedings on which the determination or action was based, as provided in section 2112 of title 28, United States Code.

(3) SCOPE OF REVIEW.—The findings of fact of the National Health Board, if supported by substantial evidence, shall be conclusive; but the court, for good cause shown, may remand the case to the Board to take further evidence, and the Board may make new or modified findings of fact and may mod-

ify its previous action, and shall certify to the court the record of the further proceedings. Such new or modified findings of fact shall likewise be conclusive if supported by substantial evidence.

## SEC. 5232. ADMINISTRATIVE AND JUDICIAL REVIEW RELATING TO COST CONTAINMENT.

There shall be no administrative or judicial review of any determination by the National Health Board respecting any matter under subtitle A of title VI.

## SEC. 5233. CIVIL ENFORCEMENT.

Unless otherwise provided in this Act, the district courts of the United States shall have jurisdiction of civil actions brought by—

(1) the Secretary of Labor to enforce any final order of such Secretary or to collect any civil monetary penalty assessed by such Secretary under this Act; and

(2) the Secretary of Health and Human Services to enforce any final order of such Secretary or to collect any civil monetary penalty assessed by such Secretary under this Act.

## SEC. 5234. PRIORITY OF CERTAIN BANKRUPTCY CLAIMS.

Section 507(a)(8) of title 11, United States Code, is amended to read as follows:

"(8) Eighth, allowed unsecured claims—

"(A) based upon any commitment by the debtor to the Federal Deposit Insurance Corporation, the Resolution Trust Corporation, the Director of the Office of Thrift Supervision, the Comptroller of the Currency, or the Board of Governors of the Federal Reserve System, or their predecessors or successors, to maintain the capital of an insured depository institution;

"(B) for payments under subtitle B of title IV of the Health Security Act owed to a regional alliance (as defined in section 1301 of such Act);

"(C) for payments owed to a corporate alliance health plan under trusteeship of the Secretary of Labor under section 1395 of the Health Security Act; or

"(D) for assessments and related amounts owed to the Secretary of Labor under section 1397 of the Health Security Act.".

## SEC. 5235. PRIVATE RIGHT TO ENFORCE STATE RESPONSIBILITIES.

The failure of a participating State to carry out a responsibility applicable to participating States under this Act constitutes a deprivation of rights secured by this Act for the purposes of section 1977 of the Revised Statutes of the United States (42 U.S.C. 1983). In an action brought under such section, the court shall exercise jurisdiction without regard to whether the aggrieved person has exhausted any administrative or other remedies that may be provided by law.

## SEC. 5236. PRIVATE RIGHT TO ENFORCE FEDERAL RESPONSIBILITIES IN OPERATING A SYSTEM IN A STATE.

(a) IN GENERAL.—The failure of the Secretary of Health and Human Services to carry out a responsibility under section 1522 (relating to operation of an alliance system in a State) confers an enforceable right of action on any person who is aggrieved by such failure. Such a person may commence a civil action against the Secretary in an appropriate State court or district court of the United States.

(b) EXHAUSTION OF REMEDIES.—In an action under subsection (a), the court shall exercise jurisdiction without regard to whether the aggrieved person has exhausted any administrative or other remedies that may be provided by law.

(c) RELIEF.—In an action under subsection (a), if the court finds that a failure described in such subsection has occurred, the aggrieved person may recover compensatory and punitive damages and the court may order any other appropriate relief.

(d) ATTORNEY'S FEES.—In an action under subsection (a), the court, in its discretion, may allow the prevailing party, other than the United States, a reasonable attorney's fee (including expert fees) as part of the costs, and the United States shall be liable for costs the same as a private person.

## SEC. 5237. PRIVATE RIGHT TO ENFORCE RESPONSIBILITIES OF ALLIANCES.

(a) IN GENERAL.—The failure of a regional alliance or a corporate alliance to carry out a responsibility applicable to the alliance under this Act confers an enforceable right of action on any person who is aggrieved by such failure. Such a person may commence a civil action against the alliance in an appropriate State court or district court of the United States.

(b) EXHAUSTION OF REMEDIES.—

(1) IN GENERAL.—Except as provided in paragraph (2), in an action under subsection (a) the court may not exercise jurisdiction until the aggrieved person has exhausted any administrative remedies that may be provided by law.

(2) NO EXHAUSTION REQUIRED.—In an action under subsection (a), the court shall exercise juris-

diction without regard to whether the aggrieved person has exhausted any administrative or other remedies that may be provided by law if the action relates to—

    (A) whether the person is an eligible individual within the meaning of section 1001(c);

    (B) whether the person is eligible for a premium discount under subpart A of part 1 of subtitle B of title VI;

    (C) whether the person is eligible for a reduction in cost sharing under subpart D of part 3 of subtitle D of title I; or

    (D) enrollment or disenrollment in a health plan.

(c) RELIEF.—In an action under subsection (a), if the court finds that a failure described in such subsection has occurred, the aggrieved person may recover compensatory and punitive damages and the court may order any other appropriate relief.

(d) ATTORNEY'S FEES.—In any action under subsection (a), the court, in its discretion, may allow the prevailing party, other than the United States, a reasonable attorney's fee (including expert fees) as part of the costs, and the United States shall be liable for costs the same as a private person.

## SEC. 5238. DISCRIMINATION CLAIMS.

(a) CIVIL ACTION BY AGGRIEVED PERSON.—

(1) IN GENERAL.—Any person who is aggrieved by the failure of a health plan to comply with section 1402(c) may commence a civil action against the plan in an appropriate State court or district court of the United States.

(2) STANDARDS.—The standards used to determine whether a violation has occurred in a complaint alleging discrimination under section 1402(c) shall be the standards applied under the Age Discrimination Act of 1973 (42 U.S.C. 6102 et seq.) and the Americans with Disabilities Act of 1990 (42 U.S.C. 12101 et seq.).

(3) RELIEF.—In an action under paragraph (1), if the court finds that the health plan has failed to comply with section 1402(c), the aggrieved person may recover compensatory and punitive damages and the court may order any other appropriate relief.

(4) ATTORNEY'S FEES.—In any action under paragraph (1), the court, in its discretion, may allow the prevailing party, other than the United States, a reasonable attorney's fee (including expert fees) as part of the costs, and the United States shall be liable for costs the same as a private person.

(c) ACTION BY SECRETARY.—Whenever the Secretary of Health and Human Services finds that the health plan has failed to comply with section 1402(c), or with an applicable regulation issued under such section, the Secretary shall notify the plan. If within a reasonable period of time the health plan fails or refuses to comply, the Secretary may—

    (1) refer the matter to the Attorney General with a recommendation that an appropriate civil action be instituted;

    (2) terminate the participation of the health plan in an alliance; or

    (3) take such other action as may be provided by law.

(d) ACTION BY ATTORNEY GENERAL.—When a matter is referred to the Attorney General under subsection (c)(1), the Attorney General may bring a civil action in a district court of the United States for such relief as may be appropriate, including injunctive relief. In a civil action under this section, the court—

    (1) may grant any equitable relief that the court considers to be appropriate;

    (2) may award such other relief as the court considers to be appropriate, including compensatory and punitive damages; and

(3) may, to vindicate the public interest when requested by the Attorney General, assess a civil money penalty against the health plan in an amount—

    (A) not exceeding $50,000 for a first violation; and

    (B) not exceeding $100,000 for any subsequent violation.

## SEC. 5239. NONDISCRIMINATION IN FEDERALLY ASSISTED PROGRAMS.

Federal payments to regional alliances under part 2 of subtitle C of title VI shall be treated as Federal financial assistance for purposes of section 504 of the Rehabilitation Act of 1973 (29 U.S.C. 794), section 303 of the Age Discrimination Act of 1975 (42 U.S.C. 6102), and section 601 of the Civil Rights Act of 1964 (42 U.S.C. 2000d).

## SEC. 5240. CIVIL ACTION BY ESSENTIAL COMMUNITY PROVIDER.

(a) IN GENERAL.—An electing essential community provider (as defined in section 1431(d)) who is aggrieved by the failure of a health plan to fulfill a duty imposed on the plan by section 1431 may commence a civil action against the plan in an appropriate State court or district court of the United States.

1 (b) RELIEF.—In an action under subsection (a), if
2 the court finds that the health plan has failed to fulfill
3 a duty imposed on the plan by section 1431, the electing
4 essential community provider may recover compensatory
5 damages and the court may order any other appropriate
6 relief.

7 (c) ATTORNEY'S FEES.—In any action under sub-
8 section (a), the court, in its discretion, may allow the pre-
9 vailing party, other than the United States, a reasonable
10 attorney's fee (including expert fees) as part of the costs,
11 and the United States shall be liable for costs the same
12 as a private person.

13 **SEC. 5241. FACIAL CONSTITUTIONAL CHALLENGES.**

14 (a) JURISDICTION.—The United States District
15 Court for the District of Columbia shall have original and
16 exclusive jurisdiction of any civil action brought to invali-
17 date this Act or a provision of this Act on the ground of
18 its being repugnant to the Constitution of the United
19 States on its face and for every purpose. In any action
20 described in this subsection, the district court may not
21 grant any temporary order or preliminary injunction re-
22 straining the enforcement, operation, or execution of this
23 Act or any provision of this Act.

(b) STATUTE OF LIMITATIONS.—An action described in subsection (a) shall be commenced not later than 1 year after the date of the enactment of this Act.

(c) CONVENING OF THREE-JUDGE COURT.—An action described in subsection (a) shall be heard and determined by a district court of three judges in accordance with section 2284 of title 28, United States Code.

(d) CONSOLIDATION.—When actions described in subsection (a) involving a common question of law or fact are pending before a district court, the court shall order all the actions consolidated.

(e) DIRECT APPEAL TO SUPREME COURT.—In any action described in subsection (a), an appeal may be taken directly to the Supreme Court of the United States from any final judgment, decree, or order in which the district court—

 (1) holds this Act or any provision of this Act invalid; and

 (2) makes a determination that its holding will materially undermine the application of the Act as whole.

(f) CONSTRUCTION.—This section does not limit—

 (1) the right of any person—

  (A) to a litigation concerning the Act or any portion of the Act; or

(B) to petition the Supreme Court for review of any holding of a district court by writ of certiorari at any time before the rendition of judgment in a court of appeals; or

(2) the authority of the Supreme Court to grant a writ of certiorari for the review described in paragraph (1)(B).

SEC. 5242. TREATMENT OF PLANS AS PARTIES IN CIVIL ACTIONS.

(a) IN GENERAL.—A health plan may sue or be sued under this Act as an entity. Service of summons, subpoena, or other legal process of a court or hearing officer upon a trustee or an administrator of any such plan in his capacity as such shall constitute service upon the plan. In a case where a plan has not designated in applicable plan documents an individual as agent for the service of legal process, service upon the Secretary of Health and Human Services (in the case of a regional alliance health plan) or the Secretary of Labor (in the case of a corporate alliance health plan) shall constitute such service. The Secretary, not later than 15 days after receipt of service under the preceding sentence, shall notify the administrator or any trustee of the plan of receipt of such service.

(b) OTHER PARTIES.—Any money judgment under this Act against a plan referred to in subsection (b) shall be enforceable only against the plan as an entity and shall not be enforceable against any other person unless liability against such person is established in his individual capacity under this Act.

### SEC. 5243. GENERAL NONPREEMPTION OF EXISTING RIGHTS AND REMEDIES.

Nothing in this title shall be construed to deny, impair, or otherwise adversely affect a right or remedy available under law to any person on the date of the enactment of this Act or thereafter, except to the extent the right or remedy is inconsistent with this title.

## Subtitle D—Medical Malpractice

### PART 1—LIABILITY REFORM

### SEC. 5301. FEDERAL TORT REFORM.

(a) APPLICABILITY.—

(1) IN GENERAL.—Except as provided in section 5302, this part shall apply with respect to any medical malpractice liability action brought in any State or Federal court, except that this part shall not apply to a claim or action for damages arising from a vaccine-related injury or death to the extent that title XXI of the Public Health Service Act applies to the claim or action.

(2) PREEMPTION.—The provisions of this part shall preempt any State law to the extent such law

is inconsistent with the limitations contained in such provisions. The provisions of this part shall not preempt any State law that provides for defenses or places limitations on a person's liability in addition to those contained in this subtitle, places greater limitations on the amount of attorneys' fees that can be collected, or otherwise imposes greater restrictions than those provided in this part.

(3) EFFECT ON SOVEREIGN IMMUNITY AND CHOICE OF LAW OR VENUE.—Nothing in paragraph (2) shall be construed to—

    (A) waive or affect any defense of sovereign immunity asserted by any State under any provision of law;

    (B) waive or affect any defense of sovereign immunity asserted by the United States;

    (C) affect the applicability of any provision of the Foreign Sovereign Immunities Act of 1976;

    (D) preempt State choice-of-law rules with respect to claims brought by a foreign nation or a citizen of a foreign nation; or

    (E) affect the right of any court to transfer venue or to apply the law of a foreign nation or to dismiss a claim of a foreign nation or of a citizen of a foreign nation on the ground of inconvenient forum.

(4) FEDERAL COURT JURISDICTION NOT ESTABLISHED ON FEDERAL QUESTION GROUNDS.—Nothing in this part shall be construed to establish any jurisdiction in the district courts of the United States over medical malpractice liability actions on the basis of section 1331 or 1337 of title 28, United States Code.

(b) DEFINITIONS.—In this subtitle, the following definitions apply:

(1) ALTERNATIVE DISPUTE RESOLUTION SYSTEM; ADR.—The term "alternative dispute resolution system" or "ADR" means a system that provides for the resolution of medical malpractice claims in a manner other than through medical malpractice liability actions.

(2) CLAIMANT.—The term "claimant" means any person who alleges a medical malpractice claim, and any person on whose behalf such a claim is alleged, including the decedent in the case of an action brought through or on behalf of an estate.

(3) HEALTH CARE PROFESSIONAL.—The term "health care professional" means any individual who provides health care services in a State and who is

required by the laws or regulations of the State to be licensed or certified by the State to provide such services in the State.

(4) HEALTH CARE PROVIDER.—The term "health care provider" means any organization or institution that is engaged in the delivery of health care services in a State and that is required by the laws or regulations of the State to be licensed or certified by the State to engage in the delivery of such services in the State.

(5) INJURY.—The term "injury" means any illness, disease, or other harm that is the subject of a medical malpractice liability action or a medical malpractice claim.

(6) MEDICAL MALPRACTICE LIABILITY ACTION.—The term "medical malpractice liability action" means a civil action brought in a State or Federal court against a health care provider or health care professional (regardless of the theory of liability on which the claim is based) in which the plaintiff alleges a medical malpractice claim.

(7) MEDICAL MALPRACTICE CLAIM.—The term "medical malpractice claim" means a claim in a civil action brought against a health care provider or health care professional in which a claimant alleges

that injury was caused by the provision of (or the failure to provide) health care services, except that such term does not include—

    (A) any claim based on an allegation of an intentional tort; or

    (B) any claim based on an allegation that a product is defective that is brought against any individual or entity that is not a health care professional or health care provider.

## SEC. 5302. PLAN-BASED ALTERNATIVE DISPUTE RESOLUTION MECHANISMS.

(a) APPLICATION TO MALPRACTICE CLAIMS UNDER PLANS.—In the case of any medical malpractice claim arising from the provision of (or failure to provide) health care services to an individual enrolled in a regional alliance plan or a corporate alliance plan, no medical malpractice liability action may be brought with respect to such claim until the final resolution of the claim under the alternative dispute resolution system adopted by the plan under subsection (b).

(b) ADOPTION OF MECHANISM BY PLANS.—Each regional alliance plan and corporate alliance plan shall—

    (1) adopt at least one of the alternative dispute resolution methods specified under subsection (c) for the resolution of medical malpractice claims arising

from the provision of health care services to individuals enrolled in the plan; and

(2) disclose to enrollees (and potential enrollees), in a manner specified by the regional alliance or the corporate alliance, the availability and procedures for consumer grievances under the plan, including the alternative dispute resolution method or methods adopted under this subsection.

(c) SPECIFICATION OF PERMISSIBLE ALTERNATIVE DISPUTE RESOLUTION METHODS.—

(1) IN GENERAL.—The National Health Board shall, by regulation, develop alternative dispute resolution methods for the use by regional alliance and corporate alliance plans in resolving medical malpractice claims under subsection (a). Such methods shall include at least the following:

(A) ARBITRATION.—The use of arbitration.

(B) MEDIATION.—The use of required mediation.

(C) EARLY OFFERS OF SETTLEMENT.—The use of a process under which parties are required to make early offers of settlement.

(2) STANDARDS FOR ESTABLISHING METHODS.—In developing alternative dispute resolution

methods under paragraph (1), the National Health Board shall assure that the methods promote the resolution of medical malpractice claims in a manner that—

    (A) is affordable for the parties involved;

    (B) provides for timely resolution of claims;

    (C) provides for the consistent and fair resolution of claims; and

    (D) provides for reasonably convenient access to dispute resolution for individuals enrolled in plans.

(d) FURTHER REDRESS.—A plan enrollee dissatisfied with the determination reached as a result of an alternative dispute resolution method applied under this section may, after the final resolution of the enrollee's claim under the method, bring a cause of action to seek damages or other redress with respect to the claim to the extent otherwise permitted under State law.

## SEC. 5303. REQUIREMENT FOR CERTIFICATE OF MERIT.

(a) REQUIRING SUBMISSION WITH COMPLAINT.—No medical malpractice liability action may be brought by any individual unless, at the time the individual brings the action (except as provided in subsection (b)(2)), the individual submits an affidavit—

(1) declaring that the individual (or the individual's attorney) has consulted and reviewed the facts of the action with a qualified medical specialist (as defined in subsection (c));

(2) including a written report by a qualified medical specialist that clearly identifies the individual and that includes the medical specialist's determination that, after a review of the medical record and other relevant material, there is a reasonable and meritorious cause for the filing of the action against the defendant; and

(3) on the basis of the qualified medical specialist's review and consultation, that the individual (or the individual's attorney) has concluded that there is a reasonable and meritorious cause for the filing of the action.

(b) EXTENSION IN CERTAIN INSTANCES.—

(1) IN GENERAL.—Subject to paragraph (2), subsection (a) shall not apply with respect to an individual who brings a medical malpractice liability action without submitting an affidavit described in such subsection if—

(A) the individual is unable to obtain the affidavit before the expiration of the applicable statute of limitations; or

(B) at the time the individual brings the action, the individual has been unable to obtain medical records or other information necessary to prepare the affidavit requested pursuant to any applicable law.

(2) DEADLINE FOR SUBMISSION WHERE EXTENSION APPLIES.—In the case of an individual who brings an action for which paragraph (1) applies, the action shall be dismissed unless the individual submits the affidavit described in subsection (a) not later than—

(A) in the case of an action for which subparagraph (A) of paragraph (1) applies, 90 days after bringing the action; or

(B) in the case of an action for which subparagraph (B) of paragraph (1) applies, 90 days after obtaining the information described in such subparagraph.

(c) QUALIFIED MEDICAL SPECIALIST DEFINED.—In subsection (a), a "qualified medical specialist" means, with respect to a defendant to a medical malpractice liability action, a health care professional who—

(1) is knowledgeable of, and has expertise in, the same specialty area of medical practice that is the subject of the action; and

(2) is reasonably believed by the individual bringing the action (or the individual's attorney)—

    (A) to be knowledgeable in the relevant issues involved in the particular action,

    (B) to practice (or to have practiced within the preceding 6 years) or to teach (or to have taught within the preceding 6 years) in the same area of health care or medicine that is at issue in the action, and

    (C) to be qualified by experience or demonstrated competence in the subject of the case.

(d) SANCTIONS FOR SUBMITTING FALSE ALLEGATIONS.—Upon the motion of any party or its own initiative, the court in a medical malpractice liability action may impose a sanction on a party or the party's attorney (or both), including a requirement that the party reimburse the other party to the action for costs and reasonable attorney's fees, if any information contained in an affidavit described in subsection (a) is submitted without reasonable cause and is found to be untrue.

## SEC. 5304. LIMITATION ON AMOUNT OF ATTORNEY'S CONTINGENCY FEES.

(a) IN GENERAL.—An attorney who represents, on a contingency fee basis, a plaintiff in a medical malpractice liability action may not charge, demand, receive, or collect for services rendered in connection with such action (including the resolution of the claim that is the subject of the action under any alternative dispute resolution) in excess of 33⅓ of the total amount recovered by judgment or settlement in such action.

(b) CALCULATION OF PERIODIC PAYMENTS.—In the event that a judgment or settlement includes periodic or future payments of damages, the amount recovered for purposes of computing the limitation on the contingency fee under subsection (a) shall be based on the cost of the annuity or trust established to make the payments. In any case in which an annuity or trust is not established to make such payments, such amount shall be based on the present value of the payments.

(c) CONTINGENCY FEE DEFINED.—As used in this section, the term "contingency fee" means any fee for professional legal services which is, in whole or in part, contingent upon the recovery of any amount of damages, whether through judgment or settlement.

**SEC. 5305. REDUCTION OF AWARDS FOR RECOVERY FROM COLLATERAL SOURCES.**

The total amount of damages recovered by a plaintiff in a medical malpractice liability action shall be reduced by the amount of any past or future payment which the claimant has received or for which the claimant is eligible on account of the same injury for which the damages are awarded, including payment under—

 (1) Federal or State disability or sickness programs;

 (2) Federal, State, or private health insurance programs;

 (3) private disability insurance programs;

 (4) employer wage continuation programs; and

 (5) any other program, if the payment is intended to compensate the claimant for the same injury for which damages are awarded.

## SEC. 5306. PERIODIC PAYMENT OF AWARDS.

At the request of any party to a medical malpractice liability action, the defendant shall not be required to pay damages in a single, lump-sum payment, but shall be permitted to make such payments periodically based on such schedule as the court considers appropriate, taking into account the periods for which the injured party will need medical and other services.

## PART 2—OTHER PROVISIONS RELATING TO MEDICAL MALPRACTICE LIABILITY

### SEC. 5311. ENTERPRISE LIABILITY DEMONSTRATION PROJECT.

(a) ESTABLISHMENT.—Not later than January 1, 1996, the Secretary of Health and Human Services shall establish a demonstration project under which the Secretary shall provide funds (in such amount as the Secretary considers appropriate) to one or more eligible States to demonstrate whether substituting liability for medical malpractice on the part of the health plan in which a physician participates for the personal liability of the physician will result in improvements in the quality of care provided under the plan, reductions in defensive medical practices, and better risk management.

(b) ELIGIBILITY OF STATE.—A State is eligible to participate in the demonstration project established under subsection (a) if the State submits an application to the Secretary (at such time and in such form as the Secretary may require) containing such information and assurances as the Secretary may require, including assurances that the State—

    (1) has entered into an agreement with a health plan (other than a fee-for-service plan) operating in the State under which the plan assumes legal liability with respect to any medical malpractice claim arising from the provision of (or failure to provide) services under the plan by any physician participating in the plan;

    (2) has provided that, under the law of the State, a physician participating in a plan that has

entered into an agreement with the State under paragraph (1) may not be liable in damages or otherwise for such a claim and the plan may not require such physician to indemnify the plan for any such liability; and

(3) will provide the Secretary with such reports on the operation of the project as the Secretary may require.

(c) AUTHORIZATION OF APPROPRIATIONS.—There are authorized to be appropriated such sums as may be necessary to carry out demonstration projects under this section.

### SEC. 5312. PILOT PROGRAM APPLYING PRACTICE GUIDELINES TO MEDICAL MALPRACTICE LIABILITY ACTIONS.

(a) ESTABLISHMENT.—Not later than 1 year after the Secretary of Health and Human Services determines that appropriate practice guidelines are available, the Secretary shall establish a pilot program under which the Secretary shall provide funds (in such amount as the Secretary considers appropriate) to one or more eligible States to determine the effect of applying practice guidelines in the resolution of medical malpractice liability actions.

(b) ELIGIBILITY OF STATE.—A State is eligible to participate in the pilot program established under subsection (a) if the State submits an application to the Secretary (at such time and in such form as the Secretary may require) containing—

> (1) assurances that, under the law of the State, in the resolution of any medical malpractice liability action, it shall be a complete defense to any allegation that a party against whom the action is filed was negligent that, in the provision of (or the failure to provide) the services that are the subject of the action, the party followed the appropriate practice guideline established by the National Quality Management Program under subtitle A; and
>
> (2) such other information and assurances as the Secretary may require.

(c) REPORTS TO CONGRESS.—Not later than 3 months after each year for which the pilot program established under subsection (a) is in effect, the Secretary shall submit a report to Congress describing the operation of the program during the previous year and containing such recommendations as the Secretary considers appropriate, including recommendations relating to revisions to the laws governing medical malpractice liability.

# Subtitle E—Fraud and Abuse

## PART 1—ESTABLISHMENT OF ALL-PAYER HEALTH CARE FRAUD AND ABUSE CONTROL PROGRAM

### SEC. 5401. ALL-PAYER HEALTH CARE FRAUD AND ABUSE CONTROL PROGRAM.

(a) IN GENERAL.—Not later than January 1, 1996, the Secretary of Health and Human Services (acting through the Office of the Inspector General of the Department of Health and Human Services) and the Attorney General shall establish a program—

    (1) to coordinate the functions of the Attorney General, the Secretary, and other organizations with respect to the prevention, detection, and control of health care fraud and abuse,

    (2) to conduct investigations, audits, evaluations, and inspections relating to the delivery of and payment for health care in the United States, and

    (3) to facilitate the enforcement of this subtitle and other statutes applicable to health care fraud and abuse.

(b) COORDINATION WITH LAW ENFORCEMENT AGENCIES.—In carrying out the program under subsection (a), the Secretary and Attorney General shall consult with, and arrange for the sharing of data and resources with Federal, State and local law enforcement agencies, State Medicaid Fraud Control Units, and State agencies responsible for the licensing and certification of health care providers.

(c) COORDINATION WITH HEALTH ALLIANCES AND HEALTH PLANS.—In carrying out the program under subsection (a), the Secretary and Attorney General shall consult with, and arrange for the sharing of data with representatives of health alliances and health plans.

(d) AUTHORITIES OF ATTORNEY GENERAL, SECRETARY, AND INSPECTOR GENERAL.—In carrying out duties established under subsection (a), the Attorney General, the Secretary, and the Inspector General are authorized—

> (1) to conduct, supervise, and coordinate audits, civil and criminal investigations, inspections, and evaluations relating to the program established under such subsection; and

> (2) to have access (including on-line access as requested and available) to all records available to health alliances and health plans that relate to ongoing investigations or the imposition of sanctions under such program (subject to restrictions based on the confidentiality of certain information under subtitle B).

(e) QUALIFIED IMMUNITY FOR PROVIDING INFORMATION.—The provisions of section 1157(a) of the Social Security Act (relating to limitation on liability) shall apply to a person providing information or communications to the Secretary or Attorney General in conjunction with their performance of duties under this section, in the same manner as such section applies to information provided to organizations with a contract under part B of title XI of such Act.

(f) AUTHORIZATIONS OF APPROPRIATIONS FOR INVESTIGATORS AND OTHER PERSONNEL.—In addition to any other amounts authorized to be appropriated to the Secretary and the Attorney General for health care anti-fraud and abuse activities for a fiscal year, there are authorized to be appropriated such additional amounts as may be necessary to enable the Secretary and the Attorney General to conduct investigations, audits, evaluations, and inspections of allegations of health care fraud and abuse and otherwise carry out the program established under subsection (a) in a fiscal year.

(g) USE OF POWERS UNDER INSPECTOR GENERAL ACT OF 1978.—In carrying out duties and responsibilities under the program established under subsection (a), the Inspector General is authorized to exercise all powers granted under the Inspector General Act of 1978 to the same manner and extent as provided in that Act.

(h) DEFINITIONS.—In this part and part 2—

(1) the term "Inspector General" means the Inspector General of the Department of Health and Human Services; and

(2) the term "Secretary" means Secretary of Health and Human Services.

## SEC. 5402. ESTABLISHMENT OF ALL-PAYER HEALTH CARE FRAUD AND ABUSE CONTROL ACCOUNT.

(a) ESTABLISHMENT.—

(1) IN GENERAL.—There is hereby created on the books of the Treasury of the United States an account to be known as the "All-Payer Health Care Fraud and Abuse Control Account" (in this section referred to as the "Anti-Fraud Account"). The Anti-Fraud Account shall consist of such gifts and bequests as may be made as provided in paragraph (2) and such amounts as may be deposited in such Anti-Fraud Account as provided in subsection (b)(4) and title XI of the Social Security Act. It shall also include the following:

(A) All criminal fines imposed in cases involving a Federal health care offense (as defined in subsection (e)).

(B) Penalties and damages imposed under the False Claims Act (31 U.S.C. 3729 et seq.), in cases involving claims related to the provision of health care items and services (other than funds awarded to a relator or for restitution).

(C) Administrative penalties and assessments imposed under titles XI, XVIII and XIX of the Social Security Act and section 5412 (except as otherwise provided by law).

(D) Amounts resulting from the forfeiture of property by reason of a Federal health care offense.

Any such funds received on or after the date of the enactment of this Act shall be deposited in the Anti-Fraud Account.

(2) AUTHORIZATION TO ACCEPT GIFTS.—The Anti-Fraud Account is authorized to accept on behalf of the United States money gifts and bequests made unconditionally to the Anti-Fraud Account, for the benefit of the Anti-Fraud Account, or any activity financed through the Anti-Fraud Account.

(b) USE OF FUNDS.—

(1) IN GENERAL.—Amounts in the Anti-Fraud Account shall be available without appropriation and until expended to assist the Secretary and Attorney

General in carrying out the All-Payer Health Care Fraud and Abuse Control Program established under section 5401 (including the administration of the Program), and may be used to cover costs incurred in operating the Program, including—

>(A) costs of prosecuting health care matters (through criminal, civil and administrative proceedings);

>(B) costs of investigations (including equipment, salaries, administratively uncontrollable work, travel and training of law enforcement personnel);

>(C) costs of financial and performance audits of health care programs and operations;

>(D) costs of inspections and other evaluations.

>(2) FUNDS USED TO SUPPLEMENT AGENCY APPROPRIATIONS.—It is intended that disbursements made from the Anti-Fraud Account to any Federal agency be used to increase and not supplant the recipient agency's appropriated operating budget.

(c) ANNUAL REPORT.—The Secretary and the Attorney General shall submit an annual report to Congress on the amount of revenue which is generated and disbursed by the Anti-Fraud Account in each fiscal year.

(d) FEDERAL HEALTH CARE OFFENSE DEFINED.—
The term "Federal health care offense" means a violation
of, or a criminal conspiracy to violate—

    (1) sections 226, 668, 1033, or 1347 of title
18, United States Code;

    (2) section 1128B of the Social Security Act;

    (3) sections 287, 371, 664, 666, 1001, 1027,
1341, 1343, or 1954 of title 18, United States Code,
if the violation or conspiracy relates to health care
fraud;

    (4) sections 501 or 511 of the Employee Retirement Income Security Act of 1974, if the violation
or conspiracy relates to health care fraud;

    (5) sections 301, 303(a)(2), or 303(b) or (e) of
the Federal Food Drug and Cosmetic Act, if the violation or conspiracy relates to health care fraud.

**SEC. 5403. USE OF FUNDS BY INSPECTOR GENERAL.**

(a) REIMBURSEMENTS FOR INVESTIGATIONS.—

    (1) IN GENERAL.—The Inspector General is authorized to receive and retain for current use reimbursement for the costs of conducting investigations,
when such restitution is ordered by a court, voluntarily agreed to by the payor, or otherwise.

    (2) CREDITING.—Funds received by such Office
as reimbursement for costs of conducting investiga-

tions shall be deposited to the credit of such Office appropriation from which initially paid, or to appropriations for similar purposes currently available at the time of deposit, and shall remain available for obligation for 365 days from the date of their deposit.

(3) EXCEPTION FOR FORFEITURES.—This subsection does not apply to investigative costs paid to such Office from the Health Care Asset Forfeiture Fund, which monies shall be deposited and expended in accordance with subsection (b).

(b) HHS OFFICE OF INSPECTOR GENERAL ASSET FORFEITURE PROCEEDS FUND.—

(1) IN GENERAL.—There is established in the Treasury of the United States the "HHS Office of Inspector General Asset Forfeiture Proceeds Fund," to be administered by the Inspector General, which shall be available to such Office without fiscal year limitation for expenses relating to the investigation of matters within the jurisdiction of such Office.

(2) DEPOSITS.—There shall be deposited in the Fund all proceeds from forfeitures that have been transferred to the Office of Inspector General from the Department of Justice Asset Forfeiture Fund

under section 524(d)(1) of title 28, United States Code.

## PART 2—APPLICATION OF FRAUD AND ABUSE AUTHORITIES UNDER THE SOCIAL SECURITY ACT TO ALL PAYERS

### SEC. 5411. EXCLUSION FROM PARTICIPATION.

(a) MANDATORY EXCLUSION.—The Secretary shall exclude an individual or entity from participation in any applicable health plan if the individual or entity is described in section 1128(a) of the Social Security Act (relating to individuals and entities convicted of health care-related crimes or patient abuse).

(b) PERMISSIVE EXCLUSION.—The Secretary may exclude an individual or entity from participation in any applicable health plan if the individual or entity is described in section 1128(b) of the Social Security Act (other than paragraphs (6)(A), (6)(C), (6)(D), (10), or (13) of such section).

(c) NOTICE, EFFECTIVE DATE, AND PERIOD OF EXCLUSION.— (1) An exclusion under this section or section 5412(b)(3) shall be effective at such time and upon such reasonable notice to the public and to the individual or entity excluded as may be specified in regulations consistent with paragraph (2).

(2) Such an exclusion shall be effective with respect to services furnished to an individual on or after the effective date of the exclusion.

(3)(A) The Secretary shall specify, in the notice of exclusion under paragraph (1) and the written notice under section 5412 of this Act, the minimum period (or, in the case of an exclusion of an individual described in section 1128(b)(12) of the Social Security Act, the period) of the exclusion.

(B) In the case of a mandatory exclusion under subsection (a), the minimum period of exclusion shall be not less than 5 years.

(C) In the case of an exclusion of an individual described in paragraph (1), (2), or (3) of section 1128(b) of the Social Security Act, the period of exclusion shall be a minimum of 3 years, unless the Secretary determines that a longer period is necessary because of aggravating circumstances.

(D) In the case of an exclusion of an individual or entity described in paragraph (4) or (5) of sections 1128(b) of the Social Security Act, the period of the exclusion shall not be less than the period during which the individual's or entity's license to provide health care is revoked, suspended or surrendered, or the individual or the entity is excluded or suspended from a Federal or State health care program.

(E) In the case of an exclusion of an individual or entity described in paragraph (6)(B) of section 1128(b) of the Social Security Act, the period of the exclusion shall be not less than 1 year.

(F) In the case of an exclusion of an individual described in paragraph (12) of section 1128(b) of the Social Security Act, the period of the exclusion shall be equal to the sum of—

   (i) the length of the period in which the individual failed to grant the immediate access described in that paragraph, and

   (ii) an additional period, not to exceed 90 days, set by the Secretary.

(d) NOTICE TO ENTITIES ADMINISTERING PUBLIC PROGRAMS FOR THE DELIVERY OF OR PAYMENT FOR HEALTH CARE ITEMS OR SERVICES.—(1) The Secretary shall exercise the authority under this section in a manner that results in an individual's or entity's exclusion from all applicable health plans for the delivery of or payment for health care items or services.

(2) The Secretary shall promptly notify each sponsor of an applicable health plan and each entity that administers a State health care program described in section

1128(h) of the Social Security Act of the fact and circumstances of each exclusion effected against an individual or entity under this section or under section 5412.

(e) NOTICE TO STATE LICENSING AGENCIES.—The provisions of section 1128(e) of the Social Security Act shall apply to this section in the same manner as such provisions apply to sections 1128 and 1128A of such Act.

(f) NOTICE, HEARING, AND JUDICIAL REVIEW.—(1) Subject to paragraph (2), any individual or entity that is excluded (or directed to be excluded) from participation under this section is entitled to reasonable notice and opportunity for a hearing thereon by the Secretary to the same extent as is provided in section 205(b) of the Social Security Act, and to judicial review of the Secretary's final decision after such hearing as is provided in section 205(g) of such Act, except that such action shall be brought in the Court of Appeals of the United States for the judicial circuit in which the individual or entity resides, or has a principal place of business, or, if the individual or entity does not reside or have a principal place of business within any such judicial circuit, in the United States Court of Appeals for the District of Columbia Circuit.

(2) Unless the Secretary determines that the health or safety of individuals receiving services warrants the exclusion taking effect earlier, any individual or entity that

is the subject of an adverse determination based on paragraphs (3), (4), (5), (6), (7), (8), (9), or (14) of section 1128(b) of the Social Security Act, shall be entitled to a hearing by an administrative law judge (as provided under section 205(b) of the Social Security Act) on the determination before any exclusion based upon the determination takes effect. If a hearing is requested, the exclusion shall be effective upon the issuance of an order by the administrative law judge upholding the determination of the Secretary to exclude.

(3) The provisions of section 205(h) of the Social Security Act shall apply with respect to this section to the same extent as such provisions apply with respect to title II of such Act.

(g) APPLICATION FOR TERMINATION OF EXCLUSION.—(1) An individual or entity excluded (or directed to be excluded) from participation under this section or section 5412(b)(3) may apply to the Secretary, in the manner specified by the Secretary in regulations and at the end of the minimum period of exclusion (or, in the case of an individual or entity described in section 1128(b)(8), the period of exclusion) provided under this section and a such other times as the Secretary may provide, for termination of the exclusion.

(2) The Secretary may terminate the exclusion if the Secretary determines, on the basis of the conduct of the applicant which occurred after the date of the notice of exclusion or which was unknown to the Secretary at the time of the exclusion, that—

>(A) there is no basis under this section or section 5412(b)(3) for a continuation of the exclusion, and
>
>(B) there are reasonable assurances that the types of actions which formed the basis for the original exclusion have not recurred and will not recur.

(3) The Secretary shall promptly notify each sponsor of an applicable health plan entity that administers a State health care program described in section 1128(h) of the Social Security Act of each termination of exclusion made under this subsection.

(h) CONVICTED DEFINED.—In this section, the term "convicted" has the meaning given such term in section 1128(i) of the Social Security Act.

(i) REQUEST FOR EXCLUSION.—The sponsor of any applicable health plan (including a State in the case of a regional alliance health plan and the Secretary of Labor in the case of a corporate alliance health plan) may request that the Secretary of Health and Human Services exclude an individual or entity with respect to actions under such a plan in accordance with this section.

SEC. 5412. CIVIL MONETARY PENALTIES.

(a) ACTIONS SUBJECT TO PENALTY.—Any person who is determined by the Secretary to have committed any of the following actions with respect to an applicable health plan shall be subject to a penalty in accordance with subsection (b):

(1) ACTIONS SUBJECT TO PENALTY UNDER MEDICARE, MEDICAID, AND OTHER SOCIAL SECURITY HEALTH PROGRAMS.—Any action that would subject the person to a penalty under paragraphs (1) through (12) of section 1128A of the Social Security Act if the action was taken with respect to title V, XVIII, XIX or XX of such Act.

(2) TERMINATION OF ENROLLMENT.—The termination of an individual's enrollment (including the refusal to re-enroll an individual) in violation of subtitle E of title I or State law.

(3) DISCRIMINATING ON BASIS OF MEDICAL CONDITION.—The engagement in any practice that would reasonably be expected to have the effect of denying or discouraging the initial or continued enrollment in a health plan by individuals whose medi-

cal condition or history indicates a need for substantial future medical services.

(4) INDUCING ENROLLMENT ON FALSE PRETENSES.—The engagement in any practice to induce enrollment in an applicable health plan through representations to individuals which the person knows or should know are false or fraudulent.

(5) PROVIDING INCENTIVES TO ENROLL.—The offer or payment of remuneration to any individual eligible to enroll in an applicable health plan that such person knows or should know is likely to influence such individual to enroll in a particular plan.

(b) PENALTIES DESCRIBED.—

(1) GENERAL RULE.—Any person who the Secretary determines has committed an action described in paragraphs (2) through (6) of subsection (a) shall be subject to a civil monetary penalty in an amount not to exceed $50,000 for each such determination.

(2) ACTIONS SUBJECT TO PENALTIES UNDER SOCIAL SECURITY ACT.—In the case of a person who the Secretary determines has committed an action described in paragraph (1) of subsection (a), the person shall be subject to the civil monetary penalty (together with any additional assessment) to which the person would be subject under section 1128A of

the Social Security Act if the action on which the determination is based had been committed with respect to title V, XVIII, XIX or XX of such Act.

(3) DETERMINATIONS TO EXCLUDE PERMITTED.—In addition to any civil monetary penalty imposed under this subsection, the Secretary may make a determination in the same proceeding to exclude the person from participation in all applicable health plans for the delivery of or payment for health care items or services (in accordance with section 5411(c)).

(c) PROCEDURES FOR IMPOSITION OF PENALTIES.—

(1) APPLICABILITY OF PROCEDURES UNDER SOCIAL SECURITY ACT.—Except as otherwise provided in paragraphs (2) and (3), the provisions of subsections (c), (d), (e), (g), (j), (k), and (l) of section 1128A of the Social Security Act shall apply with respect to the imposition of penalties under this section in the same manner as such provisions apply with respect to the imposition of civil monetary penalties under section 1128A of such Act.

(2) LIMITATION ON TIME FOR ATTORNEY GENERAL TO ACT.—The first sentence of section 1128A(c) of the Social Security Act shall be applied with respect to civil monetary penalties under this

section as if the reference in such section to "one year" was a reference to "60 days".

(3) AUTHORITY OF STATES TO IMPOSE PENALTIES.—If no proceeding to impose a civil monetary penalty under this section with respect to actions relating to a regional alliance health plan has been initiated (by either the Attorney General or the Secretary) within 120 days after the Secretary presents a case to the Attorney General for consideration of the imposition of such a penalty, the State in which the alliance is located may initiate proceedings to impose a civil monetary penalty under this section with respect to the action in the same manner as the Secretary may initiate such proceedings.

(d) TREATMENT OF AMOUNTS RECOVERED.—Any amounts recovered under this section shall be paid to the Secretary and disposed of as follows:

(1) Such portions of the amounts recovered as is determined to have been improperly paid from an applicable health plan for the delivery of or payment for health care items or services shall be repaid to such plan.

(2) The remainder of the amounts recovered shall be deposited in the All-Payer Health Care

Fraud and Abuse Control Account established under section 5402.

(e) NOTIFICATION OF LICENSING AUTHORITIES.—Whenever the Secretary's determination to impose a penalty, assessment, or exclusion under this section becomes final, the Secretary shall notify the appropriate State or local licensing agency or organization (including the agency specified in section 1864(a) and 1902(a)(33) of the Social Security Act) that such a penalty, assessment, or exclusion has become final and the reasons therefor.

**SEC. 5413. LIMITATIONS ON PHYSICIAN SELF-REFERRAL.**

The provisions of section 1877 of the Social Security Act shall apply—

    (1) to items and services (and payments and claims for payment for such items and services) furnished under any applicable health plan in the same manner as such provisions apply to designated health services (and payments and claims for payment for such services) under title XVIII of the Social Security Act; and

    (2) to a State (with respect to an item or service furnished or payment made under a regional alliance health plan) and to the Secretary of Labor (with respect to a an item or service furnished or payment made under a corporate alliance health

plan) in the same manner as such provisions apply to the Secretary.

### SEC. 5414. CONSTRUCTION OF SOCIAL SECURITY ACT REFERENCES.

(a) INCORPORATION OF OTHER AMENDMENTS.—Any reference in this part to a provision of the Social Security Act shall be considered a reference to the provision as amended under title IV.

(b) EFFECT OF SUBSEQUENT AMENDMENTS.—Except as provided in subsection (a), any reference to a provision of the Social Security Act in this part shall be deemed to be a reference to such provision as in effect on the date of the enactment of this Act, and (except as Congress may otherwise provide) any amendments made to such provisions after such date shall not be taken into account in determining the applicability of such provisions to individuals and entities under this Act.

## PART 3—AMENDMENTS TO ANTI-FRAUD AND ABUSE PROVISIONS UNDER THE SOCIAL SECURITY ACT

### SEC. 5421. REFERENCE TO AMENDMENTS.

For provisions amending the anti-fraud and abuse provisions existing under the Social Security Act, see part 5 of subtitle A of title IV.

# PART 4—AMENDMENTS TO CRIMINAL LAW

## SEC. 5431. HEALTH CARE FRAUD.

(a) IN GENERAL.—Chapter 63 of title 18, United States Code, is amended by adding at the end the following:

**"§ 1347. Health care fraud**

"(a) Whoever knowingly executes, or attempts to execute, a scheme or artifice—

"(1) to defraud any health alliance, health plan, or other person, in connection with the delivery of or payment for health care benefits, items, or services;

"(2) to obtain, by means of false or fraudulent pretenses, representations, or promises, any of the money or property owned by, or under the custody or control of, any health alliance, health plan, or person in connection with the delivery of or payment for health care benefits, items, or services;

shall be fined under this title or imprisoned not more than 10 years, or both. If the violation results in serious bodily injury (as defined in section 1365 of this title) such person shall be imprisoned for life or any term of years.

"(b) As used in this section, the terms 'health alliance' and 'health plan' have the meanings given those terms in title I of the Health Security Act.".

(b) CLERICAL AMENDMENT.—The table of sections at the beginning of chapter 63 of title 18, United States Code, is amended by adding at the end the following:

"1347. Health care fraud.".

## SEC. 5432. FORFEITURES FOR VIOLATIONS OF FRAUD STATUTES.

(a) IN GENERAL.—Section 982(a) of title 18, United States Code, is amended by inserting after paragraph (5) the following:

"(6) If the court determines that a Federal health care offense (as defined in section 5402(e) of the Health Security Act) is of a type that poses a serious threat to the health of any person or has a significant detrimental impact on the health care system, the court, in imposing sentence on a person convicted of that offense, shall order that person to forfeit property, real or personal, that—

"(A)(i) is used in the commission of the offense; or

"(ii) constitutes or is derived from proceeds traceable to the commission of the offense; and

"(B) is of a value proportionate to the seriousness of the offense.".

(b) PROCEEDS OF HEALTH CARE FRAUD FORFEITURES.—Section 524(c)(4)(A) of title 28, United States Code, is amended by inserting "all proceeds of forfeitures relating to Federal health care offenses (as defined in section 5402(e) of the Health Security Act), and" after "except".

**SEC. 5433. FALSE STATEMENTS.**

(a) IN GENERAL.—Chapter 47 of title 18, United States Code, is amended by adding at the end the following:

**"§ 1033. False statements relating to health care matters**

"(a) Whoever, in any matter involving a health alliance or health plan, knowingly and willfully falsifies, conceals, or covers up by any trick, scheme, or device a material fact, or makes any false, fictitious, or fraudulent statements or representations, or makes or uses any false writing or document knowing the same to contain any false, fictitious, or fraudulent statement or entry, shall be fined under this title or imprisoned not more than 5 years, or both.

"(b) As used in this section the terms 'health alliance' and 'health plan' have the meanings given those terms in title I of the Health Security Act.".

(b) CLERICAL AMENDMENT.—The table of sections at the beginning of chapter 47 of title 18, United States Code, is amended by adding at the end the following:

"1033. False statements relating to health care matters.".

**Health Security Act**  *Title V, Subtitle E*

**SEC. 5434. BRIBERY AND GRAFT.**

(a) IN GENERAL.—Chapter 11 of title 18, United States Code, is amended by adding at the end the following:

**"§ 226. Bribery and graft in connection with health care**

"(a) Whoever—

"(1) directly or indirectly, corruptly gives, offers, or promises anything of value to a health care official, or offers or promises a health care official to give anything of value to any other person, with intent—

"(A) to influence, or for or because of, any of the health care official's actions, decisions, or duties relating to a health alliance or health plan;

"(B) to influence such an official to commit or aid in the committing, or collude in or allow, any fraud, or make opportunity for the commission of any fraud, on a health alliance or health plan, or for or because of any such conduct on the part of such an official; or

"(C) to induce such an official to engage in any conduct in violation of the lawful duty of such official, or for or because of such conduct; or

"(2) being a health care official, directly or indirectly, corruptly demands, seeks, receives, accepts, or agrees to accept anything of value personally or for any other person or entity, the giving of which violates paragraph (1) of this subsection.

"(b) As used in this section—

"(1) the term 'health care official' means—

"(A) an administrator, officer, trustee, fiduciary, custodian, counsel, agent, or employee of any health care alliance or health plan;

"(B) an officer, counsel, agent, or employee, of an organization that provides services under contract to any health alliance or health plan;

"(C) an official or employee of a State agency having regulatory authority over any health alliance or health plan;

"(D) an officer, counsel, agent, or employee of a health care sponsor; and

"(2) the term 'health care sponsor' means any individual or entity serving as the sponsor of a health alliance or health plan for purposes of the Health Security Act, and includes the joint board of trustees or other similar body used by two or more employers to administer a health alliance or health plan for purposes of such Act.".

(b) CLERICAL AMENDMENT.—The table of chapters at the beginning of chapter 11 of title 18, United States Code, is amended by adding at the end the following:

"226. Bribery and graft in connection with health care.".

## SEC. 5435. INJUNCTIVE RELIEF RELATING TO HEALTH CARE OFFENSES.

Section 1345(a)(1) of title 18, United States Code, is amended—

(1) by striking "or" at the end of subparagraph (A);

(2) by inserting "or" at the end of subparagraph (B); and

(3) by adding at the end the following:

"(C) committing or about to commit a Federal health care offense (as defined in section 5402(e) of the Health Security Act);".

## SEC. 5436. GRAND JURY DISCLOSURE.

Section 3322 of title 18, United States Code, is amended—

(1) by redesignating subsections (c) and (d) as subsections (d) and (e), respectively; and

(2) by inserting after subsection (b) the following:

"(c) A person who is privy to grand jury information concerning a health law violation—

   "(1) received in the course of duty as an attorney for the Government; or

   "(2) disclosed under rule 6(e)(3)(A)(ii) of the Federal Rules of Criminal Procedure;

may disclose that information to an attorney for the Government to use in any civil proceeding related to a Federal health care offense (as defined in section 5402(e) of the Health Security Act), or for use in connection with civil forfeiture under section 981(a)(1)(C) of this title.".

SEC. 5437. THEFT OR EMBEZZLEMENT.

(a) IN GENERAL.—Chapter 31 of title 18, United States Code, is amended by adding at the end the following:

"§ 668. Theft or embezzlement in connection with health care

"(a) Whoever embezzles, steals, willfully and unlawfully converts to the use of any person other than the rightful owner, or intentionally misapplies any of the moneys, securities, premiums, credits, property, or other assets of a health alliance, health plan, or of any fund connected with such an alliance or plan, shall be fined under this title or imprisoned not more than 10 years, or both.

"(b) As used in this section, the terms 'health alliance' and 'health plan' have the meanings given those terms under title I of the Health Security Act.".

(b) CLERICAL AMENDMENT.—The table of sections at the beginning of chapter 31 of title 18, United States Code, is amended by adding at the end the following:

"668. Theft or embezzlement in connection with health care.".

## SEC. 5438. MISUSE OF HEALTH SECURITY CARD OR UNIQUE IDENTIFIER.

(a) IN GENERAL.—Chapter 33 of title 18, United States Code, is amended by adding at the end the following new section:

**"§ 716. Misuse of health security card or unique identifier**

"Whoever—

"(1) requires the display of, requires the use of, or uses a health security card that is issued under section 1001(b) of the American Health Security Act for any purpose other than a purpose described in section 5105(a) of such Act; or

"(2) requires the disclosure of, requires the use of, or uses a unique identifier number provided pursuant to section 5104 of such Act for any purpose that is not authorized by the National Health Board pursuant to such section;

shall be fined under this title or imprisoned not more than 2 years, or both.".

(b) CLERICAL AMENDMENTS TO TABLE OF SECTIONS.—The table of sections at the beginning of chapter 33, United States Code, is amended—

 (1) by amending the catchline to read as follows:

### "CHAPTER 33—EMBLEMS, INSIGNIA, IDENTIFIERS, AND NAMES";

and

 (2) by adding at the end the following new item:

"716. Misuse of health security card or unique identifier.".

(c) CLERICAL AMENDMENT TO TABLE OF CHAPTERS.—The item relating to chapter 33 in the table of chapters at the beginning of part 1 of title 18, United States Code, is amended to read as follows:

"33. Emblems, insignia, identifiers, and names ................... 701".

## PART 5—AMENDMENTS TO CIVIL FALSE CLAIMS ACT

**SEC. 5441. AMENDMENTS TO CIVIL FALSE CLAIMS ACT.**

Section 3729 of title 31, United States Code, is amended—

 (1) in subsection (a)(7), by inserting "or to a health plan," after "property to the Government,";

(2) in the matter following subsection (a)(7), by inserting "or health plan" before "sustains because of the act of that person,";

(3) at the end of the first sentence of subsection (a), by inserting "or health plan" before "sustains because of the act of the person.";

(4) in subsection (c)—

(A) by inserting "the term" after "section,"; and

(B) by adding at the end the following: "The term also includes any request or demand, whether under contract of otherwise, for money or property which is made or presented to a health plan."; and

(5) by adding at the end the following:

"(f) HEALTH PLAN DEFINED.—For purposes of this section, the term 'health plan' has the meaning given such term under section 1400 of the Health Security Act.".

# Subtitle F—McCarran-Ferguson Reform

SEC. 5501. REPEAL OF EXEMPTION FOR HEALTH INSURANCE.

(a) IN GENERAL.—Section 3 of the Act of March 9, 1945 (15 U.S.C. 1013), known as the McCarran-Ferguson Act, is amended by adding at the end the following:

"(c) Notwithstanding that the business of insurance is regulated by State law, nothing in this Act shall limit the applicability of the following Acts to the business of insurance to the extent that such business relates to the provision of health benefits:

"(1) The Sherman Act (15 U.S.C. 1 et seq.).

"(2) The Clayton Act (15 U.S.C. 12 et seq.).

"(3) Federal Trade Commission Act (15 U.S.C. 41 et seq.).

"(4) The Act of June 19, 1936 (49 Stat. 1526; 15 U.S.C. 21a et seq.), known as the Robinson-Patman Antidiscrimination Act.".

(b) EFFECTIVE DATE.—The amendment made by subsection (a) shall take effect on the first day of the sixth month beginning after the date of the enactment of this Act.

Health Security Act  Title VI

# TITLE VI—PREMIUM CAPS; PREMIUM-BASED FINANCING; AND PLAN PAYMENTS

TABLE OF CONTENTS OF TITLE

Sec. 6000. General definitions.

### Subtitle A—Premium Caps

PART 1—REGIONAL ALLIANCE HEALTH EXPENDITURES

SUBPART A—COMPUTATION OF TARGETS AND ACCEPTED BIDS

Sec. 6001. Computation of regional alliance inflation factors.
Sec. 6002. Board determination of national per capita baseline premium target.
Sec. 6003. Determination of alliance per capita premium targets.
Sec. 6004. Alliance initial bidding and negotiation process.
Sec. 6005. State financial incentives.
Sec. 6006. Recommendations to eliminate regional variations in alliance targets due to variation in practice patterns; congressional consideration.
Sec. 6007. Reference to limitation on administrative and judicial review of certain determinations.

SUBPART B—PLAN AND PROVIDER PAYMENT REDUCTIONS TO MAINTAIN EXPENDITURES WITHIN TARGETS

Sec. 6011. Plan payment reduction.
Sec. 6012. Provider payment reduction.

PART 2—CORPORATE ALLIANCES HEALTH EXPENDITURES

Sec. 6021. Calculation of premium equivalents.
Sec. 6022. Termination of corporate alliance for excess increase in expenditures.

PART 3—TREATMENT OF SINGLE-PAYER STATES

Sec. 6031. Special rules for single-payer States.

PART 4—TRANSITION PROVISIONS

Sec. 6041. Monitoring prices and expenditures.

### Subtitle B—Premium-Related Financing

PART 1—FAMILY PREMIUM PAYMENTS

SUBPART A—FAMILY SHARE

Sec. 6101. Family share of premium.
Sec. 6102. Amount of premium.
Sec. 6103. Alliance credit.
Sec. 6104. Premium discount based on income.

Sec. 6105. Excess premium credit.
Sec. 6106. Corporate alliance opt-in credit.
Sec. 6107. Family collection shortfall add-on.

SUBPART B—REPAYMENT OF ALLIANCE CREDIT BY CERTAIN FAMILIES

Sec. 6111. Repayment of alliance credit by certain families.
Sec. 6112. No liability for families employed full-time; reduction in liability for part-time employment.
Sec. 6113. Limitation of liability based on income.
Sec. 6114. Special treatment of certain retirees and qualified spouses and children.
Sec. 6115. Special treatment of certain medicare beneficiaries.

PART 2—EMPLOYER PREMIUM PAYMENTS

SUBPART A—REGIONAL ALLIANCE EMPLOYERS

Sec. 6121. Employer premium payment required.
Sec. 6122. Computation of base employment monthly premium.
Sec. 6123. Premium discount for certain employers.
Sec. 6124. Payment adjustment for large employers electing coverage in a regional alliance.
Sec. 6125. Employer collection shortfall add-on.
Sec. 6126. Application to self-employed individuals.

SUBPART B—CORPORATE ALLIANCE EMPLOYERS

Sec. 6131. Employer premium payment required.

Subtitle C—Payments to Regional Alliance Health Plans

Sec. 6201. Computation of blended plan per capita payment amount.
Sec. 6202. Computation of plan bid, AFDC, and SSI proportions.

## SEC. 6000. GENERAL DEFINITIONS.

(a) DEFINITIONS RELATING TO BIDS.—In this title:

(1) ACCEPTED BID.—The term "accepted bid" means the bid which is agreed to between a regional alliance health plan and a regional alliance for coverage of the comprehensive benefit package in the alliance area under part 1.

(2) FINAL ACCEPTED BID.—The term "final accepted bid" means the accepted bid, taking into account any voluntary reduction in such bid made under section 6004(e).

(3) WEIGHTED AVERAGE ACCEPTED BID.—The term "weighted average accepted bid" means, for a regional alliance for a year, the average of the accepted bids for all regional alliance health plans offered by such alliance, weighted to reflect the relative enrollment of regional alliance eligible individuals among such plans.

(4) REDUCED WEIGHTED AVERAGE ACCEPTED BID.—The term "reduced weighted average accepted bid", for a health plan offered by a regional alliance for a year, is the lesser of—

(A) the weighted average accepted bid for the regional alliance for the year (determined using the final accepted bids as the accepted bids), or

(B) the regional alliance per capita target for the year.

(b) WEIGHTED AVERAGE PREMIUM.—In this title, the term "weighted average premium" means, for a class of family enrollment and with respect to a regional alliance for a year, the product of—

(1) reduced weighted average accepted bid (as defined in subsection (a)(4));

(2) the uniform per capita conversion factor (established under section 1341(b)) for the alliance; and

(3) the premium class factor established by the Board for that class under section 1531.

(c) INCORPORATION OF OTHER DEFINITIONS.—Except as otherwise provided in this title, the definitions of terms in subtitle J of title I of this Act shall apply to this title.

# Subtitle A—Premium Caps

## PART 1—REGIONAL ALLIANCE HEALTH EXPENDITURES

### Subpart A—Computation of Targets and Accepted Bids

### SEC. 6001. COMPUTATION OF REGIONAL ALLIANCE INFLATION FACTORS.

(a) COMPUTATION.—

(1) IN GENERAL.—This section provides for the computation of a factors that limit the growth of premiums for the comprehensive benefit package in regional alliance health plans. The Board shall compute and publish, not later than March 1 of each year (beginning with 1995) the regional alliance inflation factor (as defined in paragraph (2)) for each regional alliance for the following year.

(2) REGIONAL ALLIANCE INFLATION FACTOR.—In this part, the term "regional alliance inflation factor" means, for a year for a regional alliance—

    (A) the general health care inflation factor for the year (as defined in paragraph (2));

    (B) adjusted under subsection (c) (to take into account material changes in the demographic and socio-economic characteristics of the population of alliance eligible individuals);

    (C) decreased by the percentage adjustment (if any) provided with respect to the regional alliance under subsection (d) (relating to adjustment for previous excess expenditures); and

    (D) in the case of the year 2001, increased by a factor that the Board determines to reflect the ratio of (i) the actuarial value of the increase in benefits provided in that year under the comprehensive benefit package to (ii) the actuarial value of the benefits that would have been in such package in the year without regard to the increase.

(3) GENERAL HEALTH CARE INFLATION FACTOR.—

(A) 1996 THROUGH 1999his part, the term "general health care inflation factor", for a year, means the percentage increase in the CPI (as specified under subsection (b)) for the year plus the following:

(i) For 1996, 1.5 percentage points.

(ii) For 1997, 1.0 percentage points.

(iii) For 1998, 0.5 percentage points.

(iv) For 1999, 0 percentage points.

(B) YEARS AFTER 1999.—

(i) RECOMMENDATION TO CONGRESS.—In 1998, the Board shall submit to Congress recommendations on what the general health care inflation factor should be for years beginning with 2000.

(ii) FAILURE OF CONGRESS TO ACT.— If the Congress fails to enact a law specifying the general health care inflation factor for a year after 1999, the Board, in January of the year before the year involved, shall compute such factor for the year involved. Such factor shall be the product of the factors described in subparagraph (C) for that fiscal year.

(C) FACTOR.—The factor described in this subparagraph for a year is 1 plus the following:

(i) CPI.—The percentage change in the CPI for the year, determined based upon the percentage change in the average of the CPI for the 12-month period ending with August 31 of the previous fiscal year over such average for the preceding 12-month period.

(ii) POPULATION.—The average annual percentage change in the population of the United States during the 3-year period ending in the calendar year, determined by the Board based on data supplied by the Bureau of the Census.

(iii) REAL GDP PER CAPITA.—The average annual percentage change in the real, per capita gross domestic product of the United States during the 3-year period ending in the preceding calendar year, determined by the Board based on data supplied by the Department of Commerce.

(b) PROJECTION OF INCREASE IN CPI.—

(1) IN GENERAL.—For purposes of this section, the Board shall specify, as of the time of publica-

tion, the annual percentage increase in the CPI (as defined in section 1902(9)) for the following year.

(2) DATA TO BE USED.—Such increase shall be the projection of the CPI contained in the budget of the United States transmitted by the President to the Congress in the year.

(c) SPECIAL ADJUSTMENT FOR MATERIAL CHANGES IN DEMOGRAPHIC CHARACTERISTICS OF POPULATION.—

(1) ADJUSTMENT FOR CORPORATE ALLIANCE OPT-IN.—

(A) IN GENERAL.—The Board shall develop a method for adjusting the regional alliance inflator factor for each regional alliance in order to reflect material changes in the demographic characteristics of regional alliance eligible individuals residing in the alliance area (in comparison with such characteristics for the previous year) as a result of one or more corporate alliances terminating an election under section 1313.

(B) BASIS FOR ADJUSTMENTS.—Adjustments under this paragraph (whether an increase or decrease) shall be based on the characteristics and factors used for making adjustments in payments under section 6124.

(2) ADJUSTMENT FOR REGIONAL TREND COMPARED TO NATIONAL TREND.—

(A) IN GENERAL.—The Board shall develop a method for adjusting the regional alliance inflator factor for each regional alliance in order to reflect material changes in the demographic characteristics (including at least age, gender, and socio-economic status) and health status of regional alliance eligible individuals residing in the alliance area in comparison with the average change in such characteristics for such individuals residing in the United States. The adjustment under this paragraph shall be for changes not taken into account in the adjustment under paragraph (1).

(B) NEUTRAL ADJUSTMENT.—Such method (and any annual adjustment under this paragraph) shall be designed to result in the adjustment effected under this paragraph for a year not changing the weighted average of the regional alliance inflation factors.

(3) APPLICATION.—The Board shall provide, on an annual basis, for an adjustment of regional alliance inflation factors under this subsection using such method.

(d) ADJUSTMENT FOR PREVIOUS EXCESS RATE OF INCREASE IN EXPENDITURES.—

(1) IN GENERAL.—If actual weighted average accepted bid for a regional alliance for a year (as determined by the Board based on actual enrollment in the first month of the year) exceeds the regional alliance per capita premium target (determined under section 6003(a)) for the year, then the regional alliance inflation factor—

(A) for the succeeding year shall be reduced by the product of—

(i) ½ of the excess percentage (described in paragraph (3)) for the previous year, and

(ii) the adjustment factor (described in paragraph (2)(A)) for such succeeding year; and

(B) in the second succeeding year shall be reduced by the product of—

(i) ½ of such excess percentage, and

(ii) the adjustment factor (described in paragraph (2)(B)) for such second succeeding year.

(2) ADJUSTMENT FACTORS.—

(A) SUCCEEDING YEAR.—With respect to a succeeding year, the adjustment factor described in this subparagraph is 1 plus the regional alliance inflation factor for such year.

(B) SECOND SUCCEEDING YEAR.—With respect to a second succeeding year, the adjustment factor described in this subparagraph is the product of—

(i) 1 plus the regional alliance inflation factor for such year, and

(ii) 1 plus the regional alliance inflation factor for the previous year.

(C) NO ADJUSTMENT IN FACTOR CONSIDERED.—For purposes of subparagraphs (A) and (B), the regional alliance inflation factor for a year shall not take into account any adjustment under this subsection.

(3) EXCESS PERCENTAGE.—The excess percentage described in this paragraph for a year is the percentage by which—

(A) actual weighted average accepted bid (referred to in paragraph (1)) for a regional alliance for the year, exceeds

(B) the regional alliance per capita premium target (determined under section 6003(a)) for the year.

(e) CONSULTATION PROCESS.—The Board shall have a process for consulting with representatives of States and regional alliances before establishing the regional alliance inflation factors for each year under this section.

## SEC. 6002. BOARD DETERMINATION OF NATIONAL PER CAPITA BASELINE PREMIUM TARGET.

(a) IN GENERAL.—Not later than January 1, 1995, the Board shall determine a national per capita baseline premium target. Such target is equal to—

    (1) the national average per capita current coverage health expenditures (determined under subsection (b)),

    (2) updated under subsection (c).

(b) DETERMINATION OF NATIONAL AVERAGE PER CAPITA CURRENT COVERAGE HEALTH EXPENDITURES.—

    (1) IN GENERAL.—The Board shall determine the national average per capita current coverage health expenditures equal to—

        (A) total covered current health care expenditures (described in paragraph (2)), divided by

(B) the estimated population in the United States of regional alliance eligible individuals (as determined by the Board as of the 1993 under subsection (c)(3)) for whom such expenditures were determined.

The population under subparagraph (B) shall not include SSI recipients or AFDC recipients.

(2) CURRENT HEALTH CARE EXPENDITURES.—For purposes of paragraph (1)(A), the Board shall determine current health care expenditures as follows:

(A) DETERMINATION OF TOTAL EXPENDITURES.—The Board shall first determine the amount of total payments made for items and services included in the comprehensive benefit package (determined without regard to cost sharing) in the United States in 1993.

(B) REMOVAL OF CERTAIN EXPENDITURES NOT TO BE COVERED THROUGH REGIONAL ALLIANCES.—The amount so determined shall be decreased by the proportion of such amount that is attributable to any of the following:

(i) Medicare beneficiaries (other than such beneficiaries who are regional alliance eligible individuals).

(ii) AFDC recipients or SSI recipients.

(iii) Expenditures which are paid for through workers' compensation or automobile or other liability insurance.

(iv) Expenditures by parties (including the Federal Government) that the Board determines will not be payable by regional alliance health plans for coverage of the comprehensive benefit package under this Act.

(C) ADDITION OF PROJECTED EXPENDITURES FOR UNINSURED AND UNDERINSURED INDIVIDUALS.—The amount so determined and adjusted shall be increased to take into account increased utilization of, and expenditures for, items and services covered under the comprehensive benefit package likely to occur, as a result of coverage under a regional alliance health plan of individuals who, as of 1993 were uninsured or underinsured with respect to the comprehensive benefit package. In making such determination, such expenditures shall be based on the estimated average cost for such services in 1993 (and not on private payment rates established for such services). In making such determination, the estimated amount of uncompensated care in 1993 shall be removed.

(D) ADDITION OF HEALTH PLAN AND ALLIANCE COSTS OF ADMINISTRATION.—

(i) IN GENERAL.—The amount so determined and adjusted shall be increased by an estimated percentage (determined by the Board, but no more than 15 percent) that reflects the proportion of premiums that are required for health plan and regional alliance administration (including regional alliance costs for administration of income-related premium discounts and cost sharing reductions) and for State premium taxes (which taxes shall be limited to such amounts in 1993 as are attributable to the health benefits to be included in the comprehensive benefit package).

(E) DECREASE FOR COST SHARING.—The amount so determined and adjusted shall be decreased by a percentage that reflects (i) the estimated average percentage of total amounts payable for items and services covered under the comprehensive benefit package that will be payments in the form of cost sharing under a high cost sharing plan, and (ii) the percentage reduction in utilization estimated to result from the application of high cost sharing.

(3) SPECIAL RULES.—

(A) BENEFITS USED.—The determinations under this section shall be based on the comprehensive benefit package as in effect in 1996.

(B) ASSUMING NO CHANGE IN EXPENDITURE PATTERN.—The determination under paragraph (2) shall be made without regard to any change in the pattern of expenditures that may result from the enrollment of AFDC recipients and SSI recipients in regional alliance health plans.

(C) ELIGIBLE INDIVIDUALS.—In this subsection, the determination of who are regional alliance eligible individuals under this subsection shall be made as though this Act was fully in effect in each State as of 1993.

(c) UPDATING.—

(1) IN GENERAL.—Subject to paragraph (3), the Board shall update the amount determined under subsection (b)(1) for each of 1994, 1995, and

1996 by the appropriate update factor described in paragraph (2) for the year.

(2) APPROPRIATE UPDATE FACTOR.—In paragraph (1), the appropriate update factor for a year is 1 plus the annual percentage increase for the year (as determined by the Administrator of the Health Care Financing Administration, based on actual or projected information) in private sector health care spending for items and services included in the comprehensive benefit package (as of 1996).

(3) LIMIT.—The total, cumulative update under this subsection shall not exceed 15 percent.

## SEC. 6003. DETERMINATION OF ALLIANCE PER CAPITA PREMIUM TARGETS.

(a) INITIAL DETERMINATION.—Not later than January 1, 1995, the Board shall determine, for each regional alliance for 1996, a regional alliance per capita premium target. Such target shall equal—

(1) the national per capita baseline premium target (determined by the Board under section 6002),

(2) updated by the regional alliance inflation factor (as determined under section 6001(a)(2)) for 1996, and

(3) adjusted by the adjustment factor for the regional alliance (determined under subsection (c)).

(b) SUBSEQUENT DETERMINATIONS.—

(1) DETERMINATION.—Not later than March 1 of each year (beginning with 1996) the Board shall determine, for each regional alliance for the succeeding year a regional alliance per capita premium target.

(2) GENERAL RULE.—Subject to paragraph (3), such target shall equal—

(A) the regional alliance per capita target determined under this section for the regional alliance for the previous year, and

(B) updated by the regional alliance inflation factor (as determined in section 6001(a)) for the year.

(c) ADJUSTMENT FACTORS FOR REGIONAL ALLIANCES FOR INITIAL DETERMINATION.—

(1) IN GENERAL.—The Board shall establish an adjustment factor for each regional alliance in a manner consistent with this subsection.

(2) CONSIDERATIONS.—In establishing the factor for each regional alliance, the Board shall consider, using information of the type described in paragraph (3), the difference between the national

average of the factors taken into account in determining the national per capita baseline premium target and such factors for the regional alliance, including variations in health care expenditures and in rates of uninsurance and underinsurance in the different alliance areas and including variations in the proportion of expenditures for services provided by academic health centers in the different alliance areas.

(3) TYPES OF INFORMATION.—The type of information described in this paragraph is—

(A) information on variations in premiums across States and across alliance areas within a State (based on surveys and other data);

(B) information on variations in per capita health spending by State, as measured by the Health Care Financing Administration;

(C) information on variations across States in per capita spending under the medicare program and in such spending among alliance areas within a State under such program; and

(D) area rating factors commonly used by actuaries.

(4) APPLICATION OF FACTORS IN NEUTRAL MANNER.—The application of the adjustment factors

under this subsection for 1996 shall be done in a manner so that the weighted average of the regional alliance per capita premium targets for 1996 is equal to the national per capita baseline premium target determined under section 6002. Such weighted average shall be based on the Board's estimate of the expected distribution of alliance eligible individuals (taken into account under section 6002) among the regional alliances.

(5) CONSULTATION PROCESS.—The Board shall have a process for consulting with representatives of States and regional alliances before establishing the adjustment for regional alliances under this subsection.

(d) TREATMENT OF CERTAIN STATES.—

(1) NON-ALLIANCE STATES.—In the case of a State that is not a participating State or otherwise has not established regional alliances, the entire State shall be treated under the provisions of this part as composing a single regional alliance.

(2) CHANGES IN ALLIANCE BOUNDARIES.—In the case of a State that changes the boundaries of its regional alliances (including the establishment of such alliances after 1996), the Board shall provide a method for computing a regional alliance per cap-

ita premium target for each regional alliance affected by such change in a manner that—

(A) reflects the factors taken into account in establishing the adjustment factors for regional alliances under subsection (c), and

(B) results in the weighted average of the newly computed regional targets for the regional alliances affected by the change equal to the weighted average of the regional targets for the regional alliances as previously established.

## SEC. 6004. ALLIANCE INITIAL BIDDING AND NEGOTIATION PROCESS.

(a) BIDDING PROCESS.—

(1) OBTAINING BIDS.—

(A) IN GENERAL.—Not later than July 1 before the first year, and not later than August 1 of each succeeding year, the regional alliance shall have obtained premium bids from each plan seeking to participate as a regional alliance health plan with respect to the alliance in the following year.

(B) DISCLOSURE.—In obtaining such bids, a regional alliance may determine to disclose (or not to disclose) the regional alliance per capita premium target for the regional alliance (determined under section 6003) for the year involved.

(C) CONDITION.—Each bid submitted by a plan under this subsection shall be conditioned upon the plan's agreement to accept any premium payment reduction that may be imposed under section 6011.

(2) NEGOTIATION PROCESS.—Following the bidding process under paragraph (1), a State may provide for negotiations with health plans relating to the premiums to be charged by such plans. Such negotiations may result in the resubmission of bids, but in no case shall a health plan resubmit a bid that exceeds its prior bid.

(3) LEGALLY BINDING BIDS.—All bids submitted under this subsection must be legally binding with respect to the plans involved.

(4) ACCEPTANCE.—The final bid submitted by a plan under this subsection shall be considered to be the accepted bid, except as provided in subsection (e).

(5) ASSISTANCE.—The Board shall provide regional alliances with such information and technical assistance as may assist such alliances in the bidding process under this subsection.

(b) SUBMISSION OF INFORMATION TO BOARD.—By not later than September 1 of each year for which bids are obtained under subsection (a), each regional alliance shall submit to the Board a report that discloses—

    (1) information regarding the final bids obtained under subsection (a) by the different plans;

    (2)(A) for the first year, any information the Board may request concerning an estimation of the enrollment likely in each such plan of alliance eligible individuals who will be offered enrollment in a health plan by alliance in the first year, or

    (B) for a succeeding year, the actual distribution of enrollment of alliance eligible individuals in regional alliance health plans in the year in which the report is transmitted; and

    (3) limitations on capacity of regional alliance health plans.

(c) COMPUTATION OF WEIGHTED AVERAGE ACCEPTED BID.—

    (1) IN GENERAL.—For each regional alliance the Board shall determine a weighted average accepted bid for each year for which bids are obtained under subsection (a). Such determination shall be based on information on accepted bids for the year, submitted under subsection (b)(1), and shall take

into account, subject to paragraph (2), the information on enrollment distribution submitted under subsection (b)(2).

(2) ENROLLMENT DISTRIBUTION RULES.—In making the determination under paragraph (1) for a regional alliance, the Board shall establish rules respecting the treatment of enrollment in plans that are discontinued or are newly offered.

(d) NOTICE TO CERTAIN ALLIANCES.—

(1) IN GENERAL.—By not later than October 1 of each year for which bids are obtained, the Board shall notify a regional alliance—

(A) if the weighted average accepted bid (determined under subsection (c)) for the alliance is greater than the regional alliance per capita premium target for the alliance (determined under section 6002) for the year, and

(B) the reduced weighted average accepted bid for the alliance.

(2) NOTICE OF PREMIUM REDUCTIONS.—If notice is provided to a regional alliance under paragraph (1), the Board shall notify the regional alliance and each noncomplying plan of any plan payment reduction computed under section 6011 for such a plan and the opportunity to voluntarily re-

duce the accepted bid under subsection (e) in order to avoid such a reduction.

(e) VOLUNTARY REDUCTION OF ACCEPTED BID (FINAL ACCEPTED BID).—After the Board has determined under subsection (c) the weighted average accepted bid for a regional alliance and the Board has determined preliminary plan payment reductions, before such date as the Board may specify (in order to provide for an open enrollment period), a noncomplying plan has the opportunity to voluntarily reduce its accepted bid by the amount of the plan payment reduction that would otherwise apply to the plan. Such reduction shall not affect the amount of the plan payment reduction for any other plan for that year.

## SEC. 6005. STATE FINANCIAL INCENTIVES.

(a) ELECTION.—Any participating State may elect to assume responsibility for containment of health care expenditures in the State consistent with this part. Such responsibility shall include submitting annual reports to the Board on any activities undertaken by the State to contain such expenditures.

(b) FINANCIAL INCENTIVE.—In the case of a State that has made an election under subsection (a), if Board determines for a particular year (beginning with the first year) that the statewide weighted average of the reduced weighted average accepted bids (based on actual average enrollment for the year), for regional alliances in the State, is less than the statewide weighted average of the regional alliance per capita premium targets (based upon such enrollment) for such alliances for the year, then the amount of the State maintenance-of-effort payment under section 9001(b), for the following year, shall be reduced by ½ of the product of—

>   (1)(A) the amount by which the amount of such target exceeds the amount of such premium, divided by (B) the amount of such target; and

>   (2) the total of the amount of the Federal payments made in that particular year to regional alliances in the State under subtitle B of title IX.

## SEC. 6006. RECOMMENDATIONS TO ELIMINATE REGIONAL VARIATIONS IN ALLIANCE TARGETS DUE TO VARIATION IN PRACTICE PATTERNS; CONGRESSIONAL CONSIDERATION.

(a) ESTABLISHMENT OF ADVISORY COMMISSION ON REGIONAL VARIATIONS IN HEALTH EXPENDITURES.—The chair of the Board shall establish, by not later than 60 days after the date of appointment of the first chair, an advisory commission on regional variations in health expenditures.

(b) COMPOSITION.—The advisory commission shall be composed of consumers, employers, providers, representatives of health plans, States, regional alliances, individuals with expertise in the financing of health care, individuals with expertise in the economics of health care, and representatives of diverse geographic areas.

(c) REGIONAL VARIATIONS.—

(1) INFORMATION.—The advisory commission shall provide the Board, States, and regional alliances with information about regional differences in health care costs and practice patterns.

(2) METHODS FOR ELIMINATION OF REGIONAL VARIATION DUE TO PRACTICE PATTERN.—The advisory commission shall examine methods of eliminating variation in regional alliance per capita premium targets due to variation in practice patterns, not due to other factors (such as health care input prices and demographic factors), by 2002.

(3) METHODS FOR REDUCING REGIONAL VARIATION IN PREMIUM PAYMENTS FOR AFDC AND SSI RECIPIENTS DUE TO HISTORICAL VARIATION IN CHARACTERISTICS OF STATE MEDICAID PLANS.— The advisory commission shall examine methods of reducing the variation in Federal and State payments under sections 9011 and 9101. In addition to

the factors considered in paragraph (2), the commission shall examine methods of reducing variation due to historical differences in the rates of reimbursement to providers and in the amount, duration, and scope of benefits covered under State medicaid plans.

(4) METHODS FOR REDUCTION OF REGIONAL VARIATION IN STATE MAINTENANCE-OF-EFFORT PAYMENTS FOR NON-CASH ASSISTANCE RECIPIENTS.—The advisory commission shall study the reasons for variation among State in the level of maintenance of effort payments for non-cash assistance recipients and shall examine methods of reducing variation across States in the level of maintenance of effort payments compared to the population of the State. The commission shall link consideration of the variation in premium targets under paragraph (2) with the variation in State and Federal payments described in this paragraph.

(5) OTHER FACTORS.—The advisory commission shall examine methods of reducing variations in spending among States for health care services that are attributable to historical differences.

(d) RECOMMENDATIONS TO BOARD.—The advisory commission shall submit to the Board a report that specifies—

(1) one or more methods for eliminating the variation described in subsection (c)(2), and

(2) one or more methods for reducing variations described in subsection (c)(4) across States.

(e) REPORT TO CONGRESS.—

(1) IN GENERAL.—The Board shall submit to Congress, by not later July 1, 1995, detailed recommendations respecting the specific method to be used to achieve each of the following:

(A) The elimination of the variation in the regional alliance per capita premium (as described in subsection (b)(2)) by 2002.

(B) Reducing the variation in State payments under sections 9001 and 9011 (taking into account any interaction between these payments), in a manner that is budget neutral with respect to total government payments and payments by the Federal Government.

In making recommendations in subparagraph (B), the Board shall consider the fiscal capacity of the States.

(2) SUBSEQUENT REPORT.—If a joint resolution described in subsection (f) does not become law, the Board shall submit to Congress revised detailed recommendations respecting the specific method to be used to achieve the elimination of such variation by 2002. Such recommendations shall be submitted not later than 90 days after the date such resolution is disapproved by either House (or vetoed by the President) or, if earlier, 150 days after the date of submission of the recommendations under paragraph (1).

(f) CONGRESSIONAL CONSIDERATION.—

(1) IN GENERAL.—Detailed recommendations submitted under paragraph (1)(A) or (1)(B) or (2) of subsection (e) shall apply under this subtitle only if a joint resolution (described in paragraph (2)) approving such recommendations is enacted, in accordance with the provisions of paragraph (3), before the end of the 60-day period beginning on the date on which such recommendations were submitted. For purposes of applying the preceding sentence and paragraphs (2) and (3), the days on which either

House of Congress is not in session because of an adjournment of more than three days to a day certain shall be excluded in the computation of a period.

(2) JOINT RESOLUTION OF APPROVAL.—A joint resolution described in this paragraph means only a joint resolution which is introduced within the 10-day period beginning on the date on which the Board submits recommendations under paragraph (1)(A), (1)(B), or (2) of subsection (e) and—

(A) which does not have a preamble;

(B) the matter after the resolving clause of which is either of the following 2 clauses:

(i) For recommendations under paragraph (1)(A): "That Congress approves the recommendations of the National Health Board concerning elimination of regional variation in regional alliance per capita premium targets under subtitle A of title VI of the Health Security Act, as submitted by the Board on _____.", the blank space being filled in with the appropriate date; or

(ii) For recommendations under paragraph (1)(B): "That Congress approves the recommendations of the National Health Board concerning reducing the variation in State payments under sections 9001 and 9011 of the Health Security Act, as submitted by the Board on _____.", the blank space being filled in with the appropriate date; and

(C) the title of which, respectively, is either of the following:

(i) For recommendations under paragraph (1)(A): "Joint resolution approving recommendations of the National Health Board concerning elimination of regional variation in regional alliance per capita premium targets under subtitle A of title VI of the Health Security Act, as submitted by the Board on _____.", the blank space being filled in with the appropriate date; or

(ii) For recommendations under paragraph (1)(B): "Joint resolution approving recommendations of the National Health Board concerning reducing the variation in State payments under sections 9001 and 9011 of the Health Security Act, as submitted by the Board on _____.", the blank space being filled in with the appropriate date..

(3) PROCEDURES FOR CONSIDERATION OF RESOLUTION OF APPROVAL.—Subject to paragraph (4), the provisions of section 2908 (other than subsection (a)) of the Defense Base Closure and Realignment Act of 1990 shall apply to the consideration of a joint resolution described in paragraph (2) in the same manner as such provisions apply to a joint resolution described in section 2908(a) of such Act.

(4) SPECIAL RULES.—For purposes of applying paragraph (3) with respect to such provisions—

(A) any reference to the Committee on Armed Services of the House of Representatives shall be deemed a reference to an appropriate Committee of the House of Representatives (specified by the Speaker of the House of Representatives at the time of submission of recommendations under subsection (e)) and any reference to the Committee on Armed Services of the Senate shall be deemed a reference to an appropriate Committee of the House of Representatives (specified by the Majority Leader of the Senate at the time of submission of recommendations under subsection (e)); and

(B) any reference to the date on which the President transmits a report shall be deemed a reference to the date on which the Board submits a recommendation under paragraph (1)(A), (1)(B), or (2) of subsection (e).

## SEC. 6007. REFERENCE TO LIMITATION ON ADMINISTRATIVE AND JUDICIAL REVIEW OF CERTAIN DETERMINATIONS.

For limitation on administrative and judicial review of certain determinations under this part, see section 5232.

## Subpart B—Plan and Provider Payment Reductions to Maintain Expenditures within Targets

## SEC. 6011. PLAN PAYMENT REDUCTION.

(a) PLAN PAYMENT REDUCTION.—In order to assure that payments to regional alliance health plans by a regional alliance are consistent with the applicable regional alliance per capita target for the alliance (computed under this subtitle), each noncomplying plan (as defined in subsection (b)(2)) for a year is subject to a reduction in plan payment (under section 1351) by the amount equal to plan payment reduction specified in subsection (c) for the year.

(b) NONCOMPLYING ALLIANCE AND NONCOMPLYING PLAN DEFINED.—In this part:

(1) NONCOMPLYING ALLIANCE.—The term "noncomplying alliance" means, for a year, a regional alliance for which the weighted average accepted bid (computed under section 6004(c)) exceeds the regional alliance per capita target for the year.

(2) NONCOMPLYING PLAN.—The term "noncomplying plan" means, for a year, a regional alliance health plan offered through a noncomplying alliance if the final accepted bid for the year exceeds the maximum complying bid (as defined in subsection (d)) for the year. No plan shall be a noncomplying plan for a year before the first year in which the plan is offered by a regional alliance.

(c) AMOUNT OF PLAN PAYMENT REDUCTION.—

(1) IN GENERAL.—The amount of the plan payment reduction, for a noncomplying plan offered by an alliance, is the alliance-wide reduction percentage (as defined in paragraph (2)) of the excess bid amount (as defined in paragraph (3)).

(2) ALLIANCE-WIDE REDUCTION PERCENTAGE.—

(A) IN GENERAL.—In paragraph (1), the term "alliance-wide reduction percentage" means, for a noncomplying plan offered by an alliance for a year—

(i) the amount by which (I) the weighted average accepted bid (computed under section 6004(c)(1)) for the alliance for the year, exceeds the regional alliance per capita target for the alliance for the year; divided by

(ii) the sum, for noncomplying plans offered by the alliance, of the plan proportions of alliance excess bid amount (described in subparagraph (B)(i)) for the year.

(B) PLAN PROPORTION OF ALLIANCE EXCESS BID AMOUNT DESCRIBED.—

(i) IN GENERAL.—The "plan proportion of alliance excess bid amount" described in this clause, for a noncomplying plan, is the product of—

(I) the excess bid amount (as defined in paragraph (4)) for the plan, and

(II) the plan enrollment proportion (as defined in clause (ii)) for the plan.

(ii) PLAN ENROLLMENT PROPORTION.—In clause (i)(II), the term "plan enrollment proportion" means, with respect to a health plan offered by a regional alliance, the total enrollment of alliance eligible individuals enrolled in such plan expressed as a percentage of the total enrollment of alliance eligible individuals in all regional alliance plans offered by the alliance. Such proportion shall be computed based on the information used in computing the weighted average accepted bid for the alliance under section 6004(c)(1).

(3) EXCESS BID AMOUNT.—In this subsection, the "excess bid amount", with respect to a non-complying plan for a year, is the amount by which—

(i) the accepted bid for the year (not taking into account any voluntary reduction under section 6004(e)), exceeds

(ii) the maximum complying bid (as defined in subsection (d)) for the plan for the year.

(d) MAXIMUM COMPLYING BID.—

(1) FIRST YEAR.—In this part, subject to paragraph (3), for the first year, the "maximum comply-

ing bid" for each plan offered by a regional alliance, is the regional alliance per capita premium target for the alliance (determined under section 6002) for the year.

(2) SUBSEQUENT YEARS.—In this part, subject to paragraph (3), for a subsequent year, the "maximum complying bid", for a plan offered by an alliance for a year, is the sum of the following:

(A) NET PREVIOUS YEAR ACCEPTED BID FOR PLAN.—The accepted bid for the previous year (not taking into account any voluntary reduction under section 6004(e)), minus the amount of any plan payment reduction for the plan for that year.

(B) ALLIANCE-WIDE INFLATION ALLOWANCE.—The amount by which—

(i) regional alliance per capita premium target for the year, exceeds

(ii) such target for the previous year, or, if less, the weighted average accepted bid (computed under section 6004(c)(1)) for such year.

(3) SPECIAL RULES FOR NEW PLANS.—

(A) IN GENERAL.—Subject to subparagraph (B), in the case of a plan that is first offered by a regional alliance in a year after the first year the maximum complying bid shall be the regional alliance per capita premium target for the year.

(B) AUTHORITY.—The Board or a State may establish rules to modify the application of subparagraph (A) for regional alliance health plans in the State in order—

(i) to prevent abusive premium practices by entities previously offering plans, or

(ii) to encourage the availability of all types of plans in the State and to permit establishment of new plans.

## SEC. 6012. PROVIDER PAYMENT REDUCTION.

(a) PARTICIPATING PROVIDERS.—

(1) IN GENERAL.—Each regional alliance health plan, as part of its contract under section 1406(e) with any participating provider (as defined in section 1407(c), or group of participating providers) shall—

(A) include a provision that provides that if the plan is a noncomplying plan for a year, payments to the provider (or group) shall be reduced by the applicable network reduction percentage (described in paragraph (2)) for the year, and

(B) not include any provision which the State determines otherwise varies the payments to such providers (or group) because of, or in relation to, a plan payment reduction under section 6011 or otherwise is intended to nullify the effect of subparagraph (A).

The Board may issue regulations relating to the requirements of this paragraph.

(2) APPLICABLE NETWORK REDUCTION PERCENTAGE.—

(A) IN GENERAL.—Subject to subparagraphs (B) and (C), the "adjusted plan reduction percentage", with respect to network providers of a noncomplying plan for a year is—

(i) the plan payment reduction amount for the plan for the year (as determined under section 6011(c)), divided by

(ii) the final accepted bid for the plan for the year,

adjusted under subparagraph (B).

(B) INDUCED VOLUME OFFSET.—The Board shall provide for an appropriate increase of the percentage reduction computed under subparagraph (A) to take into account any estimated increase in volume of services provided that may reasonably be anticipated as a consequence of applying a reduction in payment under this subsection. The Board may compute and apply such increase differently for different classes of providers or services or different types of health plans (as the Board may define).

(b) OTHER PROVIDERS.—

(1) IN GENERAL.—Each regional alliance health plan that is a noncomplying plan in a year shall provide for a reduction in the amount of payments to providers (or groups of providers) that are not participating providers under the applicable alliance fee schedule under section 1406(c)(3) by the applicable nonnetwork reduction percentage (described in paragraph (2)) for the year.

(2) APPLICABLE NONNETWORK REDUCTION PERCENTAGE.—

(A) IN GENERAL.—Subject to subparagraph (B), the "adjusted plan reduction percentage", with respect to nonnetwork providers of a noncomplying plan for a year is—

(i) the plan payment reduction amount for the plan for the year (as determined under section 6011(c)), divided by

(ii) the final accepted bid for the plan for the year,

adjusted under subparagraph (B).

(B) INDUCED VOLUME OFFSET.—The Board shall provide for an appropriate adjustment of the percentage reduction computed under subparagraph (A) to take into account any estimated increase in volume of services provided that may reasonably be anticipated as a consequence of applying a reduction in payment under this subsection.

(c) APPLICATION TO COST SHARING AND TO BALANCE BILLING RESTRICTIONS.—For purposes of applying section 1406(d) (relating to balance billing limitations) and part 3 of subtitle B of title I (relating to computation of cost sharing), the payment basis otherwise used for computing any limitation on billing or cost sharing shall be such payment basis as adjusted by any reductions effected under this section.

# PART 2—CORPORATE ALLIANCES HEALTH EXPENDITURES

## SEC. 6021. CALCULATION OF PREMIUM EQUIVALENTS.

(a) IN GENERAL.—By January 1, 1997, the Board shall develop a methodology for calculating an annual per capita expenditure equivalent for amounts paid for coverage for the comprehensive benefit package within a corporate alliance.

(b) ADJUSTMENT PERMITTED.—Such methodology shall permit a corporate alliance to petition the Secretary of Labor for an adjustment of the inflation adjustment that would otherwise apply to compensate for material changes in the demographic characteristics of the eligible individuals receiving coverage through the alliance.

(c) REPORTING.—In 2000 and each subsequent year, each corporate alliance shall report to the Secretary of Labor, in a form and manner specified by the Secretary, the average of the annual per capita expenditure equivalent for the previous 3-year period.

## SEC. 6022. TERMINATION OF CORPORATE ALLIANCE FOR EXCESS INCREASE IN EXPENDITURES.

(a) TERMINATION.—

(1) IN GENERAL.—If a corporate alliance has two excess years (as defined in subsection (b)) in a 3-year-period, then, effective beginning with the sec-

ond year following the second excess year in such period—

 (A) the Secretary of Labor shall terminate the corporate alliance, and

 (B) employers that were corporate alliance employers with respect to such corporate alliance shall become regional alliance employers (unless, in the case of a corporate alliance with a plan sponsor described in subparagraph (B) or (C) of section 1311(b)(1), the employers become corporate alliance employers of another such corporate alliance).

(2) INITIAL 3-YEAR-PERIOD.—Paragraph (1) shall first apply to the 3-year-period beginning with 1997.

(3) SPECIAL SUBSEQUENT TREATMENT FOR LARGE EMPLOYERS.—In the case of corporate alliance employers described in paragraph (1)(B) that are large employers, the employer premium payments under section 6121 are subject to adjustment under section 6124.

(4) NO FURTHER ELECTION.—If a corporate alliance of a large employer is terminated under this subsection, no employer that is a corporate alliance

employer for that alliance is eligible to be a sponsor of a corporate alliance.

(b) EXCESS YEAR.—

(1) IN GENERAL.—In subsection (a), the term "excess year" means, for a corporate alliance, a year (beginning on or after 2000) for which—

(A) the rate of increase for the corporate alliance (specified in paragraph (2)) for the year, exceeds

(B) the national corporate inflation factor (specified in paragraph (3)) for the year.

(2) RATE OF INCREASE FOR CORPORATE ALLIANCE.—The rate of increase for a corporate alliance for a year, specified in this paragraph, is the percentage by which—

(A) the average of the annual per capita expenditure equivalent for the corporate alliance (reported under section 6021(c)) for the 3-year period ending with such year, exceeds

(B) the average of the annual per capita expenditure equivalent for the corporate alliance (reported under such subsection) for the 3-year period ending with the previous year.

(3) NATIONAL CORPORATE INFLATION FACTOR.—The national corporate inflation factor for a

year, specified in this paragraph, is the average of the general health care inflation factors (as defined in section 6001(a)(3)) for each of the 3 years ending with such year.

## PART 3—TREATMENT OF SINGLE-PAYER STATES

### SEC. 6031. SPECIAL RULES FOR SINGLE-PAYER STATES.

In the case of a Statewide single-payer State, for purposes of section 1222(6), the Board shall compute a Statewide per capita premium target for each year in the same manner as a regional alliance per capita premium target is determined under section 6003.

## PART 4—TRANSITION PROVISIONS

### SEC. 6041. MONITORING PRICES AND EXPENDITURES.

(a) IN GENERAL.—The Secretary shall establish a program to monitor prices and expenditures in the health care system in the Unites States.

(b) REPORTS.—The Secretary shall periodically report to the President on—

(1) the rate of increase in expenditures in each sector of the health care system, and

(2) how such rates compare with rate of overall increase in health care spending and rate of increase in the consumer price index.

(c) ACCESS TO INFORMATION.—

(1) IN GENERAL.—The Secretary may obtain, through surveys or otherwise, information on prices and expenditures for health care services. The Secretary may compel health care providers and third party payers to disclose such information as is necessary to carry out the program under this section.

(2) CONFIDENTIALITY.—Non-public information obtained under this subsection with respect to individual patients is confidential.

(d) PERIODIC REPORTS.—The Secretary shall periodically issue public reports on the matters described in subsection (b).

# Subtitle B—Premium-Related Financings

## PART 1—FAMILY PREMIUM PAYMENTS

### Subpart A—Family Share

SEC. 6101. FAMILY SHARE OF PREMIUM.

(a) REQUIREMENT.—Each family enrolled in a regional alliance health plan or in a corporate alliance health plan in a class of family enrollment is responsible for payment of the family share of premium payable respecting such enrollment. Such premium may be paid by an employer or other person on behalf of such a family.

(b) FAMILY SHARE OF PREMIUM DEFINED.—

(1) IN GENERAL.—In this subtitle, the term "family share of premium" means, with respect to enrollment of a family—

 (A) in a regional alliance health plan, the amount specified in paragraph (2) for the class, or

 (B) in a corporate alliance health plan, the amount specified in paragraph (3) for the class.

(2) REGIONAL ALLIANCE.—

 (A) IN GENERAL.—The amount specified in this paragraph for a health plan based on a class of family enrollment is the sum of the base amounts described in subparagraph (B) reduced (but not below zero) by the sum of the amounts described in subparagraph (C).

 (B) BASE.—The base amounts described in this subparagraph (for a plan for a class of enrollment) are as follows:

  (i) REGIONAL ALLIANCE PREMIUM.—The premium specified in section 6102(a) with respect to such class of enrollment.

  (ii) FAMILY COLLECTION SHORTFALL.—20 percent of the family collection shortfall add-on (computed under section 6107 for such class).

(C) CREDITS AND DISCOUNTS.—The amounts described in this subparagraph (for a plan for a class of enrollment) are as follows:

(i) ALLIANCE CREDIT.—The amount of the alliance credit under section 6103(a).

(ii) INCOME RELATED DISCOUNT.—The amount of any income-related discount provided under section 6104(a)(1).

(iii) EXCESS PREMIUM CREDIT.—The amount of any excess premium credit provided under section 6105.

(iv) CORPORATE ALLIANCE OPT-IN CREDIT.—The amount of any corporate alliance opt-in credit provided under section 6106.

(v) ADDITIONAL CREDIT FOR SSI AND AFDC RECIPIENTS.—In the case of an SSI or AFDC family or for whom the amount described in clause (ii) is equal to the amount described in section 6104(b)(1)(A), the amount described in subparagraph (B)(ii).

(D) LIMIT ON MISCELLANEOUS CREDITS.—In no case shall the family share, due to credits under subparagraph (C), be less than zero.

(3) CORPORATE ALLIANCE.—

(A) IN GENERAL.—The amount specified in this paragraph for a health plan based on a class of family enrollment is the sum of the premium described in subparagraph (B) reduced (but not below zero) by the sum of the amounts described in subparagraph (C).

(B) PREMIUM.—The premium described in this subparagraph (for a plan for a class of enrollment) is premium specified under section 1364 with respect to the plan and class of enrollment involved.

(C) CREDITS AND DISCOUNTS.—The amounts described in this subparagraph (for a plan for a class of enrollment) are as follows:

(i) ALLIANCE CREDIT.—The amount of the alliance credit under section 6103(b).

(ii) INCOME RELATED DISCOUNT.—The amount of any income-related discount provided under section 6104(a)(2).

## SEC. 6102. AMOUNT OF PREMIUM.

(a) REGIONAL ALLIANCE.—The amount of the premium charged by a regional alliance for all families in a class of family enrollment under a regional alliance health plan offered by the alliance is equal to the product of—

(1) the final accepted bid for the plan (as defined in section 6000(a)(2)),

(2) the uniform per capita conversion factor (established under section 1341(b)) for the alliance; and

(3) the premium class factor established by the Board for that class under section 1531.

(b) REFERENCE TO CORPORATE ALLIANCE PREMIUM PROVISIONS.—The amount of the premium charged by a corporate alliance for all families in a class of family enrollment under a corporate alliance health plan offered by the alliance is specified under section 1364.

(c) SPECIAL RULES FOR DIVIDED FAMILIES.—In the case of an individual who is a qualifying employee of an employer and the individual has a spouse or child who is not treated as part of the individual's family because of section 1012—

(1) the combined premium for both families under this section shall be computed as though such section had not applied,

(2) the regional alliance shall divide such premium between the families proportionally (consistent with rules established by the Board), and

(3) credits and other amounts shall be prorated in a manner consistent with rules established by the Board.

**SEC. 6103. ALLIANCE CREDIT.**

(a) REGIONAL ALLIANCES.—The credit provided under this section for a family enrolled in a regional alliance health plan through a regional alliance for a class of family enrollment is equal to 80 percent of the weighted average premium (as defined in section 6000(c)) for health plans offered by the alliance for the class.

(b) CORPORATE ALLIANCES.—The credit provided under this section for a family enrolled in a health corporate alliance health plan for a class of family enrollment is equal to the minimum employer premium payment required under section 6131 with respect to the family.

**SEC. 6104. PREMIUM DISCOUNT BASED ON INCOME.**

(a) IN GENERAL.—

(1) ENROLLEES IN REGIONAL ALLIANCE HEALTH PLANS.—Each family enrolled with a regional alliance health plan is entitled to a premium discount under this section, in the amount specified in subsection (b), if the family—

(A) is an AFDC or SSI family,

(B) is determined, under subpart B of part 2 of subtitle B of title D of title I, to have family adjusted income below 150 percent of the applicable poverty level, or

(C) is a family described in subsection (c)(3) for which the family obligation amount under this subsection for the year would otherwise exceed a specified percent of family adjusted income described in such subsection.

(2) ENROLLEES IN CORPORATE ALLIANCE HEALTH PLANS.—

(A) IN GENERAL.—Subject to subparagraph (B), each family enrolled with a corporate alliance health plan in a class of family enrollment by virtue of the full-time employment of a low-wage employee (as defined in subparagraph (B)) is entitled to a premium discount under this section in the amount (if any) by which—

(i) 95 percent of the premium (specified in section 1364) for the least expensive corporate alliance health plan that is offered to the employee and that is a low or combination cost sharing plan (as defined in section 1903( )) for that class, exceeds

(ii) the alliance credit under section 6103 for that class.

(B) LOW-WAGE EMPLOYEE DEFINED.—

(i) IN GENERAL.—In this paragraph, the term "low-wage employee" means, with respect to an employer, an employee who is employed on a full-time basis and who is receiving wages (as defined in section 1902( )) for employment for the employer, as determined under clause (ii), at an annual rate of less than $15,000 (as adjusted under clause (ii)).

(ii) INDEXING.—For a year after 1994, the dollar amount specified in clause (i) shall be increased or decreased by the same percentage as the percentage increase or decrease by which the average CPI (described in section 1902( )) for the 12-month-period ending with August 31 of the preceding year exceeds such average for the 12-month period ending with August 31, 1993.

(C) TIMING OF DETERMINATION.—

(i) IN GENERAL.—The determination of whether or not an employee is a low-wage employee shall be made, in accordance with rules of the Secretary of Labor, at the time of initial enrollment and shall also be made at the time of each subsequent open enrollment period, on the basis of the wages payable by the employer at that time.

(ii) EFFECTIVE DATE.—Such determination shall apply as of the effective date of the initial enrollment, or, in the case of an open enrollment period, as of the effective date of changes in enrollment during such period.

(3) NO LIABILITY FOR INDIANS AND CERTAIN VETERANS AND MILITARY PERSONNEL.—

(A) IN GENERAL.—In the case of an individual described in subparagraph (B), because the applicable health plan does not impose any premium for such an individual, the individual is not eligible for any premium discount under this section.

(B) INDIVIDUALS DESCRIBED.—An individual described in this subparagraph is—

(i) an electing veteran (as defined in section 1012(d)(1)) who is enrolled under a health plan of the Department of Veterans Affairs and who, under the laws and rules as in effect as of December 31, 1994, has a service-connected disability or who is unable to defray the expenses of necessary care as determined under section 1722(a) of title 38, United States Code,

(ii) active duty military personnel (as defined in section 1012(d)(2)), and

(iii) an electing Indian (described in section 1012(d)(3)).

(b) AMOUNT OF PREMIUM DISCOUNT FOR REGIONAL ALLIANCE HEALTH PLANS.—

(1) IN GENERAL.—Subject to the succeeding paragraphs of this subsection, the amount of premium discount under this subsection for a family enrolled in a regional alliance health plan under a class of family enrollment is equal to—

(A) 20 percent of the weighted average premium for regional alliance health plans offered by the regional alliance for that class of enrollment, increased by any amount provided under paragraph (2); reduced (but not below zero) by

 (B) the sum of—

  (i) the family obligation amount described in subsection (c), and

  (ii) the amount of any employer payment (not required under part 2) towards the family share of premiums for covered members of the family.

(2) INCREASE TO ASSURE ENROLLMENT IN LOWER-THAN-AVERAGE-COST PLAN.—If a regional alliance determines that a family eligible for a discount under this section is unable to enroll in a lower-than-average-cost plan (as defined in paragraph (3)) that serves the area in which the family resides, the amount of the premium discount under this subsection is increased but only to such amount as will permit the family to enroll in a regional alliance health plan without the need to pay a family share of premium under this part in excess of the sum described in paragraph (1)(B).

(3) LOWER-THAN-AVERAGE-COST PLAN DEFINED.—In this section, the term "lower-than-average-cost plan" means a regional alliance health plan the premium for which does not exceed, for the class

of family enrollment involved, the weighted average premium for the regional alliance.

(c) FAMILY OBLIGATION AMOUNT.—

(1) DETERMINATION.—Subject to paragraphs (2) and (3), the family obligation amount under this subsection is determined as follows:

(A) NO OBLIGATION IF INCOME BELOW INCOME THRESHOLD AMOUNT OR IF AFDC OR SSI FAMILY.—If the family adjusted income (as determined under section 1332(a)) of the family is less than the income threshold amount (specified in paragraph (4)) or if the family is an AFDC or SSI family, the family obligation amount is zero.

(B) INCOME ABOVE INCOME THRESHOLD AMOUNT.—If such income is at least such income threshold amount and the family is not an AFDC or SSI family, the family obligation amount is the sum of the following:

(i) FOR INCOME (ABOVE INCOME THRESHOLD AMOUNT) UP TO THE POVERTY LEVEL.—The product of the initial marginal rate (specified in paragraph (2)(A)) and the amount by which—

(I) the family adjusted income (not including any portion that exceeds the applicable poverty level for the class of family involved), exceeds

(II) such income threshold amount.

(ii) GRADUATED PHASE OUT OF DISCOUNT UP TO 150 PERCENT OF POVERTY LEVEL.—The product of the final marginal rate (specified in paragraph (2)(B)) and the amount by which the family adjusted income exceeds 100 percent (but is less than 150 percent) of the applicable poverty level.

(2) MARGINAL RATES.—In paragraph (1)—

(A) INDIVIDUAL MARGINAL RATES.—For a year for an individual class of enrollment—

(i) INITIAL MARGINAL RATE.—The initial marginal rate is the ratio of—

(I) 3 percent of the applicable poverty level for the individual class of enrollment for the year, to

(II) the amount by which such poverty level exceeds such income threshold amount.

(ii) FINAL MARGINAL RATE.—The final marginal rate is the ratio of—

(I) the amount by which the general family share (as defined in subparagraph (C)) for an individual class of enrollment exceeds 3 percent of the applicable poverty level (for an individual class of enrollment for the year); to

(ii) 50 percent of such poverty level.

(B) FAMILY MARGINAL RATES.—For a year for a family class of enrollment (as defined in section 1011(c)(2)(A))—

(i) INITIAL MARGINAL RATE.—The initial marginal rate is the ratio of—

(I) 3 percent of the applicable poverty level for a dual parent class of enrollment for the year, to

(II) the amount by which such poverty level exceeds such income threshold amount.

(ii) FINAL MARGINAL RATE.—The final marginal rate is the ratio of—

(I) the amount by which the general family share (as defined in subparagraph (C)) for a dual parent class of enrollment exceeds 3 percent of the applicable poverty level (for such a class for the year); to

(ii) 50 percent of such poverty level.

(C) GENERAL FAMILY SHARE.—In subparagraphs (A) and (B), the term "general family share" means, for a class, the weighted average premium for the class minus the alliance credit (determined without regard to this section).

(3) LIMITATION TO 3.9 PERCENT FOR ALL FAMILIES.—

(A) IN GENERAL.—In the case of a family with family adjusted income of less than $40,000 (adjusted under subparagraph (B)) for a year, in no case shall the family obligation amount under this subsection for the year exceed 3.9 percent (adjusted under subparagraph (C)) of the amount of such adjusted income.

(B) INDEXING OF DOLLAR AMOUNTS.—

(i) IN GENERAL.—For a year after 1994, the dollar amounts specified in subparagraph (A) and in section 6113(d)(1)(B) shall be increased or decreased by the same percentage as the percentage increase or decrease by which the average CPI (described in section 1902( )) for the 12-month-period ending with August 31 of the preceding year exceeds such average for the 12-month period ending with August 31, 1993.

(ii) ROUNDING.—The dollar amounts adjusted under this subparagraph shall be rounded each year to the nearest multiple of $100.

(C) INDEXING OF PERCENTAGE.—

(i) IN GENERAL.—The percentage specified in subparagraph (A) shall be adjusted for any year after 1994 so that the percentage for the year bears the same ratio to the percentage so specified as the ratio of—

(I) 1 plus general health care inflation factor (as defined in section 6001(a)(3)) for the year, bears to

(II) 1 plus the percentage increase or decrease specified in section 1136(b) (relating to indexing of dollar amounts related to cost sharing) for the year.

(ii) ROUNDING.—Any adjustment under clause (i) for a year shall be rounded to the nearest multiple of 1/10 of 1 percentage point.

(4) INCOME THRESHOLD AMOUNT.—

(A) IN GENERAL.—For purposes of this subtitle, the income threshold amount specified in this paragraph is $1,000 (adjusted under subparagraph (B)).

(B) INDEXING.—For a year after 1994, the income threshold amount specified in subparagraph (A) shall be increased or decreased by the same percentage as the percentage increase or decrease by which the average CPI (described in section 1902( )) for the 12-month-period ending with August 31 of the preceding year exceeds such average for the 12-month period ending with August 31, 1993.

(C) ROUNDING.—Any increase or decrease under subparagraph (B) for a year shall be rounded to the nearest multiple of $10.

SEC. 6105. EXCESS PREMIUM CREDIT.

(a) IN GENERAL.—If plan payment reductions are made for one or more regional alliance health plans offered by a regional alliance for plan payments in a year under section 6021, the alliance shall provide for a credit under this section, in the amount described in subsection (b), in the case of each family enrolled in a regional alliance health plan offered by the alliance for premiums in the year.

(b) AMOUNT OF CREDIT.—

(1) IN GENERAL.—Subject to paragraph (2), the amount of the credit under this subsection, for a family enrolled in a class of family enrollment for a regional alliance for a year, is the amount that would be the weighted average premium for such alliance, class, and year, if the per capita excess premium amount (determined under subsection (c)) for the alliance for the year were substituted for the reduced weighted average accepted bid for the regional alliance for the year.

(2) ADJUSTMENT TO ACCOUNT FOR USE OF ESTIMATES.—Subject to section 1361(b)(3), if the total payments made by a regional alliance to all regional alliance health plans in a year under section 1351(b) exceeds (or is less than) the total of such payments estimated by the alliance (based on the re-

duced weighted average accepted bid under subsection (c)(1)), because of a difference between—

> (A) the alliance's estimate of the distribution of enrolled families between excess premium plans and other plans, and
>
> (B) the actual distribution of such enrolled families among such plans,

the amount of the credit under this section in the second succeeding year shall be reduced (or increased, respectively) by the amount of such excess (or deficit) in the total of such payments made by the alliance to all such plans.

(c) PER CAPITA EXCESS PREMIUM AMOUNT.—The per capita excess premium amount, for a regional alliance for a year, is the amount by which—

> (1) the reduced weighted average accepted bid for the alliance for the year, exceeds
>
> (2) the regional alliance per capita target for the alliance for the year.

### SEC. 6106. CORPORATE ALLIANCE OPT-IN CREDIT.

(a) IN GENERAL.—If a regional alliance is owed a payment adjustment under section 6124 for a year, then the alliance shall provide for a credit under this section, equal to 20 percent of the amount described in subsection (b), in the case of each family enrolled in a regional alliance plan offered by the alliance.

(b) AMOUNT OF CREDIT.—The amount described in this subsection, for a family enrolled in a class of family enrollment for a regional alliance for a year, is the amount that would be the weighted average premium for such alliance, class, and year, if the per capita corporate alliance opt-in amount (determined under subsection (c)) for the alliance for the year were substituted for the reduced weighted average accepted bid for the regional alliance for the year.

(c) PER CAPITA CORPORATE ALLIANCE OPT-IN AMOUNT.—The per capita corporate alliance opt-in amount, for a regional alliance for a year, is—

>    (1) the total amount of the payment adjustments owed for the year under section 6124, divided by

>    (2) the estimated average number of regional alliance eligible individuals in the regional alliance during the year (reduced by the average number of such individuals whose family share of premiums, determined without regard to this section and section 6107, is zero).

## SEC. 6107. FAMILY COLLECTION SHORTFALL ADD-ON.

(a) IN GENERAL.—The family collection shortfall add-on, for a regional alliance for a class of enrollment for a year, is the amount that would be the weighted average premium for such alliance, class, and year, if the per capita collection shortfall amount (determined under subsection (b)) for the alliance for the year were substituted for the reduced weighted average accepted bid for the regional alliance for the year.

(b) COMPUTATION OF PER CAPITA ADJUSTMENT FOR COLLECTION SHORTFALLS.—

(1) PER CAPITA COLLECTION SHORTFALL AMOUNT.—The per capita collection shortfall amount, for a regional alliance for a year, under this subsection is equal to—

(A) the amount estimated under paragraph (2)(A) for the year, divided by

(B) the estimated average number of regional alliance eligible individuals in the regional alliance during the year (reduced by the average number of such individuals whose family share of premiums, determined without regard to this section and section 6106, is zero).

(2) AGGREGATE COLLECTION SHORTFALL.—

(A) IN GENERAL.—Each regional alliance shall estimate, for each year (beginning with the first year) the total amount of payments which the alliance can reasonably identify as owed to the alliance under this Act (taking into account any premium reduction or discount under this subtitle and including amounts owed under subpart B and not taking into account any penalties) for the year and not likely to be collected (after making collection efforts described in section 1345) during a period specified by the Secretary beginning on the first day of the year.

(B) EXCLUSION OF GOVERNMENT DEBTS.—The amount under subparagraph (A) shall not include any payments owed to a regional alliance by the Federal, State, or local governments.

(C) ADJUSTMENT FOR PREVIOUS SHORTFALL ESTIMATION DISCREPANCY.—Subject to section 1361(b)(3), the amount estimated under this paragraph for a year shall be adjusted to reflect over (or under) estimations in the amounts so computed under this paragraph for previous years (based on actual collections), taking into account interest payable based upon

## Subpart B—Repayment of Alliance Credit by Certain Families

### SEC. 6111. REPAYMENT OF ALLIANCE CREDIT BY CERTAIN FAMILIES.

(a) IN GENERAL.—Subject to the succeeding provisions of this subpart, each family which is provided an alliance credit under section 6103 for a class of enrollment is liable to the regional alliance for repayment of the amount of such credit in accordance with section 1343.

(b) REDUCTION FOR SELF-EMPLOYMENT PAYMENTS.—The liability of a family under this section for a year shall be reduced (but not below zero) by the amount of any employer payments made in the year under section 6126 based on the net earnings from self-employment of a family member.

### SEC. 6112. NO LIABILITY FOR FAMILIES EMPLOYED FULL-TIME; REDUCTION IN LIABILITY FOR PART-TIME EMPLOYMENT.

(a) IN GENERAL.—The amount of any liability under section 6111 shall be reduced, in accordance with rules established by the National Health Board consistent with this section, based on employer premiums payable, under section 6121, with respect to the employment of a family member who is a qualifying employee or with respect to a family member. In no case shall the reduction under this section result in any payment owing to a family.

(b) CREDIT FOR FULL-TIME AND PART-TIME EMPLOYMENT.—

    (1) IN GENERAL.—Under such rules, in the case of a family enrolled under a class of family enrollment, if a family member is a qualifying employee for a month and the employer is liable for payment under section 6121 based on such employment—

        (A) FULL-TIME EMPLOYMENT CREDIT.—If the employment is on a full-time basis (as defined in section 1902(b)(2)) the liability under section 6111 shall be reduced by the credit amount described in subparagraph (C).

        (B) PART-TIME EMPLOYMENT CREDIT.—If the employment is on a part-time basis (as defined in section 6121(d)) the liability under section 6111 shall be reduced by the employment ratio (as defined in section 6121(d)) of the credit amount described in subparagraph (C).

        (C) FULL-TIME MONTHLY CREDIT.—The amount of the credit under this subparagraph, with respect to employment by an employer in a month, is 1/12 (or, if applicable, the fraction described in paragraph (2)) the amount owed under section 6111, based on the class of enrollment, for the year.

(2) COVERAGE DURING ONLY PART OF A YEAR.—In the case of a family that is not enrolled in a regional alliance health plan for all the months in a year, the fraction described in this paragraph is 1 divided by the number of months in the year in which the family was enrolled in such a plan.

(3) AGGREGATION OF CREDITS.—

(A) INDIVIDUALS.—In the case of an individual who is a qualifying employee of more than one employer in a month, the credit for the month shall equal the sum of the credits earned with respect to employment by each employer. Such sum may exceed the credit amount described in paragraph (1)(C).

(B) COUPLES.—In the case of a couple each spouse of which is a qualifying employee in a month, the credit for the month shall equal the sum of the credits earned with respect to employment by each spouse. Such sum may exceed the credit amount described in paragraph (1)(C).

(c) TREATMENT OF CHANGE OF ENROLLMENT STATUS.—In the case of a family for which the class of family enrollment changes during a year, the Board shall establish rules for appropriate conversion and allocation of the credit amounts under the previous provisions of this section in a manner that reflects the relative values of the base employment monthly premiums (as determined under section 6122) among the different classes of family enrollment.

## SEC. 6113. LIMITATION OF LIABILITY BASED ON INCOME.

(a) IN GENERAL.—In the case of an eligible family described in subsection (b), the repayment amount required under this subpart (after taking into account any work credit earned under section 6112) with respect to a year shall not exceed the amount of liability described in subsection (c) for the year.

(b) ELIGIBLE FAMILY DESCRIBED.—An eligible family described in this subsection is a family which is determined, under subpart B of part 2 of subtitle D of title I by the regional alliance for the alliance area in which the family resides, to have wage-adjusted income (as defined in subsection (d)) below 250 percent of the applicable poverty level.

(c) AMOUNT OF LIABILITY.—

(1) DETERMINATION.—Subject to paragraph (2), in the case of a family enrolled in a class of enrollment with wage-adjusted income (as defined in subsection (d)), the amount of liability under this subsection is determined as follows:

(A) NO OBLIGATION IF INCOME BELOW INCOME THRESHOLD AMOUNT OR IF AFDC OR SSI FAMILY.—If such income is than the income threshold amount (specified in section 6104(c)(4)) or if the family is an AFDC or SSI family, the amount of liability is zero.

(B) INCOME ABOVE INCOME THRESHOLD AMOUNT.—If such income is at least such income threshold amount and the family is not an AFDC or SSI family, the amount of liability is the sum of the following:

(i) 5.5 PERCENT OF INCOME (ABOVE INCOME THRESHOLD AMOUNT) UP TO THE POVERTY LEVEL.—The initial marginal rate (specified in paragraph (2)(A)) of the amount by which—

(I) the wage-adjusted income (not including any portion that exceeds the applicable poverty level for the class of family involved), exceeds

(II) such income threshold amount.

(ii) GRADUATED PHASE OUT OF DISCOUNT UP TO 250 PERCENT OF POVERTY LEVEL.—The final marginal rate (specified in paragraph (2)(B)) of the amount by which the wage-adjusted income exceeds 100 percent of the applicable poverty level.

(2) MARGINAL RATES.—In paragraph (1)—

(A) INITIAL MARGINAL RATE.—The initial marginal rate, for a year for a class of enrollment, is the ratio of—

(i) 5.5 percent of the applicable poverty level for the class of enrollment for the year, to

(ii) the amount by which such poverty level exceeds such income threshold amount.

(B) FINAL MARGINAL RATE.—The final marginal rate, for a year for a class of enrollment, is the ratio of—

(i) the amount by which (I) the amount of the alliance credit exceeds (II) 5.5 percent of the applicable poverty (for the class and year); to

(ii) 150 percent of such poverty level.

(C) APPLICATION FOR FAMILY ENROLLMENT BASED ON BASED ON DUAL PARENT ENROLLMENT.—The marginal rates under this paragraph for any family class of enrollment shall be determined based on the applicable poverty level for a dual parent class of enrollment.

(d) WAGE-ADJUSTED INCOME DEFINED.—In this subtitle, the term "wage-adjusted income" means, for a family, family adjusted income of the family (as defined in section 1372(d)(1)), reduced by the sum of the following:

(1)(A) Subject to subparagraph (B), the amount of any wages included in such family's income that is received for employment which is taken into account in the computation of the amount of employer premiums under section 6121 (without consideration of section 6126).

(B) The reduction under subparagraph (A) shall not exceed for a year $5,000 (adjusted under section 6104(c)(3)(B)) multiplied by the number of months (including portions of months) of employment with respect to which employer premiums were payable under section 6121 (determined in a manner consistent with section 6121(e)).

(2) The amount of net earnings from self employment of the family taken into account under section 6126).

(3) The amount of unemployment compensation included in income under section 85 of the Internal Revenue Code of 1986.

(e) DETERMINATIONS.—A family's wage-adjusted income and the amount of liability under subsection (c) shall be determined by the applicable regional alliance upon application by a family under under subpart B of part 2 of subtitle D of title I.

(f) NO LIABILITY FOR INDIANS AND CERTAIN VETERANS AND MILITARY PERSONNEL.—The provisions of paragraph (3) of section 6104(a) shall apply to the reduction in liability under this section in the same manner as such paragraph applies to the premium discount under section 6104.

SEC. 6114. SPECIAL TREATMENT OF CERTAIN RETIREES AND QUALIFIED SPOUSES AND CHILDREN.

(a) TREATMENT AS FULL-TIME EMPLOYEE.—Subject to subsection (d), an individual who is an eligible retiree (as defined in susection (b)) or a qualified spouse or child (as defined in subsection (c)) for a month in a year (beginning with 1998) is considered, for purposes of section 6112, to be a full-time employee described in such section in such month.

(b) ELIGIBLE RETIREE DEFINED.—In subsection (a), the term "eligible retiree" means, for a month, an individual who establishes to the satisfaction of the regional alliance (for the alliance area in which the individual resides), pursuant to rules of the Secretary, that the individual, as of the first day of the month—

 (1) is at least 55, but less than 65, years of age,

 (2) is not employed on a full-time basis (as defined in section 6121(d)(1)(A)),

 (3) would be eligible (under section 226(a) of the Social Security Act) for hospital insurance benefits under part A of title XVIII of such Act if the individual were 65 years of age based only on the employment of the individual, and

 (4) is not a medicare-eligible individual.

(c) QUALIFIED SPOUSE OR CHILD DEFINED.—In subsection (a), the term "qualified spouse or child" means, in relation to an eligible retiree for a month, an individual who establishes to the satisfaction of the regional alliance (for the alliance area in which the individual resides) under rules of the Secretary that the requirements in one of the following paragraphs is met with respect to the individual:

    (1) The individual (A) is under 65 years of age and is (and has been for a period of at least one year) married to an eligible retiree or (B) is a child of the eligible retiree.

    (2) In the case of a person who was an eligible retiree at the time of the person's death—

        (A) the individual was (and had for a period of at least one year been) married to the retiree at the time of the person's death,

        (B) the individual is under 65 years of age,

        (C) the individual is not employed on a full-time basis (as defined in section 6121(d)(1)(A)),

        (D) the individual is not remarried, and

        (E) the deceased spouse would still be an eligible retiree in the month if such spouse had not died.

(3) The individual is a child of an individual described in paragraph (2).

(d) INDIVIDUALS DISQUALIFIED.—Subsection (a) shall not apply to an individual for a month in a year if the individual would be subject to section 59B of the Internal Revenue Code of 1986 as a taxpayer in the year if the individual were covered under Medicare part B for any month during the year.

(e) APPLICATION.—An individual may not be determined to be an eligible retiree or qualified spouse or child unless an application has been filed with the regional alliance. Such application shall contain such information as the Secretary may require to establish such status and verify information in the application. Any material misrepresentation in the application is subject to a penalty in the same manner as a misrepresentation described in section 1374(h)(2).

**SEC. 6115. SPECIAL TREATMENT OF CERTAIN MEDICARE BENEFICIARIES.**

In the case of an individual who would be a medicare-eligible individual in a month but for the application of section 1012(a) on the basis of employment (in the month or a previous month) of the individual or the individual's spouse, the individual (or spouse, as the case may be) so employed is considered, for purposes of section 6112, to be a full-time employee described in such section in such month.

## PART 2—EMPLOYER PREMIUM PAYMENTS

### Subpart A—Regional Alliance Employers

**SEC. 6121. EMPLOYER PREMIUM PAYMENT REQUIRED.**

(a) REQUIREMENT.—

(1) IN GENERAL.—Each regional alliance employer described in paragraph (2) for a month shall pay to the regional alliance that provides health coverage to a qualifying employee of the employer an employer premium in a amount at least equal to the amount specified in subsection (b). Such payments shall be made in accordance with section 1345.

(2) EMPLOYER DESCRIBED.—An employer described in this paragraph for a month, is an employer that in the month employs one or more qualifying employees (as defined in section 1902(b)(1)).

(3) TREATMENT OF CERTAIN EMPLOYMENT BY CORPORATE ALLIANCE EMPLOYERS.—A corporate alliance employer shall be deemed, for purposes of this subpart, to be a regional alliance employer with respect to qualifying employees who are not corporate alliance eligible individuals.

(b) PREMIUM PAYMENT AMOUNT.—

(1) IN GENERAL.—Except as provided in section 6123 (relating to a discount for certain employers), section 6124 (relating to large employers electing coverage in a regional alliance), and section 6125 (relating to the employer collection shortfall add-on), the amount of the employer premium payment, for a month for qualifying employees of the employer who reside in an alliance area, is the sum of the payment amounts computed under paragraph (2) for each class of family enrollment with respect to such employees in such area.

(2) PAYMENT AMOUNT FOR ALL EMPLOYEES IN A CLASS OF FAMILY ENROLLMENT.—Subject to paragraph (3), the payment amount under this paragraph, for an employer for a class of family enrollment for a month for qualifying employees residing in an alliance area, is the product of—

(A) the base employer monthly premium determined under section 6122 for the class of family enrollment for the previous month for the regional alliance, and

(B) the number of full-time equivalent employees (determined under section 1901(b)(2)) enrolled in that class of family enrollment for the previous month and residing in the alliance area.

(3) TREATMENT OF CERTAIN EMPLOYEES.—In applying this subpart in the case of a qualifying employee (other than a medicare-eligible individual) who is not enrolled in any alliance health plan—

(A) the employee is deemed enrolled in a regional alliance health plan (for the alliance area in which the individual resides) in the dual parent class of enrollment, and

(B) if the employee's residence is not known, the employee is deemed to reside in the alliance area in which the employee principally is employed for the employer.

(4) TRANSITIONAL RULES FOR FIRST MONTH IN FIRST YEAR FOR A STATE.—In the case of an employer for a State in the first month of the State's first year—

(A) the premium amount for such month shall be computed by substituting "month" for "previous month" in paragraph (2);

(B) payment for such month shall be made on the first of the month based on an estimate of the payment for such month;

(C) an adjustment shall be made to the payment in the following month to reflect the difference between the payment in the first month and the payment in the following month (calculated without regard to the adjustment under this subparagraph); and

(D) the reconciliation of premiums for such first month under section 1602(c) shall be included in the reconciliation of premiums for the following 12 months.

(5) SPECIAL RULES FOR DIVIDED FAMILIES.—In the case of an individual who is a qualifying employee of an employer and the individual has a spouse or child who is not treated as part of the individual's family because of section 1012—

(A) the employer premium payment under this section shall be computed as though such section had not applied, and

(B) the regional alliance shall make proportional payments (consistent with rules established by the Secretary) to the health plans (if different) of the qualifying employee and of the employee's spouse and children.

(c) APPLICATION DURING TRANSITION PERIOD.—

(1) IN GENERAL.—For purposes of applying this subpart in the case of an employer described in paragraph (3), there shall only be taken into account qualifying employees (and wages of such employees) who reside in a participating State.

(2) EXCEPTION.—Paragraph (1) shall not apply in determining the average number of full-time equivalent employees or whether an employer is a small employer.

(3) EMPLOYER DESCRIBED.—An employer described in this paragraph is an employer that employs one or more qualifying employees in a participating State and one or more qualifying employees in a State that is not a participating State.

## SEC. 6122. COMPUTATION OF BASE EMPLOYMENT MONTHLY PREMIUM.

(a) IN GENERAL.—Each regional alliance shall provide for the computation for each year (beginning with the first year) of a base employment monthly premium for each class of family enrollment equal to 1/12 of 80 percent of—

(1) the weighted average premium for such regional alliance and class of enrollment, reduced by the amount described in section 6106(b), divided by

(2)(A) in the case of a class of enrollment that does not include a couple, 1, or

(B) in the case of a couple class of enrollment, the average number of premium payments per family, as determined under subsection (b), for families receiving coverage within such class from regional alliance health plans offered by the regional alliance.

(b) DETERMINATION OF AVERAGE EMPLOYER PREMIUM PAYMENTS PER FAMILY FOR COUPLES CLASSES.—

(1) IN GENERAL.—Subject to paragraph (4), the regional alliance shall determine, for each couple class of family enrollment and in a manner specified by the Board, an average, annual, estimated number of premium payments per family equal to—

(A) the alliance-wide monthly average number of premium payments (as determined under paragraph (2)) for covered families (as defined in paragraph (3)) within such class of enrollment, divided by

(B) the monthly average number of covered families receiving coverage through regional alliance health plans within such class of employment.

(2) COMPUTATION OF ALLIANCE-WIDE MONTHLY AVERAGE NUMBER.—

(A) IN GENERAL.—In determining the alliance-wide monthly average number of premium payments under paragraph (1)(A), a covered family shall count for a month as 1, or, if greater, the number computed under subparagraph (B) (but in no case greater than 2).

(B) COUNTING OF FAMILIES IN WHICH BOTH SPOUSES ARE QUALIFYING EMPLOYEES.—The number computed under this subparagraph over all families within a couple class of enrollment in which both spouses are qualifying employees, is determined on an alliance-wide basis based on the following:

(i) For such a spouse, determine, using the rules under section 1902(b)(2)(A), how many full-time equivalent employees the spouse is counted as, but not to exceed 1 for either spouse.

(ii) Add the 2 numbers determined under clause (i) for spouses in such families.

(3) COVERED FAMILY DEFINED.—In this subsection, the term "covered family" means a family other than—

(A) an SSI family or AFDC family,

(B) a family in which a spouse is a medicare-eligible individual, or

(C) a family that is enrolled in a health plan other than a regional alliance health plan.

(4) ADJUSTMENT TO ACCOUNT FOR USE OF ESTIMATES.—Subject to section 1361(b)(3), if the total receipts of a regional alliance to all regional alliance health plans in a year under this subpart exceeds, or is less than, the total of such receipts estimated by the alliance (based on the base employment monthly premium under subsection (a)), because of a difference between—

(A) the alliance's estimate of the average, annual, estimated number of premium payments per family for the alliance, and

(B) the actual number of premium payments per family for the alliance,

the average, annual, estimated number of premium payments per family to be applied under this section in the second succeeding year shall be reduced, or increased, respectively, in a manner that results in total receipts of the alliance under this subpart in such succeeding year being increased or decreased by the amount of such excess (or deficit).

(c) BASIS FOR DETERMINATIONS.—

(1) PREMIUMS.—The determinations of premiums and families under plans under this section shall be made in a manner determined by the Board and based on the premiums and families used by the Board in carrying out subtitle A (relating to cost containment) and shall be based on estimates on an annualized basis.

(2) EMPLOYMENT.—

(A) FOR FIRST YEAR.—The determinations of employment under this section for the first year for a State shall be based on estimates of employment established by the regional alliance in accordance with standards promulgated by the Secretary of Labor in consultation with the National Health Board.

(B) FOR SUBSEQUENT YEARS.—The determinations of employment under this section for a year after the first year for a State shall be based on estimates of employment established by the regional alliance in accordance with standards promulgated by the Secretary of Labor in consultation with the National Health Board.

(3) REPORTS.—In accordance with rules established by the Secretary of Labor in consultation with

the National Health Board, a regional alliance may require regional alliance employers to submit such periodic information on employment as may be necessary to monitor the determinations made under subsections (a) and (c), including months and extent of employment.

(d) TIMING OF DETERMINATION.—Determinations under this section for a year shall be made by not later than December 1, or such other date as the Board may specify, before the beginning of the year.

## SEC. 6123. PREMIUM DISCOUNT FOR CERTAIN EMPLOYERS.

(a) EMPLOYER DISCOUNT.—

(1) IN GENERAL.—Subject to section 6124(c) (relating to phase in for certain large corporate alliance employers) and section 6125 (relating to the employer collection shortfall add-on), the amount of the employer premium payment required under this part for a regional alliance employer for any year shall not exceed the limiting percentage (as defined in subsection (b)) of the employer's wages for that year.

(2) EXCLUSION OF GOVERNMENTAL EMPLOYERS AND CERTAIN CORPORATE ALLIANCE EMPLOYERS.—Paragraph (1) shall not apply to—

(A) the Federal Government, a State government, or a unit of local government, or a unit or instrumentality of such government, before 2002; and

(B) a corporate alliance employer which is treated as a regional alliance employer under section 6131(a)(2).

(b) LIMITING PERCENTAGE DEFINED.—In subsection (a)—

(1) ANY EMPLOYER.—For an employer that is not a small employer (as defined in subsection (c)), the limiting percentage is 7.9 percent.

(2) SMALL EMPLOYERS.—For an employer that is a small employer and that has an average number of full-time equivalent employees and average annual wages per full-time equivalent employee (as determined under subsection (d)), the limiting percentage is the applicable percentage determined based on following table:

Limiting Percentage

| Average number of full-time equivalent employees | Employer's average annual wages per full-time equivalent employee are: ||||| 
|---|---|---|---|---|---|
| | $0–$12,000 | $12,001–$15,000 | $15,001–$18,000 | $18,001–$21,000 | $21,001–$24,000 |
| Fewer than 25 | 3.5% | 4.4% | 5.3% | 6.2% | 7.1% |
| 25 but fewer than 50 | 4.4% | 5.3% | 6.2% | 7.1% | 7.9% |
| 50 but fewer than 75 | 5.3% | 6.2% | 7.1% | 7.9% | 7.9% |

(c) SMALL EMPLOYER DEFINED.—

(1) IN GENERAL.—In this section—

 (A) the term "small employer" means an employer that does not employ, on average, more than 75 full-time equivalent employees; and

 (B) subject to subsection (b)(3)(C)(i), the average number of full-time equivalent employees shall be determined by averaging the number of full-time equivalent employees employed by the employer in each countable month during the year.

(2) COUNTABLE MONTH.—In paragraph (1), the term "countable month" means, for an employer, a month in which the employer employs any qualifying employee.

(3) DETERMINATIONS.—The number of full-time equivalent employees shall be determined using the rules under section 1902(b)(2).

(d) AVERAGE ANNUAL WAGES DEFINED.—

(1) IN GENERAL.—In this section, the term "average annual wages" means, for an employer for a year—

 (A) the total wages paid in the year to individuals who, at the time of payment of the wages, are qualifying employees of the employer; divided by

(B) the number of full-time equivalent employees of the employer in the year.

(2) DETERMINATION.—The Board may establish rules relating to the computation of the average annual wages for employers.

(e) DETERMINATIONS.—For purposes of this section, the number of employees and average wages shall be determined on an annual basis.

(f) TREATMENT OF CERTAIN SELF-EMPLOYED INDIVIDUALS.—In the case of an individual who is a partner in a partnership, is a 2-percent shareholder in an S corporation (within the meaning of section 1372 of the Internal Revenue Code of 1986), or is any other individual who carries on a trade or business as a sole proprietorship, for purposes of this section—

(1) the individual is deemed to be an employee of the partnership, S corporation, or proprietorship, and

(2) the individual's net earnings from self employment attributable to the partnership, S corporation, or sole proprietorship are deemed to be wages from the partnership, S corporation, or proprietorship.

(g) APPLICATION TO EMPLOYERS.—An employer that claims that this section applies—

    (1) shall provide notice to the regional alliance involved of the claim at the time of making payments under this part; and

    (2) shall make available such information (and provide access to such information) as the regional alliance may require (in accordance with regulations of the Secretary of Labor) to audit the determination of—

        (A) whether the employer is a small employer, and, if so, the average number of full-time equivalent employees and average annual wages of the employer; and

        (B) the total wages paid by the employer for qualifying employees.

## SEC. 6124. PAYMENT ADJUSTMENT FOR LARGE EMPLOYERS ELECTING COVERAGE IN A REGIONAL ALLIANCE.

(a) APPLICATION OF SECTION.—

    (1) IN GENERAL.—Except as otherwise provided in this subsection, this section shall apply to the employer premium payments for full-time employees in a State of an employer if—

(A)(i) the employer is an eligible sponsor described in section 1311(b)(1)(A), (ii) the employer elected to be a corporate alliance under section 1312(a)(1), and (iii) the election is terminated under section 1313;

(B)(i) the employer is such an eligible sponsor as of the first day of the first year of the State, and (ii) the employer did not provide the notice required under section 1312(a)(1) (with respect to an election to become a corporate alliance); or

(C) the employer is such an eligible sponsor, (ii) the employer subsequently became a large employer and elected to be a corporate alliance under section 1312(a)(2), and (iii) the election was terminated under section 1313.

(2) EFFECTIVE DATE.—In the case of an employer described in—

(A) paragraph (1)(A) or (1)(C), this section shall first apply on the effective date of the termination of the election under section 1313, or

(B) paragraph (1)(B), this section shall first apply as of January 1, 1996 (or, if later with respect to a State, the first day of the first year for the State).

(3) TREATMENT OF EMPLOYEES IN SMALL ESTABLISHMENTS.—This section shall not apply to the payment of premiums for full-time employees of an employer described in paragraph (1)(A) or (1)(C), if the employees are employed at an establishment with respect to which the option described in section 1311(b)(1)(C) was exercised.

(4) SUNSET.—This section shall cease applying to an employer with respect to employment in a State after the 7th year in which this section applies to the employer in the State.

(5) LARGE EMPLOYER DEFINED.—In this section, the term "large employer" has the meaning given such term in section 1311(d)(3).

(b) ADDITIONAL AMOUNT.—

(1) IN GENERAL.—If an employer subject to this section for a year has an excess risk percentage (as defined in paragraph (3)) of greater than zero with respect to an alliance area, then the employer shall provide, on a monthly basis, for payment to the regional alliance for such area of an amount equal to $1/12$ of the excess amount described in paragraph (2) for the year.

(2) EXCESS AMOUNT.—The excess amount described in this paragraph, for an employer for a year with respect to an alliance area, is equal to the product of the following:

 (A) The reduced weighted average accepted bid for the regional alliance for the area for the year.

 (B) The total average number of alliance eligible individuals who—

  (i) were full-time employees (or family members of such employees) of the employer, and

  (ii) residing in the regional alliance area,

 in the year before the first year in which this section applies to the employer.

 (C) The extra risk proportion (specified in paragraph (3)) for the employer for such area.

 (D) The phase-down percentage (specified in paragraph (4)) for the year.

(3) EXTRA RISK PROPORTION.—

 (A) IN GENERAL.—The "extra risk proportion", specified in this paragraph, with respect to an employer and an alliance area, is a percentage that reflects, for the year before the first year in which this section applies to the employer, the amount by which—

(i) the average demographic risk for employees (and family members) described in paragraph (2)(B) residing in the alliance area, exceeds

(ii) the average demographic risk for all regional alliance eligible individuals residing in the area.

(B) MEASUREMENT OF DEMOGRAPHIC RISK.—

(i) IN GENERAL.—Demographic risk under subparagraph (A) shall be measured, in a manner specified by the Board, based on the demographic characteristics described in section 6001(c)(1)(A), that relate to the actuarial value of the comprehensive benefit package.

(ii) PROVISION OF INFORMATION.—Each employer to which this section applies shall submit, to each regional alliance for which an additional payment is required under this section, such information (and at such time) as the Board may require in order to determine the demographic risk referred to in subparagraph (A)(i).

(4) PHASE-DOWN PERCENTAGE.—The phase down percentage, specified in this paragraph for an employer for—

(A) each of the first 4 years to which this section applies to the employer, is 100 percent,

(B) the fifth such year, is 75 percent,

(C) the sixth such year, is 50 percent, and

(D) the seventh such year, is 25 percent.

(c) PHASE IN OF EMPLOYER PREMIUM DISCOUNT.—For—

(1) each of the first 4 years in which this section applies to such employer, section 6123 shall not apply to the employer;

(2) the fifth such year, section 6123 shall apply to the employer but the reduction in premium payment effected by such section shall be 25 percent of the reduction that would otherwise apply (but for this subsection);

(3) the sixth such year, section 6123 shall apply to the employer but the reduction in premium payment effected by such section shall be 50 percent of the reduction that would otherwise apply (but for this subsection);

(4) the seventh such year, section 6123 shall apply to the employer but the reduction in premium payment effected by such section shall be 75 percent of the reduction that would otherwise apply (but for this subsection); or

(5) a subsequent year, section 6123 shall apply to the employer without any reduction under this subsection.

## SEC. 6125. EMPLOYER COLLECTION SHORTFALL ADD-ON.

(a) IN GENERAL.—The amount payable by an employer under this subpart shall be increased by the amount computed under subsection (b).

(b) AMOUNT.—The amount under this subsection for an employer is equal to the premium payment amount that would be computed under section 6121(b)(2) if the per capita collection shortfall amount (computed under section 6107(b)(1)) for the year were substituted for the reduced weighted average accepted bid for the year.

(c) DISCOUNT NOT APPLICABLE.—Section 6123 shall not apply to the increase in the amount payable by virtue of this section.

## SEC. 6126. APPLICATION TO SELF-EMPLOYED INDIVIDUALS.

(a) IN GENERAL.—A self-employed individual (as defined in section 1901(6)) shall be considered, for purposes of this subpart to be an employer of himself or herself and to pay wages to himself or herself equal to the amount of net earnings from self-employment (as defined in section 1901(c)(1)).

(b) CREDIT FOR EMPLOYER PREMIUMS.—

(1) IN GENERAL.—In the case of a self-employed individual, the amount of any employer premium payable by virtue of subsection (a) in a year shall be reduced (but not below zero) by the sum of the following:

(A) Subject to paragraph (2), the amount of any employer premiums payable under this subpart (determined not taking into account any adjustment in the premium amounts under section 6123 or 6124) with respect to the employment of that individual in the year.

(B) The product of (i) the number of months in the year the individual was employed on a full-time basis by a corporate alliance employer, and (ii) the employer premium that would have been payable for such months under this subpart (determined not taking into account any adjustment in the premium amounts under section 6123 or 6124) for the class of enrollment if such employer had been a regional alliance employer.

(2) SPECIAL RULE FOR CERTAIN CLOSELY-HELD BUSINESSES.—

(A) IN GENERAL.—In the case of an individual who—

(i) has wage-adjusted income (as defined in section 6113(d), determined without regard to paragraphs (1)(B) and (2) thereof) that exceeds 250 percent (or such higher percentage as the Board may establish) of the applicable poverty level, and

(ii) is both a substantial owner and an employee of a closely held business,

the amount of any reduction under paragraph (1)(A) that is attributable to the individual's employment by that business shall be appropriately reduced in accordance with rules prescribed by the Board, in order to prevent individuals from avoiding payment of the full amount owed through sham or secondary employment arrangements.

(B) CLOSELY HELD BUSINESS.—For purposes of subparagraph (A), a business is "closely held" if it is an employer that meets the requirements of section 542(a)(2) of the Internal Revenue Code of 1986 or similar requirements as appropriate in the case of a partnership or other entity.

### Subpart B—Corporate Alliance Employers

**SEC. 6131. EMPLOYER PREMIUM PAYMENT REQUIRED.**

(a) PER EMPLOYEE PREMIUM PAYMENT.—Subject to section 6124, each corporate alliance employer of a corporate alliance that in a month in a year employs a qualifying employee who is—

(1) enrolled in a corporate alliance health plan offered by the alliance, shall provide for a payment toward the premium for the plan in an amount at least equal to the corporate employer premium specified in subsection (b); or

(2) is not so enrolled, shall make employer premium payments with respect to such employment under subpart A in the same manner as if the employer were a regional alliance employer (except as otherwise provided in such subpart).

(b) CORPORATE EMPLOYER PREMIUM.—

(1) AMOUNT.—

(A) IN GENERAL.—Except as provided in paragraph (2), the amount of the corporate employer premium for a month in a year for a class of family enrollment for a family residing in a premium area (established under section

1364(b)) is 80 percent of the weighted average monthly premium of the corporate alliance health plans offered by the corporate alliance for that class of enrollment for families residing in that area.

(B) APPLICATION TO SELF-INSURED PLANS.—In applying this paragraph in the case of one or more corporate alliance health plans that are self-insured plans—

(i) the "premium" for the plan is the actuarial equivalent of such premium, based upon the methodology (or such other consistent methodology) used under section 6021(a) (relating to application of cost containment to corporate alliance health plans), and

(ii) the premium amount, for different classes and, if applicable, for different premium areas, shall be computed in a manner based on such factors as may bear a reasonable relationship to costs for the provision of the comprehensive benefit package to the different classes in such areas.

The Secretary of Labor shall establish rules to carry out this subparagraph.

(2) LOW-WAGE EMPLOYEES.—In the case of a low-wage employee entitled to a premium discount under section 6104(a)(2), the amount of the employer premium payment for a month in a year for a class of family enrollment shall be increased by the amount of such premium discount.

(c) DETERMINATIONS.—

(1) BASIS.—Determinations under this section shall be made based on such information as the Secretary of Labor shall specify.

(2) TIMING.—Determinations of the monthly premiums under this section for months in a year shall be made not later than December 1 of the previous year.

# Subtitle C—Payments to Regional Alliance Health Plans

### SEC. 6201. COMPUTATION OF BLENDED PLAN PER CAPITA PAYMENT AMOUNT.

(a) IN GENERAL.—For purposes of section 1342, the blended plan per capita payment amount for a regional alliance health plan for enrollments in an alliance for a year is equal to the sum of the 3 components described in subsection (b), multiplied by any adjustment factor applied for the year under subsection (d).

(b) SUM OF PRODUCTS.—The 3 components described in this subsection are:

(1) PLAN BID COMPONENT FOR THAT PLAN.—The product of—

(A) the final accepted bid for plan (as defined in section 6000(a)(2)) for the year, and

(B) the plan bid proportion determined under section 6202(a)(1) for the year.

(2) AFDC COMPONENT FOR ALLIANCE.—The product of—

(A) the AFDC per capita premium amount for the regional alliance for the year (determined under section 9012), and

(B) the AFDC proportion determined under section 6202(a)(2) for the year.

(3) SSI COMPONENT FOR ALLIANCE.—The product of—

(A) the SSI per capita premium amount for the regional alliance for the year (determined under section 9013) for the year, and

(B) the SSI proportion determined under section 6202(a)(3) for the year.

## SEC. 6202. COMPUTATION OF PLAN BID, AFDC, AND SSI PROPORTIONS.

(a) IN GENERAL.—For purposes of this subtitle:

(1) PLAN BID PROPORTION.—The "plan bid proportion" is, for a type of enrollment, 1 minus the sum of (A) the AFDC proportion, and (B) the SSI proportion.

(2) AFDC PROPORTION.—The "AFDC proportion" is, for a class of family enrollment for a year, the ratio of—

(A) the average of the number of AFDC recipients (as determined under subsection (c)) enrolled in regional alliance health plans in that class of enrollment for the year, to

(B) the average of the total number of individuals enrolled in regional alliance health plans in that class of enrollment for the year.

(3) SSI PROPORTION.—The "SSI proportion" is, for a class of family enrollment for a year, the ratio of—

(A) the average of the number of SSI recipients (as determined under subsection (c)) enrolled in regional alliance health plans in that class of enrollment for the year, to

(B) the average described in paragraph (2)(B).

(b) COMPUTATION.—

(1) PROJECTIONS.—The proportions described in subsection (a) shall be determined and applied by the State, based upon the best available data, at least 1 month before the date bids are submitted under section 6004 before the beginning of the calendar year involved.

(2) ACTUAL.—For purposes of making adjustments under subsection (d), the regional alliance shall determine, after the end of each year, the actual proportions described in subsection (a).

(c) COUNTING OF AFDC AND SSI RECIPIENTS.—For purposes of subsections (a)(2)(A) and (a)(3)(A), the terms "SSI recipient" and "AFDC recipient" do not include a medicare-eligible individual.

(d) ADJUSTMENTS FOR DISCREPANCIES IN ESTIMATIONS.—

(1) IN GENERAL.—If the actual AFDC proportion or SSI proportion (as determined under subsection (a)) for a year (in this subsection referred to as the "reference year"), determined after the end

of the year based upon actual number of AFDC recipients and SSI recipients in the year, is different from the projected AFDC and SSI proportions (as determined under subsection (b)(1)) used in computing the blended plan payment amount for the year, then, subject to section 1361(b)(3), the regional alliance shall adjust the blended plan payment amount in the second succeeding year (in this subsection referred to as the "applicable year") in the manner described in paragraph (2). By regulation the Secretary may apply the adjustment, based on estimated amounts, in the year before the applicable year, with final adjustment in the applicable year.

(2) ADJUSTMENT DESCRIBED.—

(A) POSITIVE CASH FLOW.—If the cash flow difference (as defined in paragraph (3)(A)) for the reference year is positive, then in the applicable year the blended plan payment amount shall be increased by the adjustment percentage described in paragraph (4).

(B) NEGATIVE CASH FLOW.—If the cash flow difference (as defined in paragraph (3)(A)) for the reference year is negative, then in the applicable year the blended plan payment amount shall be reduced by the adjustment percentage described in paragraph (4).

(3) CASH FLOW DIFFERENCE DEFINED.—In this subsection:

(A) IN GENERAL.—The term "cash flow difference" means, for a regional alliance for a reference year, the amount by which—

(i) the actual cash flow (as defined in subparagraph (B)) for the alliance for the year, exceeds

(ii) the reconciled cash flow (as defined in subparagraph (C)) for the alliance for the year.

(B) ACTUAL CASH FLOW.—The term "actual cash flow" means, for a regional alliance for a reference year, the total amount paid by the regional alliance to the regional alliance health plans in the year based on the blended plan payment amount (computed on the basis of projected AFDC and SSI proportions determined under subsection (b)(1).

(C) RECONCILED CASH FLOW.—The term "reconciled cash flow" means, for a regional alliance for a reference year, the total amount that would have been paid to regional alliance health plans in the year if such payments had been made based on the blended plan payment amount computed on the basis of the actual AFDC and SSI proportions for the year (determined under subsection (b)(2), rather than based on such payment amount computed on the basis of the projected AFDC and SSI proportions for the year (determined under subsection (b)(1)).

(4) PERCENTAGE ADJUSTMENT.—The percentage adjustment described in this paragraph for a regional alliance for an applicable year is the ratio (expressed as a percentage) of—

    (A) the cash flow difference for the reference year, to

    (B) the total payments estimated by the regional alliance to be paid to regional alliance health plans under this subtitle in the applicable year (determined without regard to any adjustment under this subsection).

# TITLE VII—REVENUE PROVISIONS

TABLE OF CONTENTS OF TITLE

Sec. 7001. Amendment of 1986 Code.

### Subtitle A—Financing Provisions

PART 1—INCREASE IN TAX ON TOBACCO PRODUCTS

Sec. 7111. Increase in excise taxes on tobacco products.
Sec. 7112. Modifications of certain tobacco tax provisions.
Sec. 7113. Imposition of excise tax on manufacture or importation of roll-your-own tobacco.

PART 2—HEALTH RELATED ASSESSMENT

Sec. 7121. Assessment on corporate alliance employers.

PART 3—RECAPTURE OF CERTAIN HEALTH CARE SUBSIDIES

Sec. 7131. Recapture of certain health care subsidies received by high-income individuals.

PART 4—OTHER PROVISIONS

Sec. 7141. Modification to self-employment tax treatment of certain S corporation shareholders and partners.
Sec. 7142. Extending medicare coverage of, and application of hospital insurance tax to, all State and local government employees.

### Subtitle B—Tax Treatment of Employer-Provided Health Care

Sec. 7201. Limitation on exclusion for employer-provided health benefits.
Sec. 7202. Health benefits may not be provided under cafeteria plans.
Sec. 7203. Increase in deduction for health insurance costs of self-employed individuals.
Sec. 7204. Limitation on prepayment of medical insurance premiums.

### Subtitle C—Employment Status Provisions

Sec. 7301. Definition of employee.
Sec. 7302. Increase in services reporting penalties.
Sec. 7303. Revision of section 530 safe harbor rules.

### Subtitle D—Tax Treatment of Funding of Retiree Health Benefits

Sec. 7401. Post-retirement medical and life insurance reserves.
Sec. 7402. Health benefits accounts maintained by pension plans.

### Subtitle E—Coordination With COBRA Continuing Care Provisions

Sec. 7501. Coordination with COBRA continuing care provisions.

## Subtitle F—Tax Treatment of Organizations Providing Health Care Services and Related Organizations

Sec. 7601. Treatment of nonprofit health care organizations.
Sec. 7602. Tax treatment of taxable organizations providing health insurance and other prepaid health care services.
Sec. 7603. Exemption from income tax for regional alliances.

## Subtitle G—Tax Treatment of Long-term Care Insurance and Services

Sec. 7701. Qualified long-term care services treated as medical care.
Sec. 7702. Treatment of long-term care insurance.
Sec. 7703. Tax treatment of accelerated death benefits under life insurance contracts.
Sec. 7704. Tax treatment of companies issuing qualified accelerated death benefit riders.

## Subtitle H—Tax Incentives for Health Services Providers

Sec. 7801. Nonrefundable credit for certain primary health services providers.
Sec. 7802. Expensing of medical equipment.

## Subtitle I—Miscellaneous Provisions

Sec. 7901. Credit for cost of personal assistance services required by employed individuals.
Sec. 7902. Denial of tax-exempt status for borrowings of health care-related entities.
Sec. 7903. Disclosure of return information for administration of certain programs under the Health Security Act.

## SEC. 7001. AMENDMENT OF 1986 CODE.

Except as otherwise expressly provided, whenever in this title an amendment or repeal is expressed in terms of an amendment to, or repeal of, a section or other provision, the reference shall be considered to be made to a section or other provision of the Internal Revenue Code of 1986.

# Subtitle A—Financing Provisions

## PART 1—INCREASE IN TAX ON TOBACCO PRODUCTS

**SEC. 7111. INCREASE IN EXCISE TAXES ON TOBACCO PRODUCTS.**

(a) CIGARETTES.—Subsection (b) of section 5701 is amended—

    (1) by striking "$12 per thousand ($10 per thousand on cigarettes removed during 1991 or 1992)" in paragraph (1) and inserting "$49.50 per thousand", and

    (2) by striking "$25.20 per thousand ($21 per thousand on cigarettes removed during 1991 or 1992)" in paragraph (2) and inserting "$103.95 per thousand".

(b) CIGARS.—Subsection (a) of section 5701 is amended—

    (1) by striking "$1.125 cents per thousand (93.75 cents per thousand on cigars removed during 1991 or 1992)" in paragraph (1) and inserting "$38.62½ per thousand", and

    (2) by striking "equal to" and all that follows in paragraph (2) and inserting "equal to 52.594 percent of the price for which sold but not more than $123.75 per thousand."

(c) CIGARETTE PAPERS.—Subsection (c) of section 5701 is amended by striking "0.75 cent (0.625 cent on cigarette papers removed during 1991 or 1992)" and inserting "3.09 cents".

(d) CIGARETTE TUBES.—Subsection (d) of section 5701 is amended by striking "1.5 cents (1.25 cents on cigarette tubes removed during 1991 or 1992)" and inserting "6.19 cents".

(e) SMOKELESS TOBACCO.—Subsection (e) of section 5701 is amended—

(1) by striking "36 cents (30 cents on snuff removed during 1991 or 1992)" in paragraph (1) and inserting "$12.86", and

(2) by striking "12 cents (10 cents on chewing tobacco removed during 1991 or 1992)" in paragraph (2) and inserting "$12.62".

(f) PIPE TOBACCO.—Subsection (f) of section 5701 is amended by striking "67.5 cents (56.25 cents on pipe tobacco removed during 1991 or 1992)" and inserting "$13.17½".

(g) EFFECTIVE DATE.—The amendments made by this section shall apply to articles removed (as defined in section 5702(k) of the Internal Revenue Code of 1986, as amended by this Act) after September 30, 1994.

(h) FLOOR STOCKS TAXES.—

(1) IMPOSITION OF TAX.—On tobacco products and cigarette papers and tubes manufactured in or imported into the United States which are removed before October 1, 1994, and held on such date for sale by any person, there is hereby imposed a tax in an amount equal to the excess of—

(A) the tax which would be imposed under section 5701 of the Internal Revenue Code of 1986 on the article if the article had been removed on such date, over

(B) the prior tax (if any) imposed under section 5701 or 7652 of such Code on such article.

(2) AUTHORITY TO EXEMPT CIGARETTES HELD IN VENDING MACHINES.—To the extent provided in regulations prescribed by the Secretary, no tax shall be imposed by paragraph (1) on cigarettes held for retail sale on October 1, 1994, by any person in any vending machine. If the Secretary provides such a benefit with respect to any person, the Secretary may reduce the $500 amount in paragraph (3) with respect to such person.

(3) CREDIT AGAINST TAX.—Each person shall be allowed as a credit against the taxes imposed by paragraph (1) an amount equal to $500. Such credit

shall not exceed the amount of taxes imposed by paragraph (1) for which such person is liable.

(4) LIABILITY FOR TAX AND METHOD OF PAYMENT.—

(A) LIABILITY FOR TAX.—A person holding cigarettes on October 1, 1994, to which any tax imposed by paragraph (1) applies shall be liable for such tax.

(B) METHOD OF PAYMENT.—The tax imposed by paragraph (1) shall be paid in such manner as the Secretary shall prescribe by regulations.

(C) TIME FOR PAYMENT.—The tax imposed by paragraph (1) shall be paid on or before December 31, 1994.

(5) ARTICLES IN FOREIGN TRADE ZONES.—Notwithstanding the Act of June 18, 1934 (48 Stat. 998, 19 U.S.C. 81a) and any other provision of law, any article which is located in a foreign trade zone on October 1, 1994, shall be subject to the tax imposed by paragraph (1) if—

(A) internal revenue taxes have been determined, or customs duties liquidated, with respect to such article before such date pursuant to a request made under the 1st proviso of section 3(a) of such Act, or

(B) such article is held on such date under the supervision of a customs officer pursuant to the 2d proviso of such section 3(a).

(6) DEFINITIONS.—For purposes of this subsection—

(A) IN GENERAL.—Terms used in this subsection which are also used in section 5702 of the Internal Revenue Code of 1986 shall have the respective meanings such terms have in such section, and such term shall include articles first subject to the tax imposed by section 5701 of such Code by reason of the amendments made by this Act.

(B) SECRETARY.—The term "Secretary" means the Secretary of the Treasury or his delegate.

(7) CONTROLLED GROUPS.—Rules similar to the rules of section 5061(e)(3) of such Code shall apply for purposes of this subsection.

(8) OTHER LAWS APPLICABLE.—All provisions of law, including penalties, applicable with respect to the taxes imposed by section 5701 of such Code shall, insofar as applicable and not inconsistent with

the provisions of this subsection, apply to the floor stocks taxes imposed by paragraph (1), to the same extent as if such taxes were imposed by such section 5701. The Secretary may treat any person who bore the ultimate burden of the tax imposed by paragraph (1) as the person to whom a credit or refund under such provisions may be allowed or made.

## SEC. 7112. MODIFICATIONS OF CERTAIN TOBACCO TAX PROVISIONS.

(a) EXEMPTION FOR EXPORTED TOBACCO PRODUCTS AND CIGARETTE PAPERS AND TUBES TO APPLY ONLY TO ARTICLES MARKED FOR EXPORT.—

(1) Subsection (b) of section 5704 is amended by adding at the end thereof the following new sentence: "Tobacco products and cigarette papers and tubes may not be transferred or removed under this subsection unless such products or papers and tubes bear such marks, labels, or notices as the Secretary shall by regulations prescribe."

(2) Section 5761 is amended by redesignating subsections (c) and (d) as subsections (d) and (e), respectively, and by inserting after subsection (b) the following new subsection:

"(c) SALE OF TOBACCO PRODUCTS AND CIGARETTE PAPERS AND TUBES FOR EXPORT.—Except as provided in subsections (b) and (d) of section 5704—

"(1) every person who sells, relands, or receives within the jurisdiction of the United States any tobacco products or cigarette papers or tubes which have been labeled or shipped for exportation under this chapter,

"(2) every person who sells or receives such relanded tobacco products or cigarette papers or tubes, and

"(3) every person who aids or abets in such selling, relanding, or receiving,

shall, in addition to the tax and any other penalty provided in this title, be liable for a penalty equal to the greater of $1,000 or 5 times the amount of the tax imposed by this chapter. All tobacco products and cigarette papers and tubes relanded within the jurisdiction of the United States, and all vessels, vehicles, and aircraft used in such relanding or in removing such products, papers, and tubes from the place where relanded, shall be forfeited to the United States."

(3) Subsection (a) of section 5761 is amended by striking "subsection (b)" and inserting "subsection (b) or (c)".

(4) Subsection (d) of section 5761, as redesignated by paragraph (2), is amended by striking "The penalty imposed by subsection (b)" and inserting "The penalties imposed by subsections (b) and (c)".

(5)(A) Subpart F of chapter 52 is amended by adding at the end thereof the following new section:

"SEC. 5754. RESTRICTION ON IMPORTATION OF PREVIOUSLY EXPORTED TOBACCO PRODUCTS.

"(a) IN GENERAL.—Tobacco products and cigarette papers and tubes previously exported from the United States may be imported or brought into the United States only as provided in section 5704(d).

"(b) CROSS REFERENCE.—

> "For penalty for the sale of cigarettes in the United States which are labeled for export, see section 5761(d)."

(B) The table of sections for subpart F of chapter 52 is amended by adding at the end thereof the following new item:

> "Sec. 5754. Restriction on importation of previously exported tobacco products."

(b) IMPORTERS REQUIRED TO BE QUALIFIED.—

(1) Sections 5712, 5713(a), 5721, 5722, 5762(a)(1), and 5763(b) and (c) are each amended by inserting "or importer" after "manufacturer".

(2) The heading of subsection (b) of section 5763 is amended by inserting "QUALIFIED IMPORTERS," after "MANUFACTURERS,".

(3) The heading for subchapter B of chapter 52 is amended by inserting "and Importers" after **"Manufacturers"**.

(4) The item relating to subchapter B in the table of subchapters for chapter 52 is amended by inserting "and importers" after "manufacturers".

(c) REPEAL OF TAX-EXEMPT SALES TO EMPLOYEES OF CIGARETTE MANUFACTURERS.—

(1) Subsection (a) of section 5704 is amended—

(A) by striking "EMPLOYEE USE OR" in the heading, and

(B) by striking "for use or consumption by employees or" in the text.

(2) Subsection (e) of section 5723 is amended by striking "for use or consumption by their employees, or for experimental purposes" and inserting "for experimental purposes".

(d) REPEAL OF TAX-EXEMPT SALES TO UNITED STATES.—Subsection (b) of section 5704 is amended by striking "and manufacturers may similarly remove such articles for use of the United States;".

(e) BOOKS OF 25 OR FEWER CIGARETTE PAPERS SUBJECT TO TAX.—Subsection (c) of section 5701 is amended by striking "On each book or set of cigarette papers containing more than 25 papers," and inserting "On cigarette papers,".

(f) STORAGE OF TOBACCO PRODUCTS.—Subsection (k) of section 5702 is amended by inserting "under section 5704" after "internal revenue bond".

(g) AUTHORITY TO PRESCRIBE MINIMUM MANUFACTURING ACTIVITY REQUIREMENTS.—Section 5712 is amended by striking "or" at the end of paragraph (1), by redesignating paragraph (2) as paragraph (3), and by inserting after paragraph (1) the following new paragraph:

"(2) the activity proposed to be carried out at such premises does not meet such minimum capacity or activity requirements as the Secretary may prescribe, or".

(h) LIMITATION ON COVER OVER OF TAX ON TOBACCO PRODUCTS.—Section 7652 is amended by adding at the end thereof the following new subsection:

"(h) LIMITATION ON COVER OVER OF TAX ON TOBACCO PRODUCTS.—For purposes of this section, with respect to taxes imposed under section 5701 or this section on any tobacco product or cigarette paper or tube, the amount covered into the treasuries of Puerto Rico and the

Virgin Islands shall not exceed the rate of tax under section 5701 in effect on the article on the day before the date of the enactment of the Health Security Act."

(i) EFFECTIVE DATE.—The amendments made by this section shall apply to articles removed (as defined in section 5702(k) of the Internal Revenue Code of 1986, as amended by this Act) after September 30, 1994.

## SEC. 7113. IMPOSITION OF EXCISE TAX ON MANUFACTURE OR IMPORTATION OF ROLL-YOUR-OWN TOBACCO.

(a) IN GENERAL.—Section 5701 (relating to rate of tax) is amended by redesignating subsection (g) as subsection (h) and by inserting after subsection (f) the following new subsection:

"(g) ROLL-YOUR-OWN TOBACCO.—On roll-your-own tobacco, manufactured in or imported into the United States, there shall be imposed a tax of $12.50 per pound (and a proportionate tax at the like rate on all fractional parts of a pound)."

(b) ROLL-YOUR-OWN TOBACCO.—Section 5702 (relating to definitions) is amended by adding at the end thereof the following new subsection:

"(p) ROLL-YOUR-OWN TOBACCO.—The term 'roll-your-own tobacco' means any tobacco which, because of its appearance, type, packaging, or labeling, is suitable for use and likely to be offered to, or purchased by, consumers as tobacco for making cigarettes."

(c) TECHNICAL AMENDMENTS.—

(1) Subsection (c) of section 5702 is amended by striking "and pipe tobacco" and inserting "pipe tobacco, and roll-your-own tobacco".

(2) Subsection (d) of section 5702 is amended—

(A) in the material preceding paragraph (1), by striking "or pipe tobacco" and inserting "pipe tobacco, or roll-your-own tobacco", and

(B) by striking paragraph (1) and inserting the following new paragraph:

"(1) a person who produces cigars, cigarettes, smokeless tobacco, pipe tobacco, or roll-your-own tobacco solely for his own personal consumption or use, and".

(3) The chapter heading for chapter 52 is amended to read as follows:

## "CHAPTER 52—TOBACCO PRODUCTS AND CIGARETTE PAPERS AND TUBES".

(4) The table of chapters for subtitle E is amended by striking the item relating to chapter 52 and inserting the following new item:

"Chapter 52. Tobacco products and cigarette papers and tubes."

(d) EFFECTIVE DATE.—

(1) IN GENERAL.—The amendments made by this section shall apply to roll-your-own tobacco removed (as defined in section 5702(k) of the Internal Revenue Code of 1986, as amended by this Act) after September 30, 1994.

(2) TRANSITIONAL RULE.—Any person who—

    (A) on the date of the enactment of this Act is engaged in business as a manufacturer of roll-your-own tobacco or as an importer of tobacco products or cigarette papers and tubes, and

    (B) before October 1, 1994, submits an application under subchapter B of chapter 52 of such Code to engage in such business,

may, notwithstanding such subchapter B, continue to engage in such business pending final action on such application. Pending such final action, all provisions of such chapter 52 shall apply to such applicant in the same manner and to the same extent as if such applicant were a holder of a permit under such chapter 52 to engage in such business.

# PART 2—HEALTH RELATED ASSESSMENT

## SEC. 7121. ASSESSMENT ON CORPORATE ALLIANCE EMPLOYERS.

(a) IN GENERAL.—Subtitle C (relating to employment taxes) is amended by inserting after chapter 24 the following new chapter:

## "CHAPTER 24A—ASSESSMENT ON CORPORATE ALLIANCE EMPLOYERS

"Sec. 3461. Assessment on corporate alliance employers.

## "SEC. 3461. ASSESSMENT ON CORPORATE ALLIANCE EMPLOYERS.

"(a) IMPOSITION OF ASSESSMENT.—Every corporate alliance employer shall pay (in addition to any other amount imposed by this subtitle) for each calendar year an assessment equal to 1 percent of the payroll of such employer.

"(b) DEFINITIONS.—For purposes of this section—

"(1) CORPORATE ALLIANCE EMPLOYER.—The term 'corporate alliance employer' means any employer if any individual, by reason of being an employee of such employer, is provided with health coverage through any corporate alliance described in section 1311 of the Health Security Act.

"(2) PAYROLL.—The term 'payroll' means the sum of—

"(A) the wages (as defined in section 3121(a) without regard to paragraph (1) thereof) paid by the employer during the calendar year, plus

"(B)(i) in the case of a sole proprietorship, the net earnings from self-employment of the proprietor from such trade or business for the taxable year ending with or within the calendar year,

"(ii) in the case of a partnership, the aggregate of the net earnings from self-employment of each partner which is attributable to such partnership for the taxable year of such partnership ending with or within the calendar year, and

"(ii) in the case of an S corporation, the aggregate of the net earnings from self-employment of each shareholder which is attributable to such corporation for the taxable year of such corporation ending with or within the calendar year.

"(3) NET EARNINGS FROM SELF-EMPLOYMENT.—The term 'net earnings from self-employment' has the meaning given such term by section 1402; except that the amount thereof—

"(A) may never be less than zero, and

"(B) shall be determined without regard to any deduction for an assessment under this section.

"(4) EMPLOYER.—

"(A) IN GENERAL.—The term 'employer' means any person for whom an individual performs services, of whatever nature, as an employee (as defined in section 3401(c)).

"(B) SPECIAL RULES.—

"(i) An individual who owns the entire interest in an unincorporated trade or business shall be treated as his own employer.

"(ii) A partnership shall be treated as the employer of each partner who is an employee within the meaning of section 401(c)(1).

"(iii) An S corporation shall be treated as the employer of each shareholder who is an employee within the meaning of section 401(c)(1).

"(c) SPECIAL RULES.—For purposes of this section—

"(1) TREATMENT OF CERTAIN EMPLOYERS.—In the case of an employer who is a corporate alliance employer solely by reason of employees who are provided with health coverage through a corporate alliance the eligible sponsor of which is a multiemployer plan described in section 1311(b)(1)(B) of the Health Security Act, the payroll of such employer shall be determined by taking into account only such employees.

"(2) CONTROLLED GROUP RULES.—All persons treated as a single employer under section 1901 of the Health Security Act (relating to employer premiums for comprehensive health care) shall be treated as a single employer.

"(3) APPLICATION OF ASSESSMENT BEGINNING IN 1996.—

"(A) IN GENERAL.—Every employer eligible to elect to be an eligible sponsor under section 1311 of the Health Security Act shall be treated as a corporate alliance employer as of January 1, 1996, unless the employer waives such employer's rights ever to be treated as such a sponsor. The waiver under this subparagraph shall be irrevocable.

"(B) EXCEPTION.—Subparagraph (A) shall not apply to any employer referred to in paragraph (1).

"(4) TREATMENT OF FEDERAL GOVERNMENT.—Nothing in any provision of law shall be construed to exempt any agency or instrumentality of the United States from the assessment under this section.

"(d) ADMINISTRATIVE PROVISIONS.—

"(1) PAYMENT.—The assessment under this section shall be paid at the same time and manner as the tax imposed by chapter 21.

"(2) COLLECTION, ETC.—For purposes of subtitle F, the assessment under this section shall be treated as if it were a tax imposed by this subtitle."

(b) CLERICAL AMENDMENT.—The table of chapters for subtitle C is amended by inserting after the item relating to chapter 24 the following new item:

"Chapter 24A. Assessment on corporate alliance employers."

(c) EFFECTIVE DATE.—The amendments made by this section shall take effect on January 1, 1996.

# PART 3—RECAPTURE OF CERTAIN HEALTH CARE SUBSIDIES

SEC. 7131. RECAPTURE OF CERTAIN HEALTH CARE SUBSIDIES RECEIVED BY HIGH-INCOME INDIVIDUALS.

(a) IN GENERAL.—Subchapter A of chapter 1 is amended by adding at the end thereof the following new part:

## "PART VIII—CERTAIN HEALTH CARE SUBSIDIES RECEIVED BY HIGH-INCOME INDIVIDUALS

"Sec. 59B. Recapture of certain health care subsidies.

"SEC. 59B. RECAPTURE OF CERTAIN HEALTH CARE SUBSIDIES.

"(a) IMPOSITION OF RECAPTURE AMOUNT.—In the case of an individual, if the modified adjusted gross income of the taxpayer for the taxable year exceeds the threshold amount, such taxpayer shall pay (in addition to any other amount imposed by this subtitle) a recapture amount for such taxable year equal to the sum of—

"(1) the aggregate of the Medicare part B recapture amounts (if any) for months during such year that a premium is paid under part B of title XVIII of the Social Security Act for the coverage of the individual under such part, and

"(2) the aggregate reductions (if any) in the individual's liability for periods after December 31, 1999, under section 6111 of the Health Security Act (relating to repayment of alliance credit by certain families) pursuant to section 6114 of such Act (relating to special treatment of certain retirees and qualified spouses and children) for months during such year.

"(b) MEDICARE PART B PREMIUM RECAPTURE AMOUNT FOR MONTH.—For purposes of this section, the Medicare part B premium recapture amount for any month is the amount equal to the excess of—

"(1) 150 percent of the monthly actuarial rate for enrollees age 65 and over determined for that calendar year under section 1839(b) of the Social Security Act, over

"(2) the total monthly premium under section 1839 of the Social Security Act (determined without regard to subsections (b) and (f) of section 1839 of such Act).

"(c) PHASEIN OF RECAPTURE AMOUNT.—If the modified adjusted gross income of the taxpayer for any taxable year exceeds the threshold amount by less than $10,000, the recapture amount imposed by this section for such taxable year shall be an amount which bears the same ratio to the recapture amount which would (but for this subsection) be imposed by this section for such taxable year as such excess bears to $10,000.

"(d) OTHER DEFINITIONS AND SPECIAL RULES.—For purposes of this section—

"(1) THRESHOLD AMOUNT.—The term 'threshold amount' means—

"(A) except as otherwise provided in this paragraph, $90,000,

"(B) $115,000 in the case of a joint return, and

"(C) zero in the case of a taxpayer who—

"(i) is married (as determined under section 7703) but does not file a joint return for such year, and

"(ii) does not live apart from his spouse at all times during the taxable year.

"(2) MODIFIED ADJUSTED GROSS INCOME.—The term 'modified adjusted gross income' means adjusted gross income—

"(A) determined without regard to sections 135, 911, 931, and 933, and

"(B) increased by the amount of interest received or accrued by the taxpayer during the taxable year which is exempt from tax.

"(3) JOINT RETURNS.—In the case of a joint return—

"(A) the recapture amount under subsection (a) shall be the sum of the recapture amounts determined separately for each spouse, and

"(B) subsections (a) and (c) shall be applied by taking into account the combined modified adjusted gross income of the spouses.

"(4) COORDINATION WITH OTHER PROVISIONS.—

"(A) TREATED AS TAX FOR SUBTITLE F.—For purposes of subtitle F, the recapture amount imposed by this section shall be treated as if it were a tax imposed by section 1.

"(B) NOT TREATED AS TAX FOR CERTAIN PURPOSES.—The recapture amount imposed by this section shall not be treated as a tax imposed by this chapter for purposes of determining—

"(i) the amount of any credit allowable under this chapter, or

"(ii) the amount of the minimum tax under section 55."

(b) TRANSFERS TO SUPPLEMENTAL MEDICAL INSURANCE TRUST FUND.—

(1) IN GENERAL.—There are hereby appropriated to the Supplemental Medical Insurance Trust Fund amounts equivalent to the aggregate increase in liabilities under chapter 1 of the Internal Revenue Code of 1986 which is attributable to the application of section 59B(a)(1) of such Code, as added by this section.

(2) TRANSFERS.—The amounts appropriated by paragraph (1) to the Supplemental Medical Insurance Trust Fund shall be transferred from time to time (but not less frequently than quarterly) from the general fund of the Treasury on the basis of estimates made by the Secretary of the Treasury of the amounts referred to in paragraph (1). Any quarterly payment shall be made on the first day of such quarter and shall take into account the recapture amounts referred to in such section 59B(a)(1) for such quarter. Proper adjustments shall be made in the amounts subsequently transferred to the extent prior estimates were in excess of or less than the amounts required to be transferred.

(c) REPORTING REQUIREMENTS.—

(1)(A) Paragraph (1) of section 6050F(a) (relating to returns relating to social security benefits) is amended by striking "and" at the end of subparagraph (B) and by inserting after subparagraph (C) the following new subparagraph:

"(D) the number of months during the calendar year for which a premium was paid under part B of title XVIII of the Social Security Act for the coverage of such individual under such part, and".

(B) Paragraph (2) of section 6050F(b) is amended to read as follows:

"(2) the information required to be shown on such return with respect to such individual."

(C) Subparagraph (A) of section 6050F(c)(1) is amended by inserting before the comma "and in the case of the information specified in subsection (a)(1)(D)".

(D) The heading for section 6050F is amended by inserting "**AND MEDICARE PART B COVERAGE**" before the period.

(E) The item relating to section 6050F in the table of sections for subpart B of part III of subchapter A of chapter 61 is amended by inserting "and Medicare part B coverage" before the period.

(2)(A) Subpart B of part III of subchapter A of chapter 61 (relating to information concerning transactions with other persons) is amended by adding at the end thereof the following new section:

"SEC. 6050Q. RETURNS RELATING TO CERTAIN RETIREE HEALTH CARE SUBSIDIES.

"(a) IN GENERAL.—Every alliance (as defined in section 1301 of the Health Security Act) that reduces an individual's liability under section 6111 of such Act (relating to repayment of alliance credit by certain families) pursuant to section 6114 of such Act (relating to special treatment of certain retirees and qualified spouses and children) shall make a return (according to the forms and regulations prescribed by the Secretary) setting forth—

"(1) the aggregate amount of such reductions by such alliance with respect to any individual during such calendar year, and

"(2) the name and address of such individual.

"(b) STATEMENTS TO BE FURNISHED TO INDIVIDUALS WITH RESPECT TO WHOM INFORMATION IS REQUIRED TO BE REPORTED.—Every alliance required to make a return under subsection (a) shall furnish to each individual whose name is required to be set forth in such return a written statement showing—

"(1) the name and address of such alliance, and

"(2) the information required to be shown on the return with respect to such individual." The written statement required under the preceding sentence shall be furnished to the individual as soon as practicable after the close of the calendar year for which the return under subsection (a) was made."

    (B) Subparagraph (B) of section 6724(d)(1) is amended by inserting after clause (viii) the following new clause (and by redesignating the following clauses accordingly):

        "(ix) section 6050Q (relating to returns relating to certain retiree health care subsidies),".

    (C) Paragraph (2) of section 6724(d) is amended by redesignating subparagraphs (Q) through (T) as subparagraphs (R) through (U), respectively, and by inserting after subparagraph (P) the following new subparagraph:

        "(Q) section 6050Q(b) (relating to returns relating to certain retiree health care subsidies),".

    (D) The table of sections for subpart B of part III of subchapter A of chapter 61 is amended by adding at the end thereof the following new item:

> "Sec. 6050Q. Returns relating to certain retiree health care subsidies."

(d) WAIVER OF ESTIMATED TAX PENALTIES FOR 1996.—No addition to tax shall be imposed under section 6654 of the Internal Revenue Code of 1986 (relating to failure to pay estimated income tax) for any period before—

(1) April 16, 1997, with respect to any underpayment to the extent that such underpayment resulted from section 59B(a)(1) of the Internal Revenue Code of 1986, as added by this section, and

(2) April 16, 2001, with respect to any underpayment to the extent that such underpayment resulted from section 59B(a)(2) of such Code, as added by this section.

(e) CLERICAL AMENDMENT.—The table of parts for subchapter A of chapter 1 is amended by adding at the end thereof the following new item:

"Part VIII. Certain health care subsidies received by high-income individuals."

(f) EFFECTIVE DATE.—The amendments made by this section shall apply to periods after December 31, 1995, in taxable years ending after such date.

# PART 4—OTHER PROVISIONS

SEC. 7141. MODIFICATION TO SELF-EMPLOYMENT TAX TREATMENT OF CERTAIN S CORPORATION SHAREHOLDERS AND PARTNERS.

(a) TREATMENT OF CERTAIN S CORPORATION SHAREHOLDERS.—

(1) AMENDMENT TO INTERNAL REVENUE CODE.—Section 1402 (relating to definitions) is amended by adding at the end thereof the following new subsection:

"(k) TREATMENT OF CERTAIN S CORPORATION SHAREHOLDERS.—

"(1) IN GENERAL.—In the case of any individual—

"(A) who is a 2-percent shareholder (as defined in section 1372(b)) of an S corporation for any taxable year of such corporation, and

"(B) who materially participates in the activities of such S corporation during such taxable year,

such shareholder's net earnings from self-employment for such shareholder's taxable year in which the taxable year of the S corporation ends shall include such shareholder's pro rata share (as determined under section 1366(a)) of the taxable income or loss of such corporation from service-related businesses carried on by such corporation.

"(2) CERTAIN EXCEPTIONS TO APPLY.—In determining the amount to be taken into account under paragraph (1), the exceptions provided in subsection (a) shall apply, except that, in the case of the exceptions provided in subsection (a)(5), the rules of subparagraph (B) thereof shall apply to shareholders in S corporations.

"(3) SERVICE-RELATED BUSINESS.—For purposes of this subsection, the term 'service-related business' means any trade or business described in subparagraph (A) of section 1202(e)(3)."

(2) AMENDMENT TO SOCIAL SECURITY ACT.—Section 211 of the Social Security Act is amended by adding at the end the following new subsection: "Treatment of Certain S Corporation Shareholders

"(k)(1) In the case of any individual—

"(A) who is a 2-percent shareholder (as defined in section 1372(b) of the Internal Revenue Code of 1986) of an S corporation for any taxable year of such corporation, and

"(B) who materially participates in the activities of such S corporation during such taxable year, such shareholder's net earnings from self-employment for such shareholder's taxable year in which the taxable year of the S corporation ends shall include such shareholder's pro rata share (as determined under section 1366(a) of such Code) of the taxable income or loss of such corporation from service-related businesses (as defined in section 1402(k)(3) of such Code) carried on by such corporation.

"(2) In determining the amount to be taken into account under paragraph (1), the exceptions provided in subsection (a) shall apply, except that, in the case of the exceptions provided in subsection (a)(5), the rules of subparagraph (B) thereof shall apply to shareholders in S corporations.".

(b) TREATMENT OF CERTAIN LIMITED PARTNERS.—

(1) AMENDMENT OF INTERNAL REVENUE CODE.—Paragraph (13) of section 1402(a) is amended by striking "limited partner, as such" and inserting "limited partner who does not materially participate in the activities of the partnership".

(2) AMENDMENT OF SOCIAL SECURITY ACT.—Paragraph (12) of section 211(a) of the Social Security Act is amended by striking "limited partner, as such" and inserting "limited partner who does not

materially participate in the activities of the partnership".

(c) EFFECTIVE DATE.—The amendments made by this section shall apply to taxable years of individuals beginning after December 31, 1995, and to taxable years of S corporations and partnerships ending with or within such taxable years of individuals.

## SEC. 7142. EXTENDING MEDICARE COVERAGE OF, AND APPLICATION OF HOSPITAL INSURANCE TAX TO, ALL STATE AND LOCAL GOVERNMENT EMPLOYEES.

(a) IN GENERAL.—

(1) APPLICATION OF HOSPITAL INSURANCE TAX.—Section 3121(u)(2) is amended by striking subparagraphs (C) and (D).

(2) COVERAGE UNDER MEDICARE.—Section 210(p) of the Social Security Act (42 U.S.C. 410(p)) is amended by striking paragraphs (3) and (4).

(3) EFFECTIVE DATE.—The amendments made by this subsection shall apply to services performed after September 30, 1995.

(b) TRANSITION IN BENEFITS FOR STATE AND LOCAL GOVERNMENT EMPLOYEES AND FORMER EMPLOYEES.—

(1) IN GENERAL.—

(A) EMPLOYEES NEWLY SUBJECT TO TAX.—For purposes of sections 226, 226A, and 1811 of the Social Security Act, in the case of any individual who performs services during the calendar quarter beginning October 1, 1995, the wages for which are subject to the tax imposed by section 3101(b) of the Internal Revenue Code of 1986 only because of the amendment made by subsection (a), the individual's medicare qualified State or local government employment (as defined in subparagraph (B)) performed before October 1, 1995, shall be considered to be "employment" (as defined for purposes of title II of such Act), but only for purposes of providing the individual (or another person) with entitlement to hospital insurance benefits under part A of title XVIII of such Act for months beginning with October 1995.

(B) MEDICARE QUALIFIED STATE OR LOCAL GOVERNMENT EMPLOYMENT DEFINED.—In this paragraph, the term "medicare qualified State or local government employment" means medicare qualified government employment described in section 210(p)(1)(B) of the Social Security Act (determined without regard to section 210(p)(3) of such Act, as in effect before its repeal under subsection (a)(2)).

(2) AUTHORIZATION OF APPROPRIATIONS.—There are authorized to be appropriated to the Federal Hospital Insurance Trust Fund from time to time such sums as the Secretary of Health and Human Services deems necessary for any fiscal year on account of—

   (A) payments made or to be made during such fiscal year from such Trust Fund with respect to individuals who are entitled to benefits under title XVIII of the Social Security Act solely by reason of paragraph (1),

   (B) the additional administrative expenses resulting or expected to result therefrom, and

   (C) any loss in interest to such Trust Fund resulting from the payment of those amounts, in order to place such Trust Fund in the same position at the end of such fiscal year as it would have been in if this subsection had not been enacted.

(3) INFORMATION TO INDIVIDUALS WHO ARE PROSPECTIVE MEDICARE BENEFICIARIES BASED ON STATE AND LOCAL GOVERNMENT EMPLOYMENT.—

Section 226(g) of the Social Security Act (42 U.S.C. 426(g)) is amended—

>(A) by redesignating paragraphs (1) through (3) as subparagraphs (A) through (C), respectively,

>(B) by inserting "(1)" after "(g)", and

>(C) by adding at the end the following new paragraph:

>"(2) The Secretary, in consultation with State and local governments, shall provide procedures designed to assure that individuals who perform medicare qualified government employment by virtue of service described in section 210(a)(7) are fully informed with respect to (A) their eligibility or potential eligibility for hospital insurance benefits (based on such employment) under part A of title XVIII, (B) the requirements for, and conditions of, such eligibility, and (C) the necessity of timely application as a condition of becoming entitled under subsection (b)(2)(C), giving particular attention to individuals who apply for an annuity or retirement benefit and whose eligibility for such annuity or retirement benefit is based on a disability."

(c) TECHNICAL AMENDMENTS.—

(1) Subparagraph (A) of section 3121(u)(2) is amended by striking "subparagraphs (B) and (C)," and inserting "subparagraph (B),".

(2) Subparagraph (B) of section 210(p)(1) of the Social Security Act (42 U.S.C. 410(p)(1)) is amended by striking "paragraphs (2) and (3)." and inserting "paragraph (2)."

(3) Section 218 of the Social Security Act (42 U.S.C. 418) is amended by striking subsection (n).

(4) The amendments made by this subsection shall apply after September 30, 1995.

## Subtitle B—Tax Treatment of Employer-Provided Health Care

SEC. 7201. LIMITATION ON EXCLUSION FOR EMPLOYER-PROVIDED HEALTH BENEFITS.

(a) GENERAL RULE.—Section 106 (relating to contributions by employer to accident and health plans) is amended to read as follows:

"SEC. 106. CONTRIBUTIONS BY EMPLOYER TO ACCIDENT AND HEALTH PLANS.

"(a) GENERAL RULE.—Except as otherwise provided in this section, gross income of an employee does not include employer-provided coverage under an accident or health plan.

"(b) INCLUSION OF CERTAIN BENEFITS NOT PART OF COMPREHENSIVE BENEFIT PACKAGE.—

"(1) IN GENERAL.—Effective on and after January 1, 2003, gross income of an employee shall include employer-provided coverage under any accident or health plan except to the extent that—

"(A) such coverage consists of comprehensive health coverage described in section 1101 of the Health Security Act, or

"(B) such coverage consists of permitted coverage.

"(2) PERMITTED COVERAGE.—For purposes of this subsection, the term 'permitted coverage' means—

"(A) any coverage providing wages or payments in lieu of wages for any period during which the employee is absent from work on account of sickness or injury,

"(B) any coverage providing for payments referred to in section 105(c),

"(C) any coverage provided to an employee or former employee after such employee has attained age 65, unless such coverage is provided by reason of the current employment of the individual (within the meaning of section

1862(b)(1)(A)(i)(I) of the Social Security Act) with the employer providing the coverage,

"(D) any coverage under a qualified long-term care insurance policy (as defined in section 7702B),

"(E) any coverage provided under Federal law to any individual (or spouse or dependent thereof) by reason of such individual being—

"(i) a member of the Armed Forces of the United States, or

"(ii) a veteran, and

"(F) any other coverage to the extent that the Secretary determines that the continuation of an exclusion for such coverage is not inconsistent with the purposes of this subsection.

"(3) SPECIAL RULES FOR FLEXIBLE SPENDING ARRANGEMENTS.—

"(A) IN GENERAL.—To the extent that any employer-provided coverage is provided through a flexible spending or similar arrangement, paragraph (1) shall be applied by substituting 'January 1, 1997,' for 'January 1, 2003'.

"(B) FLEXIBLE SPENDING ARRANGEMENT.—For purposes of this paragraph, a flexible spending arrangement is a benefit program which provides employees with coverage under which—

"(i) specified incurred expenses may be reimbursed (subject to reimbursement maximums and other reasonable conditions), and

"(ii) the maximum amount of reimbursement which is reasonably available to a participant for such coverage is less than 200 percent of the value of such coverage.

In the case of an insured plan, the maximum amount reasonably available shall be determined on the basis of the underlying coverage.

"(c) SPECIAL RULES FOR DETERMINING AMOUNT OF INCLUSION.—

"(1) IN GENERAL.—For purposes of this section, the value of any coverage shall be determined on the basis of the average cost of providing such coverage to the beneficiaries receiving such coverage.

"(2) SPECIAL RULE.—To the extent provided by the Secretary, cost determinations under paragraph (1) may be made on the basis of reasonable estimates.

"(d) POTENTIAL CASH PAYMENT NOT TO AFFECT EXCLUSION.—No amount shall be included in the gross income of an employee solely because the employee may select coverage under an accident or health plan which results in a cash payment referred to in section 1607 of the Health Security Act."

(b) EMPLOYMENT TAX TREATMENT.—

    (1) SOCIAL SECURITY TAX.—

        (A) Subsection (a) of section 3121 is amended by inserting after paragraph (21) the following new sentence:

"Nothing in paragraph (2) shall exclude from the term 'wages' any amount which is required to be included in gross income under section 106(b)."

        (B) Subsection (a) of section 209 of the Social Security Act is amended by inserting after paragraph (21) the following new sentence:

"Nothing in paragraph (2) shall exclude from the term 'wages' any amount which is required to be included in gross income under section 106(b) of the Internal Revenue Code of 1986."

    (2) RAILROAD RETIREMENT TAX.—Paragraph (1) of section 3231(e) is amended by adding at the end thereof the following new sentence: "Nothing in

clause (i) of the second sentence of this paragraph shall exclude from the term 'compensation' any amount which is required to be included in gross income under section 106(b).''

(3) UNEMPLOYMENT TAX.—Subsection (b) of section 3306 is amended by inserting after paragraph (16) the following new sentence: "Nothing in paragraph (2) shall exclude from the term 'wages' any amount which is required to be included in gross income under section 106(b).''

(4) WAGE WITHHOLDING.—Subsection (a) of section 3401 is amended by adding at the end thereof the following new sentence: "Nothing in the preceding provisions of this subsection shall exclude from the term 'wages' any amount which is required to be included in gross income under section 106(b).''

(c) EFFECTIVE DATE.—The amendments made by this section shall take effect on January 1, 1997.

**SEC. 7202. HEALTH BENEFITS MAY NOT BE PROVIDED UNDER CAFETERIA PLANS.**

(a) GENERAL RULE.—Subsection (f) of section 125 (defining qualified benefits) is amended by adding at the end thereof the following new sentence: "Such term shall not include any benefits or coverage (other than coverage described in section 106(b)(2)(A)) under an accident or health plan."

(b) CONFORMING AMENDMENT.—Subsection (g) of section 125 is amended by striking paragraph (2) and redesignating paragraphs (3) and (4) as paragraphs (2) and (3), respectively.

(c) EFFECTIVE DATE.—The amendments made by this section shall take effect on January 1, 1997.

## SEC. 7203. INCREASE IN DEDUCTION FOR HEALTH INSURANCE COSTS OF SELF-EMPLOYED INDIVIDUALS.

(a) PROVISION MADE PERMANENT.—

(1) IN GENERAL.—Subsection (l) of section 162 (relating to special rules for health insurance costs of self-employed individuals) is amended by striking paragraph (6).

(2) EFFECTIVE DATE.—The amendment made by paragraph (1) shall apply to taxable years beginning after December 31, 1993.

(b) DEDUCTION LIMITED TO BASIC COVERAGE PURCHASED FROM HEALTH ALLIANCE.—

(1) IN GENERAL.—Paragraphs (1) and (2) of section 162(l) are amended to read as follows:

"(1) IN GENERAL.—In the case of an individual who is an employee within the meaning of section

401(c), there shall be allowed as a deduction under this section an amount equal to 100 percent of the amount paid during the taxable year for insurance which constitutes medical care for the taxpayer, his spouse, and dependents; but only to the extent such insurance is comprehensive health coverage described in section 1101 of the Health Security Act purchased from a qualified alliance described in section 1311 of such Act.

"(2) LIMITATIONS.—

"(A) LOWER PERCENTAGE IN CERTAIN CASES.—If—

"(i) the taxpayer has 1 or more employees in a trade or business with respect to which such taxpayer is treated as an employee within the meaning of section 401(c), and

"(ii) the taxpayer does not pay at least 100 percent of the weighted average premium applicable under the Health Security Act for each of such employees,

paragraph (1) shall be applied by substituting for '100 percent' the lowest percentage of such weighted average premium paid by the taxpayer for any of such employees.

"(B) DEDUCTION LIMITED TO EARNED INCOME.—No deduction shall be allowed under paragraph (1) to the extent that the amount of such deduction exceeds the taxpayer's earned income (within the meaning of section 401(c)).

"(C) OTHER COVERAGE.—Paragraph (1) shall not apply to amounts paid for coverage for any individual for any calendar month if such individual is employed on a full-time basis (within the meaning of section 1901 of the Health Security Act) by an employer during such month."

(2) CONFORMING AMENDMENT.—Subparagraph (A) of section 162(l)(5) is amended by striking "shall be treated as such individual's earned income" and inserting "shall be included in such individual's earned income".

(3) EFFECTIVE DATE.—The amendments made by this subsection shall take effect on the earlier of—

(A) January 1, 1997, or

(B) the first day on which the taxpayer could purchase comprehensive health coverage from a qualified alliance.

## SEC. 7204. LIMITATION ON PREPAYMENT OF MEDICAL INSURANCE PREMIUMS.

(a) GENERAL RULE.—Subsection (d) of section 213 is amended by adding at the end thereof the following new paragraph:

"(10) LIMITATION ON PREPAYMENTS.—If the taxpayer pays a premium or other amount which constitutes medical care under paragraph (1), to the extent such premium or other amount is properly allocable to insurance coverage or care to be provided during periods more than 12 months after the month in which such payment is made, such premium shall be treated as paid ratably over the period during which such insurance coverage or care is to be provided. The preceding sentence shall not apply to any premium to which paragraph (7) applies nor to any premium paid under a qualified long-term care insurance policy."

(b) EFFECTIVE DATE.—The amendment made by subsection (a) shall apply to amounts paid after December 31, 1996.

# Subtitle C—Employment Status Provisions

**SEC. 7301. DEFINITION OF EMPLOYEE.**

(a) GENERAL RULE.—Chapter 25 (relating to general provisions applicable to employment taxes) is amended by adding at the end thereof the following new section:

"**SEC. 3510. DEFINITION OF EMPLOYEE.**

"(a) REGULATIONS.—The Secretary shall prescribe regulations setting forth rules for determining whether an individual is an employee for purposes of—

"(1) the employment taxes imposed under this subtitle, and

"(2) to the extent provided in such regulations, subtitle A.

"(b) OVERRIDE OF CURRENT RULES.—To the extent provided in the regulations prescribed in subsection (a), such regulations shall be in lieu of the rules (statutory or otherwise) otherwise applicable for the determination referred to in subsection (a). Nothing in such regulations shall override the provisions of section 3511."

(b) CLERICAL AMENDMENT.—The table of sections for chapter 25 is amended by adding at the end thereof the following new item:

"Sec. 3510. Definition of employee."

## SEC. 7302. INCREASE IN SERVICES REPORTING PENALTIES.

(a) INCREASE IN PENALTY.—Section 6721(a) (relating to imposition of penalty) is amended by adding at the end the following new paragraph:

"(3) INCREASED PENALTY FOR RETURNS INVOLVING PAYMENTS FOR SERVICES.—

"(A) IN GENERAL.—Subject to the overall limitation of paragraph (1), the amount of the penalty under paragraph (1) for any failure with respect to any applicable return shall be equal to the greater of $50 or 5 percent of the amount required to be reported correctly but not so reported.

"(B) EXCEPTION WHERE SUBSTANTIAL COMPLIANCE.—Subparagraph (A) shall not apply to failures with respect to applicable returns required to be filed by a person during any calendar year if the aggregate amount which is timely and correctly reported on applicable returns filed by the person for the calendar year is at least 97 percent of the aggregate amount which is required to be reported on applicable returns by the person for the calendar year.

"(C) APPLICABLE RETURN.—For purposes of this paragraph, the term 'applicable return' means any information return required to be filed under—

"(i) section 6041(a) which relates to payments to any person for services performed by such person (other than as an employee), or

"(ii) section 6041A(a)."

(b) CONFORMING AMENDMENT.—Section 6721(a)(1) is amended by striking "In" and inserting "Except as provided in paragraph (3), in".

(c) EFFECTIVE DATE.—The amendments made by this section shall apply to returns the due date for which (without regard to extensions) is more than 30 days after the date of the enactment of this Act.

## SEC. 7303. REVISION OF SECTION 530 SAFE HARBOR RULES.

(a) GENERAL RULE.—Chapter 25 (relating to general provisions applicable to employment taxes) is amended by adding at the end thereof the following new section:

## "SEC. 3511. PROTECTION AGAINST RETROACTIVE EMPLOYMENT TAX RECLASSIFICATIONS.

"(a) GENERAL RULE.—If—

"(1) for purposes of employment taxes, the taxpayer treats an individual as not being an employee for any period,

"(2) for such period, the taxpayer meets—

"(A) the consistency requirements of subsection (b),

"(B) the return filing requirements of subsection (c), and

"(C) the safe harbor requirement of subsection (d), and

"(3) the Secretary has not notified the taxpayer in writing before the beginning of such period that the Secretary has determined that the taxpayer should treat such individual (or any individual holding a substantially similar position) as an employee, then, for purposes of applying this subtitle for such period, the individual shall be deemed not to be an employee of the taxpayer.

"(b) CONSISTENCY REQUIREMENTS.—A taxpayer meets the consistency requirements of this subsection with respect to any individual for any period if the taxpayer treats such individual (and all other individuals holding substantially similar positions) as not being an employee for purposes of the employment taxes for such period and all prior periods.

"(c) RETURN FILING REQUIREMENTS.—

"(1) IN GENERAL.—The taxpayer meets the return filing requirements of this subsection with respect to any individual for any period if all Federal tax returns (including information returns) required to be filed by the taxpayer for such period with respect to such individual (and all other individuals holding substantially similar positions) are timely filed on a basis consistent with the taxpayer's treatment of such individuals as not being employees.

"(2) SPECIAL RULES.—For purposes of paragraph (1)—

"(A) any return filed for which the penalty under section 6721(a) is reduced or waived pursuant to subsection (b) or (c) of section 6721 shall be considered timely filed, and

"(B) a taxpayer shall not be considered as failing to meet the requirements of paragraph (1) solely because the taxpayer failed to timely file accurate information returns in respect of payments to individuals holding substantially similar positions if the taxpayer satisfies the requirements of section 6721(a)(3)(B) for such period.

"(d) SAFE HARBORS.—

"(1) IN GENERAL.—The taxpayer meets the safe harbor requirement of this subsection with respect to any individual for any period if the taxpayer's treatment of such individual as not being an employee for such period was—

"(A) in reasonable reliance on a written determination (as defined in section 6110(b)(1)) issued to or in respect of the taxpayer that addressed the employment status of the individual or an individual holding a substantially similar position;

"(B) in reasonable reliance on a concluded Internal Revenue Service audit of the taxpayer—

"(i) which was for a period in which the rules for determining employment status were the same as for the period in question, and

"(ii) in which the employment status of the individual or any individual holding a substantially similar position was examined without change to any such individual's status;

"(C) in reasonable reliance on a longstanding recognized practice of a significant segment of the industry in which the individual is engaged; or

"(D) supported by substantial authority.

For purposes of subparagraph (D), the term 'substantial authority' has the same meaning as when used in section 6662(d)(2)(B)(i); except that such term shall not include any private letter ruling issued to a person other than the taxpayer.

"(2) SPECIAL RULES.—

"(A) SUBSEQUENT AUTHORITY.—The taxpayer shall not be considered to meet the safe harbor requirement of paragraph (1)(B) with respect to any individual for any period if the treatment of such individual as not being an employee is inconsistent with any regulation, Revenue Ruling, Revenue Procedure, or other authority published by the Secretary before the beginning of such period and after the conclusion of the audit referred to in paragraph (1)(B).

"(B) TERMINATION OF INDUSTRY PRACTICE SAFE HARBOR.—The taxpayer shall not be considered to meet the safe harbor requirement of paragraph (1)(C) with respect to any individual for—

"(i) any period beginning after the date on which the Secretary prescribes regulations pursuant to section 3510, or "(ii) any period if the treatment of such individual as not being an employee is inconsistent with any regulation, Revenue Ruling, Revenue Procedure, or other authority published by the Secretary before the beginning of such period.

"(e) DEFINITIONS AND SPECIAL RULES.—For purposes of this section—

"(1) EMPLOYMENT TAX.—The term 'employment tax' means any tax imposed by this subtitle.

"(2) TAXPAYER.—The term 'taxpayer' includes any person or entity (including a governmental entity) which is (or would be but for this section) liable for any employment tax. Such term includes any predecessor or successor to the taxpayer.

"(f) REGULATIONS.—The Secretary shall prescribe such regulations as may be appropriate to carry out the purposes of this section."

(b) RULES TO APPLY FOR INCOME TAX PURPOSES.—Part I of subchapter B of chapter 1 is amended by adding at the end thereof the following new section:

"SEC. 69. DETERMINATION OF EMPLOYMENT STATUS.

"For purposes of this subtitle, an individual shall be treated as a self-employed individual with respect to any services performed by such individual for another person if, under the rules of section 3511, such individual is treated as not being an employee of such other person with respect to such services."

(c) CONFORMING AMENDMENT.—Section 530 of the Revenue Act of 1978 is hereby repealed.

(d) CLERICAL AMENDMENTS.—

(1) The table of sections for chapter 25 is amended by adding at the end thereof the following new item:

"Sec. 3511. Protection against retroactive employment tax reclassifications."

(2) The table of sections for part I of subchapter B of chapter 1 is amended by adding at the end thereof the following new item:

"Sec. 69. Determination of employment status."

(e) EFFECTIVE DATE.—

(1) IN GENERAL.—Except as provided in paragraph (2), the amendments made by this section shall apply to all periods beginning after December 31, 1995.

(2) REPEAL OF LIMITATIONS ON REGULATIONS AND RULINGS.—The repeal made by subsection (c), insofar as it relates to section 530(b) of the Revenue Act of 1978, shall take effect on the date of the enactment of this Act.

# Subtitle D—Tax Treatment of Funding of Retiree Health Benefits

### SEC. 7401. POST-RETIREMENT MEDICAL AND LIFE INSURANCE RESERVES.

(a) MINIMUM PERIOD FOR WORKING LIVES.—Section 419A(c)(2) (relating to additional reserves for post-retirement medical and life insurance benefits) is amended by inserting "(but not less than 10 years)" after "working lives of the covered employees".

(b) SEPARATE ACCOUNTING.—

(1) REQUIREMENT.—Section 419A(c)(2) is amended by adding at the end the following new flush sentence:

"Such reserve shall be maintained as a separate account."

(2) USE OF RESERVE FOR OTHER PURPOSES.—Paragraph (1) of section 4976(b) (defining disqualified benefit) is amended by striking "and" at the end of subparagraph (B), by striking the period at the end of subparagraph (C) and inserting ", and", and by adding after subparagraph (C) the following new subparagraph:

"(D) any payment to which subparagraph (C) does not apply which is out of an account described in section 419A(c)(2) and which is not used to provide a post-retirement medical benefit or life insurance benefit."

(c) SPECIAL LIMITATIONS.—Section 419A(e) (relating to special limitations on reserves) is amended by adding at the end the following new paragraph:

"(3) BENEFITS MUST BE EXCLUDABLE.—Post-retirement medical benefits and life insurance benefits shall not be taken into account under subsection (c)(2) to the extent it may be reasonably anticipated that such benefits will be required to be included in gross income when provided."

(d) EFFECTIVE DATES.—

(1) IN GENERAL.—Except as provided in paragraph (2), the amendments made by this section shall apply to contributions paid or accrued after December 31, 1994, in taxable years ending after such date.

(2) SEPARATE ACCOUNTING.—The amendments made by subsection (b) shall apply to contributions paid or accrued after the date of the enactment of this Act, in taxable years ending after such date.

## SEC. 7402. HEALTH BENEFITS ACCOUNTS MAINTAINED BY PENSION PLANS.

(a) TERMINATION OF ACCOUNTS.—

(1) IN GENERAL.—Section 401(h) (relating to medical, etc., benefits for retired employees and their spouses and dependents) is amended by adding at the end the following new paragraph:

"(2) TERMINATION.—

"(A) IN GENERAL.—In the case of a pension or annuity plan to which paragraph (1) applies—

"(i) no contributions may be made to the separate account described in paragraph (1)(C) other than allowable contributions, and

"(ii) such plan may pay benefits described in paragraph (1) only from funds attributable to allowable contributions and earnings allocable to such contributions.

"(B) ALLOWABLE CONTRIBUTION.—For purposes of subparagraph (A), the term 'allowable contribution' means—

"(i) any contribution made before January 1, 1995,

"(ii) in the case of a plan maintained pursuant to 1 or more collective bargaining agreements between employee representatives and 1 or more employees ratified on or before October 29, 1993, any contribution under such plan made before the earlier of—

"(I) the date on which the last of such agreements terminates (determined without regard to any extension after October 29, 1993), or, if later, January 1, 1995, or

"(II) January 1, 1998, or

"(iii) any qualified transfer under section 420."

(2) CONFORMING AMENDMENTS.—Section 401(h) is amended—

(A) by striking "Under" and inserting: "(1) IN GENERAL.—Under",

(B) by redesignating paragraphs (1) through (6) as subparagraphs (A) through (F), respectively,

(C) by striking "paragraph (6)" and inserting "subparagraph (F)", and

(D) by striking "paragraph (1)" and inserting "subparagraph (A)".

(b) MINIMUM COST REQUIREMENTS OF EMPLOYER.—Paragraph (3) of section 420(c) (relating to minimum cost requirements) is amended by adding at the end the following new subparagraph:

"(E) ADJUSTMENT FOR COST SAVINGS UNDER HEALTH SECURITY ACT.—To the extent provided by the Secretary, a plan shall not be treated as failing to meet the requirements of this section to the extent such failure is attributable to a reduction in qualified current retiree health liabilities by reason of the enactment of the Health Security Act."

## Subtitle E—Coordination With COBRA Continuing Care Provisions

### SEC. 7501. COORDINATION WITH COBRA CONTINUING CARE PROVISIONS.

(a) PERIOD OF COVERAGE.—Clause (iv) of section 4980B(f)(2)(B) (defining period of coverage) is amended—

(1) by striking "or" at the end of subclause (I), by striking the period at the end of subclause (II) and inserting ", or", and by adding at the end the following new subclause:

"(III) eligible for comprehensive health coverage described in section 1101 of the Health Security Act.", and

(2) by striking "OR MEDICARE ENTITLEMENT" in the heading and inserting ", MEDICARE ENTITLEMENT, OR HEALTH SECURITY ACT ELIGIBILITY".

(b) QUALIFIED BENEFICIARY.—Section 4980B(g)(1) (defining qualified beneficiary) is amended by adding at the end the following new subparagraph:

"(E) SPECIAL RULE FOR INDIVIDUALS COVERED BY HEALTH SECURITY ACT.—The term 'qualified beneficiary' shall not include any individual who, upon termination of coverage under a group health plan, is eligible for comprehensive health coverage described in section 1101 of the Health Security Act."

(c) REPEAL UPON IMPLEMENTATION OF HEALTH SECURITY ACT.—

(1) IN GENERAL.—Section 4980B (relating to failure to satisfy continuation coverage requirements of group health care plans) is hereby repealed.

(2) CONFORMING AMENDMENTS.—

(A) Section 414(n)(3)(C) is amended by striking "505, and 4980B" and inserting "and 505".

(B) Section 414(t)(2) is amended by striking "505, or 4980B" and inserting "or 505".

(C) The table of sections for chapter 43 is amended by striking the item relating to section 4980B.

(3) EFFECTIVE DATE.—The amendments made by this subsection shall take effect on the earlier of—

(A) January 1, 1998, or

(B) the first day of the first calendar year following the calendar year in which all States have in effect plans under which individuals are eligible for comprehensive health coverage described in section 1101 of this Act.

Such amendments shall not apply in determining the amount of any tax under section 4980B of the Internal Revenue Code of 1986 with respect to any failure occurring before the date determined under the preceding sentence.

# Subtitle F—Tax Treatment of Organizations Providing Health Care Services and Related Organizations

SEC. 7601. TREATMENT OF NONPROFIT HEALTH CARE ORGANIZATIONS.

(a) TREATMENT OF HOSPITALS AND OTHER ENTITIES PROVIDING HEALTH CARE SERVICES.—Section 501 (relating to exemption from tax on corporations, certain trusts, etc.) is amended by redesignating subsection (n) as subsection (o) and by inserting after subsection (m) the following new subsection:

"(n) QUALIFICATION OF ORGANIZATIONS PROVIDING HEALTH CARE SERVICES AS CHARITABLE ORGANIZATIONS.—For purposes of subsection (c)(3), the provision of health care services shall not be treated as an activity that accomplishes a charitable purpose unless the organization providing such services, on a periodic basis (no less frequently than annually), and with the participation of community representatives—

"(1) assesses the health care needs of its community, and

"(2) develops a plan to meet those needs.

In the case of a health maintenance organization, the provision of health care services shall not be treated as an activity that accomplishes a charitable purpose for purposes of subsection (c)(3) unless, in addition to meeting the requirement of the preceding sentence, such services are provided as described in subsection (m)(3)(B)(i)."

(b) TREATMENT OF HEALTH MAINTENANCE ORGANIZATIONS.—Section 501(m) is amended by adding at the end thereof the following new paragraph:

"(6) INSURANCE PROVIDED BY HEALTH MAINTENANCE ORGANIZATIONS.—

"(A) CERTAIN INSURANCE NOT TREATED AS COMMERCIAL-TYPE INSURANCE.—Health insurance provided by a health maintenance organization shall not be treated as commercial-type insurance if such insurance relates to care provided other than pursuant to a pre-existing arrangement with such organization. In applying the preceding sentence, care described in subparagraph (B)(iv) shall not be taken into account.

"(B) CERTAIN INSURANCE TREATED AS COMMERCIAL-TYPE INSURANCE.—Health insurance provided by a health maintenance organization shall be treated as commercial-type insurance if it relates to—

"(i) care provided by such organization to its members at its own facilities through health care professionals who do not provide substantial health care services other than on behalf of such organization,

"(ii) primary care provided by a health care professional to a member of such organization on a basis under which the amount paid to such professional does not vary with the amount of care provided to such member,

"(iii) services other than primary care provided pursuant to a pre-existing arrangement with such organization, or

"(iv) emergency care provided to a member of such organization at a location outside such member's area of residence."

(c) TREATMENT OF PARENT ORGANIZATIONS OF HEALTH CARE PROVIDERS.—Section 509(a) (defining private foundation) is amended by striking "and" at the end of paragraph (3), by redesignating paragraph (4) as paragraph (5), and by inserting after paragraph (3) the following new paragraph:

"(4) an organization which is organized and operated for the benefit of, and which directly or indirectly controls, an organization described in section 170(b)(1)(A)(iii), and".

(d) EFFECTIVE DATES.—

(1) IN GENERAL.—Except as provided in paragraph (2), the amendments made by this section shall take effect on January 1, 1995.

**Health Security Act** *Title VII, Subtitle F*

1138

(2) SUBSECTIONS (b) AND (c).—The amendments made by subsections (b) and (c) shall take effect on the date of the enactment of this Act.

**SEC. 7602. TAX TREATMENT OF TAXABLE ORGANIZATIONS PROVIDING HEALTH INSURANCE AND OTHER PREPAID HEALTH CARE SERVICES.**

(a) GENERAL RULE.—Section 833 is amended to read as follows:

**"SEC. 833. TREATMENT OF ORGANIZATIONS PROVIDING HEALTH INSURANCE AND OTHER PREPAID HEALTH CARE SERVICES.**

"(a) GENERAL RULE.—Any organization to which this section applies shall be taxable under this part in the same manner as if it were an insurance company other than a life insurance company.

"(b) ORGANIZATIONS TO WHICH SECTION APPLIES.—This section shall apply to any organization—

　　"(1) which is not exempt from taxation under this subtitle, and

　　"(2) the primary and predominant business activity of which during the taxable year consists of 1 or more of the following:

　　　　"(A) Issuing accident and health insurance contracts or the reinsuring of risks undertaken by other insurance companies under such contracts.

"(B) Operating as a health maintenance organization.

"(C) Entering into arrangements under which—

"(i) fixed payments or premiums are received as consideration for the organization's agreement to provide or arrange for the provision of health care services, regardless of how the health care services are provided or arranged to be provided, and

"(ii) such fixed payments or premiums do not vary depending on the amount of health care services provided."

(b) CONFORMING AMENDMENTS.—

(1) Subsection (c) of section 56 is amended by striking paragraph (3).

(2) The table of sections for part II of subchapter L of chapter 1 is amended by striking the item relating to section 833 and inserting the following:

"Sec. 833. Treatment of organizations providing health insurance and other prepaid health care services."

(c) EFFECTIVE DATES.—

(1) IN GENERAL.—Except as otherwise provided in this subsection, the amendments made by this section shall apply to taxable years beginning after December 31, 1996.

(2) TRANSITION RULES FOR BLUE CROSS AND BLUE SHIELD ORGANIZATIONS.—

(A) PRIOR FRESH START PRESERVED.—The adjusted basis of any asset determined under section 1012(c)(3)(A)(ii) of the Tax Reform Act of 1986 shall not be affected by the amendments made by this section nor by reason of any failure to qualify in taxable years beginning after December 31, 1996, as an existing Blue Cross or Blue Shield organization (as defined in section 833(c)(2) of the Internal Revenue Code of 1986, as in effect on the day before the date of the enactment of this Act).

(B) RECOUPMENT OF PRIOR RESERVE BENEFIT.—In the case of any organization entitled to the benefits of section 833(a)(3) of the Internal Revenue Code of 1986 (as in effect on the day before the date of the enactment of this Act) for such organization's last taxable year beginning before January 1, 1997, the amount determined under paragraph (4) of section

832(b) of such Code for each of such organization's first 6 taxable years beginning after December 31, 1996, shall be increased by an amount equal to 3 ⅓ percent of its unearned premiums on outstanding business as of the close of such organization's last taxable year beginning before January 1, 1997.

(C) PHASE-OUT OF SPECIAL DEDUCTION FOR CERTAIN ORGANIZATIONS.—

(i) IN GENERAL.—In the case of an organization which meets the requirements of clause (ii)—

(I) such organization shall continue to be entitled to the deduction provided under section 833(b) of the Internal Revenue Code of 1986 (as in effect on the day before the date of the enactment of this Act) for its first 2 taxable years beginning after December 31, 1996, except that

(II) the amount of such deduction for such organization's taxable year beginning in 1997 shall be 67 percent of the amount which would have been determined under such section 833(b) as so in effect, and the amount of such deduction for organization's taxable year beginning in 1998 shall be 33 percent of the amount which would have been so determined.

Notwithstanding the amendment made by subsection (b)(1), any deduction under the preceding sentence shall not be allowable in computing alternative minimum taxable income.

(ii) REQUIREMENTS.—An organization meets the requirements of this clause if, for each of its taxable years beginning in 1995 and 1996, such organization—

(I) was an organization to which section 833 of such Code (as so in effect) applied, and

(II) met the requirements of subparagraph (A) of section 833(c)(3) of such Code (as so in effect).

(3) TRANSITIONAL RULES FOR OTHER COMPANIES.—

(A) ORGANIZATIONS TO WHICH PARAGRAPH APPLIES.—This paragraph shall apply to any organization to which section 833 of the Internal Revenue Code of 1986 (as amended by subsection (a)) applies for such organization's first taxable year beginning after December 31, 1996; except that this paragraph shall not apply if such organization treated itself as an insurance company taxable under part II of subchapter L of chapter 1 of such Code on its original Federal income tax return for its taxable year beginning in 1992 and for all of its taxable years thereafter beginning before January 1, 1997.

(B) TREATMENT OF CURRENTLY TAXABLE COMPANIES.—Except as provided in subparagraph (C), in the case of any organization to which this paragraph applies—

(i) the amendments made by this section shall be treated as a change in the method of accounting, and

(ii) all adjustments required to be taken into account under section 481 of the Internal Revenue Code of 1986, shall be taken into account for such company's first taxable year beginning after December 31, 1996.

(C) TREATMENT OF CURRENTLY TAX EXEMPT COMPANIES.—In the case of any organization to which this paragraph applies and which was exempt from tax under chapter 1 of the Internal Revenue Code of 1986 for such organization's last taxable year beginning before January 1, 1997—

(i) no adjustment shall be made under section 481 (or any other provision) of such Code on account of a change in its method of accounting required by this section for its first taxable year beginning after December 31, 1996, and

(ii) for purposes of determining gain or loss, the adjusted basis of any asset held by such organization on the first day of such taxable year shall be treated as equal to its fair market value as of such day.

## SEC. 7603. EXEMPTION FROM INCOME TAX FOR REGIONAL ALLIANCES.

(a) IN GENERAL.—Subsection (c) of section 501 (relating to exemption from tax on corporations, certain trusts, etc.) is amended by adding at the end thereof the following new paragraph:

"(26) Any regional alliance described in section 1301 of the Health Security Act. Such an alliance shall be treated as not described in any other paragraph of this subsection."

(b) EFFECTIVE DATE.—The amendment made by subsection (a) shall apply to taxable years beginning after the date of the enactment of this Act.

# Subtitle G—Tax Treatment of Long-term Care Insurance and Services

### SEC. 7701. QUALIFIED LONG-TERM CARE SERVICES TREATED AS MEDICAL CARE.

(a) GENERAL RULE.—Paragraph (1) of section 213(d) (defining medical care) is amended by striking "or" at the end of subparagraph (B), by redesignating subparagraph (C) as subparagraph (D), and by inserting after subparagraph (B) the following new subparagraph:

"(C) for qualified long-term care services (as defined in subsection (g)), or".

(b) QUALIFIED LONG-TERM CARE SERVICES DEFINED.—Section 213 (relating to the deduction for medical, dental, etc., expenses) is amended by adding at the end thereof the following new subsection:

"(g) QUALIFIED LONG-TERM CARE SERVICES.—For purposes of this section—

"(1) IN GENERAL.—The term 'qualified long-term care services' means necessary diagnostic, curing, mitigating, treating, preventive, therapeutic, and rehabilitative services, and maintenance and personal care services (whether performed in a residential or nonresidential setting) which—

"(A) are required by an individual during any period the individual is an incapacitated individual (as defined in paragraph (2)),

"(B) have as their primary purpose—

"(i) the provision of needed assistance with 1 or more activities of daily living (as defined in paragraph (3)), or

"(ii) protection from threats to health and safety due to severe cognitive impairment, and

"(C) are provided pursuant to a continuing plan of care prescribed by a licensed professional (as defined in paragraph (4)).

"(2) INCAPACITATED INDIVIDUAL.—The term 'incapacitated individual' means any individual who—

"(A) is unable to perform, without substantial assistance from another individual (including assistance involving cueing or substantial supervision), at least 2 activities of daily living as defined in paragraph (3), or

"(B) has severe cognitive impairment as defined by the Secretary in consultation with the Secretary of Health and Human Services.

Such term shall not include any individual otherwise meeting the requirements of the preceding sentence unless a licensed professional within the preceding 12-month period has certified that such individual meets such requirements.

"(3) ACTIVITIES OF DAILY LIVING.—Each of the following is an activity of daily living:

"(A) Eating.

"(B) Toileting.

"(C) Transferring.

"(D) Bathing.

"(E) Dressing.

"(4) LICENSED PROFESSIONAL.—The term 'licensed professional' means—

"(A) a physician or registered professional nurse, or

"(B) any other individual who meets such requirements as may be prescribed by the Secretary after consultation with the Secretary of Health and Human Services.

"(5) CERTAIN SERVICES NOT INCLUDED.—The term 'qualified long-term care services' shall not include any services provided to an individual—

"(A) by a relative (directly or through a partnership, corporation, or other entity) unless the relative is a licensed professional with respect to such services, or

"(B) by a corporation or partnership which is related (within the meaning of section 267(b) or 707(b)) to the individual.

For purposes of this paragraph, the term 'relative' means an individual bearing a relationship to the individual which is described in paragraphs (1) through (8) of section 152(a)."

(c) TECHNICAL AMENDMENTS.—

(1) Subparagraph (D) of section 213(d)(1) (as redesignated by subsection (a)) is amended to read as follows:

"(D) for insurance (including amounts paid as premiums under part B of title XVIII of the Social Security Act, relating to supplementary medical insurance for the aged) covering medical care referred to in—

"(i) subparagraphs (A) and (B), or

"(ii) subparagraph (C), but only if such insurance is provided under a qualified long-term care insurance policy (as defined in section 7702B(b)) and the amount paid for such insurance is not disallowed under section 7702B(d)(4)."

(2) Paragraph (6) of section 213(d) is amended—

(A) by striking "subparagraphs (A) and (B)" and inserting "subparagraph (A), (B), and (C)", and

(B) by striking "paragraph (1)(C)" in subparagraph (A) and inserting "paragraph (1)(D)".

(d) EFFECTIVE DATE.—The amendments made by this section shall apply to taxable years beginning after December 31, 1995.

SEC. 7702. TREATMENT OF LONG-TERM CARE INSURANCE.

(a) GENERAL RULE.—Chapter 79 (relating to definitions) is amended by inserting after section 7702A the following new section:

"SEC. 7702B. TREATMENT OF LONG-TERM CARE INSURANCE.

"(a) IN GENERAL.—For purposes of this title—

"(1) a qualified long-term care insurance policy (as defined in subsection (b)) shall be treated as an accident and health insurance contract,

"(2) amounts (other than policyholder dividends (as defined in section 808) or premium refunds) received under a qualified long-term care insurance policy shall be treated as amounts received for personal injuries and sickness and shall be treated as reimbursement for expenses actually incurred for medical care (as defined in section 213(d)),

"(3) any plan of an employer providing coverage under a qualified long-term care insurance policy shall be treated as an accident and health plan with respect to such coverage,

"(4) amounts paid for a qualified long-term care insurance policy providing the benefits described in subsection (b)(6)(B) shall be treated as payments made for insurance for purposes of section 213(d)(1)(D), and

"(5) a qualified long-term care insurance policy shall be treated as a guaranteed renewable contract subject to the rules of section 816(e).

"(b) QUALIFIED LONG-TERM CARE INSURANCE POLICY.—For purposes of this title—

"(1) IN GENERAL.—The term 'qualified long-term care insurance policy' means any long-term care insurance policy (as defined in section 2304 of the Health Security Act) that—

"(A) satisfies the requirements of subpart B of part 3 of subtitle B of title II of the Health Security Act,

"(B) limits benefits under such policy to individuals who are certified by a licensed professional (as defined in section 213(g)(4)) within the preceding 12-month period as being unable to perform, without substantial assistance from another individual (including assistance involving cueing or substantial supervision), 2 or more activities of daily living (as defined in section 213(g)(3)), or who have a severe cognitive impairment (as defined in section 213(g)(2)(B)), and

"(C) satisfies the requirements of paragraphs (2), (3), (4), (5), and (6).

"(2) PREMIUM REQUIREMENTS.—The requirements of this paragraph are met with respect to a policy if such policy provides that premium payments may not be made earlier than the date such payments would have been made if the contract provided for level annual payments over the life expectancy of the insured or 20 years, whichever is shorter. A policy shall not be treated as failing to meet the requirements of the preceding sentence solely by reason of a provision in the policy providing for a waiver of premiums if the insured becomes an individual certified in accordance with paragraph (1)(B).

"(3) PROHIBITION OF CASH VALUE.—The requirements of this paragraph are met if the policy does not provide for a cash value or other money that can be paid, assigned, pledged as collateral for a loan, or borrowed, other than as provided in paragraph (4).

"(4) REFUNDS OF PREMIUMS AND DIVIDENDS.—The requirements of this paragraph are met with respect to a policy if such policy provides that—

"(A) policyholder dividends are required to be applied as a reduction in future premiums or, to the extent permitted under paragraph (6), to increase benefits described in subsection (a)(2), and

"(B) refunds of premiums upon a partial surrender or a partial cancellation are required to be applied as a reduction in future premiums, and

"(C) any refund on the death of the insured, or on a complete surrender or cancellation of the policy, cannot exceed the aggregate premiums paid under the contract.

Any refund on a complete surrender or cancellation of the policy shall be includible in gross income to the extent that any deduction or exclusion was allowable with respect to the premiums.

"(5) COORDINATION WITH OTHER ENTITLEMENTS.—The requirements of this paragraph are met with respect to a policy if such policy does not cover expenses incurred to the extent that such expenses are also covered under title XVIII of the Social Security Act or are covered under comprehensive health coverage described in section 1101 of the Health Security Act.

"(6) MAXIMUM BENEFIT.—

"(A) IN GENERAL.—The requirements of this paragraph are met if the benefits payable under the policy for any period (whether on a periodic basis or otherwise) shall not exceed the dollar amount in effect for such period.

"(B) NONREIMBURSEMENT PAYMENTS PERMITTED.—Benefits shall include all payments described in subsection (a)(2) to or on behalf of an insured individual without regard to the expenses incurred during the period to which the payments relate. For purposes of section 213(a), such payments shall be treated as compensation for expenses paid for medical care.

"(C) DOLLAR AMOUNT.—The dollar amount in effect under this paragraph shall be $150 per day (or the equivalent amount within the calendar year in the case of payments on other than a per diem basis).

"(D) ADJUSTMENTS FOR INCREASED COSTS.—

"(i) IN GENERAL.—In the case of any calendar year after 1996, the dollar amount in effect under subparagraph (C) for any period or portion thereof occurring during such calendar year shall be equal to the sum of—

"(I) the amount in effect under subparagraph (C) for the preceding calendar year (after application of this subparagraph), plus

"(II) the product of the amount referred to in subclause (I) multiplied by the cost-of-living adjustment for the calendar year of the amount under subclause (I).

"(ii) COST-OF-LIVING ADJUSTMENT.—For purposes of clause (i), the cost-of-living adjustment for any calendar year is the percentage (if any) by which the cost index under clause (iii) for the preceding calendar year exceeds such index for the second preceding calendar year.

"(iii) COST INDEX.—The Secretary, in consultation with the Secretary of Health and Human Services, shall before January 1, 1997, establish a cost index to measure increases in costs of nursing home and similar facilities. The Secretary may from time to time revise such index to the extent necessary to accurately measure increases or decreases in such costs.

"(iv) SPECIAL RULE FOR CALENDAR YEAR 1997.—Notwithstanding clause (ii), for purposes of clause (i), the cost-of-living adjustment for calendar year 1997 is the sum of 1 ½ percent plus the percentage by which the CPI for calendar year 1996 (as defined in section 1(f)(4)) exceeds the CPI for calendar year 1995 (as so defined).

"(E) PERIOD.—For purposes of this paragraph, a period begins on the date that an individual has a condition which would qualify for certification under subsection (b)(1)(B) and ends on the earlier of the date upon which—

"(i) such individual has not been so certified within the preceding 12-months, or

"(ii) the individual's condition ceases to be such as to qualify for certification under subsection (b)(1)(B).

"(F) AGGREGATION RULE.—For purposes of this paragraph, all policies issued with respect to the same insured shall be treated as one policy.

"(c) TREATMENT OF LONG-TERM CARE INSURANCE POLICIES.—For purposes of this title, any amount received or coverage provided under a long-term care insurance policy that is not a qualified long-term care insurance policy shall not be treated as an amount received for personal injuries or sickness or provided under an accident and health plan and shall not be treated as excludible from gross income under any provision of this title.

"(d) TREATMENT OF COVERAGE PROVIDED AS PART OF A LIFE INSURANCE CONTRACT.—Except as otherwise provided in regulations prescribed by the Secretary, in the case of any long-term care insurance coverage (whether or not qualified) provided by rider on a life insurance contract—

"(1) IN GENERAL.—This section shall apply as if the portion of the contract providing such coverage is a separate contract or policy.

"(2) PREMIUMS AND CHARGES FOR LONG-TERM CARE COVERAGE.—Premium payments for coverage under a long-term care insurance policy and charges against the life insurance contract's cash surrender value (within the meaning of section 7702(f)(2)(A)) for such coverage shall be treated as premiums for purposes of subsection (b)(2).

"(3) APPLICATION OF 7702.—Section 7702(c)(2) (relating to the guideline premium limitation) shall be applied by increasing the guideline premium limitation with respect to a life insurance contract, as of any date—

"(A) by the sum of any charges (but not premium payments) described in paragraph (2) made to that date under the contract, less

"(B) any such charges the imposition of which reduces the premiums paid for the contract (within the meaning of section 7702(f)(1)).

"(4) APPLICATION OF SECTION 213.—No deduction shall be allowed under section 213(a) for charges against the life insurance contract's cash surrender value described in paragraph (2), unless such charges are includible in income as a result of the application of section 72(e)(10) and the coverage provided by the rider is a qualified long-term care insurance policy under subsection (b).

For purposes of this subsection, the term 'portion' means only the terms and benefits under a life insurance contract that are in addition to the terms and benefits under the contract without regard to the coverage under a long-term care insurance policy.

"(e) PROHIBITION OF DISCRIMINATION.—

"(1) IN GENERAL.—Notwithstanding subsection (a)(3), any plan of an employer providing coverage under a qualified long-term care insurance policy shall qualify as an accident and health plan with respect to such coverage only if—

"(A) the plan allows all employees, except as provided in paragraph (2), to participate, and

"(B) the benefits provided under the plan are identical for all employees that choose to participate.

"(2) EXCLUSION OF CERTAIN EMPLOYEES.—For purposes of paragraph (1), there may be excluded from consideration—

"(A) employees who have not completed 3 years of service;

"(B) employees who have not attained age 25;

"(C) part-time or seasonal employees; and

"(D) employees who are nonresident aliens and who receive no earned income (within the meaning of section 911(d)(2)) from the employer which constitutes income from sources within the United States (within the meaning of section 861(a)(3)).

"(f) REGULATIONS.—The Secretary shall prescribe such regulations as may be necessary to carry out the requirements of this section, including regulations to prevent the avoidance of this section by providing long-term care insurance coverage under a life insurance contract and to provide for the proper allocation of amounts between the long-term care and life insurance portions of a contract.".

(b) CLERICAL AMENDMENT.—The table of sections for chapter 79 is amended by inserting after the item relating to section 7702A the following new item:

"Sec. 7702B. Treatment of long-term care insurance.".

(c) EFFECTIVE DATE.—

(1) IN GENERAL.—The amendments made by this section shall apply to policies issued after December 31, 1995. Solely for purposes of the preceding sentence, a policy issued prior to January 1, 1996, that satisfies the requirements of a qualified long-term care insurance policy as set forth in section 7702B(b) shall, on and after January 1, 1996, be treated as being issued after December 31, 1995.

(2) TRANSITION RULE.—If, after the date of enactment of this Act and before January 1, 1996, a policy providing for long-term care insurance coverage is exchanged solely for a qualified long-term care insurance policy (as defined in section 7702B(b)), no gain or loss shall be recognized on the exchange. If, in addition to a qualified long-term care insurance policy, money or other property is received in the exchange, then any gain shall be rec-

ognized to the extent of the sum of the money and the fair market value of the other property received. For purposes of this paragraph, the cancellation of a policy providing for long-term care insurance coverage and reinvestment of the cancellation proceeds in a qualified long-term care insurance policy within 60 days thereafter shall be treated as an exchange.

"(3) ISSUANCE OF CERTAIN RIDERS PERMITTED.—For purposes of determining whether section 7702 or 7702A of the Internal Revenue Code of 1986 applies to any contract, the issuance, whether before, on, or after December 31, 1995, of a rider on a life insurance contract providing long-term care insurance coverage shall not be treated as a modification or material change of such contract.

## SEC. 7703. TAX TREATMENT OF ACCELERATED DEATH BENEFITS UNDER LIFE INSURANCE CONTRACTS.

(a) GENERAL RULE.—Section 101 (relating to certain death benefits) is amended by adding at the end thereof the following new subsection:

"(g) TREATMENT OF CERTAIN ACCELERATED DEATH BENEFITS.—

"(1) IN GENERAL.—For purposes of this section, any amount distributed to an individual under a life insurance contract on the life of an insured who is a terminally ill individual (as defined in paragraph (3)) shall be treated as an amount paid by reason of the death of such insured.

"(2) NECESSARY CONDITIONS.—

"(A) Paragraph (1) shall not apply to any distribution unless—

"(i) the distribution is not less than the present value (determined under subparagraph (B)) of the reduction in the death benefit otherwise payable in the event of the death of the insured, and

"(ii) the percentage derived from dividing the cash surrender value of the contract, if any, immediately after the distribution by the cash surrender value of the contract immediately before the distribution is equal to or greater than the percentage derived by dividing the death benefit immediately after the distribution by the death benefit immediately before the distribution.

"(B) The present value of the reduction in the death benefit occurring on the distribution must be determined by—

"(i) using as the discount rate a rate not to exceed the highest rate set forth in subparagraph (C), and

"(ii) assuming that the death benefit (or the portion thereof) would have been paid at the end of a period that is no more than the insured's life expectancy from the date of the distribution or 12 months, whichever is shorter.

"(C) RATES.—The rates set forth in this subparagraph are the following:

"(i) the 90-day Treasury bill yield,

"(ii) the rate described as Moody's Corporate Bond Yield Average-Monthly Average Corporates as published by Moody's Investors Service, Inc., or any successor thereto for the calendar month ending 2 months before the date on which the rate is determined,

"(iii) the rate used to compute the cash surrender values under the contract during the applicable period plus 1 percent per annum, and "(iv) the maximum permissible interest rate applicable to policy loans under the contract.

"(3) TERMINALLY ILL INDIVIDUAL.—For purposes of this subsection, the term 'terminally ill individual' means an individual who the insurer has determined, after receipt of an acceptable certification by a licensed physician, has an illness or physical condition which can reasonably be expected to result in death within 12 months of the date of certification.

"(4) APPLICATION OF SECTION 72(e)(10).—For purposes of section 72(e)(10) (relating to the treatment of modified endowment contracts), section 72(e)(4)(A)(i) shall not apply to distributions described in paragraph (1).

(b) EFFECTIVE DATE.—The amendment made by subsection (a) shall apply to taxable years beginning after December 31, 1993.

## SEC. 7704. TAX TREATMENT OF COMPANIES ISSUING QUALIFIED ACCELERATED DEATH BENEFIT RIDERS.

(a) QUALIFIED ACCELERATED DEATH BENEFIT RIDERS TREATED AS LIFE INSURANCE.—Section 818 (relating to other definitions and special rules) is amended by adding at the end thereof the following new subsection:

"(g) QUALIFIED ACCELERATED DEATH BENEFIT RIDERS TREATED AS LIFE INSURANCE.—For purposes of this part—

"(1) IN GENERAL.—Any reference to a life insurance contract shall be treated as including a reference to a qualified accelerated death benefit rider on such contract.

"(2) QUALIFIED ACCELERATED DEATH BENEFIT RIDERS.—For purposes of this subsection, the term 'qualified accelerated death benefit rider' means any rider on a life insurance contract which provides for a distribution to an individual upon the insured becoming a terminally ill individual (as defined in section 101(g)(3)).

(b) DEFINITIONS OF LIFE INSURANCE AND MODIFIED ENDOWMENT CONTRACTS.—Paragraph (5)(A) of section 7702(f) is amended by striking "or" at the end of clause (iv), by redesignating clause (v) as clause (vi), and by inserting after clause (iv) the following new clause:

"(v) any qualified accelerated death benefit rider (as defined in section 818(g)), or".

(c) EFFECTIVE DATE.—

1    (1) IN GENERAL.—The amendments made by
2 this section shall apply to contracts issued after December 31, 1993.

4    (2) TRANSITIONAL RULE.—For purposes of determining whether section 7702 or 7702A of the Internal Revenue Code of 1986 applies to any contract, the issuance, whether before, on, or after December 31, 1993, of a rider on a life insurance contract permitting the acceleration of death benefits (as described in section 101(g) of such Code) shall not be treated as a modification or material change of such contract.

# Subtitle H—Tax Incentives for Health Services Providers

## SEC. 7801. NONREFUNDABLE CREDIT FOR CERTAIN PRIMARY HEALTH SERVICES PROVIDERS.

(a) IN GENERAL.—Subpart A of part IV of subchapter A of chapter 1 (relating to nonrefundable personal credits) is amended by inserting after section 22 the following new section:

## "SEC. 23. PRIMARY HEALTH SERVICES PROVIDERS.

"(a) ALLOWANCE OF CREDIT.—There shall be allowed as a credit against the tax imposed by this chapter for the taxable year an amount equal to the product of—

"(1) the number of months during such taxable year—

"(A) during which the taxpayer is a qualified primary health services provider, and

"(B) which are within the taxpayer's mandatory service period, and

"(2) $1,000 ($500 in the case of a qualified practitioner who is not a physician).

"(b) QUALIFIED PRIMARY HEALTH SERVICES PROVIDER.—For purposes of this section, the term 'qualified primary health services provider' means, with respect to any month, any qualified practitioner who—

"(1) has in effect a certification by the Bureau as a provider of primary health services and such certification is, when issued, for a health professional shortage area in which the qualified practitioner is commencing the providing of primary health services,

"(2) is providing primary health services full time in the health professional shortage area identified in such certification, and

"(3) has not received a scholarship under the National Health Service Corps Scholarship Program or any loan repayments under the National Health Service Corps Loan Repayment Program.

For purposes of paragraph (2), a provider shall be treated as providing services in a health professional shortage area when such area ceases to be such an area if it was such an area when the provider commenced providing services in the area.

"(c) MANDATORY SERVICE PERIOD.—For purposes of this section, the term 'mandatory service period' means the period of 60 consecutive calendar months beginning with the first month the taxpayer is a qualified primary health services provider. A taxpayer shall not have more than 1 mandatory service period.

"(d) DEFINITIONS AND SPECIAL RULES.—For purposes of this section—

"(1) BUREAU.—The term 'Bureau' means the Bureau of Primary Health Care, Health Resources and Services Administration of the United States Public Health Service.

"(2) QUALIFIED PRACTITIONER.—The term 'qualified practitioner' means a physician, a physician assistant, a nurse practitioner, or a certified nurse-midwife.

"(3) PHYSICIAN.—The term 'physician' has the meaning given to such term by section 1861(r) of the Social Security Act.

"(4) PHYSICIAN ASSISTANT; NURSE PRACTITIONER.—The terms 'physician assistant' and 'nurse practitioner' have the meanings given to such terms by section 1861(aa)(5) of the Social Security Act.

"(5) CERTIFIED NURSE-MIDWIFE.—The term 'certified nurse-midwife' has the meaning given to such term by section 1861(gg)(2) of the Social Security Act.

"(6) PRIMARY HEALTH SERVICES.—The term 'primary health services' has the meaning given such term by section 330(b)(1) of the Public Health Service Act.

"(7) HEALTH PROFESSIONAL SHORTAGE AREA.—The term 'health professional shortage area' has the meaning given such term by section 332(a)(1)(A) of the Public Health Service Act.

"(e) RECAPTURE OF CREDIT.—

"(1) IN GENERAL.—If there is a recapture event during any taxable year, then—

"(A) no credit shall be allowed under subsection (a) for such taxable year and any succeeding taxable year, and

"(B) the tax of the taxpayer under this chapter for such taxable year shall be increased by an amount equal to the product of—

"(i) the applicable percentage, and

"(ii) the aggregate unrecaptured credits allowed to such taxpayer under this section for all prior taxable years.

"(2) APPLICABLE RECAPTURE PERCENTAGE.—

"(A) IN GENERAL.—For purposes of this subsection, the applicable recapture percentage shall be determined from the following table:

| If the recapture event occurs during: | The applicable recapture percentage is: |
|---|---|
| Months 1–24 | 100 |
| Months 25–36 | 75 |
| Months 37–48 | 50 |
| Months 49–60 | 25 |
| Months 61 and thereafter | 0. |

"(B) TIMING.—For purposes of subparagraph (A), month 1 shall begin on the first day of the mandatory service period.

"(3) RECAPTURE EVENT DEFINED.—

"(A) IN GENERAL.—For purposes of this subsection, the term 'recapture event' means the failure of the taxpayer to be a qualified primary health services provider for any month during the taxpayer's mandatory service period.

"(B) CESSATION OF DESIGNATION.—The cessation of the designation of any area as a health professional shortage area after the beginning of the mandatory service period for any taxpayer shall not constitute a recapture event.

"(C) SECRETARIAL WAIVER.—The Secretary, in consultation with the Secretary of Health and Human Services, may waive any recapture event caused by extraordinary circumstances.

"(4) NO CREDITS AGAINST TAX; MINIMUM TAX.—Any increase in tax under this subsection shall not be treated as a tax imposed by this chapter for purposes of determining the amount of any credit under subpart A, B, or D of this part or for purposes of section 55."

(b) CLERICAL AMENDMENT.—The table of sections for subpart A of part IV of subchapter A of chapter 1 is amended by inserting after the item relating to section 22 the following new item:

"Sec. 23. Primary health services providers."

(c) EFFECTIVE DATE.—The amendments made by this section shall apply to taxable years beginning after December 31, 1994.

**SEC. 7802. EXPENSING OF MEDICAL EQUIPMENT.**

(a) IN GENERAL.—Paragraph (1) of section 179(b) (relating to dollar limitation on expensing of certain depreciable business assets) is amended to read as follows:

"(1) DOLLAR LIMITATION.—

"(A) GENERAL RULE.—The aggregate cost which may be taken into account under subsection (a) for any taxable year shall not exceed $17,500.

"(B) HEALTH CARE PROPERTY.—The aggregate cost which may be taken into account under subsection (a) shall be increased by the lesser of—

"(i) the cost of section 179 property which is health care property placed in service during the taxable year, or

"(ii) $10,000."

(b) DEFINITION.—Section 179(d) (relating to definitions) is amended by adding at the end the following new paragraph:

"(11) HEALTH CARE PROPERTY.—For purposes of this section, the term 'health care property' means section 179 property—

"(A) which is medical equipment used in the screening, monitoring, observation, diagnosis, or treatment of patients in a laboratory, medical, or hospital environment,

"(B) which is owned (directly or indirectly) and used by a physician (as defined in section 1861(r) of the Social Security Act) in the active conduct of such physician's full-time trade or business of providing primary health services (as defined in section 330(b)(1) of the Public Health Service Act) in a health professional shortage area (as defined in section 332(a)(1)(A) of the Public Health Service Act), and

"(C) substantially all the use of which is in such area."

(c) EFFECTIVE DATE.—The amendments made by this section shall apply to property placed in service after December 31, 1994.

## Subtitle I—Miscellaneous Provisions

### SEC. 7901. CREDIT FOR COST OF PERSONAL ASSISTANCE SERVICES REQUIRED BY EMPLOYED INDIVIDUALS.

(a) IN GENERAL.—Subpart A of part IV of subchapter A of chapter 1 (relating to nonrefundable personal credits) is amended by inserting after section 23 the following new section:

"SEC. 24. COST OF PERSONAL ASSISTANCE SERVICES REQUIRED BY EMPLOYED INDIVIDUALS.

"(a) ALLOWANCE OF CREDIT.—

"(1) IN GENERAL.—In the case of an eligible individual, there shall be allowed as a credit against the tax imposed by this chapter for the taxable year an amount equal to the applicable percentage of the personal assistance expenses paid or incurred by the taxpayer during such taxable year.

"(2) APPLICABLE PERCENTAGE.—For purposes of paragraph (1), the term 'applicable percentage' means 50 percent reduced (but not below zero) by 10 percentage points for each $5,000 by which the modified adjusted gross income (as defined in section 59B(d)(2)) of the taxpayer for the taxable year exceeds $45,000. In the case of a married individual filing a separate return, the preceding sentence shall be applied by substituting '$2,500' for '$5,000' and '$22,500' for '$45,000'.

"(b) LIMITATION.—The amount of personal assistance expenses incurred for the benefit of an individual which may be taken into account under subsection (a) for the taxable year shall not exceed the lesser of—

"(1) $15,000, or

"(2) such individual's earned income (as defined in section 32(c)(2)) for the taxable year.

In the case of a joint return, the amount under the preceding sentence shall be determined separately for each spouse.

"(c) ELIGIBLE INDIVIDUAL.—For purposes of this section, the term 'eligible individual' means any individual (other than a nonresident alien) who, by reason of any medically determinable physical impairment which can be expected to result in death or which has lasted or can be expected to last for a continuous period of not less than 12 months, is unable to engage in any substantial gainful activity without personal assistance services appropriate to carry out activities of daily living. An individual shall not be treated as an eligible individual unless such individual furnishes such proof thereof (in such form and manner, and at such times) as the Secretary may require.

"(d) OTHER DEFINITIONS.—For purposes of this section—

"(1) PERSONAL ASSISTANCE EXPENSES.—The term 'personal assistance expenses' means expenses for—

"(A) personal assistance services appropriate to carry out activities of daily living in or outside the home,

"(B) homemaker/chore services incidental to the provision of such personal assistance services,

"(C) in the case of an individual with a cognitive impairment, assistance with life skills,

"(D) communication services,

"(E) work-related support services,

"(F) coordination of services described in this paragraph,

"(G) assistive technology and devises, including assessment of the need for particular technology and devices and training of family members, and

"(H) modifications to the principal place of abode of the individual to the extent the expenses for such modifications would (but for subsection (e)(2)) be expenses for medical care (as defined by section 213) of such individual.

"(2) ACTIVITIES OF DAILY LIVING.—The term 'activities of daily living' means the activities referred to in section 213(g)(3).

"(e) SPECIAL RULES.—

"(1) PAYMENTS TO RELATED PERSONS.—No credit shall be allowed under this section for any amount paid by the taxpayer to any person who is related (within the meaning of section 267 or 707(b)) to the taxpayer.

"(2) COORDINATION WITH MEDICAL EXPENSE DEDUCTION.—Any amount taken into account in determining the credit under this section shall not be taken into account in determining the amount of the deduction under section 213.

"(3) BASIS REDUCTION.—For purposes of this subtitle, if a credit is allowed under this section for any expense with respect to any property, the increase in the basis of such property which would (but for this paragraph) result from such expense shall be reduced by the amount of the credit so allowed.

"(f) COST-OF-LIVING ADJUSTMENT.—In the case of any taxable year beginning after 1996, the $45,000 and $22,500 amounts in subsection (a)(2) and the $15,000 amount in subsection (b) shall be increased by an amount equal to—

"(1) such dollar amount, multiplied by

"(2) the cost-of-living adjustment determined under section 1(f)(3) for the calendar year in which the taxable year begins by substituting 'calendar year 1995' for 'calendar year 1992' in subparagraph (B) thereof.

If any increase determined under the preceding sentence is not a multiple of $1,000, such increase shall be rounded to the nearest multiple of $1,000."

(b) TECHNICAL AMENDMENT.—Subsection (a) of section 1016 is amended by striking "and" at the end of paragraph (24), by striking the period at the end of paragraph (25) and inserting ", and", and by adding at the end thereof the following new paragraph:

"(26) in the case of any property with respect to which a credit has been allowed under section 23, to the extent provided in section 23(e)(3)."

(c) CLERICAL AMENDMENT.—The table of sections for subpart A of part IV of subchapter A of chapter 1 is amended by inserting after the item relating to section 22 the following new item:

"Sec. 23. Cost of personal assistance services required by employed individuals."

(d) EFFECTIVE DATE.—The amendments made by this section shall apply to taxable years beginning after December 31, 1995.

## SEC. 7902. DENIAL OF TAX-EXEMPT STATUS FOR BORROWINGS OF HEALTH CARE-RELATED ENTITIES.

(a) IN GENERAL.—Paragraph (6) of section 141(b) (relating to private business use) is amended by adding at the end thereof the following new subparagraph:

"(C) CERTAIN HEALTH CARE-RELATED ENTITIES.—Use by—

"(i) any regional alliance described in section 1301 of the Heath Security Act,

"(ii) any corporate alliance described in section 1311 of such Act, and "(iii) any guaranty fund described in section 1204 of such Act,

shall be treated as private business use by an organization that is not a 501(c)(3) organization."

(b) EFFECTIVE DATE.—The amendment made by subsection (a) shall apply to obligations issued after the date of the enactment of this Act.

## SEC. 7903. DISCLOSURE OF RETURN INFORMATION FOR ADMINISTRATION OF CERTAIN PROGRAMS UNDER THE HEALTH SECURITY ACT.

(a) IN GENERAL.—Subparagraph (D) of section 6103(l)(7) (relating to disclosure of return information to Federal, State, and local agencies administering certain programs) is amended by striking "and" at the end of clause (viii), by striking the period at the end of clause (ix) and inserting "; and", and by inserting after clause (ix) the following new clause:

"(x) assistance provided under the Health Security Act."

(b) INFORMATION NOT AVAILABLE TO LOCAL AGENCIES.—Subparagraph (D) of section 6103(l)(7) is amended by adding at the end thereof the following new sentence: "Subparagraphs (A) and (B) shall be applied with-

**Health Security Act**  *Title VII, Subtitle I*

1 out regard to any reference to any local agency with re-
2 spect to the program referred to in clause (x).''

# TITLE VIII—HEALTH AND HEALTH-RELATED PROGRAMS OF THE FEDERAL GOVERNMENT

TABLE OF CONTENTS OF TITLE

### Subtitle A—Military Health Care Reform

Sec. 8001. Uniformed services health plans.

### Subtitle B—Department of Veterans Affairs

Sec. 8101. Benefits and eligibility through Department of Veterans Affairs Medical System.
Sec. 8102. Organization of Department of Veterans Affairs facilities as health plans.

### Subtitle C—Federal Employees Health Benefits Program

Sec. 8201. Definitions.
Sec. 8202. FEHBP termination.
Sec. 8203. Treatment of Federal employees, annuitants, and other individuals (who would otherwise have been eligible for fehbp) under health plans.
Sec. 8204. Treatment of individuals residing abroad.
Sec. 8205. Transition and savings provisions.
Sec. 8206. Regulations.
Sec. 8207. Technical and conforming amendments.

### Subtitle D—Indian Health Service

Sec. 8301. Definitions.
Sec. 8302. Eligibility and health service coverage of Indians.
Sec. 8303. Supplemental Indian health care benefits.
Sec. 8304. Health plan and health alliance requirements.
Sec. 8305. Exemption of tribal governments and tribal organizations from employer payments.
Sec. 8306. Provision of health services to non-enrollees and non-Indians.
Sec. 8307. Payment by other payors.
Sec. 8308. Contracting authority.
Sec. 8309. Consultation.
Sec. 8310. Infrastructure.
Sec. 8311. Financing.
Sec. 8312. Rule of construction.
Sec. 8313. Authorizations regarding Public Health Service Initiatives fund.

### Subtitle E—Amendments to the Employee Retirement Income Security Act of 1974

Sec. 8401. Group health plan defined.

Sec. 8402. Limitation on coverage of group health plans under title I of ERISA.
Sec. 8403. Amendments relating to continuation coverage.
Sec. 8404. Additional amendments relating to group health plans.
Sec. 8405. Plan claims procedures.
Sec. 8406. Effective dates.

**Subtitle F—Special Fund for WIC Program**

Sec. 8501. Additional funding for special supplemental food program for women, infants, and children (WIC).

# Subtitle A—Military Health Care Reform

**SEC. 8001. UNIFORMED SERVICES HEALTH PLANS.**

(a) ESTABLISHMENT OF PLANS.—(1) Chapter 55 of title 10, United States Code, is amended by inserting after section 1073 the following new section:

**"§ 1073a. Uniformed Services Health Plans: establishment and coordination with national health care reform**

"(a) ESTABLISHMENT AUTHORIZED.—(1) The Secretary of Defense, in consultation with the other administering Secretaries, may establish one or more Uniformed Services Health Plans pursuant to this section in order to provide health care services to members of the uniformed services on active duty for a period of more than 30 days and persons described in subsection (e)(2).

"(2) The establishment and operation of a Uniformed Services Health Plan shall be carried out in accordance with regulations prescribed by the Secretary of Defense, in consultation with the other administering Secretaries.

The Secretary shall assure that such regulations conform, to the maximum extent practicable, to the requirements for health plans set forth in the Health Security Act.

"(b) USE OF UNIFORMED SERVICES FACILITIES AND OTHER HEALTH CARE PROVIDERS.—(1) A Uniformed Services Health Plan may rely upon the use of facilities of the uniformed services for the provision of health care services to persons enrolled in the plan, supplemented by the use of civilian health care providers or health plans under agreements entered into by the Secretary of Defense.

"(2) An agreement with a civilian health care provider or a health plan under paragraph (1) may be entered into without regard to provisions of law requiring the use of competitive procedures. An agreement with a health plan may provide for the sharing of resources with the health plan that is a party to the agreement.

"(c) HEALTH CARE SERVICES UNDER A PLAN.—(1) Subject to paragraph (2), a Uniformed Services Health Plan shall provide to persons enrolled in the plan the items and services in the comprehensive benefit package under the Health Security Act.

"(2)(A) In addition, a Uniformed Services Health Plan shall guarantee to each person described in subparagraph (B) who is enrolled in the plan those health care services that the person would be entitled to receive under this chapter in the absence of this section. In the case of a person described in subparagraph (B) who is a covered beneficiary, such health care services shall consist of the types of health care services described in section 1079(a) of this title.

"(B) A person referred to in subparagraph (A) is a member of the uniformed services on active duty for a period of more than 30 days as of December 31, 1994, or any person who is a covered beneficiary as of that date, who is (or afterwards becomes) enrolled in a Uniformed Services Health Plan.

"(d) PREEMPTION OF CONFLICTING STATE REQUIREMENTS.—In carrying out responsibilities under the Health Security Act, a State (or State-established entity)—

> "(1) may not impose any standard or requirement on a Uniformed Services Health Plan that is inconsistent with this section or any regulation prescribed under this section or other Federal law regarding the operation of this section; and
>
> "(2) may not deny certification of a Uniformed Services Health Plan as a health plan under the Health Security Act on the basis of a conflict between a rule of a State or health alliance and this

section or any regulation prescribed under this section or other Federal law regarding the operation of this section.

"(e) ENROLLMENT.—(1) Except as authorized by the administering Secretary concerned, each member of a uniformed service on active duty for a period of more than 30 days shall be required to enroll in a Uniformed Services Health Plan available to the member.

"(2) After enrolling members described in paragraph (1), opportunities for further enrollment in a Uniformed Services Health Plan shall be offered by the administering Secretaries to covered beneficiaries in the following order of priority:

"(A) Spouses and children of members of the uniformed services who are on active duty for a period of more than 30 days.

"(B) Persons described in subsection (c) of section 1086 of this title. The administering Secretary concerned may disregard the exclusion set forth in subsection (d)(1) of such section in the case of a person described in subsection (c) of such section who is enrolled in the supplementary medical insurance program under part B of title XVIII of the Social Security Act (42 U.S.C. 1395j et seq.).

"(3) With respect to a member described in paragraph (1) or a covered beneficiary described in paragraph (2) who enrolls in a Uniformed Services Health Plan, participation in such a plan shall be the exclusive source of health care services available to the member or person under this chapter.

"(f) EFFECT OF FAILURE TO ENROLL.—(1) Except as provided in paragraph (2), if a person described in subsection (e)(2) declines the opportunity offered by the administering Secretaries to enroll in a Uniformed Services Health Plan, the person shall not be entitled or eligible for health care services in facilities of the uniformed services or pursuant to a contract entered into under this chapter. However, nothing in this paragraph shall be construed to effect the right of a person to a premium payment by the Secretary of Defense if the person is enrolled in another health plan under the Health Security Act and is otherwise entitled to such a payment under subsection (h).

"(2) A person described in subsection (e)(2) who is enrolled with a health plan that is not a Uniformed Services Health Plan may receive the items and services in the comprehensive benefit package in a facility of the uniformed services only if—

"(A) the Secretary of Defense authorizes the provision of a particular item or service in the package to the person;

"(B) the Secretary determines that the provision of the item or service involved will not interfere with the provision of health care services to members of the uniformed services or persons enrolled in a Uniformed Services Health Plan; and

"(C) the health plan in which the person is enrolled agrees to pay the actual and full cost of the items and services in the package actually provided to the person.

"(3) The administering Secretaries shall assure that all rights and entitlements under this chapter of any person described in subsection (e)(2) are fully preserved if the person—

"(A) is not offered the opportunity to enroll in a Uniformed Services Health Plan; and

"(B) is not otherwise enrolled in a health plan provided through a health alliance under the Health Security Act.

"(g) SPECIAL RULE FOR OTHER PAYERS.—(1)(A) In the case of a person who is enrolled in the supplementary medical insurance program under part B of title XVIII of the Social Security Act (42 U.S.C. 1395j et seq.) and who is also enrolled in a Uniformed Services Health Plan, Medicare shall be responsible for making a premium payment on behalf of the person. The Secretary of Defense and the Secretary of Health and Human Services shall enter into an agreement specifying the payment responsibilities of Medicare under this paragraph, except that the amount of the premium payment may not exceed the expected per capita costs that Medicare would bear for the person if the person remained in the Medicare program. A premium payment by Medicare under this paragraph shall be the person's exclusive benefit under Medicare.

"(B) In this paragraph, the term 'Medicare' means any plan administered under title XVIII of the Social Security Act (42 U.S.C. 1395c et seq.).

"(2) Nothing in this section shall affect the payment of the retiree discount under the Health Security Act on behalf of a person who is enrolled in a Uniformed Services Health Plan if the person is otherwise eligible for the retiree discount.

"(h) PAYMENT RESPONSIBILITIES OF THE SECRETARY.—(1) In the case of a person described in subsection (e)(2) who is not enrolled in a Uniformed Services Health Plan, the Secretary may make a premium payment for the person's enrollment through a health alliance in another health plan. In determining the amount of the payment, the Secretary shall consider the amount of any retiree discount payable under the Health Security Act on behalf of the person and the amount of any premium credits attributable to employer payments with respect to employment of the person.

"(2) The Secretary shall not make a payment pursuant to this subsection in connection with any person enrolled in a health plan of the Department of Veterans Affairs or a health program of the Indian Health Service.

"(i) PAYMENT RESPONSIBILITIES OF PERSONS ENROLLED IN A UNIFORMED SERVICES HEALTH PLAN.—(1) In the case of an active duty member who is enrolled in a Uniformed Services Health Plan, the administering Secretaries may not impose or collect from the member a cost-share charge of any kind (whether a premium, copayment, deductible, coinsurance charge, or other charge) other than subsistence charges authorized under section 1075 of this title.

"(2) Subject to paragraph (3), persons described in subsection (e)(2) who are enrolled in a Uniformed Services Health Plan shall be required to pay a family share under section 1342 of a premium and cost sharing. Payment obligations established under this paragraph may not exceed those obligations otherwise required under the national standards for health plans established pursuant to the Health Security Act.

"(3)(A) Persons described in subsection (e)(2) who enroll in a Uniformed Services Health Plan and who (in the absence of this section) would be covered beneficiaries under section 1079 or 1086 of this title continuously since December 31, 1994, shall have, as a group, out-of-pocket costs in 1995 no greater than the lesser of—

"(i) the out-of-pocket costs in effect for such beneficiaries under section 1075, 1078, 1079(b), or 1086(b) of this title (whichever applies) on December 31, 1994; and

"(ii) those obligations otherwise required under the national standards for health plans established pursuant to the Health Security Act.

"(B) Members of the uniformed services on active duty as of December 31, 1994, who afterward become covered beneficiaries under section 1079 or 1086 of this title (or would become covered beneficiaries in the absence of this section) without a break in eligibility for health care services under this chapter shall have, as a group, out-of-pocket costs as covered beneficiaries no higher than the out-of-pocket costs in effect for similarly situated covered beneficiaries described in subparagraph (A).

"(C) The limitation on out-of-pocket costs established pursuant to subparagraph (A) may be adjusted for years after 1995 by an appropriate economic index, as determined by the Secretary of Defense.

"(4) The Secretary of Defense shall establish the payment requirements under paragraph (2), and enforce the limitations on such requirements specified in paragraph (3), in regulations prescribed pursuant to subsection (a).

"(j) FINANCIAL ACCOUNT.—There is hereby established in the Department of Defense a financial account to which shall be credited all premium payments and other receipts from other payers and beneficiaries made in connection with any person enrolled in a Uniformed Services Health Plan. The account shall be administered by the Secretary of Defense, and funds in the account may be used by the Secretary for any purpose directly related to the delivery and financing of health care services under this chapter, including operations, maintenance, personnel, procurement, contributions toward construction projects, and related costs. Funds in the account shall remain available until expended.".

(2) The table of sections at the beginning of such chapter is amended by inserting after the item relating to section 1073 the following new item:

"1073a. Uniformed Services Health Plans: establishment and coordination with national health care reform.".

(b) DEFINITION.—Section 1072 of such title is amended by adding at the end the following new paragraph:

"(6) The term 'Uniformed Services Health Plan' means a plan established by the Secretary of Defense under section 1073a(a) of this title in order to provide health care services to members of the uniformed services on active duty and other covered beneficiaries under this chapter.".

(c) REPORT ON ESTABLISHMENT.—If the Secretary of Defense determines to establish any Uniformed Services Health Plan under section 1073a of title 10, United States Code, as added by subsection (a), the Secretary shall submit to Congress a report describing the Plans proposed to be initially offered under such section. The report required by this subsection shall be submitted not later than 30 days before the date on which the Secretary first issues proposed rules under subsection (a) of such section to establish any such Plan.

# Subtitle B—Department of Veterans Affairs

## SEC. 8101. BENEFITS AND ELIGIBILITY THROUGH DEPARTMENT OF VETERANS AFFAIRS MEDICAL SYSTEM.

(a) DVA AS A PARTICIPANT IN HEALTH CARE REFORM.—

(1) IN GENERAL.—Title 38, United States Code, is amended by inserting after chapter 17 the following new chapter:

**"CHAPTER 18—ELIGIBILITY AND BENEFITS UNDER HEALTH SECURITY ACT**

"SUBCHAPTER I—GENERAL

"1801. Definitions.

"SUBCHAPTER II—ENROLLMENT

"1811. Enrollment: veterans.
"1812. Enrollment: CHAMPVA eligibles.
"1813. Enrollment: family members.

"SUBCHAPTER III—BENEFITS

"1821. Benefits for VA enrollees.
"1822. Chapter 17 benefits described.
"1823. Entitlement to chapter 17 benefits for certain veterans.
"1824. Supplemental benefits packages and policies.
"1825. Limitation regarding veterans enrolled with health plans outside Department.

"SUBCHAPTER IV—FINANCIAL MATTERS

"1831. Premiums, copayments, etc..
"1832. Medicare coverage and reimbursement.
"1833. Recovery of cost of certain care and services.
"1834. Health Plan Funds.

## "SUBCHAPTER I—GENERAL

### "§ 1801. Definitions

"For purposes of this chapter:

"(1) The term 'health plan' means an entity that has been certified under the Health Security Act as a health plan.

"(2) The term 'VA health plan' means a health plan that is operated by the Secretary under section 7341 of this title.

"(3) The term 'VA enrollee' means an individual enrolled under the Health Security Act in a VA health plan.

## "SUBCHAPTER II—ENROLLMENT

### "§ 1811. Enrollment: veterans

"Each veteran who is an eligible individual within the meaning of section 1001 of the Health Security Act may enroll with a VA health plan. A veteran who wants to receive the comprehensive benefit package through the Department shall enroll with a VA health plan.

### "§ 1812. Enrollment: CHAMPVA eligibles

"An individual who is eligible for benefits under section 1713 of this title and who is eligible to enroll in a health plan pursuant to section 1001 of the Health Security Act may enroll under that Act with a VA health plan in the same manner as a veteran.

### "§ 1813. Enrollment: family members

"(a) The Secretary may authorize a VA health plan to enroll members of the family of an enrollee under section 1811 or 1812 of this title, subject to payment of premiums, deductibles, copayments, and coinsurance as required under the Health Security Act.

"(b) For purposes of subsection (a), an enrollee's family is those individuals (other than the enrollee) included within the term 'family' as defined in section 1011(b) of the Health Security Act.

"SUBCHAPTER III—BENEFITS

### "§ 1821. Benefits for VA enrollees

"The Secretary shall ensure that each VA health plan provides to each individual enrolled with it the items and services in the comprehensive benefit package under the Health Security Act.

### "§ 1822. Chapter 17 benefits described

"The Secretary shall provide to each veteran described in section 1823(a) of this title the care and services that are authorized to be provided under chapter 17 of this title in accordance with the terms and conditions applicable to that care under such chapter, notwithstanding that such care and services are not included in the comprehensive benefit package.

## "§ 1823. Entitlement to chapter 17 benefits for certain veterans

"(a) The following veterans are eligible for additional care and services as described in section 1822 of this title:

"(1) Any veteran with a service-connected disability.

"(2) Any veteran whose discharge or release from the active military, naval or air service was for a disability incurred or aggravated in the line of duty.

"(3) Any veteran who is in receipt of, or who, but for a suspension pursuant to section 1151 of this title (or both such a suspension and the receipt of retired pay), would be entitled to disability compensation, but only to the extent that such a veteran's continuing eligibility for such care is provided for in the judgment or settlement provided for in such section.

"(4) Any veteran who is a former prisoner of war.

"(5) Any veteran of the Mexican border period or World War I.

"(6) Any veteran who is unable to defray the expenses of necessary care as determined under section 1722(a) of this title.

"(b) In the case of a veteran who is eligible to receive care or services under section 1710(a)(1)(G) of this title for a disability which may be associated with exposure to a toxic substance, radiation, or environmental hazard, the Secretary shall furnish such care or services to that veteran.

"(c) A veteran covered by subsection (a) or (b)—

　"(1) is eligible for care and services described in that subsection whether or not such veteran is a VA enrollee; and

　"(2) shall not be subject to any charge or any other cost for such care and services.

**"§ 1824. Supplemental benefits packages and policies**

"(a)(1) In order to meet the special needs of veterans, the Secretary may offer to veterans supplemental health benefits packages for health care services not included in the comprehensive benefit package. A veteran eligible under section 1823 of this title to receive the health care services described in section 1822 of this title may not be offered a supplemental health benefits package under this subsection. The supplemental health benefits packages offered under this subsection may consist of any or all of the benefits that the Secretary may provide under chapter 17 of this title that are not included in the comprehensive benefit package.

"(2) The Secretary shall charge a premium for a supplemental health benefits package under this subsection. The amount of such premium shall be established so as to cover the actual and full costs of such care.

"(b) A VA health plan may offer supplemental health benefits policies for health care services not provided under chapter 17 of this title and cost sharing policies consistent with the requirements of part 2 of subtitle E of title I of the Health Security Act.

"**§ 1825. Limitation regarding veterans enrolled with health plans outside Department**

"A veteran who is residing in a regional alliance area in which the Department operates a health plan and who is enrolled in a health plan that is not operated by the Department may be provided the items and services in the comprehensive benefit package by a VA health plan only if the plan is reimbursed for the actual and full cost of the care provided.

"SUBCHAPTER IV—FINANCIAL MATTERS

"**§ 1831. Premiums, copayments, etc.**

"(a) In the case of a veteran described in section 1823(a) of this title who is a VA enrollee, the Secretary may not impose or collect from the veteran a cost-share charge of any kind (whether a premium, copayment, deductible, coinsurance charge, or other charge). The Secretary shall make such arrangements as necessary with health alliances in order to carry out this subsection.

"(b) For other VA enrollees, the Secretary shall charge premiums and establish copayments, deductibles, and coinsurance amounts. The premium rate, and the rates for deductibles and copayments, for each VA health plan shall be established by that health plan based on rules established by the health alliance under which it is operating.

**"§ 1832. Medicare coverage and reimbursement**

"(a) For purposes of any program administered by the Secretary of Health and Human Services under title XVIII of the Social Security Act, a VA health plan or Department facility shall be deemed to be a Medicare provider.

"(b)(1) The Secretary of Health and Human Services shall enter into an agreement with a VA health plan or Department health-care facility to treat such plan or facility as a Medicare HMO in any case in which that health plan or facility seeks to enter into such an agreement.

"(2) For purposes of this section, the term 'Medicare HMO' means an eligible organization under section 1876 of the Social Security Act.

"(c) In the case of care provided to a veteran other than a veteran described in section 1823(a) of this title who is eligible for benefits under the Medicare program under title XVIII of the Social Security Act, the Secretary of Health and Human Services shall reimburse a VA health plan or Department health-care facility providing services as a Medicare provider or Medicare HMO on the same basis as that Secretary reimburses other Medicare providers or Medicare HMOs, respectively. The Secretary of Health and Human Services shall include with each such reimbursement a Medicare explanation of benefits.

"(d) When the Secretary provides care to a veteran for which the Secretary receives reimbursement under this section, the Secretary shall require the veteran to pay to the Department any applicable deductible or copayment that is not covered by Medicare.

"**§ 1833. Recovery of cost of certain care and services**

"(a) In the case of an individual provided care or services through a VA health plan who has coverage under a supplemental health insurance policy pursuant to part 2 of subtitle E of title I of the Health Security Act or under any other provision of law, or who has coverage under a Medicare supplemental health insurance plan (as defined in the Health Security Act) or under any other provision of law, the Secretary has the right to recover or collect charges for care or services (as determined by the Secretary, but not including care or services for a service-connected disability) from the party providing that coverage to the extent that the individual (or the provider of the care or services) would be eligible to receive payment for such care or services from such party if the care or services had not been furnished by a department or agency of the United States.

"(b) The provisions of subsections (b) through (f) of section 1729 of this title shall apply with respect to claims by the United States under subsection (a) in the same manner as they apply to claims under subsection (a) of that section.

## "§ 1834. Health Plan Funds

"(a) The Secretary shall establish for each VA health plan a separate revolving fund.

"(b) Any amount received by the Department by reason of the furnishing of health care by a VA health plan or the enrollment of an individual with a VA health plan (including amounts received as premiums, premium discount payments, copayments or coinsurance, and deductibles, amounts received as third-party reimbursements, and amounts received as reimbursements from another health plan for care furnished to one of its enrollees) shall be credited to the revolving fund of that health plan.

"(c) Notwithstanding subsection (b), a VA health plan may not retain amounts received for care furnished to a VA enrollee in a case in which the costs of such care have been covered by appropriations. Such amounts shall be deposited in the General Fund of the Treasury.

"(d) Each revolving fund for a health plan shall be managed by that health plan.

"(e) Amounts in a revolving fund for a health plan are hereby made available for the expenses of the delivery of the items and services in the comprehensive benefit package by the health plan.".

(2) The table of chapters at the beginning of part II of title 38, United States Code, is amended by inserting after the item relating to chapter 17 the following new item:

"18. Benefits and Eligibility Under Health Security Act ............... 1801.".

(b) PRESERVATION OF EXISTING BENEFITS FOR FACILITIES NOT OPERATING AS HEALTH PLANS.—(1) Chapter 17 of title 38, United States Code, is amended by inserting after section 1704 the following new section:

**"§ 1705. Facilities not operating within health plans; veterans not eligible to enroll in health plans**

"The provisions of this chapter shall apply with respect to the furnishing of care and services—

"(1) by any facility of the Department that is not operating as or within a health plan certified as a health plan under the Health Security Act; and

"(2) to any veteran who is an eligible individual with the meaning of section 1001 of the Health Security Act.".

(2) The table of sections at the beginning of such chapter is amended by inserting after the item relating to section 1704 the following new item:

"1705. Facilities not operating within health plans; veterans not eligible to enroll in health plans.".

## SEC. 8102. ORGANIZATION OF DEPARTMENT OF VETERANS AFFAIRS FACILITIES AS HEALTH PLANS.

(a) IN GENERAL.—Chapter 73 of title 38, United States Code, is amended—

    (1) by redesignating subchapter IV as subchapter V; and

    (2) by inserting after subchapter III the following new subchapter:

"SUBCHAPTER IV—PARTICIPATION AS PART OF NATIONAL HEALTH CARE REFORM

"**§ 7341. Organization of health care facilities as health plans**

"(a) The Secretary shall organize health plans and operate Department facilities as or within health plans under the Health Security Act. The Secretary shall prescribe regulations establishing standards for the operation of Department health care facilities as or within health plans under that Act. In prescribing those standards, the

Secretary shall assure that they conform, to the maximum extent practicable, to the requirements for health plans generally set forth in part 1 of subtitle E of title I of the Health Security Act.

"(b) Within a geographic area or region, health care facilities of the Department located within that area or region may be organized to operate as a single health plan encompassing all Department facilities within that area or region or may be organized to operate as several health plans.

"(c) In carrying out responsibilities under the Health Security Act, a State (or a State-established entity)—

"(1) may not impose any standard or requirement on a VA health plan that is inconsistent with this section or any regulation prescribed under this section or other Federal laws regarding the operation of this section; and

"(2) may not deny certification of a VA health plan under the Health Security Act on the basis of a conflict between a rule of a State or health alliance and this section or regulations prescribed under this section or other Federal laws regarding the operation of this section.

**"§ 7342. Contract authority for facilities operating as or within health plans**

"The Secretary may enter into a contract (without regard to provisions of law requiring the use of competitive procedures) for the provision of services by a VA health plan in any case in which the Secretary determines that such contracting is more cost-effective than providing such services directly through Department facilities or when such contracting is necessary because of geographic inaccessibility.

**"§ 7343. Resource sharing authority: facilities operating as or within health plans**

"The Secretary may enter into agreements under section 8153 of this title with other health care plans, with health care providers, and with other health industry organizations, and with individuals, for the sharing of resources of the Department through facilities of the Department operating as or within health plans.

**"§ 7344. Administrative and personnel flexibility**

"(a) In order to carry out this subchapter, the Secretary may—

"(1) carry out administrative reorganizations of the Department without regard to those provisions of section 510 of this title following subsection (a) of that section; and

"(2) enter into contracts for the performance of services previously performed by employees of the Department without regard to section 8110(c) of this title.

"(b) The Secretary may establish alternative personnel systems or procedures for personnel at facilities operating as or with health plans under the Health Security Act whenever the Secretary considers such action necessary in order to carry out the terms of that Act.

"(c) Subject to the provisions of section 1404 of the Health Security Act, the Secretary may carry out appropriate promotional, advertising, and marketing activities to inform individuals of the availability of facilities of the Department operating as or within health plans. Such activities may only be carried out using nonappropriated funds.

"**§ 7345. Funding provisions: grants and other sources of assistance**

"The Secretary may apply for and accept, if awarded, any grant or other source of funding that is intended to meet the needs of special populations and that but for this section is unavailable to facilities of the Department or to health plans operated by the Government if funds obtained through the grant or other source of funding will be used through a facility of the Department operating as or within a health plan.".

(b) CLERICAL AMENDMENT.—The table of sections at the beginning of chapter 73 is amended by striking out the item relating to the heading for subchapter IV and inserting in lieu thereof the following:

> "SUBCHAPTER IV—PARTICIPATION AS PART OF NATIONAL HEALTH CARE REFORM
>
> "7341. Organization of health care facilities as health plans.
> "7342. Contract authority for facilities operating as or within health plans.
> "7343. Resource sharing authority: facilities operating as or within health plans.
> "7344. Administrative and personnel flexibility.
> "7345. Funding provisions: grants and other sources of assistance.
>
> "SUBCHAPTER V—RESEARCH CORPORATIONS".

# Subtitle C—Federal Employees Health Benefits Program

SEC. 8201. DEFINITIONS.

Except as otherwise specifically provided, in this subtitle:

(1) ABROAD.—The term "abroad" means outside the United States.

(2) ANNUITANT, ETC.—The terms "annuitant", "employee", and "Government", have the same respective meanings as are given such terms by section 8901 of title 5, United States Code.

(3) EMPLOYEES HEALTH BENEFITS FUND.—The term "Employees Health Benefits Fund" means

the fund under section 8909 of title 5, United States Code.

(4) FEHBP.—The term "FEHBP" means the health insurance program under chapter 89 of title 5, United States Code.

(5) FEHBP PLAN.—The term "FEHBP plan" has the same meaning as is given the term "health benefits plan" by section 8901(6) of title 5, United States Code.

(6) FEHBP TERMINATION DATE.—The term "FEHBP termination date" means the date (specified in section 8202) after which FEHBP ceases to be in effect.

(7) RETIRED EMPLOYEES HEALTH BENEFITS FUND.—The term "Retired Employees Health Benefits Fund" means the fund under section 8 of the Retired Federal Employees Health Benefits Act (Public Law 86-724; 74 Stat. 851).

(8) RFEHBP.—The term "RFEHBP" means the health insurance program under the Retired Federal Employees Health Benefits Act.

**SEC. 8202. FEHBP TERMINATION.**

Chapter 89 of title 5, United States Code, is repealed effective as of December 31, 1997, and all contracts under such chapter shall terminate not later than such date.

## SEC. 8203. TREATMENT OF FEDERAL EMPLOYEES, ANNUITANTS, AND OTHER INDIVIDUALS (WHO WOULD OTHERWISE HAVE BEEN ELIGIBLE FOR FEHBP) UNDER HEALTH PLANS.

(a) APPLICABILITY.—This section sets forth rules applicable, after the FEHBP termination date, with respect to individuals who—

(1) are eligible individuals under section 1001; and

(2) but for this subtitle, would be eligible to enroll in a FEHBP plan.

(b) FEDERAL EMPLOYEES.—

(1) SAME TREATMENT AS NON–FEDERAL EMPLOYEES.—A Federal employee shall be treated in the same way, for purposes of provisions of this Act outside of this subtitle, as if that individual were a non-Federal employee, including for purposes of any requirements relating to enrollment, individual or family premium payments, and employer premium payments.

(2) EMPLOYER PREMIUM PAYMENTS.—Any employer premium payment required with respect to the employment of a Federal employee shall be payable from the appropriation or fund from which any Government contribution on behalf of such employee would have been payable under FEHBP.

(3) OPTIONAL OFFER OF FEHBP SUPPLEMENTAL PLANS.—The Federal Government may, but is not required to—

(A) offer to Federal employees one or more FEHBP supplemental plans developed under subsection (f)(1); and

(B) make a Government contribution with respect to the premium for such a plan.

Any Government contribution under subparagraph (B) shall be payable from the same appropriation or fund as would a Government contribution under paragraph (2) on behalf of the Federal employee involved.

(4) DEFINITIONS.—In this subsection:

(A) FEDERAL EMPLOYEE.—The term "Federal employee" means an "employee" as defined by section 8201.

(B) NON-FEDERAL EMPLOYEE.—The term "non–Federal employee" means an "employee" as defined by section 1901.

(c) ANNUITANTS.—

(1) HEALTH PLAN.—

(A) AUTHORITY TO MAKE CERTAIN WITHHOLDINGS FROM ANNUITIES.—The Office of Personnel Management may, on the request of an annuitant enrolled in a health plan, withhold from the annuity of such annuitant any premiums required for such enrollment. The Office shall forward any amounts so withheld to the appropriate fund or as otherwise indicated in the request. A request under this subparagraph shall contain such information, and otherwise be made in such form and manner, as the Office shall by regulation prescribe.

(B) PAYMENT OF ALLIANCE CREDIT LIABILITY FOR ANNUITANTS BELOW AGE 55.—In the case of an annuitant who does not satisfy the eligibility requirements under section 6115, a Government contribution shall be made equal to such amount as is necessary to reduce the employee's liability under section 6111 to zero.

(2) FEHBP SUPPLEMENTAL PLAN.—

(A) CURRENT ANNUITANTS.—

(i) IN GENERAL.—Each current annuitant—

(I) shall be eligible to enroll in FEHBP supplemental plans developed under subsection (f)(1); and

(II) shall be eligible for the Government contribution amount described in clause (ii) toward the premium for such a plan.

(ii) GOVERNMENT CONTRIBUTION AMOUNT.—The Office of Personnel Management shall specify a level of Government contribution under this paragraph for a FEHBP supplemental plan. Such level—

(I) shall reasonably reflect the portion of the Government contributions (last provided under FEHBP) attributable to the portion of FEHBP benefits which the plan is designed to replace; and

(II) shall be applied toward premiums for such a plan.

(B) FUTURE ANNUITANTS.—In the case of a future annuitant, the Federal Government may, but is not required—

(i) to offer to such an annuitant one or more FEHBP supplemental plans developed under subsection (f)(1); and

(ii) to make a Government contribution with respect to the premium for such a plan.

(C) DEFINITIONS.—In this paragraph:

(i) CURRENT ANNUITANT.—The term "current annuitant" means an individual who is residing in a State on January 1, 1998, and, on the day before such date, was—

(I) enrolled in a FEHBP plan as an annuitant; or

(II) covered under a FEHBP plan as a family member (but only if such individual would otherwise have been eligible to enroll in a FEHBP plan as an annuitant).

(ii) FUTURE ANNUITANT.—The term "future annuitant" means an annuitant who is not a current annuitant.

(d) INDIVIDUALS WHO WOULD NOT BE ELIGIBLE FOR A GOVERNMENT CONTRIBUTION UNDER FEHBP.—

(1) IN GENERAL.—In the case of an individual described in paragraph (2)—

(A) the Federal Government may, but is not required to, offer one or more FEHBP supplemental plans developed under subsection (f)(1); and

(B) no Government contribution shall be payable with respect to the premium for such a plan.

(2) APPLICABILITY.—This subsection shall apply with respect to any individual who (but for this subtitle) would be eligible to enroll in a FEHBP plan, but would not be eligible for a Government contribution toward any such plan.

(e) MEDICARE-ELIGIBLE INDIVIDUALS.—

(1) CURRENT MEDICARE-ELIGIBLE INDIVIDUALS.—

(A) IN GENERAL.—Each current medicare-eligible individual—

(i) shall be eligible to enroll in medicare supplemental plans developed under subsection (f)(2); and

(ii) if such individual would (but for this subtitle) have been eligible for a Government contribution under FEHBP (assuming such individual were then enrolled thereunder), shall be eligible for the Government medicare contribution amount described in subparagraph (B) toward the premium for such a plan or toward the premium of a medicare select plan (as defined in paragraph (3)).

(B) MEDICARE CONTRIBUTION AMOUNT.—The Office of Personnel Management shall specify a level of Government contribution under this paragraph for a FEHBP medicare supplemental plan. Such level—

(i) shall reasonably reflect the portion of the Government contributions (last provided under FEHBP) attributable to the portion of FEHBP benefits which the plan is designed to replace; and

(ii) except as otherwise provided in paragraph (3), shall be applied toward premiums for such a plan.

(2) FUTURE MEDICARE-ELIGIBLE INDIVIDUALS.—In the case of a future medicare-eligible individual, the Federal Government may, but is not required to—

(A) offer to such a medicare-eligible individual one or more FEHBP medicare supplemental plans developed under subsection (f)(2); and

(B) make a Government contribution with respect to the premium for such a plan.

(3) APPLICATION OF CONTRIBUTION TOWARD MEDICARE HMO OPTION.—

(A) ELECTION.—A medicare-eligible individual may elect to have the amount of the Government contribution described in paragraph (1)(B) or referred to in paragraph (2)(B) applied toward premiums for enrollment with an eligible organization under a risk-sharing contract under section 1876 of the Social Security Act.

(B) LEVEL CONTRIBUTION RULE.—The level of such Government contribution on behalf of an individual shall be determined without taking into account any election under subparagraph (A).

(4) DEFINITIONS.—In this subsection:

(A) CURRENT MEDICARE-ELIGIBLE INDIVIDUAL.—The term "current medicare-eligible individual" means an individual who is residing in a State on January 1, 1998, and, on the day before such date, was a medicare-eligible individual.

(B) FUTURE MEDICARE-ELIGIBLE INDIVIDUAL.—The term "future medicare-eligible individual" means a medicare-eligible individual who is not a current medicare-eligible individual.

(5) INAPPLICABILITY.—Subsections (b) through (d) shall not apply with respect to a medicare-eligible individual.

(f) DEVELOPMENT OF SUPPLEMENTAL PLANS.—

(1) FEHBP SUPPLEMENTAL PLANS.—The Office of Personnel Management shall develop one or more FEHBP supplemental plans which are supplemental health benefit policies or cost sharing policies (as defined in section 1421(b)). Each such plan shall—

>(A) be consistent with the applicable requirements of part 2 of subtitle E of title I (including the requirements under section 1423(f)); and

>(B) reflect (taking into consideration the benefits in the comprehensive benefit package) the overall level of benefits generally afforded under FEHBP (as last in effect).

(2) FEHBP MEDICARE SUPPLEMENTAL PLANS.—The Office of Personnel Management shall develop one or more medicare supplemental plans. Each such plan shall—

    (A) offer benefits which shall include the core group of basic benefits identified under section 1882(p)(2) of the Social Security Act; and

    (B) reflect (taking into consideration the benefits provided under the medicare program) the overall level of benefits generally afforded under FEHBP (as last in effect).

 (g) AUTHORIZATION OF APPROPRIATIONS.—The Government contributions authorized by this section on behalf of an annuitant (including an annuitant who is a medicare-eligible individual) shall be paid from annual appropriations which are authorized to be made for that purpose and which may be made available until expended.

 (h) FUND.—

  (1) ESTABLISHMENT.—There shall be established in the Treasury of the United States a fund into which shall be paid all contributions relating to any—

    (A) FEHBP supplemental plan developed under subsection (f)(1);

    (B) FEHBP medicare supplemental plan developed under subsection (f)(2); or

    (C) health insurance program established under section 8204.

(2) ADMINISTRATION AND USE.—The fund shall be administered by the Office of Personnel Management, and any monies in the fund shall be available for purposes of the plan or program (referred to in paragraph (1)) to which they are attributable.

## SEC. 8204. TREATMENT OF INDIVIDUALS RESIDING ABROAD.

(a) IN GENERAL.—After the FEHBP termination date, individuals residing abroad who (but for this subtitle) would be eligible to enroll in a FEHBP plan shall be eligible for health insurance under a program which the Office of Personnel Management shall by regulation establish.

(b) REQUIREMENT.—To the extent practicable, coverage and benefits provided to individuals under such program shall be equal to the coverage and benefits which would be available to them if they were residing in the United States.

(c) GOVERNMENT CONTRIBUTIONS.—Any Government contribution payable under such program shall be made from the appropriation or fund from which any Government contribution would have been payable under FEHBP (if any) on behalf of the individual involved, except that, in the case of an annuitant, any such contribution shall be payable from amounts appropriated pursuant to section 8203(g).

**SEC. 8205. TRANSITION AND SAVINGS PROVISIONS.**

(a) EMPLOYEES HEALTH BENEFITS FUND.—

(1) TEMPORARY CONTINUED AVAILABILITY.—Notwithstanding section 8202, the Employees Health Benefits Fund shall be maintained, and amounts in such Fund shall remain available, after the FEHBP termination date, for such period of time as the Office of Personnel Management considers necessary in order to satisfy any outstanding claims.

(2) FINAL DISBURSEMENT.—After the end of the period referred to in paragraph (1), any amounts remaining in the Fund shall be disbursed (between the Government and former participants in FEHBP) in accordance with a plan which the Office shall prepare, consistent with the cost-sharing ratio between the Government and plan enrollees during the final contract term. The details of any such plan shall be submitted to the President and the Congress at least 1 year before the date of its proposed implementation.

(b) PROCEEDINGS.—After the FEHBP termination date, chapter 89 of title 5, United States Code (as last in effect) shall be considered to have remained in effect for purposes of any suit, action, or other proceeding with respect to any liability incurred or violation which occurred on or before such date.

(c) RFEHBA.—

(1) REPEAL.—The Retired Federal Employees Health Benefits Act (Public Law 86-724; 74 Stat. 849) is repealed effective as of the FEHBP termination date.

(2) RELATED PROVISIONS.—After the FEHBP termination date—

(A) the Retired Employees Health Benefits Fund shall temporarily remain available, and amounts in that fund shall subsequently be disbursed, in a manner comparable to that provided for under subsection (a); and

(B) retired employees who, but for this subtitle, would be eligible for coverage under the Retired Federal Employees Health Benefits Act shall be treated, for purposes of this subtitle, as if they were annuitants (subject to any differences in the overall level of coverage or benefits generally afforded them under FEHBP and RFEHBP, respectively, as last in effect).

(3) REGULATIONS.—Regulations prescribed under section 8206 to carry out this subsection shall include any necessary provisions relating to individuals residing abroad.

**SEC. 8206. REGULATIONS.**

The Office of Personnel Management shall prescribe any regulations which may be necessary to carry out this subtitle.

**SEC. 8207. TECHNICAL AND CONFORMING AMENDMENTS.**

(a) OPM's ANNUAL REPORT ON FEHBP.—Subsection (c) of section 1308 of title 5, United States Code, is repealed.

(b) OTHER REFERENCES TO FEHBP.—Any reference in any provision of law to the health insurance program under chapter 89 of title 5, United States Code (or any aspect of such program) shall be considered to be a reference to the health insurance program under subtitle C of title VIII of the Health Security Act (or corresponding aspect), subject to such clarification as may be provided, or except as may otherwise be provided, in regulations prescribed by the agency or other authority responsible for the administration of such provision.

(c) OMNIBUS BUDGET RECONCILIATION ACT OF 1993.—Effective as of the date of the enactment of this Act, section 11101(b)(3) of the Omnibus Budget Reconciliation Act of 1993 (Public Law 103-66; 107 Stat. 413) is amended by striking "September 30, 1998" and inserting "December 31, 1997".

(d) EFFECTIVE DATE.—Except as provided in subsection (c), this section and the amendments made by this section shall take effect on the day after the FEHBP termination date.

# Subtitle D—Indian Health Service

**SEC. 8301. DEFINITIONS.**

For the purposes of this subtitle—

(1) the term "health program of the Indian Health Service" means a program which provides health services under this Act through a facility of the Indian Health Service, a tribal organization under the authority of the Indian Self-Determination Act or a self-governance compact, or an urban Indian program;

(2) the term "reservation" means the reservation of any federally recognized Indian tribe, former Indian reservations in Oklahoma, and lands held by incorporated Native groups, regional corporations, and village corporations under the provisions of the Alaska Native Claims Settlement Act (43 U.S.C. 1601 et seq.);

(3) the term "urban Indian program" means any program operated pursuant to title V of the Indian Health Care Improvement Act; and

(4) the terms "Indian", "Indian tribe", "tribal organization", "urban Indian", "urban Indian organization", and "service unit" have the same meaning as when used in the Indian Health Care Improvement Act (25 U.S.C. 1601 et seq.).

## SEC. 8302. ELIGIBILITY AND HEALTH SERVICE COVERAGE OF INDIANS.

(a) ELIGIBILITY.—An eligible individual, as defined in section 1001(c), is eligible to enroll in a health program of the Indian Health Service if the individual is—

(1) an Indian, or a descendent of a member of an Indian tribe who belongs to and is regarded as an Indian by the Indian community in which the individual lives, who resides on or near an Indian reservation or in a geographical area designated by statute as meeting the requirements of being on or near an Indian reservation notwithstanding the lack of an Indian reservation;

(2) an urban Indian; or

(3) an Indian described in section 809(b) of the Indian Health Care Improvement Act (25 U.S.C. 1679(b)).

(b) ELECTION.—An individual described in subsection (a) may elect a health program of the Indian Health Service instead of a health plan.

(c) ENROLLMENT FOR BENEFITS.—An individual who elects a health program of the Indian Health Service under subsection (b) shall enroll in such program through a service unit, tribal organization, or urban Indian program. An individual who enrolls in such program is not subject to any charge for health insurance premiums, deductibles, copayments, coinsurance, or any other cost for health services provided under such program.

(d) PAYMENTS BY INDIVIDUALS WHO DO NOT ENROLL.—If an individual described in subsection (a) does not enroll in a health program of the Indian Health Service, no payment shall be made by the Indian Health Service to the individual (or on behalf of the individual) with respect to premiums charged for enrollment in an applicable health plan or any other cost of health services under the applicable health plan which the individual is required to pay.

**SEC. 8303. SUPPLEMENTAL INDIAN HEALTH CARE BENEFITS.**

(a) IN GENERAL.—All individuals described in sections 8302(a) remain eligible for such benefits under the laws administered by the Indian Health Service as supplement the comprehensive benefit package. The individual shall not be subject to any charge or any other cost for such benefits.

(b) AUTHORIZATION OF APPROPRIATIONS.—In addition to amounts otherwise authorized to be appropriated, there is authorized to be appropriated to carry out this section $180,000,000 for fiscal year 1995, $200,000,000 for each of the fiscal years 1996 through 1999, and such sums as may be necessary for fiscal year 2000 and each fiscal year thereafter.

## SEC. 8304. HEALTH PLAN AND HEALTH ALLIANCE REQUIREMENTS.

(a) COMPREHENSIVE BENEFIT PACKAGE.—The Secretary shall ensure that the comprehensive benefit package is provided by all health programs of the Indian Health Service effective January 1, 1999, notwithstanding section 1001(a).

(b) APPLICABLE REQUIREMENTS OF HEALTH PLANS.—In addition to subsection (a), the Secretary shall determine which other requirements relating to health plans apply to health programs of the Indian Health Service.

(c) CERTIFICATION.—Effective January 1, 1999, all health programs of the Indian Health Service must meet the certification requirements for health plans, as required by the Secretary under this section, as certified from time to time by the Secretary. Before January 1, 1999, all such health programs shall, to the extent practicable, meet such certification requirements.

(d) HEALTH ALLIANCE REQUIREMENTS.—The Secretary shall determine which requirements relating to health alliances apply to the Indian Health Service.

## SEC. 8305. EXEMPTION OF TRIBAL GOVERNMENTS AND TRIBAL ORGANIZATIONS FROM EMPLOYER PAYMENTS.

A tribal government and a tribal organization under the Indian Self-Determination and Educational Assistance Act or a self-governance compact shall be exempt from making employer premium payments as an employer under section 6121.

## SEC. 8306. PROVISION OF HEALTH SERVICES TO NON-ENROLLEES AND NON-INDIANS.

(a) CONTRACTS WITH HEALTH PLANS.—

(1) IN GENERAL.—A health program of the Indian Health Service, a service unit, a tribal organization, or an urban Indian organization operating within a health program may enter into a contract with a health plan for the provision of health care services to individuals enrolled in such health plan if the program, unit, or organization determines that

the provision of such health services will not result in a denial or diminution of health services to any individual described in section 8302(a) who is enrolled for health services provided by such program, unit, or organization.

(2) REIMBURSEMENT.—Any contract entered into pursuant to paragraph (1) shall provide for reimbursement to such program, unit, or organization in accordance with the essential community provider provisions of section 1431(c), as determined by the Secretary.

(b) FAMILY TREATMENT.—

(1) DETERMINATION TO OPEN ENROLLMENT.—A health program of the Indian Health Service may open enrollment to family members of individuals described in section 8302(a).

(2) ELECTION.—If a health program of the Indian Health Service opens enrollment to family members of individuals described in section 8302(a), an individual described in that section may elect family enrollment in the health program instead of in a health plan.

(3) ENROLLMENT.—

(A) IN GENERAL.—An individual who elects family enrollment under paragraph (2) in a health program of the Indian Health Service shall enroll in such program.

(B) APPLICABLE INDIVIDUAL CHARGES.—The individual who enrolls in such program under subparagraph (A) is not subject to any charge for health insurance premiums, deductibles, copayments, coinsurance, or any other cost for health services provided under such program attributable to the individual, but the family members who are not eligible for a health program of the Indian Health Service under section 8302(a) are subject to all such charges.

(C) APPLICABLE EMPLOYER CHARGES.—Employers, other than tribal governments and tribal organizations exempt under section 8305, are liable for making employer premium payments as an employer under section 6121 in the case of any family member enrolled under this subsection who is not eligible for a health program of the Indian Health Service under section 8302(a).

(4) PREMIUM.—

(A) ESTABLISHMENT AND COLLECTION.—The Secretary shall establish a premium for all family members enrolled in a health program of the Indian Health Service under this paragraph who are not eligible for a health program of the Indian Health Service under section 8302(a). The Secretary shall collect each premium payment owed under this paragraph.

(B) REDUCTION.—The Secretary shall provide for a process for premium reduction which is the same as the process, and uses the same standards, used by regional alliances for the areas in which individuals described in subparagraph (A), except that in computing the family share of the premiums the Secretary shall use the lower of the premium quoted or the reduced weighted average accepted bid for the reference regional alliance.

(C) PAYMENT BY SECRETARY.—The Secretary shall pay to each health program of the Indian Health Service, in the same manner as payments under section 6201, amounts equivalent to the amount of payments that would have been made to a regional alliance if the individuals described in subparagraph (A) were enrolled in a regional alliance health plan (with a final accepted bid equal to the reduced weighted average accepted bid premium for the regional alliance).

(c) ESSENTIAL COMMUNITY PROVIDER.—

(1) HEALTH SERVICES.—If a health program of the Indian Health Service, a service unit, a tribal organization, or an urban Indian organization operating within a health program elects to be an essential community provider under section 1431, an individual described in paragraph (2) enrolled in a health plan other than a health program of the Indian Health Service may receive health services from that essential community provider.

(2) INDIVIDUAL COVERED.—An individual referred to in paragraph (1) is an individual who—

(A) is described in section 8303(a)(1); or

(B) is a family member described in subsection (b) who does not enroll in a health program of the Indian Health Service.

**SEC. 8307. PAYMENT BY OTHER PAYORS.**

(a) PAYMENT FOR SERVICES PROVIDED BY INDIAN HEALTH SERVICE PROGRAMS.—Nothing in this subtitle shall be construed as amending section 206, 401, or 402 of the Indian Health Care Improvement Act (relating to payments on behalf of Indians for health services from other Federal programs or from other third party payors).

(b) PAYMENT FOR SERVICES PROVIDED BY CONTRACTORS.—Nothing in this subtitle shall be construed as affecting any other provision of law, regulation, or judicial or administrative interpretation of law or policy concerning the status of the Indian Health Service as the payor of last resort for Indians eligible for contract health services under a health program of the Indian Health Service.

### SEC. 8308. CONTRACTING AUTHORITY.

Section 601(d)(1)(B) of the Indian Health Care Improvement Act (25 U.S.C. 1661(d)(1)(B)) is amended by inserting "(including personal services for the provision of direct health care services)" after "goods and services".

### SEC. 8309. CONSULTATION.

The Secretary shall consult with representatives of Indian tribes, tribal organizations, and urban Indian organizations annually concerning health care reform initiatives that affect Indian communities.

### SEC. 8310. INFRASTRUCTURE.

(a) FACILITIES.—The Secretary, acting through the Indian Health Service, may expend amounts appropriated pursuant to section 8313 for the construction and renovation of hospitals, health centers, health stations, and other facilities for the purpose of improving and expanding such facilities to enable the delivery of the full array of items and services guaranteed in the comprehensive benefit package.

(b) CAPITAL FINANCING.—There is established in the Indian Health Service a revolving loan program. Under the program, the Secretary, acting through the Indian Health Service, shall provide guaranteed loans under such terms and conditions as the Secretary may prescribe to providers within the Indian Health System to improve and expand health care facilities to enable the delivery of the full array of items and services guaranteed in the comprehensive benefit package.

**SEC. 8311. FINANCING.**

(a) ESTABLISHMENT OF FUND.—Each health program of the Indian Health Service shall establish a comprehensive benefit package fund (hereafter in this section referred to as the "fund").

(b) DEPOSITS.—There shall be deposited into the fund the following:

(1) All amounts received as employer premium payments pursuant to section 1351(e)(3).

(2) All amounts received as family premium payments and premium discount payments pursuant to section 8306(b)(4).

(3) All amounts appropriated for the fund for the purpose of providing the comprehensive benefit

package to individuals enrolled in a health program of the Indian Health Service.

(4) Any other amount received with respect to health services for the comprehensive benefit package.

(c) ADMINISTRATION AND EXPENDITURES.—

(1) MANAGEMENT.—The fund shall be managed by the health program of the Indian Health Service.

(2) EXPENDITURES.—Expenditures may be made from the fund to provide for the delivery of the items and services of the comprehensive benefit package under the health program of the Indian Health Service.

(3) AVAILABILITY OF FUNDS.—Amounts in the fund established by a service unit of the Indian Health Service under this section shall be available without further appropriation and shall remain available until expended for payments for the delivery of the items and services in the comprehensive benefit package.

**SEC. 8312. RULE OF CONSTRUCTION.**

Unless otherwise provided by this Act, no part of this Act shall be construed to rescind or otherwise modify any obligations, findings, or purposes contained in the Indian

Health Care Improvement Act (25 U.S.C. 1601 et seq.) and in the Indian Self-Determination and Education Assistance Act.

**SEC. 8313. AUTHORIZATIONS REGARDING PUBLIC HEALTH SERVICE INITIATIVES FUND.**

(a) AUTHORIZATION OF APPROPRIATIONS.—For the purpose of carrying out this subtitle, there are authorized to be appropriated from the Public Health Service Initiatives Fund (established in section 3701) $40,000,000 for fiscal year 1995, $180,000,000 for fiscal year 1996, and $200,000,000 for each of the fiscal years 1997 through 2000.

(b) RELATION TO OTHER FUNDS.—The authorizations of appropriations established in subsection (a) are in addition to any other authorizations of appropriations that are available for the purposes described in such subsection.

# Subtitle E—Amendments to the Employee Retirement Income Security Act of 1974

**SEC. 8401. GROUP HEALTH PLAN DEFINED.**

Section 3 of the Employee Retirement Income Security Act of 1974 (29 U.S.C. 1002) is amended by adding at the end the following new paragraph:

"(42) The term 'group health plan' means an employee welfare benefit plan which provides medical care (as defined in section 213(d) of the Internal Revenue Code of 1986) to participants or beneficiaries directly or through insurance, reimbursement, or otherwise.".

**SEC. 8402. LIMITATION ON COVERAGE OF GROUP HEALTH PLANS UNDER TITLE I OF ERISA.**

(a) IN GENERAL.—Section 4 of the Employee Retirement Income Security Act of 1974 (29 U.S.C. 1003) is amended—

(1) in subsection (a), by striking "subsection (b)" and inserting "subsections (b) and (c)";

(2) in subsection (b), by striking "The provisions" and inserting "Except as provided in subsection (c), the provisions"; and

(3) by adding at the end the following new subsection:

"(c) COVERAGE OF GROUP HEALTH PLANS.—

"(1) LIMITED INCLUSION.—This title shall apply to a group health plan only to the extent provided in this subsection.

"(2) COVERAGE UNDER CERTAIN PROVISIONS WITH RESPECT TO CERTAIN PLANS.—

"(A) IN GENERAL.—Except as provided in subparagraph (B), parts 1 and 4 of subtitle B shall apply to—

"(i) a group health plan which is maintained by—

"(I) a corporate alliance (as defined in section 1311(a) of the Health Security Act), or

"(II) a member of a corporate alliance (as so defined) whose eligible sponsor is described in section 1311(b)(1)(C) (relating to rural electric cooperatives and rural telephone cooperative associations), and

"(ii) a group health plan not described in subparagraph (A) which provides benefits which are permitted under paragraph (4) of section 1003 of the Health Security Act.

"(B) INAPPLICABILITY WITH RESPECT TO STATE-CERTIFIED HEALTH PLANS.—Subparagraph (A) shall not apply with respect to any plan or portion thereof which consists of a State-certified health plan (as defined in section 1400(c) of the Health Security Act). The Secretary shall provide by regulation for treatment as a separate group health plan of any arrangement which would otherwise be treated under this title as part of a group health plan to the extent necessary to carry out the purposes of this title.

"(3) CIVIL ACTIONS BY CORPORATE ALLIANCE PARTICIPANTS, BENEFICIARIES, AND FIDUCIARIES AND BY THE SECRETARY.—

"(A) IN GENERAL.—Except as provided in subparagraph (B), in the case of a group health plan to which parts 1 and 4 of subtitle B apply under paragraph (2), section 502 shall apply with respect to a civil action described in such section brought—

"(i) by a participant, beneficiary, or fiduciary under such plan, or

"(ii) by the Secretary.

"(B) EXCEPTION WHERE REVIEW IS OTHERWISE AVAILABLE UNDER HEALTH SECURITY ACT.—Subparagraph (A) shall not apply with respect to any cause of action for which, under section 5202(d) of the Health Security Act, proceedings under sections 5203 and 5204 of such Act pursuant to complaints filed under section 5202(b) of such Act, and review under section 5205 of such Act of determinations made under such section 5204, are the exclusive means of review.

"(4) DEFINITIONS AND ENFORCEMENT PROVISIONS.—Sections 3, 501, 502, 503, 504, 505, 506, 507, 508, 509, 510, and 511 and the preceding provisions of this section shall apply to a group health plan to the extent necessary to effectively carry out, and enforce the requirements under, the provisions of this title as they apply pursuant to this subsection.

"(5) APPLICABILITY OF PREEMPTION RULES.—Section 514 shall apply in the case of any group health plan to which parts 1 and 4 of subtitle B apply under paragraph (2).".

(b) REPORTING AND DISCLOSURE REQUIREMENTS APPLICABLE TO GROUP HEALTH PLANS.—

(1) IN GENERAL.—Part 1 of subtitle B of title I of such Act is amended—

(A) in the heading for section 110, by adding "BY PENSION PLANS" at the end;

(B) by redesignating section 111 as section 112; and

(C) by inserting after section 110 the following new section:

"SPECIAL RULES FOR GROUP HEALTH PLANS

"SEC. 111. IN GENERAL.—The Secretary may by regulation provide special rules for the application of this part to group health plans which are consistent with the purposes of this title and the Health Security Act and which take into account the special needs of participants, beneficiaries, and health care providers under such plans.

"(b) EXPEDITIOUS REPORTING AND DISCLOSURE.—Such special rules may include rules providing for—

"(1) reductions in the periods of time referred to in this part,

"(2) increases in the frequency of reports and disclosures required under this part, and

"(3) such other changes in the provisions of this part as may result in more expeditious reporting and disclosure of plan terms and changes in such terms to the Secretary and to plan participants and beneficiaries,

to the extent that the Secretary determines that the rules described in this subsection are necessary to ensure timely reporting and disclosure of information consistent with the purposes of this part and the Health Security Act as they relate to group health plans.

"(c) ADDITIONAL REQUIREMENTS.—Such special rules may include rules providing for reporting and disclosure to the Secretary and to participants and beneficiaries of additional information or at additional times with respect to group health plans to which this part applies under section 4(c)(2), if such reporting and disclosure would be comparable to and consistent with similar requirements applicable under the Health Security Act with respect to plans maintained by regional alliances (as defined in such section 1301 of such Act) and applicable regulations of the Secretary of Health and Human Services prescribed thereunder.".

(2) CLERICAL AMENDMENT.—The table of contents in section 1 of such Act is amended by striking the items relating to sections 110 and 111 and inserting the following new items:

"Sec. 110. Alternative methods of compliance by pension plans.
"Sec. 111. Special rules for group health plans.
"Sec. 112. Repeal and effective date.".

(d) EXCLUSION OF PLANS MAINTAINED BY REGIONAL ALLIANCES FROM TREATMENT AS MULTIPLE EMPLOYER WELFARE ARRANGEMENTS.—Section 3(40)(A) of such Act (29 U.S.C. 1002(40)(A)) is amended—

(1) in clause (ii), by striking "or";

(2) in clause (iii), by striking the period and inserting ", or"; and

		(3) by adding after clause (iii) the following new clause:

		"(iv) by a regional alliance (as defined in section 1301 of the Health Security Act).".

**SEC. 8403. AMENDMENTS RELATING TO CONTINUATION COVERAGE.**

(a) PERIOD OF COVERAGE.—Subparagraph (D) of section 602(2) of the Employee Retirement Income Security Act of 1974 (29 U.S.C. 1161(2)) is amended—

		(1) by striking "or" at the end of clause (i), by striking the period at the end of clause (ii) and inserting ", or", and by adding at the end the following new clause:

			"(iii) eligible for coverage under a comprehensive benefit package described in section 1101 of the Health Security Act.", and

		(2) by striking "OR MEDICARE ENTITLEMENT" in the heading and inserting ", MEDICARE ENTITLEMENT, OR HEALTH SECURITY ACT ELIGIBILITY".

(b) QUALIFIED BENEFICIARY.—Section 607(3) of such Act (29 U.S.C. 1167(2)) is amended by adding at the end the following new subparagraph:

		"(D) SPECIAL RULE FOR INDIVIDUALS COVERED BY HEALTH SECURITY ACT.—The term 'qualified beneficiary' shall not include any individual who, upon termination of coverage under a group health plan, is eligible for coverage under a comprehensive benefit package described in section 1101 of the Health Security Act."

(c) REPEAL UPON IMPLEMENTATION OF HEALTH SECURITY ACT.—

(1) IN GENERAL.—Part 6 of subtitle B of title I of such Act (29 U.S.C. 601 et seq.) is amended by striking sections 601 through 608 and by redesignating section 609 as section 601.

(2) CONFORMING AMENDMENTS.—

(A) Section 502(a)(7) of such Act (29 U.S.C. 1132(a)(7)) is amended by striking "609(a)(2)(A)" and inserting "601(a)(2)(A)".

(B) Section 502(c)(1) is amended by striking "paragraph (1) or (4) of section 606".

(C) Section 514 of such Act (29 U.S.C. 1144) is amended by striking "609" each place it appears in subsections (b)(7) and (b)(8) and inserting "601".

(D) The table of contents in section 1 of such Act is amended by striking the items relating to sections 601 through 609 and inserting the following new item:

"Sec. 601. Additional standards for group health plans."

(d) EFFECTIVE DATE.—

(1) SUBSECTIONS (a) AND (b).—The amendments made by subsections (a) and (b) shall take effect on the date of the enactment of this Act.

(2) SUBSECTION (c).—The amendments made by subsection (c) shall take effect on the earlier of—

(A) January 1, 1998, or

(B) the first day of the first calendar year following the calendar year in which all States have in effect plans under which individuals are eligible for coverage under a comprehensive benefit package described in section 1101 of this Act.

## SEC. 8404. ADDITIONAL AMENDMENTS RELATING TO GROUP HEALTH PLANS.

(a) REGULATIONS OF THE NATIONAL HEALTH BOARD REGARDING CASES OF ADOPTION.—Section 601(c) of such Act (as redesignated by section 8403) is amended by adding at the end the following new subsection:

"(4) REGULATIONS BY NATIONAL HEALTH BOARD.—The preceding provisions of this subsection shall apply except to the extent otherwise provided in regulations of the National Health Board under the Health Security Act.".

(b) COVERAGE OF PEDIATRIC VACCINES.—Section 601(d) of such Act (as redesignated by section 8403) is amended by adding at the end the following new sentence: "The preceding sentence shall cease to apply to a group health plan upon becoming a corporate alliance health plan pursuant to an effective election of the plan sponsor to be a corporate alliance under section 1311 of the Health Security Act.".

(c) TECHNICAL CORRECTIONS.—

(1) Subsection (a)(2)(B)(ii) of section 601 of such Act (as redesignated by section 8403) is amended by striking "section 13822" and inserting "section 13623".

(2) Subsection (a)(4) of such section 601 is amended by striking "section 13822" and inserting "section 13623".

(3) Subsection (d) of such section 601 is amended by striking "section 13830" and inserting "section 13631".

**SEC. 8405. PLAN CLAIMS PROCEDURES.**

Section 503 of the Employee Retirement Income Security Act of 1974 (29 U.S.C. 1133) is amended—

(1) by inserting "(a) IN GENERAL.—" after "SEC. 503."; and

(2) by adding at the end the following new subsection:

"(b) GROUP HEALTH PLANS.—In addition to the requirements of subsection (a), a group health plan to which parts 1 and 4 apply under section 4(c)(2) shall comply with the requirements of section 5201 of the Health Security Act (relating to health plan claims procedure).".

**SEC. 8406. EFFECTIVE DATES.**

Except as otherwise provided in this subtitle, the amendments made by this subtitle shall take effect on the earlier of—

(1) January 1, 1998, or

(2) such date or dates as may be prescribed in regulations of the National Health Board in connection with plans whose participants or beneficiaries reside in any State which becomes a participating State under the Health Security Act before January 1, 1998.

# Subtitle F—Special Fund for WIC Program

**SEC. 8501. ADDITIONAL FUNDING FOR SPECIAL SUPPLEMENTAL FOOD PROGRAM FOR WOMEN, INFANTS, AND CHILDREN (WIC).**

(a) AUTHORIZATION OF ADDITIONAL APPROPRIATIONS.—There is hereby authorized to be appropriated for the special supplemental food program for women, infants, and children (WIC) under section 17 of the Child Nutrition Act of 1966, in addition to amounts otherwise authorized to be appropriated for such program, such amounts as are necessary for the Secretary of the Treasury to fulfill the requirements of subsection (b).

(b) WIC FUND.—

(1) CREDIT.—For each of fiscal years 1996 through 2000, the Secretary of the Treasury shall credit to a special fund of the Treasury an amount equal to—

(A) $254,000,000 for fiscal year 1996,

(B) $407,000,000 for fiscal year 1997,

(C) $384,000,000 for fiscal year 1998,

(D) $398,000,000 for fiscal year 1999, and

(E) $411,000,000 for fiscal year 2000.

(2) AVAILABILITY.—Subject to paragraph (3), amounts in such fund—

 (A) shall be available only for the program authorized under section 17 of the Child Nutrition Act of 1966, exclusive of activities authorized under section 17(m) of such Act, and

 (B) shall be paid to the Secretary of Agriculture for such purposes.

(3) LIMITATION.—For a fiscal year specified in paragraph (1), the amount credited to such fund for the fiscal year shall be available for use in such program only if appropriations Acts for the fiscal year, without the addition of amounts provided under subsection (a) for the fund, provide new budget authority for the program of no less than—

 (A) $3,660,000,000 for fiscal year 1996,

 (B) $3,759,000,000 for fiscal year 1997,

 (C) $3,861,000,000 for fiscal year 1998,

 (D) $3,996,000,000 for fiscal year 1999, and

 (E) $4,126,000,000 for fiscal year 2000.

# TITLE IX—AGGREGATE GOVERNMENT PAYMENTS

TABLE OF CONTENTS OF TITLE

## Subtitle A—Aggregate State Payments

### PART 1—STATE MAINTENANCE OF EFFORT PAYMENT

Sec. 9001. State maintenance-of-effort payment relating to non-cash assistance recipients.
Sec. 9002. Non-cash baseline amounts.
Sec. 9003. Updating of baseline amounts.
Sec. 9004. Non-cash assistance child and adult defined.

### PART 2—STATE PREMIUM PAYMENTS

Sec. 9011. State premium payment relating to cash assistance recipients.
Sec. 9012. Determination of AFDC per capita premium amount for regional alliances.
Sec. 9013. Determination of SSI per capita premium amount for regional alliances.
Sec. 9014. Determination of number of AFDC and SSI recipients.
Sec. 9015. Regional alliance adjustment factors.

### PART 3—GENERAL AND MISCELLANEOUS PROVISIONS

Sec. 9021. Timing and manner of payments.
Sec. 9022. Review of payment level.
Sec. 9023. Special rules for Puerto Rico and other territories.

## Subtitle B—Aggregate Federal Alliance Payments

Sec. 9101. Federal premium payments for cash assistance recipients.
Sec. 9102. Capped Federal alliance payments.

## Subtitle C—Borrowing Authority to Cover Cash-flow Shortfalls

Sec. 9201. Borrowing authority to cover cash-flow shortfalls.

# Subtitle A—Aggregate State Payments

## PART 1—STATE MAINTENANCE OF EFFORT PAYMENT

### SEC. 9001. STATE MAINTENANCE-OF-EFFORT PAYMENT RELATING TO NON-CASH ASSISTANCE RECIPIENTS.

(a) PAYMENT.—

(1) IN GENERAL.—Subject to paragraph (2), each participating State shall provide for each year (beginning with State's first year) for payment to regional alliances in the State in the amounts specified in subsection (b).

(2) EXCEPTION.—The amounts specified in subsection (b) that are attributable to the element of the non-cash, non-DSH baseline amount described in section 9002(a)(1)(C) shall be paid to the Federal Government.

(b) AMOUNT.—Subject to sections 6005, 9023, and 9201(c)(2), the total amount of such payment for a year shall be equal to the following:

(1) FIRST YEAR.—In the case of the first year for a State, the sum of—

(A) the State non-cash, non-DSH baseline amount for the State, determined under section

9002(a)(1) and updated under section 9003(a)(1), and

 (B) the State non-cash, DSH baseline amount for the State, determined under section 9002(a)(2) and updated under section 9003(a)(2).

 (2) SUBSEQUENT YEAR.—In the case of any succeeding year, the sum computed under paragraph (1) for the first year updated to the year involved under section 9003(b).

(c) DIVISION AMONG REGIONAL ALLIANCES.—In the case of a State with more than one regional alliance, the payment required to be made under this section shall be distributed among the regional alliances in an equitable manner (determined by the State) that takes into account, for each regional alliance, the proportion of the non-cash baseline amount (described in section 9002) that is attributable to individuals who resided in the alliance area of the regional alliance.

## SEC. 9002. NON-CASH BASELINE AMOUNTS.

(a) BASELINE AMOUNTS.—

 (1) NON-DSH AMOUNT.—The Secretary shall determine a non-cash, non-DSH baseline amount which is equal to the sum of the following:

(A) EXPENDITURES FOR COMPREHENSIVE BENEFIT PACKAGE FOR NON-CASH ASSISTANCE CHILDREN.—The aggregate State medicaid expenditures in fiscal year 1993 (as defined in subsection (b)(1)) for the comprehensive benefit package for non-cash assistance children (as defined in section 9004(a)).

(B) EXPENDITURES FOR COMPREHENSIVE BENEFIT PACKAGE FOR NON-CASH ASSISTANCE ADULTS.—The aggregate State medicaid expenditures in fiscal year 1993 for the comprehensive benefit package for non-cash assistance adults (as defined in section 9004(b)).

(C) EXPENDITURES FOR ADDITIONAL BENEFITS FOR CERTAIN CHILDREN.—The aggregate medicaid expenditures in fiscal year 1993 for all medically necessary items and services described in section 1905(a) (including items and services described in section 1905(r) but excluding long-term care services described in section 1933(c)) for qualified children described in section 1934(b)(1).

(2) DSH AMOUNT.—The Secretary shall determine a non-cash, DSH baseline amount which is

equal to the DSH expenditures in fiscal year 1993 (as defined in subsection (b)(2)).

(b) STATE MEDICAID EXPENDITURES AND DSH EXPENDITURES DEFINED.—

(1) AGGREGATE STATE MEDICAID EXPENDITURES.—

(A) IN GENERAL.—In this section, the term "aggregate State medicaid expenditures" means, with respect to specified individuals and a State in fiscal year 1993, the amount of payments under the State medicaid plan with respect to medical assistance furnished for such individuals for calendar quarters in fiscal year 1993, less the amount of Federal financial participation paid to the State with respect to such assistance, and not including any DSH expenditures.

(B) LIMITED TO PAYMENTS FOR SERVICES.—In applying subparagraph (A), payments under the State medicaid plan shall not be included unless Federal financial participation is provided with respect to such payments under section 1903(a)(1) of the Social Security Act and such payments shall not include payments for medicare cost-sharing (as defined in section 1905(p)(3) of the Social Security Act).

(2) DSH EXPENDITURES.—In this section, the term "DSH expenditures" means, with respect to fiscal year 1993, payments made under section 1923 of the Social Security Act in fiscal year 1993 multiplied by proportion of payments for medical assistance for hospital services (including psychiatric hospital services) under the State medicaid plan in fiscal year 1993 that is attributable to non-cash assistance adults and non-cash asssistance children.

(3) ADJUSTMENT AUTHORIZED TO TAKE INTO ACCOUNT CASH FLOW VARIATIONS.—If the Secretary finds that a State took an action that had the effect of shifting the timing of medical assistance payments under the State medicaid plan between quarters or fiscal years in a manner so that the payments made in fiscal year 1993 do not accurately reflect the value of the medical assistance provided with respect to items and services furnished in that fiscal year, the Secretary may provide for such adjustment in the amounts computed under this subsection as may be necessary so that the non-cash baseline amounts determined under this section accurately reflects such value.

(4) TREATMENT OF DISALLOWANCES.—The amounts determined under this subsection shall take into account amounts (or an estimate of amounts) disallowed.

(c) APPLICATION TO PARTICULAR ITEMS AND SERVICES IN COMPREHENSIVE BENEFIT PACKAGE.—For purposes of subsection (a)(1), in determining the aggregate State medicaid expenditures for a category of items and services (within the comprehensive benefit package) furnished in a State, there shall be counted only that proportion of such expenditures that were attributable to items and services included in the comprehensive benefit package (taking into account any limitation on amount, duration, or scope of items and services included in such package).

## SEC. 9003. UPDATING OF BASELINE AMOUNTS.

(a) INITIAL UPDATE THROUGH THE FIRST YEAR.—

(1) NON-CASH, NON-DSH BASELINE AMOUNT.—The Secretary shall update the non-cash, non-DSH baseline amount determined under section 9002(a)(1) for each State from fiscal year 1993 through the first year, by the following percentage:

(A) If such first year is 1996, the applicable percentage is 56.6 percent.

(B) If such first year is 1997, the applicable percentage is 78.1 percent.

(C) If such first year is 1998, the applicable percentage is 102.2 percent.

(2) NON-CASH, DSH BASELINE AMOUNT.—The Secretary shall update the non-cash, DSH baseline amount determined under section 9002(a)(2) for each State from fiscal year 1993 through the first year, by the following percentage:

(A) If such first year is 1996, the applicable percentage is 45.9 percent.

(B) If such first year is 1997, the applicable percentage is 61.8 percent.

(C) If such first year is 1998, the applicable percentage is 79.0 percent.

(3) ADJUSTMENT AUTHORIZED TO TAKE INTO ACCOUNT CASH FLOW VARIATIONS.—In determining the updates under paragraphs (1) and (2), the Secretary may provide for an adjustment in a manner similar to the adjustment permitted under section 9002(b)(3).

(b) UPDATE FOR SUBSEQUENT YEARS.—For each State for each year after the first year, the Board shall update the non-cash baseline amount (as previously updated under this subsection) by the product of—

(1) 1 plus the general health care inflation factor (as defined in section 6001(a)(3)) for the year, and

(2) 1 plus the annual percentage increase in the population of the United States of individuals who are under 65 years of age (as estimated by the Board based on projections made by the Bureau of Labor Statistics of the Department of Labor) for the year.

**SEC. 9004. NON-CASH ASSISTANCE CHILD AND ADULT DEFINED.**

(a) NON-CASH ASSISTANCE CHILD.—In this part, the term "non-cash assistance child" means a child described in section 1934(b)(1) of the Social Security Act (as inserted by section 4221(c)) who is not a medicare-eligible individual.

(b) NON-CASH ASSISTANCE ADULT.—In this part, the term "non-cash assistance adult" means an individual who is—

(1) over 21 years,

(2) is a citizen or national of the United States or an alien who is lawfully admitted for permanent residence or otherwise permanently residing in the United States under color of law, and

(3) is not an AFDC or SSI recipient or a medicare-eligible individual.

## PART 2—STATE PREMIUM PAYMENTS

### SEC. 9011. STATE PREMIUM PAYMENT RELATING TO CASH ASSISTANCE RECIPIENTS.

(a) IN GENERAL.—Each participating State shall provide in each year (beginning with the State's first year) for payment to each regional alliance in the State of an amount equal to the State medical assistance percentage (as defined in subsection (b)) of 95 percent of the sum of the following products:

(1) AFDC PORTION.—The product of—

(A) the AFDC per capita premium amount for the regional alliance for the year (determined under section 9012(a)), and

(B) the number of AFDC recipients residing in the alliance area in the year (as determined under section 9014(b)(1)).

(2) SSI PORTION.—The product of—

(A) the SSI per capita premium amount for the regional alliance for the year (determined under section 9013), and

(B) the number of SSI recipients residing in the alliance area in the year (as determined under section 9014(b)(1)).

(b) STATE MEDICAL ASSISTANCE PERCENTAGE DEFINED.—In subsection (a), the term "State medical assistance percentage" means, for a State for a quarter in a fiscal year, 100 percent minus the Federal medical assistance percentage (as defined in section 1905(b) of the Social Security Act) for the State for the fiscal year.

## SEC. 9012. DETERMINATION OF AFDC PER CAPITA PREMIUM AMOUNT FOR REGIONAL ALLIANCES.

(a) IN GENERAL.—For each regional alliance in a State for each year, the Secretary shall determine an AFDC per capita premium amount in accordance with this section. Such amount is equal to—

(1) the per capita State medicaid expenditures for the comprehensive benefit package for AFDC recipients for the State for the year (as determined under subsection (b)), multiplied by

(2) the adjustment factor (determined under section 9015) for the year for the regional alliance.

(b) PER CAPITA STATE MEDICAID EXPENDITURES DEFINED.—The "per capita State medicaid expenditures for the comprehensive benefit package for AFDC recipients" for a State for a year is equal to the base per capita expenditures (described in subsection (c)), updated to the year involved under subsection (d)).

(c) BASE PER CAPITA EXPENDITURES.—The "base per capita expenditures" described in this subsection, for a State for a year, is—

(1) the baseline medicaid expenditures (as defined in subsection (e)) for the State, divided by

(2) the number of AFDC recipients enrolled in the State medicaid plan in fiscal year 1993, as determined under section 9014(a).

(d) UPDATING.—

(1) INITIAL UPDATE THROUGH YEAR BEFORE FIRST YEAR.—

(A) IN GENERAL.—The Secretary shall update the base per capita expenditures described in subsection (c) for each State from fiscal year 1993 through the year before first year, by the applicable percentage specified in paragraph (2).

(B) APPLICABLE PERCENTAGE.—For purposes of paragraph (1), the applicable percentage specified in this paragraph, in the case of a State in which the first year is—

(i) 1996 is 32.2 percent,

(ii) 1997 is 46.6 percent, or

(iii) 1998 is 62.1 percent.

(C) ADJUSTMENT AUTHORIZED TO TAKE INTO ACCOUNT CASH FLOW VARIATIONS.—In determining the update under paragraph (1), the Secretary may provide for an adjustment in a manner similar to the adjustment permitted under section 9002(b)(3).

(2) UPDATE FOR SUBSEQUENT YEARS.—For each State for the first year and for each year after the first year, the Board shall update the base per capita expenditures described in subsection (c) (as previously updated under this subsection) by a factor equal to 1 plus the general health care inflation factor (as defined in section 6001(a)(3)) for the year.

(e) DETERMINATION OF BASELINE MEDICAID EXPENDITURES.—

(1) IN GENERAL.—For purposes of subsection (c)(1), the "baseline medicaid expenditures" for a State is the gross amount of payments under the State medicaid plan with respect to medical assistance furnished, for items and services included in the comprehensive benefit package, for AFDC recipients for calendar quarters in fiscal year 1993, but does not include such expenditures for which no

Federal financial participation is provided under such plan.

(2) DISPROPORTIONATE SHARE PAYMENTS NOT INCLUDED.—In applying paragraph (1), payments made under section 1923 of the Social Security Act shall not be counted in the gross amount of payments.

(3) TREATMENT OF DISALLOWANCES.—The amount determined under this subsection shall take into account amounts (or an estimate of amounts) disallowed.

(f) APPLICATION TO PARTICULAR ITEMS AND SERVICES IN COMPREHENSIVE BENEFIT PACKAGE.—For purposes of this section, in determining the per capita State medicaid expenditures for a category of items and services (within the comprehensive benefit package) furnished in a State, there shall be counted only that proportion of such expenditures (determined only with respect to medical assistance furnished to AFDC recipients) that were attributable to items and services included in the comprehensive benefit package (taking into account any limitation on amount, duration, or scope of items and services included in such package).

## SEC. 9013. DETERMINATION OF SSI PER CAPITA PREMIUM AMOUNT FOR REGIONAL ALLIANCES.

For each regional alliance in a State for each year, the Secretary shall determine an SSI per capita premium amount for each regional alliance in accordance with this section. Such amount shall be determined in the same manner as the AFDC per capita premium amount for the regional alliance is determined under section 9012 except that, for purposes of this section—

(1) any reference in such section (or in sections referred to in such section) to an "AFDC recipient" is deemed a reference to an "SSI recipient", and

(2) the following percents shall be substituted for the percents specified in section 9012(d)(1)(B):

(A) For 1996, 29.4 percent.

(B) For 1997, 43.7 percent.

(C) For 1998, 58.8 percent.

## SEC. 9014. DETERMINATION OF NUMBER OF AFDC AND SSI RECIPIENTS.

(a) BASELINE.—For purposes of section 9012 and section 9013, the number of AFDC recipients and SSI recipients for a State for fiscal year 1993 shall be determined based on actual reports submitted by the State to the Secretary. In the case of individuals who were not recipients for the entire fiscal year, the number shall take into account only the portion of the year in which they were such recipients. The Secretary may audit such reports.

(b) SUBSEQUENT YEARS.—

(1) PAYMENTS.—For purposes of section 9011(b), the number of AFDC and SSI recipients enrolled in regional alliance health plans for a regional alliance shall be determined on a monthly basis based on actual enrollment.

(2) COMPUTATION OF REGIONAL ADJUSTMENT FACTORS AND BLENDED PLAN PAYMENT RATES.—For purposes of computing regional alliance adjustment factors under section 9015 and the AFDC and SSI proportions under section 6202, the number of AFDC and SSI recipients for a regional alliance in a State for a year (beginning with 1997) shall be determined by the State before the date the State is required to compute AFDC and SSI proportions under section 6202 based on the best available estimate of such proportion in the previous year.

SEC. 9015. REGIONAL ALLIANCE ADJUSTMENT FACTORS.

(a) IN GENERAL.—If a State—

(1) has more than one regional alliance operating in the State for a year, the State shall compute under this section a regional alliance adjustment fac-

tor for each such regional alliance for the year in accordance with subsection (b), or

(2) has only one regional alliance for a year, the regional alliance adjustment factor under this section is 1.

(b) RULES.—The adjustment factors under subsection (a)(1) for a year shall be computed in a manner so that—

   (1) such factors for the different regional alliances reflect—

      (A) the variation in regional alliance per capita premium targets (determined under section 6003), and

      (B) the variation in baseline per capita medicaid expenditures across regional alliances; and

   (2) the weighted average of such factors is 1.

(c) USE OF SAME DATA.—The weighted average under subsection (b)(2) shall be determined based on the number of AFDC recipients or SSI recipients (as the case may be) enrolled in each regional alliance in a State (as determined for each regional alliance under section 9014(b)(2)).

(d) CLARIFICATION OF SEPARATE COMPUTATIONS.—Determinations of adjustment factors under this section shall be made separately for AFDC recipients and for SSI recipients.

## PART 3—GENERAL AND MISCELLANEOUS PROVISIONS

**SEC. 9021. TIMING AND MANNER OF PAYMENTS.**

The provisions of paragraphs (1) and (2) of section 9101(b) apply to payments by a State under this subtitle in the same manner as they apply to payments by the Secretary under section 9101, and any reference in such provisions to the Secretary is deemed a reference to the State.

**SEC. 9022. REVIEW OF PAYMENT LEVEL.**

(a) IN GENERAL.—The National Health Board shall review from time to time the appropriateness of the levels of payments required of States under this subtitle.

(b) REPORT.—The Board may report to the Congress on such adjustments as should be made to assure an equitable distribution of State payments under this Act, taking into account the revenue base in each of the States.

(c) LIMIT ON AUTHORITY.—Nothing in this subtitle shall be construed as permitting the Board to change the amount of the payments required by States under the the previous sections in this subtitle.

### SEC. 9023. SPECIAL RULES FOR PUERTO RICO AND OTHER TERRITORIES.

(a) WAIVER AUTHORITY.—Notwithstanding any other requirement of this title or title VI, the Secretary may waive or modify any requirement of this title or title VI (other than financial contribution and subsidy requirements) with respect to Puerto Rico, the Virgin Islands, Guam, American Samoa, and the Northern Mariana Islands, consistent with this section, to accommodate their unique geographic and social conditions and features of their health care systems.

(b) TERRITORIAL MAINTENANCE OF EFFORT AND DIVISION OF FINANCIAL RESPONSIBILITY.—

(1) IN GENERAL.—In the case of such a territory, the Secretary shall determine an appropriate allocation of the payments described in paragraph (2) based on—

(A) payments that qualify for Federal financial participation under the medicaid program,

(B) payments would would qualify for such participation in the absence of section 1108(c) of the Social Security Act, and

(C) other factors that the Secretary may consider.

(2) PAYMENTS DESCRIBED.—The payments described in this paragraph are—

(A) State cash assistance payments under section 9011;

(B) State maintenance of effort payments under section 9001;

(C) Federal payments under section 9101; and

(D) Federal payments under section 9111.

(3) CASH ASSISTANCE RECIPIENTS.—With respect to such territories, in this Act, the term "SSI recipient" means an individual receiving aid under a territorial program for the aged, blind, or disabled under the Social Security Act.

# Subtitle B—Aggregate Federal Alliance Payments

SEC. 9101. FEDERAL PREMIUM PAYMENTS FOR CASH ASSISTANCE RECIPIENTS.

(a) AMOUNT.—

(1) IN GENERAL.—The Secretary shall provide each year (beginning with a State's first year) for payment to each regional alliance of an amount equal to the Federal medical assistance percentage (as defined in section 1905(b) of the Social Security Act) of 95 percent of the sum of the products de-

scribed in section 9011(a) for that State for that fiscal year.

(2) SPECIAL RULES FOR SINGLE-PAYER STATES.—In determining the products referred to in paragraph (1) in the case of a single-payer State, the State is deemed to be a single regional alliance and the regional alliance adjustment factor (under section 9015) is deemed to be 1.

(b) TIMING AND MANNER OF PAYMENT.—

(1) IN GENERAL.—Amounts required to be paid under this section shall be paid on a periodic basis that reflects the cash flow requirements of regional alliances for payments under this section in order to meet obligations established under this Act.

(2) PERIODIC PROVISION OF INFORMATION.—Each regional alliance shall periodically transmit to the Secretary such information as the Secretary may require to make such payments.

(3) RECONCILIATION.—

(A) PRELIMINARY.—At such time after the end of each year as the Secretary shall specify, the State shall submit to the Secretary such information as the Secretary may require to do a preliminary reconciliation of the amounts paid under this section and the amounts due.

(B) FINAL.—No later than June 30 of each year, the Secretary shall provide for a final reconciliation for such payments for quarters in the previous year. Amounts subsequently payable are subject to adjustment to reflect the results of such reconciliation.

(C) AUDIT.—Payments under this section are subject to audits by the Secretary in accordance with rules established by the Secretary.

## SEC. 9102. CAPPED FEDERAL ALLIANCE PAYMENTS.

(a) CAPPED ENTITLEMENT.—

(1) PAYMENT.—The Secretary shall provide for each calendar quarter (beginning on or after January 1, 1996) for payment to each regional alliance of an amount equal to the capped Federal alliance payment amount (as defined in subsection (b)(1)) for the regional alliance for the quarter.

(2) ENTITLEMENT.—This section constitutes budget authority in advance of appropriations Acts, and represents the obligation of the Federal Government to provide for the payment to regional alliances of the capped Federal alliance payment under this section.

(b) CAPPED FEDERAL ALLIANCE PAYMENT AMOUNT.—

(1) IN GENERAL.—In this section, the term "capped Federal alliance payment amount" means, for a regional alliance for a calendar quarter in a year and subject to subsection (e), the amount by which—

    (A) ¼ of the total payment obligation (described in paragraph (2)) for the alliance for the year, exceeds

    (B) ¼ of the total amounts receivable (described in paragraph (3)) by the alliance for the year.

(2) TOTAL PAYMENT OBLIGATION.—The total payment obligation described in this paragraph for an alliance for a year is the total amount payable by the alliance for the following:

    (A) PLAN PAYMENTS (AND CERTAIN COST SHARING REDUCTIONS).—Payments to regional alliance health plans under section 1351 (including amounts attributable to cost sharing reductions under section 1371, not including a reduction under subsection (c)(2) thereof) not otherwise counted.

    (B) ALLIANCE ADMINISTRATIVE EXPENSES.—Payments retained by the regional alliance for administration (in accordance with section 1352).

(3) TOTAL AMOUNTS RECEIVABLE.—The total amounts receivable by a regional alliance for a year is the sum of the following:

(A) PREMIUMS.—The amount payable to the regional alliance for the family share of premiums, employer premiums, and liabilities owed the alliance under subpart B of part 1, not taking into account any failure to make or collect such payments.

(B) OTHER GOVERNMENT PAYMENTS.—The amounts payable to the regional alliance under sections 9001, 9011, and 9101, and payable under section 1895 of the Social Security Act during the year.

(4) NO PAYMENT FOR CERTAIN AMOUNTS.—

(A) UNCOLLECTED ALLIANCE PREMIUMS.—Each regional alliance is responsible, under section 1345(a), for the collection of all amounts owed the alliance (whether by individuals, employers, or others and whether on the basis of premiums owed, incorrect amounts of discounts or premium, cost sharing, or other reductions made, or otherwise), and no amounts are payable by the Federal Goverment under this section with respect to the failure to collect any such amounts.

(B) ADMINISTRATIVE ERRORS.—

(i) IN GENERAL.—Each participating State is responsible, under section 1202(g), for the payment to regional alliances in the State of amounts attributable to administrative errors (described in clause (ii)).

(ii) ADMINISTRATIVE ERRORS DESCRIBED.—The administrative errors described in this clause include the following:

(I) An eligibility error rate for premium discounts, liability reductions, and cost sharing reductions under sections 6104 and 6123, section 6113, and section 1371, respectively, to the extent the applicable error rate exceeds the maximum permissible error rate, specified by the applicable Secretary under section 1361(b)(1)(C), with respect to the section involved.

(II) Misappropriations or other regional alliance expenditures that the

Secretary finds are attributable to malfeasance or misfeasance by the regional alliance or the State.

(5) SPECIAL RULES FOR SINGLE-PAYER STATES.—In applying this subsection in the case of a single-payer State, the Secretary shall develop and apply a methodology for computing an amount of payment (with respect to each calendar quarter) that is equivalent to the amount of payment that would have been made to all regional alliances in the State for the quarter if the State were not a single-payer State.

(c) DETERMINATION OF CAPPED FEDERAL ALLIANCE PAYMENT AMOUNTS.—

(1) REPORTS.—At such time as the Secretary may require before the beginning of each fiscal year, each regional alliance shall submit to the Secretary such information as the Secretary may require to estimate the capped Federal alliance payment amount under this section for the succeeding calendar year (and the portion of such year that falls in such fiscal year).

(2) ESTIMATION.—Before the beginning of each year, the Secretary shall estimate for each regional alliance the capped Federal alliance payment amount

for calendar quarters in such year. Such estimate shall be based on factors including prior financial experience in the alliance, future estimates of income, wages, and employment, and other characteristics of the area found relevant by the Secretary. The Secretary shall transmit to Congress, on a timely basis consistent with the timely appropriation of funds under this section, a report that specifies an estimate of the total capped Federal alliance payment amounts owed to States under this section for the fiscal and calendar year involved.

(d) PAYMENTS TO REGIONAL ALLIANCES.—Subject to subsection (e), the provisions of section 9101(b) apply to payments under this section in the same manner as they apply to payments under section 9101.

(e) CAP ON PAYMENTS.—

(1) IN GENERAL.—The total amount of the capped Federal alliance payments made under this section for quarters in a fiscal year may not exceed the cap specified under paragraph (2) for the fiscal year.

(2) CAP.—Subject to paragraphs (4) and (6)—

(A) FISCAL YEARS 1996 THROUGH 2000.—The cap under this paragraph—

(i) for fiscal year 1996, is $10.3 billion,

(ii) for fiscal year 1997, is $28.3 billion,

(iii) for fiscal year 1998, is $75.6 billion,

(iv) for fiscal year 1999, is $78.9 billion, and

(v) for fiscal year 2000, is $81.0 billion.

(B) SUBSEQUENT FISCAL YEAR.—The cap under this paragraph for a fiscal year after fiscal year 2000 is the cap under this paragraph for the previous fiscal year (not taking into account paragraph (4)) multiplied by the product of the factors described in subparagraph (C) for that fiscal year and for each previous year after fiscal year 2000.

(C) FACTOR.—The factor described in this subparagraph for a fiscal year is 1 plus the following:

(i) CPI.—The percentage change in the CPI for the fiscal year, determined based upon the percentage change in the average of the CPI for the 12-month period ending with May 31 of the previous fiscal year over such average for the preceding 12-month period.

(ii) POPULATION.—The average annual percentage change in the population of the United States during the 3-year period ending in the preceding calendar year, determined by the Board based on data supplied by the Bureau of the Census.

(iii) REAL GDP PER CAPITA.—The average annual percentage change in the real, per capita gross domestic product of the United States during the 3-year period ending in the preceding calendar year, determined by the Board based on data supplied by the Department of Commerce.

(3) CARRYFORWARD.—If the total of the capped Federal alliance payment amounts for all regional alliances for all calendar quarters in a fiscal year is less than the cap specified in paragraph (2) for the fiscal year, then the amount of such surplus shall be accumulated and will be available in the case of a year in which the cap would otherwise be breached.

(4) NOTIFICATION.—

(A) IN GENERAL.—If the Secretary anticipates that the amount of the cap, plus any carryforward from a previous year accumulated under paragraph (3), will not be sufficient for a fiscal year, the Secretary shall notify the President, the Congress, and each regional alliance. Such notification shall include information about the anticipated amount of the shortfall and the anticipated time when the shortfall will first occur.

(B) REQUIRED ACTION.—Within 30 days after receiving such a notice, the President shall submit to Congress a report containing specific legislative recommendations for actions which would eliminate the shortfall.

(5) CONGRESSIONAL CONSIDERATION.—

(A) EXPEDITED CONSIDERATION.—If a joint resolution the substance of which approves the specific recommendations submitted under paragraph (4)(A) is introduced, subject to subparagraph (B), the provisions of section 2908 (other than subsection (a)) of the Defense Base Closure and Realignment Act of 1990 shall apply to the consideration of the joint resolution in the same manner as such provisions apply to a joint resolution described in section 2908(a) of such Act.

(B) SPECIAL RULES.—For purposes of applying subparagraph (A) with respect to such provisions, any reference to the Committee on Armed Services of the House of Representatives shall be deemed a reference to an appropriate Committee of the House of Representatives (specified by the Speaker of the House of Representatives at the time of submission of recommendations under paragraph (4)) and any reference to the Committee on Armed Services of the Senate shall be deemed a reference to an appropriate Committee of the House of Representatives (specified by the Majority Leader of the Senate at the time of submission of such recommendations).

(6) METHOD FOR ADJUSTING THE CAP FOR CHANGES IN INFLATION.—If the inflation rate, as measured by the percentage increase in the CPI, is projected to be significantly different from the inflation rate projected by the Council of Economic Advisors to the President as of October 1993, the Secretary may adjust the caps under paragraph (2) so as to reflect such deviation from the projection.

tenance-of-effort payment required under section 9001.

(d) REPORTS.—The Secretary shall annually report to Congress on the loans made (and loan amounts repaid) under this section.

(e) SOURCES OF ERROR DESCRIBED.—

(1) ESTIMATION DISCREPANCIES.—The estimation discrepancies described in this paragraph are discrepancies in estimating the following:

(A) The average premium payments per family under section 6122(b).

(B) The AFDC and SSI proportions under section 6202.

(C) The distribution of enrolled families in different risk categories for purposes of under section 1343(b)(2).

(D) The distribution of enrollment in excess premium plans (for purposes of calculating and applying the reduced weighted average accepted bid under section 6105(c)(1)).

(E) The collection shortfalls (used in computing the family collection shortfall add-on under section 6107).

(2) ADMINISTRATIVE ERRORS.—The administrative errors described in this paragraph include the following:

(A) An eligibility error rate for premium discounts and liability reductions under sections 6104 and 6113, to the extent such rate exceeds the maximum permissible error rate established for the alliance under subpart B of part 3 of subtitle D of title I.

(B) Misappropriations or other regional alliance expenditures that are determined to be attributable to malfeasance or misfeasance by the regional alliance or the State.

(f) ESTIMATION ADJUSTMENT PROVISIONS DESCRIBED.—The estimation adjustment provisions, referred to in subsection (b)(3)) are the following adjustments (corresponding to the respective estimation discrepancies specified in subsection (d)(1)):

(1) Adjustments for average premium payments per family under section 6122(b) under section 6122(b)(4).

(2) Adjustments in the AFDC and SSI proportions under section 6202(d).

(3) Adjustments pursuant to methodology described in section 1541(b)(8).

(4) Adjustments in excess premium credit pursuant to section 6105(b)(2).

(5) Adjustment in the collection shortfall add-on under section 6017(b)(2)(C)).

# TITLE X—COORDINATION OF MEDICAL PORTION OF WORKERS COMPENSATION AND AUTOMOBILE INSURANCE

TABLE OF CONTENTS OF TITLE

### Subtitle A—Workers Compensation Insurance

Sec. 10000. Definitions.

#### PART 1—HEALTH PLAN REQUIREMENTS RELATING TO WORKERS COMPENSATION

Sec. 10001. Provision of workers compensation services.
Sec. 10002. Payment by workers compensation carrier.

#### PART 2—REQUIREMENTS OF PARTICIPATING STATES

Sec. 10011. Coordination of specialized workers compensation providers.
Sec. 10012. Preemption of State laws restricting delivery of workers compensation medical benefits.
Sec. 10013. Development of supplemental schedule.
Sec. 10014. Construction.

#### PART 3—APPLICATION OF INFORMATION REQUIREMENTS; REPORT ON PREMIUM REDUCTIONS

Sec. 10021. Application of information requirements.
Sec. 10022. Report on reduction in workers compensation premiums.

#### PART 4—DEMONSTRATION PROJECTS

Sec. 10031. Authorization.
Sec. 10032. Development of work-related protocols.
Sec. 10033. Development of capitation payment models.

### Subtitle B—Automobile Insurance

Sec. 10100. Definitions.

#### PART 1—HEALTH PLAN REQUIREMENTS RELATING TO AUTOMOBILE INSURANCE

Sec. 10101. Provision of automobile insurance medical benefits through health plans.
Sec. 10102. Payment by automobile insurance carrier.

#### PART 2—REQUIREMENT OF PARTICIPATING STATES

Sec. 10111. Development of supplemental schedule.
Sec. 10112. Construction.

PART 3—APPLICATION OF INFORMATION REQUIREMENTS.

Sec. 10121. Application of information requirements.

### Subtitle C—COMMISSION ON INTEGRATION OF HEALTH BENEFITS

Sec. 10201. Commission.

### Subtitle D—Federal Employees' Compensation Act

Sec. 10301. Application of policy.

### Subtitle E—Davis-Bacon Act and Service Contract Act

Sec. 10401. Coverage of benefits under Health Security Act.

### Subtitle F—Effective Dates

Sec. 10501. Regional alliances.
Sec. 10502. Corporate alliances.
Sec. 10503. Federal requirements.

# Subtitle A—Workers Compensation Insurance

**SEC. 10000. DEFINITIONS.**

In this subtitle:

(1) INJURED WORKER.—The term "injured worker" means, with respect to a health plan, an individual enrolled under the plan who has a work-related injury or illness for which workers compensation medical benefits are available under State law.

(2) SPECIALIZED WORKERS COMPENSATION PROVIDER.—The term "specialized workers compensation provider" means a health care provider that specializes in the provision of treatment relating to work-related injuries or illness, and includes specialists in industrial medicine, specialists in occupa-

tional therapy, and centers of excellence in industrial medicine and occupational therapy.

(3) WORKERS COMPENSATION MEDICAL BENEFITS.—The term "workers compensation medical benefits" means, with respect to an enrollee who is an employee subject to the workers compensation laws of a State, the comprehensive medical benefits for work-related injuries and illnesses provided for under such laws with respect to such an employee.

(4) WORKERS COMPENSATION CARRIER.—The term "workers compensation carrier" means an insurance company that underwrites workers compensation medical benefits with respect to one or more employers and includes an employer or fund that is financially at risk for the provision of workers compensation medical benefits.

(5) WORKERS COMPENSATION SERVICES.—The term "workers compensation services" means items and services included in workers compensation medical benefits and includes items and services (including rehabilitation services and long-term care services) commonly used for treatment of work-related injuries and illnesses.

# PART 1—HEALTH PLAN REQUIREMENTS RELATING TO WORKERS COMPENSATION

## SEC. 10001. PROVISION OF WORKERS COMPENSATION SERVICES.

(a) PROVISION OF BENEFITS.—Subject to subsection (b)—

(1) REQUIREMENT FOR CERTAIN HEALTH PLANS.—

(A) IN GENERAL.—Each health plan that provides services to enrollees through participating providers shall enter into such contracts and arrangements as are necessary (in accordance with subparagraph (B)) to provide or arrange for the provision of workers compensation services to such enrollees, in return for payment from the workers compensation carrier under section 10002.

(B) PROVISION OF SERVICES.—For purposes of this paragraph, a health plan provides (or arranges for the provision of) workers compensation services with respect to an enrollee if the services are provided by—

(i) a participating provider in the plan,

(ii) any other provider with whom the plan has entered into an agreement for the provision of such services, or

(iii) a specialized workers compensation provider (designated by the State under 10011), whether or not the provider is a provider described in clause (i) or (ii).

(2) INDIVIDUAL REQUIREMENT.—An individual entitled to workers compensation medical benefits and enrolled in a health plan (whether or not the plan is described in paragraph (1)(A)) shall receive workers compensation services through the provision (or arrangement for the provision) of such services by the health plan.

(3) EXCEPTIONS.—

(A) EMERGENCY SERVICES.—Paragraphs (1) and (2) shall not apply in the case of emergency services.

(B) ELECTING VETERANS, MILITARY PERSONNEL, INDIANS, AND PRISONERS.—Paragraphs (1) and (2) shall not apply in the case of an individual described in section 1004(b) and making an election described in such section.

(4) USE OF SPECIALIZED WORKERS COMPENSATION PROVIDERS.—If a participating State has designated under section 10011 specialized workers compensation providers with respect to one or more types of injuries or illnesses for a geographic area, either a health plan or an injured worker who has an injury or illness of such type may elect to provide or receive the benefits under this subsection through such a provider.

(b) ALTERNATIVE PERMITTED.—Subsection (a) shall not be construed as preventing an injured worker and a workers compensation carrier from agreeing that workers compensation services shall be provided other than by or through the health plan in which the worker is enrolled.

(c) COORDINATION.—

(1) DESIGNATION OF CASE MANAGER.—Each health plan shall employ or contract with one or more individuals, such as occupational nurses, with experience in the treatment of occupational illness and injury to provide case management services with respect to workers compensation services provided through the plan under this section.

(2) FUNCTIONS OF CASE MANAGER.—The health plan (through the case manager described in paragraph (1)) is responsible for ensuring that—

(A) there is plan of treatment (when appropriate) for each enrollee who is an injured worker designed to assure appropriate treatment and facilitate return to work;

(B) the plan of treatment is coordinated with the workers compensation carrier, the employer, or both;

(C) the health plan (and its providers) comply with legal duties and requirements under State workers compensation law; and

(D) if the health plan is unable to provide a workers compensation service needed to treat a work-related injury or illness, that the injured worker is referred (in consultation with the workers compensation carrier) to an appropriate provider.

## SEC. 10002. PAYMENT BY WORKERS COMPENSATION CARRIER.

(a) PAYMENT.—

(1) IN GENERAL.—Except as provided in subsection (b), each workers compensation carrier that is liable for payment for workers compensation services furnished by or through a health plan, regardless of whether or not the services are included in

the comprehensive benefit package, shall make payment for such services.

(2) USE OF REGIONAL ALLIANCE FEE SCHEDULE.—Such payment shall be made in accordance with the applicable fee schedule established under section 1322(c) or section 10013.

(b) ALTERNATIVE PAYMENT METHODOLOGIES.—Subsection (a) shall not apply—

(1) in the case of a regional alliance or participating State that establishes an alternative payment methodology (such as payment on a negotiated fee for each case) for payment for workers compensation services; or

(2) in the case in which a workers compensation carrier and the health plan negotiate alternative payment arrangements.

(c) LIMITATION OF LIABILITY OF INJURED WORKER.—Nothing in this subpart shall be construed as requiring an injured worker to make any payment (including payment of any cost sharing or any amount in excess of the applicable fee schedule) to any health plan or health care provider for the receipt of workers compensation services.

# PART 2—REQUIREMENTS OF PARTICIPATING STATES

## SEC. 10011. COORDINATION OF SPECIALIZED WORKERS COMPENSATION PROVIDERS.

(a) IN GENERAL.—Each participating State shall coordinate access to specialized workers compensation providers on behalf of health plans, providing coverage to individuals residing in the State, under part 1.

(b) OPTIONAL DESIGNATION OF SPECIALIZED WORKERS COMPENSATION PROVIDERS.—A participating State may designate such specialized workers compensation providers, as the State determines to be appropriate, to provide under part 1 workers compensation services that—

(1) are not included in the comprehensive benefit package, or

(2) are so included but are specialized services that are typically provided (as determined by the State) by specialists in occupational or rehabilitative medicine.

Injured workers and health plans may elect to use such providers under section 10001(a)(4).

## SEC. 10012. PREEMPTION OF STATE LAWS RESTRICTING DELIVERY OF WORKERS COMPENSATION MEDICAL BENEFITS.

(a) IN GENERAL.—Subject to section 10011(b), no State law shall have any effect that restricts the choice, or payment, of providers that may provide workers compensation services for individuals enrolled in a health plan.

(b) DISPUTE RESOLUTION.—A State law may provide for a method for resolving disputes among parties related to—

(1) an individual's entitlement to workers compensation medical benefits under State law,

(2) the necessity and appropriateness of workers compensation services provided to an injured worker, and

(3) subject to section 10002, the reasonableness of charges or fees charged for workers compensation services.

## SEC. 10013. DEVELOPMENT OF SUPPLEMENTAL SCHEDULE.

Each participating State shall develop a fee schedule applicable to payment for workers compensation services for which a fee is not included in the applicable fee schedule established under section 1322(c).

## SEC. 10014. CONSTRUCTION.

(a) IN GENERAL.—Nothing in this subtitle shall be construed as altering—

(1) the effect of a State workers compensation law as the exclusive remedy for work-related injuries or illnesses,

(2) the determination of whether or not a person is an injured worker and entitled to workers compensation medical benefits under State law,

(3) the scope of items and services available to injured workers entitled to workers compensation medical benefits under State law, or

(4) the eligibility of any individual or class of individuals for workers compensation medical benefits under State law.

(b) EARLY INTEGRATION.—Nothing in this subtitle shall prevent a State from integrating or otherwise coordinating the payment for workers compensation medical benefits with payment for benefits under health insurance or health benefit plans before the date the Commission submits its report under section 10201(e).

## PART 3—APPLICATION OF INFORMATION REQUIREMENTS; REPORT ON PREMIUM REDUCTIONS

### SEC. 10021. APPLICATION OF INFORMATION REQUIREMENTS.

(a) IN GENERAL.—The provisions of—

(1) part 3 of subtitle B of title V (relating to use of standard forms), and

(2) section 5101(e)(9) (relating to provision of data on quality),

apply to the provision of workers compensation services in the same manner as such provisions apply with respect to the provision of services included in the comprehensive benefit package.

(b) RULES.—The Secretary of Labor shall promulgate rules to clarify the responsibilities of health plans and workers compensation carriers in carrying out the provisions referred to in subsection (a).

**SEC. 10022. REPORT ON REDUCTION IN WORKERS COMPENSATION PREMIUMS.**

(a) STUDY AND REPORT.—

(1) STUDY.—The Secretary of Labor shall provide for a study of the impact of the provisions of this subtitle on the premium rates charged to employers for workers compensation insurance. Such study shall use information supplied by States relating to workers compensation premiums and such other information as such Secretary finds appropriate.

(2) REPORT.—Such Secretary shall submit to the Congress, by not later than 2 years after the

date that this subtitle applies in all States, a report on the findings of the study.

(b) WORKERS COMPENSATION CARRIER FILINGS.—

(1) IN GENERAL.—Within six months after the date this subtitle is effective in a participating State, each workers compensation carrier (other than a self-funded employer) providing workers compensation insurance in the State shall make a filing with an agency designated by the State. Such filing shall describe the manner in which such carrier has modified (or intends to modify) its premium rates for workers compensation insurance provided in the State to reflect the changes brought about by the provisions in this subtitle. The filing shall include such actuarial projections and assumptions as necessary to support the modifications of such rates.

(2) REPORT TO SECRETARY.—Each participating State shall provide to the Secretary of Labor such information on filings made under paragraph (1) as such Secretary may specify.

**PART 4—DEMONSTRATION PROJECTS**

**SEC. 10031. AUTHORIZATION.**

The Secretary of Health and Human Services and the Secretary of Labor are authorized to conduct demonstration projects under this part in one or more States with respect to treatment of work-related injuries and illnesses.

### SEC. 10032. DEVELOPMENT OF WORK-RELATED PROTOCOLS.

(a) IN GENERAL.—Under this part, the Secretaries, in consultation with States and such experts on work-related injuries and illnesses as the Secretaries find appropriate, shall develop protocols for the appropriate treatment of work-related conditions.

(b) TESTING OF PROTOCOLS.—The Secretaries shall enter into contracts with one or more health alliances to test the validity of the protocols developed under subsection (a).

### SEC. 10033. DEVELOPMENT OF CAPITATION PAYMENT MODELS.

Under this part, the Secretaries shall develop, using protocols developed under section 10032 if possible, methods of providing for payment by workers compensation carriers to health plans on a per case, capitated payment for the treatment of specified work-related injuries and illnesses.

## Subtitle B—Automobile Insurance

### SEC. 10100. DEFINITIONS.

In this subtitle:

(1) INJURED INDIVIDUAL.—The term "injured individual" means, with respect to a health plan, an individual enrolled under the plan who has an injury or illness sustained in an automobile accident for which automobile insurance medical benefits are available.

(2) AUTOMOBILE INSURANCE MEDICAL BENEFITS.—The term "automobile insurance medical benefits" means, with respect to an enrollee, the comprehensive medical benefits for injuries or illnesses sustained in automobile accidents.

(3) AUTOMOBILE INSURANCE CARRIER.—The term "automobile insurance carrier" means an insurance company that underwrites automobile insurance medical benefits and includes an employer or fund that is financially at risk for the provision of automobile insurance medical benefits.

(4) AUTOMOBILE INSURANCE MEDICAL SERVICES.—The term "automobile insurance medical services" means items and services included in automobile insurance medical benefits and includes items and services (such as rehabilitation services and long-term care services) commonly used for treatment of injuries and illnesses sustained in automobile accidents.

## PART 1—HEALTH PLAN REQUIREMENTS RELATING TO AUTOMOBILE INSURANCE

### SEC. 10101. PROVISION OF AUTOMOBILE INSURANCE MEDICAL BENEFITS THROUGH HEALTH PLANS.

(a) IN GENERAL.—An individual entitled to automobile insurance medical benefits and enrolled in a health plan shall receive automobile insurance medical services through the provision (or arrangement for the provision) of such services by the health plan.

(b) REFERRAL FOR SPECIALIZED SERVICES.—Each health plan shall provide for such referral for automobile insurance medical services as may be necessary to assure appropriate treatment of injured individuals.

(c) EXCEPTIONS.—Subsections (a) and (b) shall not apply in the case of an individual described in section 1004(b) and making an election described in such section.

(d) ALTERNATIVE PERMITTED.—Subsection (a) shall not be construed as preventing an injured individual and an automobile insurance carrier from agreeing that automobile insurance medical services shall be provided other than by or through the health plan in which the individual is enrolled.

### SEC. 10102. PAYMENT BY AUTOMOBILE INSURANCE CARRIER.

(a) PAYMENT.—

(1) IN GENERAL.—Except as provided in subsection (b), each automobile insurance carrier that is liable for payment for automobile insurance medical services furnished by or through a health plan, regardless of whether or not the services are included in the comprehensive benefit package, shall make payment for such services.

(2) USE OF REGIONAL ALLIANCE FEE SCHEDULE.—Such payment shall be made in accordance with the applicable fee schedule established under section 1322(c) or section 10111.

(b) ALTERNATIVE PAYMENT METHODOLOGIES.—Subsection (a) shall not apply—

(1) in the case of a regional alliance or participating State that establishes an alternative payment methodology (such as payment on a negotiated fee for each case) for payment for automobile insurance medical services; or

(2) in the case in which a automobile insurance carrier and the health plan negotiate alternative payment arrangements.

(c) LIMITATION OF LIABILITY OF INJURED INDIVIDUAL.—Nothing in this part shall be construed as requiring an injured individual to make any payment (including payment of any cost sharing or any amount in excess of the applicable fee schedule) to any health plan or health care provider for the receipt of automobile insurance medical services.

## PART 2—REQUIREMENT OF PARTICIPATING STATES

**SEC. 10111. DEVELOPMENT OF SUPPLEMENTAL SCHEDULE.**

Each participating State shall develop a fee schedule applicable to payment for automobile insurance medical services for which a fee is not included in the applicable fee schedule established under section 1322(c).

**SEC. 10112. CONSTRUCTION.**

Nothing in this subtitle shall be construed as altering—

>(1) the determination of whether or not a person is an injured individual and entitled to automobile insurance medical benefits under State law, or

>(2) the scope of items and services available to injured individuals entitled to automobile insurance medical benefits under State law.

## PART 3—APPLICATION OF INFORMATION REQUIREMENTS.

**SEC. 10121. APPLICATION OF INFORMATION REQUIREMENTS.**

(a) IN GENERAL.—The provisions of—

> (1) part 3 of subtitle B of title V (relating to use of standard forms), and
>
> (2) section 5101(e)(9) (relating to provision of data on quality),

apply to the provision of automobile insurance medical services in the same manner as such provisions apply with respect to the provision of services included in the comprehensive benefit package.

(b) RULES.—The Secretary of Labor shall promulgate rules to clarify the responsibilities of health plans and automobile insurance carriers in carrying out the provisions referred to in subsection (a).

# Subtitle C—COMMISSION ON INTEGRATION OF HEALTH BENEFITS

### SEC. 10201. COMMISSION.

(a) ESTABLISHMENT.—There is hereby created a Commission on Integration of Health Benefits (in this section referred to as the "Commission").

(b) COMPOSITION.—

> (1) IN GENERAL.—The Commission shall consist of 15 members appointed jointly by the Secretaries of Health and Human Services and the Secretary of Labor.

(2) NO COMPENSATION EXCEPT TRAVEL EXPENSES.—Members of the Commission shall serve without compensation, but the Secretaries shall provide that each member shall receive travel expenses, including per diem in lieu of subsistence, in accordance with sections 5702 and 5703 of title 5, United States Code.

(c) DUTIES.—The Commission shall study the feasibility and appropriateness of transferring financial responsibility for all medical benefits (including those currently covered under workers compensation and automobile insurance) to health plans.

(d) STAFF SUPPORT.—The Secretaries shall provide staff support for the Commission.

(e) REPORT.—The Commission shall submit a report to the President by not later than July 1, 1995. If such report recommends the integration of financial responsibility for all medical benefits in health plans, such report shall provide for a detailed plan as to how (and when) such an integration should be effected under this Act.

(f) TERMINATION.—The Commission shall terminate 90 days after the date of submission of its report under subsection (e).

(g) AUTHORIZATION OF APPROPRIATIONS.—There are authorized to be appropriated such sums as may be necessary to carry out this section.

# Subtitle D—Federal Employees' Compensation Act

SEC. 10301. APPLICATION OF POLICY.

(a) IN GENERAL.—Chapter 81 of title 5, United States Code, known as the Federal Employees' Compensation Act shall be interpreted and administered consistent with the provisions of subtitle A.

(b) CONSTRUCTION.—In applying subsection (a), subtitle A shall be applied as if the following modifications had been made in subtitle A:

>  (1) Any reference in section 10000, section 10001(c)(2)(C), section 10012(b), or section 10014 to a State law is deemed to include a reference to chapter 81 of title 5, United States Code.

>  (2) The term "workers compensation carrier" includes the Employees Compensation Fund (established under section 8147 of title 5, United States Code).

# Subtitle E—Davis-Bacon Act and Service Contract Act

## SEC. 10401. COVERAGE OF BENEFITS UNDER HEALTH SECURITY ACT.

(a) DAVIS-BACON ACT.—Section 1(b)(2) of the Davis Bacon Act (40 U.S.C. 276a(b)(2)) is amended in the matter following subparagraph (B) by inserting after "local law" the following: "(other than benefits provided pursuant to the Health Security Act)".

(b) SERVICE CONTRACT ACT OF 1965.—The second sentence of section 2(a)(2) of the Service Contract Act of 1965 (41 U.S.C. 351(a)(2)) is amended by inserting after "local law" the following: "(other than benefits provided pursuant to the Health Security Act)".

# Subtitle F—Effective Dates

## SEC. 10501. REGIONAL ALLIANCES.

The provisions of subtitles A and B of this title apply to regional alliances, and regional alliance health plans, in a State 2 years after the State's first year (as defined in section 1902(17)).

## SEC. 10502. CORPORATE ALLIANCES.

The provisions of subtitles A and B of this title apply to corporate alliances, and corporate alliance health plans, on January 1, 1998.

## SEC. 10503. FEDERAL REQUIREMENTS.

The provisions of subtitle D of this title shall take effect on January 1, 1998.

# TITLE XI—TRANSITIONAL INSURANCE REFORM

TABLE OF CONTENTS OF TITLE

Sec. 11001. Imposition of requirements.
Sec. 11002. Enforcement.
Sec. 11003. Requirements relating to preserving current coverage.
Sec. 11004. Restrictions on premium increases during transition.
Sec. 11005. Requirements relating to portability.
Sec. 11006. Requirements limiting reduction of benefits.
Sec. 11007. National transitional health insurance risk pool.
Sec. 11008. Definitions.
Sec. 11009. Termination.

## SEC. 11001. IMPOSITION OF REQUIREMENTS.

(a) IN GENERAL.—The Secretary and the Secretary of Labor shall apply the provisions of this title to assure, to the extent possible, the maintenance of current health care coverage and benefits during the period between the enactment of the Health Security Act and the dates its provisions are implemented in the various States.

(b) ENFORCEMENT.—

(1) HEALTH INSURANCE PLANS.—The Secretary shall enforce the requirements of this title with respect to health insurance plans. The Secretary shall promulgate regulations to carry out the requirements under this title health insurance plans. The Secretary shall promulgate regulations with re-

spect to section 11004 within 90 days after the date of the enactment of this Act.

(2) SELF-INSURED PLANS.—The Secretary of Labor shall enforce the requirements of this title with respect to self-insured plans. Such Secretary shall promulgate regulations to carry out the requirements under this title as they relate to self-funded plans.

(3) ARRANGEMENTS WITH STATES.—The Secretary and the Secretary of Labor may enter into arrangements with a State to enforce the requirements of this title with respect to health insurance plans and self-insured plans issued or sold, or established and maintained, in the State.

(c) PREEMPTION.—The requirements of this title do not preempt any State law unless State law directly conflicts with such requirements. The provision of additional protections under State law shall not be considered to directly conflict with such requirements. The Secretary (or, in the case of a self-insured plan, the Secretary of Labor) may issue letter determinations with respect to whether this Act preempts a provision of State law.

(d) INTERIM FINAL REGULATIONS.—Section 1911 shall apply to regulations issued to carry out this title. The Secretary may consult with States and the National

Association of Insurance Commissioners in issuing regulations and guidelines under this title.

(e) CONSTRUCTION.—The provisions of this title shall be construed in a manner that assures, to the greatest extent practicable, continuity of health benefits under health benefit plans in effect on the effective date of this Act.

(f) SPECIAL RULES FOR ACQUISITIONS AND TRANSFERS.—The Secretary may issue regulations regarding the application of this title in the case of health insurance plans (or groups of such plans) which are transferred from one insurer to another insurer through assumption, acquisition, or otherwise.

**SEC. 11002. ENFORCEMENT.**

(a) IN GENERAL.—Any health insurer or health benefit plan sponsor that violates a requirement of this title shall be subject to civil money penalties of not more than $25,000 for each such violation. The provisions of section 1128A of the Social Security Act (other than subsections (a) and (b)) shall apply to civil money penalties under this subparagraph in the same manner as they apply to a penalty or proceeding under section 1128A(a) of such Act.

(b) EQUITABLE REMEDIES.—

(1) IN GENERAL.—A civil action may be brought by the applicable Secretary—

(A) to enjoin any act or practice which violates any provision of this title, or

(B) to obtain other appropriate equitable relief (i) to redress such violations, or (ii) to enforce any provision of this title, including, in the case of a wrongful termination of (or refusal to renew) coverage, reinstating coverage effective as of the date of the violation.

### SEC. 11003. REQUIREMENTS RELATING TO PRESERVING CURRENT COVERAGE.

(a) PROHIBITION OF TERMINATION.—

(1) GROUP HEALTH INSURANCE PLANS.—Each health insurer that provides a group health insurance plan may not terminate (or fail to renew) coverage for any covered employee if the employer of the employee continues the plan, except in the case of—

(A) nonpayment of required premiums,

(B) fraud, or

(C) misrepresentation of a material fact relating to an application for coverage or claim for benefits.

(2) INDIVIDUAL HEALTH INSURANCE PLANS.—Each health insurer that provides coverage to a covered individual under an individual health insurance

plan may not terminate (or fail to renew) coverage for such individual (or a covered dependent), except in the case of—

>  (A) nonpayment of required premiums,
>
>  (B) fraud, or
>
>  (C) misrepresentation of a material fact relating to an application for coverage or claim for benefits.

(2) EFFECTIVE DATE OF TITLE.—

>  (A) IN GENERAL.—This subsection shall take effect on the effective date of this title and shall apply to coverage on or after such date.
>
>  (B) DEFINITION.—Except as otherwise provided, in this title the term "effective date of this title" means the date of the enactment of this Act.

(b) ACCEPTANCE OF NEW MEMBERS IN A GROUP HEALTH INSURANCE PLAN.—

(1) IN GENERAL.—In the case of a health insurer that provides a group health insurance plan that is in effect on the effective date of this title, the insurer is required—

>  (A) to accept all individuals, and their eligible dependents, who become full-time employ-

ees (as defined in section 1901(b)(2)(C)) of an employer covered after such effective date;

(B) to establish and apply premium rates that are consistent with section 11004(b); and

(C) to limit the application of pre-existing condition restrictions in accordance with section 11005.

(2) CONSISTENT APPLICATION OF RULES RELATING TO DEPENDENTS AND WAITING PERIODS.—In this subsection, the term "eligible dependent", with respect to a group health insurance plan, has the meaning provided under the plan as of the date of introduction of the Health Security Act or, in the case of a plan not established as of such date, as of the date of establishment of the plan.

**SEC. 11004. RESTRICTIONS ON PREMIUM INCREASES DURING TRANSITION.**

(a) DIVISION OF HEALTH INSURANCE PLANS BY SECTOR.—For purposes of this section, each health insurer shall divide its health insurance business into the following 3 sectors:

(1) Health insurance for groups with at least 100 covered lives (in this section referred to as the "large group sector")

(2) Health insurance for groups with fewer than 100 covered lives (in this section referred as the "small group sector").

(3) Health insurance for individuals, and not for groups (in this section referred to as the "individual sector").

(b) PREMIUM CHANGES TO REFLECT CHANGES IN GROUP OR INDIVIDUAL CHARACTERISTICS OR TERMS OF COVERAGE.—

(1) APPLICATION.—The provisions of this subsection shall apply to changes in premiums that reflect—

(A) changes in the number of individuals covered under a plan;

(B) changes in the group or individual characteristics (including age, gender, family composition or geographic area but not including health status, claims experience or duration of coverage under the plan) of individuals covered under a plan;

(C) changes in the level of benefits (including changes to in cost-sharing) under the plan; and

(D) changes in any material terms and conditions of the health insurance plan (other than factors related to health status, claims experience and duration).

(2) SPECIFICATION OF REFERENCE RATE FOR EACH SECTOR.—Each health insurer shall calculate a reference rate for each such sector. The reference rate for a sector shall be calculated so that, if it were applied using the rate factors specified under paragraph (3), the average premium rate for individuals and groups in that sector would approximate the average premium rate charged individuals and groups in the sector as of the effective date of this title.

(3) SINGLE SET OF RATE FACTORS WITHIN EACH SECTOR.—

(A) IN GENERAL.—Each health insurer shall develop for each sector a single set of rate factors which will be used to calculate any changes in premium that relate to the reasons described in subparagraphs (B) through (D) of paragraph (1).

(B) STANDARDS.—Such rate factors—

(i) shall relate to reasonable and objective differences in demographic characteristics, in the design and in levels of coverage, and in other terms and conditions of a contract,

(ii) shall not relate to expected health status, claims experience, or duration of coverage of the one or more groups or individuals, and

(iii) shall comply with regulations established under subsection (f).

(4) COMPUTATION OF PREMIUM CHANGES.—

(A) IN GENERAL.—Changes in premium rates that relate to the reasons described in paragraph (1) shall be calculated using the rate factors developed pursuant to paragraph (3).

(B) APPLICATION TO CHANGES IN NUMBER OF COVERED INDIVIDUALS.—In the case of a change in premium rates related to the reason described in paragraph (1)(A), the change in premium rates shall be calculated to reflect, with respect to the enrollees who enroll or disenroll in a health insurance plan, the sum of the products, for such individuals, of the reference rate (determined under paragraph (2)) and the rate factors (specified under paragraph (3)) applicable to such enrollees.

(C) APPLICATION OF OTHER FACTORS.—

(i) IN GENERAL.—In the case of a change in premium rates related to a reason described in subparagraph (B), (C), or (D) of paragraph (1), the change in premium rates with respect to each health insurance plan in each sector shall reflect the rate factors specified under paragraph (3) applicable to the reason as applied to the current premium charged for the health insurance plan. Such rate factors shall be applied in a manner so that the resulting adjustment, to the extent possible, reflects the premium that would have been charged under the plan if the reason for the change in premium had existed at the time that the current premium rate was calculated.

(ii) NO REFLECTION OF CHANGE IN HEALTH STATUS.—In applying the rate factors under this subparagraph, the adjustment shall not reflect any change in the health status, claims experience or duration of coverage with respect to any employer or individual covered under the plan.

(5) LIMITATION ON APPLICATION.—This subsection shall only apply—

 (A) to changes in premiums occurring on or after the date of the enactment of this Act to groups and individuals covered as of such date, and

 (B) with respect to groups and individuals subsequently covered, to changes in premiums subsequent to such coverage.

(6) APPLICATION TO COMMUNITY-RATED PLANS.—Nothing in this subsection shall require the application of rate factors related to individual or group characteristics with respect to community-rated plans.

(c) LIMITATIONS ON CHANGES IN PREMIUMS RELATED TO INCREASES IN HEALTH CARE COSTS AND UTILIZATION.—

(1) APPLICATION.—The provisions of this subsection shall apply to changes in premiums that reflect increases in health care costs and utilization.

(2) EQUAL INCREASE FOR ALL PLANS IN ALL SECTORS.—

 (A) IN GENERAL.—Subject to subparagraph (B), the annual percentage increase in premiums by a health insurer for health insurance plans in the individual sector, small group sector, and large group sector, to the extent such increase reflect increases in health care costs and utilization, shall be the same for all such plans in those sectors.

(B) SPECIAL RULE FOR LARGE GROUP SECTOR.—The annual percentage increase in premiums by a health insurer for health insurance plans in the large group sector may vary among such plans based on the claims experience of such employer (to the extent the experience is credible), so long as the weighted average of such increases for all such plans in the sector complies with the requirement of subparagraph (A).

(C) GEOGRAPHIC APPLICATION.—Subparagraphs (A) and (B)—

(i) may be applied on a national level, or

(ii) may vary based on geographic area, but only if (I) such areas are sufficiently large to provide credible data on which to calculate the variation and (II) the variation is due to reasonable factors related to the objective differences among such areas in costs and utilization of health services.

(D) EXCEPTIONS TO ACCOMMODATE STATE RATE REFORM EFFORTS.—Subparagraphs (A) and (B) shall not apply, in accordance with guidelines of the Secretary, to the extent necessary to permit a State to narrow the variations in premiums among health insurance plans offered by health insurers to similarly situated groups or individuals within a sector.

(E) EXCEPTION FOR RATES SUBJECT TO PRIOR APPROVAL.—Subparagraphs (A) and (B) shall not apply to premiums that are subject to prior approval by a State insurance commissioner (or similar official) and are approved by such official.

(F) OTHER REASONS SPECIFIED BY THE SECRETARY.—The Secretary may specify through regulations such other exceptions to the provisions of this subsection as the Secretary determines are required to enhance stability of the health insurance market and continued availability of coverage.

(3) EVEN APPLICATION THROUGHOUT A YEAR.—In applying the provisions of this subsection

to health insurance plans that are renewed in different months of a year, the annual percentage increase shall be applied in a consistent, even manner so that any variations in the rate of increase applied in consecutive months are even and continuous during the year.

(4) PETITION FOR EXCEPTION.—A health insurer may petition the Secretary (or a State acting under a contract with the Secretary under section 11001(b)(3)) for an exception from the application of the provisions of this subsection. The Secretary may approve such an exception if—

 (A) the health insurer demonstrates that the application of this subsection would threaten the financial viability of the insurer, and

 (B) the health insurer offers an alternative method for increasing premiums that is not substantially discriminatory to any sector or to any group or individual covered by a health insurance plan offered by the insurer.

(d) PRIOR APPROVAL FOR CERTAIN RATE INCREASES.—

(1) IN GENERAL.—If the percentage increase in the premium rate for the individual and small group sector exceeds a percentage specified by the Sec-

retary under paragraph (2), annualized over any 12-month period, the increase shall not take effect unless the Secretary (or a State acting under a contract with the Secretary under section 11001(b)(3)) has approved the increase.

(2) PERCENTAGE.—The Secretary shall specify, for each 12-month period beginning after the date of the enactment of this Act, a percentage that will apply under paragraph (1). Such percentage shall be determined taking into consideration the rate of increase in health care costs and utilization, previous trends in health insurance premiums, and the conditions in the health insurance market. Within 30 days after the date of the enactment of this Act, the Secretary shall first specify a percentage under this paragraph.

(e) DOCUMENTATION OF COMPLIANCE.—

(1) PERIOD FOR CONFORMANCE.—Effective 1 year after the date of the enactment of this Act, the premium for each policy shall be conformed in a manner that complies with the provisions of this section.

(2) METHODOLOGY.—Each health insurer shall document the methodology used in applying subsections (b) and (c) with respect to each sector (and

each applicable health plan). Such documentation shall be sufficient to permit the auditing of the application of such methodology to determine if such application was consistent with such subsections.

(3) CERTIFICATION.—For each 6-month period in which this section is effective, each health insurer shall file a certification with the Secretary (or with a State with which the Secretary has entered into an arrangement under section 11001(b)(3)) that the insurer is in compliance with such requirements.

(f) REGULATIONS.—The Secretary shall establish regulations to carry out this section. Such regulations may include guidelines relating to the permissible variation that results from the use of demographic or other characteristics in the development of rate factors. Such guidelines may be based on the guidelines currently used by States in applying rate limitations under State insurance regulations.

(g) EFFECTIVE PERIOD.—This section shall apply to premium increases occurring during the period beginning on the date of the enactment of this Act and ending, for a health insurance plan provided in a State, on the first day of the State's first year.

## SEC. 11005. REQUIREMENTS RELATING TO PORTABILITY.

(a) TREATMENT OF PREEXISTING CONDITION EXCLUSIONS.—

(1) IN GENERAL.—Subject to the succeeding provisions of this subsection, a group health benefit plan may exclude coverage with respect to services related to treatment of a preexisting condition, but the period of such exclusion may not exceed 6 months. The exclusion of coverage shall not apply to services furnished to newborns or in the case of a plan that did not apply such exclusions as of the effective date of this title.

(2) CREDITING OF PREVIOUS COVERAGE.—

(A) IN GENERAL.—A group health benefit plan shall provide that if an individual covered under such plan is in a period of continuous coverage (as defined in subparagraph (B)(i)) with respect to particular services as of the date of initial coverage under such plan, any period of exclusion of coverage with respect to a preexisting condition for such services or type of services shall be reduced by 1 month for each month in the period of continuous coverage.

(B) DEFINITIONS.—As used in this paragraph:

(i) PERIOD OF CONTINUOUS COVERAGE.—The term "period of continuous coverage" means, with respect to particular services, the period beginning on the date an individual is enrolled under a group or individual health benefit plan, self-insured plan, the medicare program, a State medicaid plan, or other health benefit arrangement which provides benefits with respect to such services and ends on the date the individual is not so enrolled for a continuous period of more than 3 months.

(ii) PREEXISTING CONDITION.—The term "preexisting condition" means, with respect to coverage under a health benefits plan, a condition which has been diagnosed or treated during the 6-month period ending on the day before the first date of such coverage (without regard to any waiting period).

(b) WAITING PERIODS.—A self-insured plan, and an employer with respect to a group health insurance plan, may not discriminate among employees in the establishment of a waiting period before making health insurance coverage available based on the health status, claims experience, receipt of health care, medical history, or lack of evidence of insurability, of the employee or the employee's dependents.

## SEC. 11006. REQUIREMENTS LIMITING REDUCTION OF BENEFITS.

(a) IN GENERAL.—A self-insured sponsor may not make a modification of benefits described in subsection (b).

(b) MODIFICATION OF BENEFITS DESCRIBED.—

(1) IN GENERAL.—A modification of benefits described in this subsection is any reduction or limitation in coverage, effected on or after the effective date of this title, with respect to any medical condition or course of treatment for which the anticipated cost is likely to exceed $5,000 in any 12-month period.

(2) TREATMENT OF TERMINATION.—A modification of benefits includes the termination of a plan if the sponsor, within a period establishes a substitute plan that reflects the reduction or limitation described in paragraph (1).

(c) REMEDY.—Any modification made in violation of this section shall not be effective and the self-insured sponsor shall continue to provide benefits as though the modification (described in subsection (b)) had not occurred.

**SEC. 11007. NATIONAL TRANSITIONAL HEALTH INSURANCE RISK POOL.**

(a) ESTABLISHMENT.—In order to assure access to health insurance during the transition, the Secretary is authorized to establish a National Transitional Health Insurance Risk Pool (in this section referred to as the "national risk pool") in accordance with this section.

(b) ADMINISTRATION.—

   (1) IN GENERAL.—The Secretary may administer the national risk pool through contracts with—

      (A) one or more existing State health insurance risk pools,

      (B) one or more private health insurers, or

      (C) such other contracts as the Secretary deems appropriate.

   (2) COORDINATION WITH STATE RISK POOLS.—The Secretary may enter into such arrangements with existing State health insurance risk pools to coordinate the coverage under such pools with the coverage under the national risk pool. Such coordination may address eligibility and funding of coverage for individuals currently covered under State risk pools.

(c) ELIGIBILITY FOR COVERAGE.—The national risk pool shall provide health insurance coverage to individuals who are unable to secure health insurance coverage from private health insurers because of their health status or condition (as determined in accordance with rules and procedures specified by the Secretary).

(d) BENEFITS.—

(1) IN GENERAL.—Benefits and terms of coverage provided through the national risk pool shall include items and services, conditions of coverage, and cost sharing (subject to out-of-pocket limits on cost sharing) comparable to the benefits and terms of coverage available in State health insurance risk pools.

(2) PAYMENT RATES.—Payments under the national risk pool for covered items and services shall be made at rates (specified by the Secretary) based on payment rates for comparable items and services under the medicare program. Providers who accept payment from the national risk pool shall accept such payment as payment in full for the service, other than for cost sharing provided under the national risk pool.

(e) PREMIUMS.—

(1) IN GENERAL.—Premiums for coverage in the national risk pool shall be set in a manner specified by the Secretary.

(2) VARIATION.—Such premiums shall vary based upon age, place of residence, and other traditional underwriting factors other than on the basis of health status or claims experience.

(3) LIMITATION.—The premiums charged individuals shall be set at a level that is no less than 150 percent of the premiums that the Secretary estimates would be charged to a population of average risk for the covered benefits.

(f) TREATMENT OF SHORTFALLS.—

(1) ESTIMATES.—The Secretary shall estimate each year the extent to which the total premiums collected under subsection (c) in the year are insufficient to cover the expenses of the national risk pool with respect to the year.

(2) TEMPORARY BORROWING AUTHORITY.—The Secretary of the Treasury is authorized to advance to the Secretary amounts sufficient to cover the amount estimated under paragraph (1) during the year before assessments are collected under paragraph (3). The Secretary shall repay such amounts, with interest at a rate specified by the Secretary of

the Treasury, from the assessments under paragraph (3).

(3) ASSESSMENTS.—

(A) IN GENERAL.—Each health benefit plan sponsor shall be liable for an assessment in the amount specified in subparagraph (C).

(B) AMOUNT.—For each year for which amounts are advanced under paragraph (2), the Secretary shall—

(i) estimate the total amount of premiums (and premium equivalents) for health benefits under health benefit plans for the succeeding year, and

(ii) calculate a percentage equal to (I) the total amounts repayable by the Secretary to the Secretary of the Treasury under paragraph (2) for the year, divided by the amount determined under clause (i).

(C) ASSESSMENT AMOUNT.—The amount of an assessment for a sponsor of a health benefit plan for a year shall be equal to the percentage calculated under subparagraph (B)(ii) (or, if less, ½ of 1 percent) of the total amount of premiums (and premium equivalents) for health benefits under the plan for the previous year.

(D) SELF-INSURED PLANS.—The amount of premiums (and premium equivalents) under this paragraph shall be estimated—

(i) by the Secretary for health insurance plans, and

(ii) by the Secretary of Labor for self-insured plans.

Such estimates may be based on a methodology that requires plans liable for assessment to file information with the applicable Secretary.

**SEC. 11008. DEFINITIONS.**

In this title:

(1) APPLICABLE SECRETARY.—The term "applicable Secretary" means—

(A) the Secretary with respect to health insurance plans and insurers, or

(B) the Secretary of labor with respect to self-insured plans and self-insured plan sponsors.

(2) COVERED EMPLOYEE.—The term "covered employee" means an employee (or dependent of such an employee) covered under a group health benefits plan.

(3) COVERED INDIVIDUAL.—The "covered individual" means, with respect to a health benefit plan, an individual insured, enrolled, eligible for benefits, or otherwise covered under the plan.

(4) GROUP HEALTH BENEFITS PLAN.—The term "group health benefits plan" means a group health insurance plan and a self-insured plan.

(5) GROUP HEALTH INSURANCE PLAN.—

(A) IN GENERAL.—The term "group health insurance plan" means a health insurance plan offered primarily to employers for the purpose of providing health insurance to the employees (and dependents) of the employer.

(B) INCLUSION OF ASSOCIATION PLANS AND MEWAS.—Such term includes—

(i) any arrangement in which coverage for health benefits is offered to employers through an association, trust, or other arrangement, and

(ii) a multiple employer welfare arrangement (as defined in section 3(40) of the Employee Retirement Income Security Act of 1974), whether funded through insurance or otherwise.

(6) HEALTH BENEFITS PLAN.—The term "health benefits plan" means health insurance plan and a self-insured health benefit plan.

(7) HEALTH BENEFIT PLAN SPONSOR.—The term "health benefit plan sponsor" means, with respect to a health insurance plan or self-insured plan, the insurer offering the plan or the self-insured sponsor for the plan, respectively.

(8) HEALTH INSURANCE PLAN.—

   (A) IN GENERAL.—Except as provided in subparagraph (B), the term "health insurance plan" means any contract of health insurance, including any hospital or medical service policy or certificate, any major medical policy or certificate, any hospital or medical service plan contract, or health maintenance organization subscriber contract offered by an insurer.

   (B) EXCEPTION.—Such term does not include any of the following—

      (i) coverage only for accident, dental, vision, disability income, or long-term care insurance, or any combination thereof,

      (ii) medicare supplemental health insurance,

(iii) coverage issued as a supplement to liability insurance,

(iv) worker's compensation or similar insurance, or

(v) automobile medical-payment insurance,

or any combination thereof.

(C) STOP LOSS INSURANCE NOT COVERED.—Such term does not include any aggregate or specific stop-loss insurance or similar coverage applicable to a self-insured plan. The Secretary may develop rules determining the applicability of this subparagraph with respect to minimum premium plans or other partially insured plans.

(9) HEALTH INSURER.—The term "health insurer" means a licensed insurance company, a prepaid hospital or medical service plan, a health maintenance organization, or other entity providing a plan of health insurance or health benefits with respect to which the State insurance laws are not preempted under section 514 of the Employee Retirement Income Security Act of 1974.

(10) INDIVIDUAL HEALTH INSURANCE PLAN.—

(A) IN GENERAL.—The term "individual health insurance plan" means any health insurance plan directly purchased by an individual or offered primarily to individuals (including families) for the purpose of permitting individuals (without regard to an employer contribution) to purchase health insurance coverage.

(B) INCLUSION OF ASSOCIATION PLANS.—Such term includes any arrangement in which coverage for health benefits is offered to individuals through an association, trust, list-billing arrangement, or other arrangement in which the individual purchaser is primarily responsible for the payment of any premium associated with the contract.

(C) TREATMENT OF CERTAIN ASSOCIATION PLANS.—In the case of a health insurance plan sponsored by an association, trust, or other arrangement that provides health insurance coverage both to employers and to individuals, the plan shall be treated as—

(i) a group health insurance plan with respect to such employers, and

(ii) an individual health insurance plan with respect to such individuals.

(11) SELF-INSURED PLAN.—The term "self-insured plan" means an employee welfare benefit plan or other arrangement insofar as the plan or arrangement provides benefits with respect to some or all of the items and services included in the comprehensive benefit package (as in effect as of January 1, 1995) that is funded in a manner other than through the purchase of one or more health insurance plans. such term shall not include a group health insurance plan (as defined in paragraph (5)(B)(ii)).

(12) SELF-INSURED SPONSOR.—The term "self-insured sponsor" includes, with respect to a self-insured plan, any entity which establishes or maintains the plan.

(13) STATE COMMISSIONER OF INSURANCE.—The term "State commissioner of insurance" includes a State superintendent of insurance.

**SEC. 11009. TERMINATION.**

(a) HEALTH INSURANCE PLANS.—The provisions of this title shall not apply to a health insurance plan provided in a State on and after the first day of the first year for the State.

(b) SELF-INSURED PLANS.—The provisions of this title shall not apply to a self-insured plan that—

1     (1) is sponsored by a sponsor that is an eligible
2 sponsor of a corporate alliance (described in section
3 1311(b)(1)), as of the effective date of the election
4 under section 1312(c).
5     (2) is sponsored by a sponsor that is not such
6 an eligible sponsor, with respect to individuals or
7 groups in a State on and after the first day of the
8 first year for the State.

# TITLE XII—TEMPORARY ASSESSMENT ON EMPLOYERS WITH RETIREE HEALTH BENEFIT COSTS

TABLE OF CONTENTS OF TITLE

Sec. 1201. Temporary assessment on employers with retiree health benefit costs.
Sec. 1202. Recapture of retiree subsidy beginning in 1998.

## SEC. 1201. TEMPORARY ASSESSMENT ON EMPLOYERS WITH RETIREE HEALTH BENEFIT COSTS.

(a) IN GENERAL.—Subtitle C (relating to employment taxes) is amended by inserting after chapter 24A the following new chapter:

## "CHAPTER 24B—TEMPORARY ASSESSMENT ON EMPLOYERS WITH RETIREE HEALTH BENEFIT COSTS

"Subchapter A. Temporary assessment.
"Subchapter B. Definitions and administrative provisions.

### "Subchapter A—Temporary Assessment

"Sec. 3463. Temporary assessment on employers with retiree health benefit costs.

## "SEC. 3463. TEMPORARY ASSESSMENT ON EMPLOYERS WITH RETIREE HEALTH BENEFIT COSTS.

"(a) IMPOSITION OF ASSESSMENT.—Every employer with base period retiree health costs shall pay (in addition to any other amount imposed by this subtitle) for each calendar year to which this section applies an assessment equal to the amount determined under subsection (b).

"(b) AMOUNT OF ASSESSMENT.—For purposes of subsection (a), the amount determined under this subsection with respect to any employer for any calendar year is 50 percent of the greater of—

"(1) the adjusted base period retiree health costs of such employer for such calendar year, or

"(2) the amount (determined in the manner prescribed by the Secretary) by which such employer's applicable retiree health costs for such calendar year were reduced by reason of the enactment of the Health Security Act.

"(c) DEFINITIONS.—For purposes of this section—

"(1) BASE PERIOD RETIREE HEALTH COSTS.—The term 'base period retiree health costs' means the average of the applicable retiree health costs of the employer for calendar years 1991, 1992, and 1993.

"(2) ADJUSTED BASE PERIOD RETIREE HEALTH COSTS.—

"(A) IN GENERAL.—The term 'adjusted base period retiree health costs' means, with respect to any employer for any calendar year, the base period retiree health costs of the employer adjusted in the manner prescribed by the Secretary to reflect increases in the medical care component of the Consumer Price Index during the period after 1992 and before such calendar year.

"(B) ADJUSTMENTS FOR ACQUISITIONS AND DISPOSITIONS.—Rules similar to the rules of subparagraphs (A) and (B) of section 41(f)(3) shall apply to acquisitions and dispositions after December 31, 1993.

"(3) APPLICABLE RETIREE HEALTH COSTS.—

"(A) IN GENERAL.—The term 'applicable retiree health costs' means, with respect to any employer for any calendar year, the aggregate cost (including administrative costs) of the health benefits or coverage provided during such calendar year (whether directly by the employer or through a plan described in section 401(h) or a welfare benefit fund as defined in section 419(e)) to individuals who are entitled to receive such benefits or coverage by reason of being retired employees of such employer (or by reason of being a spouse or other beneficiary of such an employee).

"(B) ONLY BENEFITS AND COVERAGE AFTER AGE 55 AND BEFORE AGE 65 TAKEN INTO ACCOUNT.—In applying subparagraph (A), there shall be taken into account only health benefits and coverage provided after the date the retired employee attained age 55 and before the date such employee attained (or, but for the death of such employee, would have attained) age 65.

"(d) YEARS TO WHICH ASSESSMENT APPLIES.—This section shall apply to calendar years 1998, 1999, and 2000.

## "Subchapter B—Definitions and Administrative Provisions

"SEC. 3464. DEFINITIONS AND ADMINISTRATIVE PROVISIONS

"(a) EMPLOYER.—For purposes of this chapter—

"(1) IN GENERAL.—The term 'employer' means any person or governmental entity for whom an individual performs services, of whatever nature, as an employee (as defined in section 3401(c)).

"(2) SPECIAL RULES.—

"(A) An individual who owns the entire interest in an unincorporated trade or business shall be treated as his own employer.

"(B) A partnership shall be treated as the employer of each partner who is an employee within the meaning of section 401(c)(1).

"(C) An S corporation shall be treated as the employer of each shareholder who is an employee within the meaning of section 401(c)(1).

"(b) ASSESSMENT TO APPLY TO GOVERNMENTAL AND OTHER TAX-EXEMPT ENTITIES.—Notwithstanding any other provision of law or rule of law, none of the following shall be exempt from the assessment imposed by this chapter:

"(1) The United States, any State or political subdivision thereof, the District of Columbia, and any agency or instrumentality of any of the foregoing.

"(2) Any other entity otherwise exempt from tax under chapter 1.

"(c) ADMINISTRATIVE PROVISIONS.—

"(1) PAYMENT.—Any assessment under section 3463 for any calendar year shall be paid on or before March 15 of the following calendar year; except that the Secretary may require quarterly estimated payments of such assessment in a manner similar to the requirements of section 6655.

"(2) COLLECTION, ETC.—For purposes of subtitle F, any assessment under this subchapter shall be treated as if it were a tax imposed by this subtitle."

(b) CLERICAL AMENDMENT.—The table of chapters for subtitle C is amended by inserting after the item relating to chapter 24A the following new item:

"Chapter 24B. Temporary Assessment on Employers With Retiree Health Benefit Costs."

(c) EFFECTIVE DATE.—The amendments made by this section shall take effect on January 1, 1998.

## SEC. 1202. RECAPTURE OF RETIREE SUBSIDY BEGINNING IN 1998.

(a) IN GENERAL.—Paragraph (2) of section 59B(a) (relating to recapture of certain health care subsidies), as added by title VII of this Act, is amended by striking "December 31, 1999" and inserting "December 31, 1997".

(b) TECHNICAL AMENDMENT.—Paragraph (2) of section 7131(d) of this Act is amended by striking "December 31, 2001" and inserting "December 31, 1999".